HIV/AIDS

Fourth Edition ~~████~~ 3/13/00

HIV/AIDS
A GUIDE TO PRIMARY CARE MANAGEMENT

Peter J. Ungvarski, MS, RN, ACRN, FAAN

Clinical Nurse Specialist, HIV Infection
Clinical Director, AIDS Services
Visiting Nurse Service of New York Home Care

Clinical Associate
Hunter-Bellevue School of Nursing
Hunter College
City University of New York
New York, New York

Jacquelyn Haak Flaskerud, PhD, RN, FAAN

Professor
School of Nursing
Center for Health Sciences
University of California, Los Angeles
Los Angeles, California

W.B. SAUNDERS COMPANY
A Division of Harcourt Brace & Company

Philadelphia   London   Toronto   Montreal   Sydney   Tokyo

W.B. SAUNDERS COMPANY

A Division of Harcourt Brace & Company

The Curtis Center
Independence Square West
Philadelphia, Pennsylvania 19106

Library of Congress Cataloging-in-Publication Data

HIV/AIDS : a guide to primary care management / [edited by] Peter J.
    Ungvarski, Jacquelyn H. Flaskerud. — 4th ed.
        p.   cm.
    Includes bibliographical references and index.
    ISBN 0-7216-7322-8
     1. AIDS (Disease)—Treatment.   2. AIDS (Disease)—Nursing.
I. Ungvarski, Peter J.   II. Flaskerud, Jacquelyn Haak.
    [DNLM: 1. HIV Infections—nursing.   2. Acquired Immunodeficiency
Syndrome—nursing.   WY 153.5 H675 1999]
RC607.A26H555 1999
610.73'699—dc21
DNLM/DLC

                          98-20112

HIV/AIDS: A GUIDE TO PRIMARY CARE MANAGEMENT   ISBN 0-7216-7322-8

Printed in the United States of America

Last digit is the print number: 9   8   7   6   5   4   3   2   1

To my sister JoAnn Panza for her love, humor, and support
Peter

and

To my son John Murray for his spirit, optimism, talent, and humor
Jackie

Contributors

Joyce K. Anastasi, PhD, RN, FAAN
Associate Professor of Nursing and Director, Center for AIDS Research, Columbia University School of Nursing, New York, New York
Alternative and Complementary Therapies

James Angell, MSN, RN, CNS, FNP, ACRN
Assistant Professor of Nursing, Family Nurse Practitioner Program, Arkansas State University, State University, Arkansas; Family Nurse Practitioner, Crittenden Memorial Hospital, Rural Health Network, West Memphis, Arkansas
Adolescents and Adults: HIV Disease Care Management

Mary Boland, MSN, RN
François-Xavier Bagnoud Professor of Nursing, School of Nursing, University of Medicine and Dentistry of New Jersey, Newark, New Jersey
Infants and Children: HIV Disease Care Management

Michele Crespo-Fierro, MS/MPH, RN, CRNI, ACRN
HIV-AIDS Consultant, Private Practice; Per-diem Nurse, Visiting Nurse Service of New York, New York, New York
Community-Based and Long-Term Care

Lynn Czarniecki, MSN, RNC, CNS-C, ACRN
Advanced Practice Nurse, University of Medicine and Dentistry of New Jersey, Newark, New Jersey
Infants and Children: AIDS Care Management

Richard Ferri, PhD, ANP, ACRN
HIV/AIDS Nurse Practitioner, Private Practice; President, Richard Ferri & Associates, Provincetown, Massachusetts
The Needs of Special Populations: Adolescents and Persons with Hemophilia

Jacquelyn Haak Flaskerud, PhD, RN, FAAN
Professor, School of Nursing, Center for Health Sciences, University of California, Los Angeles, Los Angeles, California
Overview and Update of HIV Disease; Health Promotion and Maintenance; Psychosocial and Neuropsychiatric Dysfunction; Culture and Ethnicity

William D. Frumkin, JD
Partner, Sapir & Frumkin LLP, White Plains, New York; Chair, Subcommittee on AIDS and the Workplace, New York State Bar Association Special Committee on AIDS and the Law; Co-Chair, National Employment Lawyers Association's ERISA Committee
Legal Issues

Arnold H. Grossman, PhD
Professor, Department of Health Studies, and Project Director, New York University AIDS/SIDA Mental Hygiene Project, School of Education, New York University, New York, New York
The Needs of Special Populations: Men Who Have Sex with Men; The Needs of Special Populations: Older Adults

Roger Herr, MPA, PT
Adjunct Faculty, Department of Physical Therapy, School of Education, New York University; Rehabilitation Manager, Visiting Nurse Service of New York Home Care, New York, New York
Adolescents and Adults: Care Management of AIDS-Indicator Diseases

Steven L. Kessler, Esq, JD
Adjunct Professor of Law, New York Law School; private practice, New York, New York; Member, American Bar Association Special Committee on AIDS; formerly Chair, New York State Bar Association Special Committee on AIDS and the Law
Legal Issues

Robert J. Kizior, BS, RPh
Educational Coordinator, Department of Pharmacy, Alexian Brothers Medical Center, Elk Grove Village, Illinois
Pharmacologic Treatment of HIV/AIDS

Ann Kurth, MPH, MSN, RN, CNM
Doctoral candidate, Department of Epidemiology, School of Public Health and Community Medicine, University of Washington, Seattle, Washington
The Needs of Special Populations: Women, Pregnant Women, Lesbians, and Transgender/Transsexual Persons

Danny J. Lancaster, MD
Clinical Associate Professor of Internal Medicine and Preventive Medicine, University of Tennessee; Codirector, Internal Medicine and Transitional Residency, Methodist Hospital, Memphis, Tennessee
Adolescents and Adults: HIV Disease Care Management

Ronnie E. Leibowitz, MA, RN, CIC
Nurse Epidemiologist, New York, New York
Legal Issues

Juliana P. Manlapaz, MA, RD, LD
Director, Food and Nutrition Services, Washington Center for Aging Services; Consultant, Women, Infant and Child Nutrition (WIC Program), Children's Hospital, Washington, District of Columbia
Adolescents and Adults: HIV Disease Care Management

Mary McCarthy, RN, NP
Nurse Practitioner Supervisor, HIV Neurobehavioral Research Center, University of California at San Diego, San Diego, California
The Needs of Special Populations: Injecting Drug Users, Incarcerated Persons, and Commercial Sex Workers

Eric N. Miller, PhD
Associate Research Psychologist, Department of Psychiatry and Biobehavioral Science, University of California Los Angeles Neuropsychiatric Institute and Hospital, Los Angeles, California
Psychosocial and Neuropsychiatric Dysfunction

Helen M. Miramontes, MSN, RN, FAAN
Associate Clinical Professor and Nurse Coordinator, Pacific AIDS Education and Training Center, School of Nursing, University of California, San Francisco; Deputy Director, The International Center for HIV/AIDS Research and Clinical Training in Nursing, San Francisco, California; Member, Presidential Advisory Council on HIV/AIDS
Personal Perspectives on Policy Issues of the HIV/AIDS Epidemic

James Oleske, MD, MPH
François-Xavier Bagnoud Professor of Pediatrics, New Jersey Medical School, University of Medicine and Dentistry of New Jersey, Newark, New Jersey
Infants and Children: HIV Disease Care Management; Infants and Children: AIDS Care Management

Pamela Rothpletz-Puglia, MS, RD
Clinical Assistant Professor, School of Health Related Professions, University of Medicine and Dentistry of New Jersey, Newark, New Jersey
Infants and Children: HIV Disease Care Management; Infants and Children: AIDS Care Management

Judith Saunders, DNSc, FAAN
Primary Care Integration Specialist, PacifiCare Behavioral Health, Van Nuys, California
Ethical Issues

Joan Schmidt, MS, MPH, RN, ACRN
Clinical Instructor, AIDS Services, Visiting Nurse Service of New York, New York, New York
Community-Based and Long-Term Care

Michael Sheran, MD
Assistant Professor of Medicine, New York Medical College, Valhalla, New York; Deputy Chief, Section of HIV Medicine, Saint Vincents Hospital and Medical Center, New York, New York
Adolescents and Adults: Care Management of AIDS-Indicator Diseases

Jo Anne Staats, MSN, ANP
Director of Primary Care and Research for Early Identification and Intervention Services, Bronx-Lebanon Hospital Center, Bronx, New York
Adolescents and Adults: Care Management of AIDS-Indicator Diseases

Peter J. Ungvarski, MS, RN, ACRN, FAAN
Clinical Nurse Specialist, HIV Infection, and Clinical Director, AIDS Services, Visiting Nurse Service of New York Home Care; Clinical Associate, Hunter-Bellevue School of Nursing, Hunter College, City University of New York, New York, New York
Overview and Update of HIV Disease; Adolescents and Adults: HIV Disease Care Management; Postexposure Prophylaxis after Exposure to HIV

John K. Weiser, MD
Associate Professor of Family Medicine, Albert Einstein College of Medicine; Attending Physician, Department of Family Practice, Beth Israel Medical Center, New York, New York

Diagnostic Testing in HIV Disease

Walter R. Weiss, BBA, BS, PA-C
Professional Science Liaison, Agouron Pharmaceuticals, Inc., La Jolla, California

Health Teaching for the Client with HIV Infection

Preface

Since the original concept for the first edition of *HIV/AIDS: A Guide to Primary Care Management* was developed in 1986, substantial progress has been made in understanding not only the behavioral aspects of HIV infection but also the pathophysiology and treatment of this disease. In the last three years alone testing techniques to monitor HIV disease activity have been developed to guide our clinical decision making, and combination antiretroviral therapies that contain the destructive forces of HIV and slow the disease progression have been identified. Today, HIV is viewed, as we had suggested in previous editions, as a chronic illness. As with any chronic disease, there is an identifiable illness trajectory with a beginning and an end. Therefore it is important to note that although great progress has been achieved, the disease does advance, and many individuals continue to die from HIV infection.

The primary goal of the fourth edition of *HIV/AIDS* is to provide health care professionals who care for people infected and affected by HIV with a clinical reference tool that can increase their understanding of HIV and assist them in their care management. To meet this goal in the fourth edition, a team of clinical experts was invited to develop a book that reflected a multidisciplinary approach to HIV disease care management. As in past editions, we have maintained our research-based approach to care and, when data are not available, utilized evidence-based practice. In this edition we have provided information covering the following subjects:

- The history of the epidemic, the changes in HIV epidemiology, and emerging clinical concerns

- Health promotion and disease prevention including variables affecting the pathogenesis of HIV disease, factors related to HIV transmission, and personal, social group, and community efforts to prevent HIV infection

- The needs of infants, children, adults, and families, which have been expanded into chapters addressing the separate needs associated with HIV disease and the definitive diagnosis of AIDS

- Symptom management, now broadened to include nonpharmacologic and pharmacologic interventions as well as complementary therapies that can be employed for symptom control

- The new guidelines for the use of highly active antiretroviral therapy (HAART) and opportunistic infection prophylaxis for both pediatric and adult clients, which are discussed along with medication self-care management and adherence

- Psychosocial and spiritual needs of persons living with HIV disease, their families, lovers, spouses, and friends, which are covered in depth along with a discussion of the common psychiatric and neuropsychiatric conditions and psychotropic medications that can be used for treatment

- Cultural and social diversity issues related to beliefs, practices, models of illness and care, prevention, and health care delivery

- The needs of special populations including men who have sex with men; older adults; adolescents and persons with hemophilia; women, pregnant women, lesbians, and transgender/transsexual persons; injecting drug users, incarcerated persons, and commercial sex workers

- Alternative and complementary therapies including mind-body medicine, alternative systems of medicine, herbal medicine, and pharmacologic and biologic treatments
- Legal and ethical concerns including access to quality HIV care, accepting or refusing treatment, assisted suicide and euthanasia, wills, trusts, estate planning, the federal Family and Medical Leave Act of 1993, and Medicaid planning
- Community-based and long-term care including case management, home care, home infusion therapy, institutional long-term care, residential care, and hospice care
- The stresses and needs of health care providers, including psychosocial stresses, psychosocial tasks in treating persons living with HIV disease, HIV exposure in health care settings and postexposure prophylaxis, risk management, discrimination, and worker protection
- The drugs most frequently prescribed to treat HIV disease and related conditions and the common laboratory tests and interpretations ordered for evaluating patient responses to HIV disease, which are presented in two appendixes that will facilitate care management

Readers of this text should be aware of two phenomena associated with HIV disease. First, a wealth of new literature in this field becomes available on a daily basis. This evolving body of information will affect the treatment and education clinicians provide to their clients. Second, there is a vast array of opinions on certain issues related to HIV care. The most currently debated issues include when to initiate HAART and which drugs to use. This is partly due to human nature and partly due to the constant and consistent change in available information and the expedited process for drug approval in the United States (drugs becoming available sooner, with less knowledge about their long-term effects). It is important that health care providers stay well informed about opinion and give accurate information so their patients can make informed choices.

This fourth edition of *HIV/AIDS* represents not only the expertise and commitment of the contributors but also the hard work of several "behind the scenes" individuals without whom this endeavor might not have been possible: Thomas Eoyang, who not only has supported but also encouraged our work from its inception, Karen Taka, who is always there with editing, computer support, and keeping us "on track," and finally to our longtime companions and best friends, Jimie Rottner and John Flaskerud, who get a special heartfelt thanks for their love, good cheer, and dedication to the detail and completion of this project.

Peter and **Jackie**

Contents

1

Overview and Update of HIV Disease

JACQUELYN HAAK FLASKERUD ▪ PETER J. UNGVARSKI

At this writing, more than 640,000 cases of acquired immunodeficiency syndrome (AIDS) have been documented in the United States (CDC, December 31, 1997). The most recent estimate of HIV prevalence indicates that between 650,000 and 900,000 Americans are living with HIV (CDC, 1997). Statistical models suggest that at least 40,000 persons in the United States are being infected each year and roughly the same number die each year of HIV-related illness. HIV is the leading cause of death of all Americans between the ages of 25 and 44 years (CDC, 1997). Among African-American men 25 to 44 years of age, one in every three deaths was due to HIV-related illness in 1995; among African-American women the rate was one in every five deaths. For the total U.S. working-age population (15 to 64 years), the elimination of HIV would result in gains in life expectancy similar to that observed with a 50% reduction of heart disease or malignant neoplasms. Among African-American men, however, the elimination of HIV deaths would be similar to a 100% elimination of heart disease or malignant neoplasm deaths (Lai et al., 1997). Estimated AIDS incidence has increased at a rate of less than 5% each year since 1992. The CDC reported that in 1996 AIDS incidence (new cases) declined by 6% (CDC, September 19, 1997). AIDS *incidence* is much lower than in the mid 1980s, when incidence increased by 65% to 96% each year (CDC, 1997). Because the number of persons infected each year was roughly the same as the number who died each year, *prevalence* since 1992 has been stable. Recently, however, because of the use of combination antiretroviral therapy, more persons living with HIV (PLWH)

are living longer, and the prevalence of AIDS increased from 1995 to 1996 (CDC, September 19, 1997). Notable shifts in the epidemic demonstrate that the gains made in estimated AIDS incidence and prevalence are not being shared by all populations, most notably persons of color, women, and heterosexuals (CDC, September 19, 1997).

To date, no cure or vaccine has been found for HIV infection, and predictions are that AIDS will be with us well into the twenty-first century. Since 1995 there have been dramatic changes in pharmacologic treatment that hold out the promise that HIV/AIDS will become a chronic, treatable disease. This promise is yet to be realized in the populations most affected by the shifting demographics of the disease (Mulder, 1996).

HISTORY OF AIDS

The history of the AIDS epidemic in the United States is very recent. In June 1981 the first description of what would soon be referred to as AIDS appeared in the CDC's *Morbidity and Mortality Weekly Report* of June 5, 1981. The report described the occurrence of *Pneumocystis carinii* pneumonia (PCP) in five previously healthy, sexually active, young homosexual men from Los Angeles. This report was quickly followed by case reports of an unusual and extremely rare tumor, Kaposi's sarcoma (KS), in a male homosexual population in New York City. Both conditions occur infrequently and had previously been seen only in severely immunosuppressed persons.

Between June 1981 and May 1982, similar cases were reported to the CDC in increasing numbers. Initially the number of cases was doubling every 6 months. In addition to PCP and KS, other unusual viral, fungal, and parasitic infections were being diagnosed in young homosexual men. Again, these diseases had previously been seen only in severely immunosuppressed persons. Laboratory studies of patients with these opportunistic infections and cancers revealed that all of them had severe immunodeficiencies; clinically, their condition deteriorated and they quickly died of these unusual infections (CDC, September 24, 1982).

At first only homosexual and bisexual men were thought to be affected, and some aspect of the gay lifestyle was hypothesized to be the probable cause of the immunodeficiency. The disease was named gay-related immunodeficiency at that time. However, as the complex of diseases became more widely recognized, other cases reported to the CDC made it obvious that this was not a disease limited to homosexuals. The same infections and tumors were reported in heterosexual injecting drug users (IDUs); Haitian immigrants; persons with hemophilia; spouses, sexual partners, and children of persons with the disease; and recipients of blood or blood components from infected persons (CDC, July 9, 1982; CDC, July 16, 1982). In September 1982 the CDC designated the disease as AIDS and defined its characteristics. With the exception of Haitian immigrants, in whom infections were found to be related to the other modes of transmission, the originally identified groups became and currently remain those most frequently exposed to the virus. It soon became apparent that AIDS was transmitted through an exchange of body fluids. Sexual transmission occurs between men and men and between men and women, but currently the largest sexual-transmission group in the United States remains men who have sex with men (MSM), 50%; the next largest group is injecting drug users (IDUs), 26%, both male and female. These two groups and a combination of the two groups (MSM and IDU) account for 76% of persons 13 years of age and older with AIDS nationwide; 85% of adolescent and adult persons with AIDS are male (CDC, December 31, 1997). The World Health Organization (WHO) has designated this pattern of transmission as pattern 1. However, the proportion of newly reported AIDS cases among adults and adolescents

in the United States attributed to use of injected drugs has increased from 17% in 1985 to 26% in 1995 (CDC, 1997). The proportion of cases related to each exposure category varies significantly among the geographic regions of the United States. These differences are addressed later in this chapter.

While the number of cases was mounting in the United States, AIDS started appearing in Europe, where an interesting phenomenon was observed. Although in many European countries transmission patterns were similar to those in the United States (pattern 1 transmission), a sizable number of cases were occurring in immigrants from Central Africa or in Europeans who had traveled the major trade routes in sub-Saharan Africa. When investigators turned their attention to Africa, they discovered an epidemic that could be traced through serologic studies to 1959 (von Reyn & Mann, 1987). HIV-1 origins in Africa have been attributed to cross-species trafficking between African primates (probably the chimpanzee and humans) (Ryan, 1997, pp. 285–300). Blood-to-blood contact from bites or scratches incurred in the hunting of primates has been proposed as the crossover mechanism. A different aspect of the epidemic in Africa is that it affects men and women equally and is widespread in the heterosexual population (WHO designation, pattern 2) (van Harmelen et al., 1997). The disease has been reported in 54 countries in Africa and has been transmitted principally through heterosexual contact, with HIV incidence higher among women than among men in sub-Saharan Africa (Anderson, 1996; Mann & Tarantola, 1996, p. 19). In Africa, in addition to HIV-1, retroviruses designated HIV-2 and HTLV-IV were isolated in 1985. The highest rates of HIV-2 infection have been reported in West Africa. HIV-2 infection also exists in Angola and Mozambique, and sporadic cases have been reported in the U.S., North and South America, the Caribbean, India, and Europe (DeCock & Brun-Vezinet, 1996). HIV-2 infection has transmission patterns, clinical features, and public health interventions similar to those of HIV-1 (CDC, August 18, 1995; DeCock & Brun-Vezinet, 1996).

HIV-1 was identified and named in stages. Not until early 1983 was there any indication that a human T-cell leukemia/lymphotropic virus might be the causative agent of AIDS (Barre-

Sinoussi et al., 1983; Ryan, 1997, pp. 247–267). Luc Montagnier and scientists at the Institut Pasteur in France named the virus *lymphadenopathy-associated virus (LAV)*. In the United States in May 1984, Robert Gallo and other investigators at the National Institutes of Health reported the isolation of a group of cytopathic retroviruses and antibodies against those viruses in persons with AIDS. They termed their discovery *human T-lymphotropic virus type III (HTLV-III)* (Popovic et al., 1984; Ryan, 1997, pp. 249–267). At the same time, West Coast scientists at the University of California San Francisco who were studying the virus named it the *AIDS-associated retrovirus (ARV)* (Levy et al., 1984). In the summer of 1986, the International Society on the Taxonomy of Viruses arbitrated, changing the name to *human immunodeficiency virus type 1 (HIV-1)*. Through legal arbitration, Montagnier and Gallo have been recognized as codiscoverers of the virus. For the sake of standardization and communication, the virus is now known worldwide as HIV-1.

Identification of the virus led to development of a test for HIV antibody in the blood. This test made it possible to determine which persons carried HIV antibody and therefore had been infected by HIV; it also permitted the screening of blood and blood products to prevent transmission by blood transfusion (Abrams, 1986; Najera et al., 1987).

Since 1981 the AIDS pandemic has assumed major proportions. It has been characterized as a global epidemic out of control (Mann & Tarantola, 1996, pp. 5–39). The Global AIDS Policy Coalition (GAPC), made up of ranking scientists, educators, and health workers around the world, has described the epidemic as volatile, dynamic, and unstable, with its major impact yet to come (Mann & Tarantola, 1996, pp. 5–39). AIDS in the World II survey estimates are that about 22 million people around the world are living with the virus and that as many as 60 to 70 million adults will become infected by the year 2000 (Mann & Tarantola, 1996, pp. 5–39). From the beginning of the pandemic until January 1, 1996, an estimated 30.6 million persons have been infected with HIV and 9 million have died. The largest numbers of HIV-infected people have been in sub-Saharan Africa (63%) and Southeast Asia (23%). The number of HIV-infected people

in Southeast Asia is now three times the total in the industrialized world. Currently there are 11.6 million living infected persons in sub-Saharan Africa, 2 million in the Americas, more than 6.6 million in Northeast and mostly (>95%) Southeast Asia, about 700,000 in Western Europe, 362,000 in the Caribbean, 32,000 in Eastern Europe, 69,000 in the Southeastern Mediterranean, and 25,000 in Oceania (Mann & Tarantola, 1996, pp. 5–39). Worldwide, about 75% of HIV infections are transmitted sexually, with four cases transmitted by male-female contact to each one case transmitted by male-male sexual contact. The remainder of infections are about equally divided between the exposure routes of injectable drug use, perinatal transmission, and transfusion transmission. From these data, it is obvious that the picture of the epidemic worldwide is very different from that in the United States.

After careful study of the global epidemic, the GAPC characterized the epidemic and its lessons:

1. No community or country already affected by AIDS has been able to stop the spread of HIV.
2. HIV is spreading rapidly to new communities and countries around the world, and HIV will reach most, if not all, human communities. Geography may delay the spread but will not protect against it.
3. The global epidemic becomes more complex as it matures and is composed of thousands of smaller, complicated subepidemics as HIV exploits every potential avenue for spread.
4. HIV has demonstrated repeatedly its ability to cross all borders—social, economic, cultural, political, and geographic—and the conditions that foster HIV spread are complex and changing.
5. A plateau of the efforts against HIV dominates the global picture while at the same time the pandemic is expanding at a dynamic pace (Mann & Tarantola, 1996, pp. 5–39; Weniger & Brown, 1996).

Current Issues

The picture of HIV infection today in the United States is more optimistic. Yet it is necessary to focus on the knowledge, commitment, and action that can make a difference. When the first edition of this text was published in 1989, the progress made against the disease from 1981 to that time was summarized: the probable causative agent of AIDS had been discovered, the virus had been cloned, a blood-screening program had been implemented, work on the development of a vaccine had begun, and therapies that extend life had been identified. By the second edition, many major changes had occurred in the progression and epidemiology of the disease, treatment and health care, and the delivery of care. These changes included increased survival time after diagnosis, a decline in Kaposi's sarcoma as a presenting diagnosis, testing of several vaccines, changes in biologic and behavioral cofactors to infection and disease progression, expanded use of zidovudine and prophylactic antibiotics, a shift in treatment and care from acute care centers to the community, changes in the cost of care, and changes in the efficacy and ethics of HIV antibody testing

By the third edition, additional changes occurred in the epidemiology of HIV infection, disease expression, treatment, costs of care, and the political climate. These changes included a revised classification system from the CDC and WHO; resurgence of a tuberculosis (TB) epidemic synergistic with the HIV epidemic and the emergence of multidrug-resistant TB; questions from scientists and clinicians about the efficacy of early retroviral treatment and hope for combination therapies, along with questions regarding the validity of the CD4+ marker for determining the efficacy of such drugs; the continuing issue of cost of care as the managed care industry gained control; and continued sociopolitical furor, anger, and discrimination, as examplified by the transmission of HIV from a dentist to a patient.

Since the third (1995) edition, several more changes have occurred in HIV treatment, disease progression, knowledge of the virus and transmission, and social/political issues surrounding these changes. An overview of changes is given here. Those that address health care practices and issues are covered in depth in later, related chapters.

Two major changes have gone hand in hand in the treatment of HIV disease: (1) the development of a laboratory assay—HIV RNA quantitation—as a marker of HIV progression through the estimation of HIV viral load or viral burden present in the blood and (2) treatment with combination antiretroviral drugs, including protease inhibitors, based on HIV viral burden.

The major change in HIV treatment that has occurred since the third edition of this text was written involves the use of protease inhibitors in combination with other antiretroviral drugs (termed a "cocktail" of drugs), which are used as treatment early in the course of HIV disease. Typically, this cocktail regimen consists of several drugs (for instance, two reverse transcriptase inhibitors plus a protease inhibitor) (Phillips, 1996; Williams, 1997). Combination therapy is the preferred treatment because these drugs, in combination, have a synergistic effect. They attack different stages of the HIV life cycle and act in different reservoirs of infection (e.g., cell, tissue). Finally, combinations may slow viral mutations and subsequent resistance to drug therapy (Phillips, 1996; Williams, 1997). Effective anti-HIV regimens are complex and individually tailored and rely on client partnership in taking prescribed medications with consistency, regularity, and diligence. Each of the antiretroviral drugs has side effects, some of which are severe and toxic. These medications can cost $600 to $1000 per month (CDC, July 1997). Taken together, combination antiretroviral drugs have worked so effectively that they have reduced plasma HIV viral burden below levels that can be detected with current HIV RNA quantitative assays. Because these drug cocktails have been so effective, the International AIDS Society–USA Panel recommended in 1997 that combination antiretroviral therapy be initiated in all HIV-infected persons who have detectable plasma HIV RNA and who are committed to a treatment regimen (Carpenter et al., 1997).

To quickly determine the most effective therapeutic management of HIV infection, clinicians must rely on an assessment of disease progression and prognosis of each person with HIV. As reported in the third edition of this text, both clinicians and researchers had become skeptical of the validity of the CD4+ count as a surrogate marker of HIV pathogenesis. A major breakthrough in assessing HIV status and prognosis came with the development of a new laboratory assay to quantitate HIV RNA in blood plasma (Ho et al., 1995). The two most common methods currently in use are the PCR (polymerase chain reaction) and bDNA (branched DNA) techniques, which have comparable detection limits (Melroe et al., 1997). The significance of HIV RNA quantitation is that it has been shown to be a highly valid marker in determining disease progression (Mellors et al., 1996). The ability to monitor disease progression allows clinicians to determine the effectiveness of treatment and to adjust antiretroviral therapy on the basis of detectable viral levels.

The development of HIV RNA quantitation has facilitated the rapid development of new therapy combinations. Current treatment with combination antiretroviral therapy has resulted in nondetectable viral plasma loads in some PLWH. The development of HIV RNA quantitation and combination antiretroviral therapies has produced a whole new set of issues surrounding HIV exposure and treatment. Many of the misunderstandings about exposure are the result of the public's not knowing what "nondetectable viral load" means. Several reports have given the impression that PLWH and the public believe that, because HIV is nondetectable in their blood, they no longer are infected with it. Interviews with HIV-infected gay men in New York City revealed that these men were engaging in unprotected anal intercourse because they were "on proteases and have no viral load" (Shernoff & Ball, 1997). Similarly, Cookie Johnson told an interviewer that she believed "the Lord has definitely healed Earvin [Magic Johnson]. . . . there is no virus left in his blood" (Randolph, 1997). Statements such as these lead to concern among clinicians and researchers that there will be a return to risky behavior in HIV-infected persons who believe that the virus is no longer in their blood. "Nondetectable viral load" means that the assay's minimum of detection could not determine the amount of virus. PLWH need to understand this and to know that HIV is still present in body tissues.

The effectiveness of combination antiretroviral therapy in lowering viral burden has also led to the belief that this treatment can be prescribed as a "morning after" treatment for exposure to HIV. Indeed, in some cities it is being given as such to persons who have engaged in risky behaviors (Gorman, 1997). Again, the concern is that with the new drug treatments people will see AIDS as more benign and start relying on pills instead of safer sex practices to guard against infection. Because of these developments, a major question has arisen: Who should get prophylactic, combination therapy?

The use of postexposure prophylaxis for health care workers with occupational exposures has been recommended by the CDC (June 7, 1996) and is standard practice in hospitals and other health care facilities (Katz & Gerberding, 1997). See Appendix IV for information on postexposure prophylaxis. The premise behind postexposure treatment is that chemoprophylaxis may prevent initial cellular infection and local propagation of HIV and allow host immune defenses to eliminate the inoculum of virus. Postexposure treatment in a case-control study reduced the odds of HIV infection by 79%; however, a randomized, controlled trial has not been conducted and may not be feasible (Katz & Gerberding, 1997). If postexposure treatment is available and is believed to be effective in treating health care workers after occupational exposure, it would seem unethical to deny it to persons exposed sexually or through contaminated injecting drug equipment. However, the concern is that some people will abandon safer behaviors and ask for these treatments repeatedly. There is a clear need for a public health policy in this area that addresses number of exposures, motivation and intention of individuals, HIV status of partner(s), and cost of treatment. Prophylaxis must be placed in the context of an overall program of health promotion.

The question of who should receive antiretroviral combination therapy involves also the complexity of the treatment protocols and the ability or willingness of persons to follow a therapeutic regimen. Many factors enter into whether a person will be able to adhere to a treatment regimen (Crespo-Fierro, 1997). These include severe side effects, complex regimens, inconvenient dosing schedules, skepticism about treatment efficacy, a culturally different world view of illness and treatment, control issues, continuing substance use, and tenuous living arrangements, among others. The reason that compliance has become an overriding concern is that any level of noncompliance will lead eventually to the development of drug resistance (Crespo-Fierro, 1997). If therapeutic levels of protease inhibitors are not maintained, drug resistance (the emergence of drug-resistant virus) can develop quickly (2 to 4 weeks) and spread to other drugs in this class (Williams, 1997). The inappropriate use of antiretroviral agents leads the virus toward selective pressure to form resistant organisms (Huebscher, 1997). The problem of drug resistance is not an individual one but, rather, a population or aggregate problem and has consequences for both infected and uninfected persons. A public health perspective of host-agent-environment interaction best explains the wide-ranging effect of not maintaining therapeutic levels of protease inhibitors. A drug-resistant agent (HIV-1) produced within an infected individual can then be transmitted to other persons (hosts), creating a new epidemic in the populations most vulnerable to infection. Therefore the question of who should get combination antiretroviral drugs must take into account which persons will follow a therapeutic regimen and which ones will not. Clinicians and researchers have recommended that postexposure prophylaxis should not be given to persons who do not follow the therapeutic regimen to completion or who continue to practice risky behaviors (Katz & Gerberding, 1997). Similarly, the International AIDS Society–USA Panel has recommended that combination treatment regimens be given to HIV-infected persons who are committed to a treatment regimen (Carpenter et al., 1997).

Finally, the question of who pays for combination antiretroviral therapy needs to be answered. The cost of postexposure prophylaxis has been estimated at about $800 to $1000 for a 4-week course of zidovudine, lamivudine, and indinavir (Katz & Gerberding, 1997). The issue of who will pay the up-front costs of prophylaxis is a concern surrounding combination antiretroviral therapy. Insurers may refuse such payment without knowing its effectiveness. Persons at risk may not be insured or may not be able to afford the therapy.

In today's managed care industry, the cost of care, access to care, and risk selection are all significant issues for PLWH who are given combination antiretroviral therapy (Volberding, 1996). The additional cost of HIV RNA quantitation is also part of a state-of-the-art approach to this treatment. The increasing cost of antiretroviral protocols means that these therapies are unavailable to the majority of people who could benefit from them in the United States (Williams, 1997). About half of all people with HIV are uninsured (Katz & Gerberding, 1997). For those on Medicaid, there is limited access to outpatient care (Medicaid Access Study Group, 1994). Many managed care companies are abandoning the Medicaid market altogether because of reduced

profitability (Center for Studying Health System Change, 1997). A health care climate that relies on outcomes, empirical data, cost containment, and reduced use challenges, if not endangers, the access of most persons with HIV to antiretroviral treatment protocols (Graham et al., 1994). Without a change in the current health care delivery business, there is the actuality of an ever-increasing underserved population of people with AIDS.

A serious and current issue removed from combination antiretroviral therapy is the dangerous synergy that exists between HIV and TB. This concern was raised in the previous edition of this text in the context of an emerging TB epidemic and multidrug-resistant TB. The facilitative nature of the relationship between HIV and TB deserves added emphasis here. Nearly one half of urban TB patients in the United States are also infected with HIV (Asch et al., 1997). Among homeless persons in Los Angeles and San Francisco, one third are infected with TB (Gelberg et al., 1997). The CDC (January 19, 1996) has recommended cross-checking of TB and HIV registries to assist in characterizing the extent of comorbidity. The increased coincidence of TB and HIV requires that health care providers become familiar with the case definition of TB and diagnostic accuracy. Lack of familiarity is evidenced by a study in Los Angeles that showed that one third of TB patients were not tested for HIV because providers considered them to be at "low risk" (Asch et al., 1997). Physicians are less likely to suspect TB in high-risk women than in men (Cegielski et al., 1997). Health care workers must be familiar with TB and HIV and the synergy between them. Persons with TB should be given HIV testing and counseling, and persons with HIV should be screened for TB, although anergy skin testing is no longer recommended (CDC, September 5, 1997). The concern over HIV and TB remains at the forefront of the HIV epidemic.

A final current issue of scientific and clinical interest is the association between HIV-1 subtypes and mode of transmission that has been identified in South Africa and Thailand (Mastro et al., 1997; van Harmelen et al., 1997). HIV subtype B predominates in industrialized western countries where transmission is through MSM and IDUs. Subtype C viruses are associated with heterosexual and vertical transmission. These data suggest that there might be two independent epidemics of HIV in the world, one heterosexual and perinatal and the other homosexual/bisexual and involving injection drug use. Currently, these epidemics are considered very dynamic, but they may imply different transmission efficiencies, a need for different vaccines for different risk groups, and the development of subtype-appropriate prevention modalities (Mastro et al., 1997; van Harmelen et al., 1997).

The epidemiology of AIDS has changed also in the past 4 years. The epidemiology of AIDS for specific populations is discussed in Chapters 3 through 9. An overview of epidemiologic changes is given here.

CHANGES IN EPIDEMIOLOGY OF HIV DISEASE

The sociodemographic characteristics of persons with HIV disease differ with geographic re-

gions in the United States. These differences have become more pronounced during the past 4 years and have come to characterize the population with AIDS in each region. The national statistics often do not adequately reflect the gender, ethnicity, or route of transmission of PLWH in a particular city or region. To mount effective prevention and treatment programs, health care workers must be aware of the sociodemographic characteristics of PLWH in their own region. The demographics of total AIDS cases in the 10 metropolitan statistical areas (MSAs) and the 10 states or commonwealths with the most AIDS cases are presented in Table 1–1.

As may be noted in Table 1–1, the geographic distribution of AIDS has changed in the past 4 years. The percentage of the total number of AIDS cases represented in the 10 leading MSAs has decreased since 1991, reflecting a spread of

Table 1–1 ▪ Demographics of Total AIDS Cases

	% of Total U.S. Cases		
	1997	1993	1991
TEN LEADING MSAs*			
New York City (1)†	15.7	16.6	19.0
Los Angeles (2)	6.0	6.4	7.0
San Francisco (3)	4.2	5.0	6.0
Miami (4)	3.4	2.9	2.4
Washington, DC (6)	2.9	2.8	2.8
Chicago (5)	2.8	2.8	2.4
Houston (7)	2.5	2.7	3.0
Philadelphia (9)	2.3	2.1	2.7
Newark (8)	2.3	2.2	2.0
Atlanta (11)	2.1	2.0	2.0
Combined % of total	44.2	43.0	49.3
TEN LEADING STATES OR COMMONWEALTHS			
New York (1)†	18.4	19.2	22.0
California (2)	16.8	18.3	19.0
Florida (3)	9.8	9.8	8.0
Texas (4)	6.8	7.0	7.0
New Jersey (5)	5.7	5.7	6.5
Puerto Rico (6)	3.2	3.2	2.9
Illinois (7)	3.2	3.2	3.0
Pennsylvania (9)	2.3	2.7	2.8
Georgia (8)	2.9	2.7	2.6
Maryland	2.6	—	—
Combined % of total	72.5	73.9‡	75.8‡

*MSA, Metropolitan Statistical Area.
†(1) Position in 1993.
‡Included Massachusetts in Position 10.
Statistics from Centers for Disease Control (June 30, 1997). *HIV/AIDS Surveillance Report.* United States AIDS Program, Atlanta, Georgia.

AIDS to smaller cities and rural areas of the United States and to the Southeast. Other than the MSAs in Table 1–1, metropolitan statistical areas with more than 10,000 cases (more than 2% of total cases) are San Juan, Puerto Rico, Baltimore, Boston, and Dallas. The 10 leading states together continue to decrease their percentage of total cases. However, there is an apparent shift to a greater percentage of total cases in the Southeastern United States. The CDC reported that although the rate of AIDS cases per 100,000 persons remains highest in the Northeast, the epidemic is spreading to other regions, with an increasing proportion of cases reported in the South (CDC, 1997). Cases in the Northeast represent a decreasing proportion of the annual total, declining from 42% in 1985 to 31% in 1995. The proportion of cases in the West has also decreased, from 28% in 1985 to 20% in 1995. However, the proportion of newly reported cases of AIDS in the South has increased from 24% in 1985 to 36% in 1995 and in the North Central region from 6% in 1985 to 10% in 1995 (CDC, 1997). From the analysis of national trends, it is apparent that AIDS has been spreading from larger metropolitan regions to smaller metropolitan areas of the nation (Mukhopadhyay, 1996). Clearly, the geographic face of AIDS is changing in the United States.

The surveillance data for route of exposure, gender, and ethnicity in the Northeastern states and MSAs differ from the national surveillance data and those in the Midwest (North Central) and West. Infection of MSM is greater in the West and among some ethnic groups; infection of IDUs, women, African-Americans, and Latinos is greater in the Northeast and Southeast.

Exposure

The proportion of newly reported AIDS cases attributed to MSM decreased from 66% of the annual total in 1985 to 42% in 1995. While the proportion of AIDS cases related to MSM is declining overall, the proportion attributable to young MSM continues to rise (Hays et al., 1997). For male adolescents 13 to 19 years of age the proportion related to MSM increased from 29% in 1994 to 34% in 1995. For the ages of 13 to 25 years between 1989 and 1994, AIDS incidence decreased 34% in young white MSM and increased 19% in young African-American MSM

and 24% in Latinos (Denning et al., 1996). There is indirect evidence that high-risk behavior among MSM may be increasing. Gonorrhea trends in MSM in eight major U.S. cities reflect an increase in unprotected anal intercourse between 1993 and 1996 (CDC, September 26, 1997). These sexual behaviors also influence the risk of HIV.

MSM with AIDS tend to be concentrated in major metropolitan areas. When AIDS emerged in the early 1980s, prevention programs were first targeted to those hardest hit—MSM in New York City, Los Angeles, and San Francisco. Partly because of sustained prevention efforts, the rate of new AIDS diagnoses among gay and bisexual men has decreased dramatically among white men in these cities, with rates declining by 20% in New York City, 16% in Los Angeles, and 3% in San Francisco between 1989 and 1994. In these same cities, however, the rate of new AIDS diagnoses among African-American MSM increased dramatically during this period, with rates increasing by 49% in New York City, 48% in Los Angeles, and 53% in San Francisco (CDC, 1997).

The AIDS epidemic in California plateaued in 1992 (Singleton et al., 1996). Cases declined in Los Angeles and San Francisco counties and increased in the rest of the state. The decline was the result of a decrease in cases among white MSM. Women, African-Americans, and Latinos (male-to-male, male-to-female, and female-to-male transmission) all experienced an increase in AIDS incidence (CDC, November 18, 1994). In addition, cases of AIDS increased in the group aged 13 to 19 years (Singleton et al., 1996). A study of MSM in New York City showed that AIDS case rates have flattened in white MSM but that case rates continued to rise in African-American and Latino MSM (Torian et al., 1996). See Table 1–2 for additional comparative data on MSM and regional distribution. HIV prevalence data suggest that the rate of infection among IDUs has stabilized at a high rate, with the highest concentration in the Northeast. By region, the Northeast accounted for 50% of adult and adolescent AIDS cases in IDUs in 1995, followed by the South (27%), and the West (10%) (CDC, 1997). AIDS cases and new infections related to IDU appear to be increasingly concentrated in ethnic people of color, especially African-Americans. See Table

1–2 for additional comparative data on injection drug use.

Injecting drug users with AIDS are concentrated in major metropolitan areas. As may be noted in Table 1–2, IDUs now account for the largest percentage of AIDS cases in New York City, Newark, New Jersey, and Washington, D.C. (Mukhopadhyay, 1996). In Chicago, AIDS cases among IDUs accounted for 21% of the cases diagnosed in 1990. This number grew to 34% in 1995. Similarly, IDU-related transmission (IDU, MSM-IDUs, sexual partners of IDUs, children of IDUs, or partners of IDUs) grew from 31% in 1990 to 44% in 1995. In 1995 IDU-related transmission accounted for as many AIDS cases as MSM transmission (Chicago Department of Public Health, 1997).

The proportion of yearly reported (incidence) AIDS cases related to heterosexual contact has increased steadily over time, from 2% in 1985 to 11% in 1995 (CDC, 1997). Heterosexuals are concentrated in the nonmetropolitan and smaller metropolitan statistical areas, which tend to have a population of less than 1 million (Mukhopadhyay, 1996).

Gender

Women account for an increasing proportion of newly reported AIDS cases. The proportion of AIDS cases in female adults and adolescents increased from 7% of the annual total in 1985 to 19% in 1995 (CDC, 1997). In contrast, the proportion of AIDS cases in male adults and adolescents decreased from 93% of the annual total in 1985 to 81% in 1995. Of heterosexual AIDS cases reported in 1995, 65% were among women. Of these cases, 37% were sex partners of IDUs. Of the remaining cases, 54% were sex partners of HIV-infected persons whose risk was not specified, 7% were sex partners of bisexual men, and 25% were sex partners of recipients of blood or blood products. The CDC conducts investigations of adults and adolescents whose risk is not specified. Among males, 58% were reclassified as MSM, 22% as IDUs, and 5% as a combination of IDUs and MSM (CDC, December 31, 1996). These data represent an explanation of partners whose risk is unspecified for heterosexual transmission to women. Dade County, Florida (including Miami), represents an extreme example of unidentified risk for women. AIDS cases

reported in 1997 from January through August included 23% of white women with risk not reported, 35% of black women, and 27% of Latino women (Dade County Health Department, August 30, 1997). If national reclassification of unidentified risk can be applied to Dade County, heterosexual exposure of these women would be attributed to sex with an MSM, IDU, or MSM/IDU. Another group of these women might be exposed through their own injection drug use practices.

In 1995, 35% of heterosexual AIDS occurred in men. Of these, 33% were sex partners of IDUs and 65% were sex partners of persons whose risk was not specified. Among females whose risk was unspecified, 27% were reclassified as IDUs (CDC, December 31, 1996). Again using Dade County, Florida, as an example, in the first 8 months of 1997, 8% of white men, 36% of black men, and 15% of Latino men had unreported risk (Dade County Health Department, August 30, 1997). For those men exposed heterosexually, the most likely exposure would be sex with an IDU. However, these men may also have been exposed through MSM, IDUs, or MSM-IDUs. In comparing the first 6 months of 1995 with the first 6 months of 1994, AIDS incidence among women who were heterosexual partners of IDUs increased 9%, and AIDS incidence increased 17% among men who were heterosexual partners of IDUs (CDC, 1997).

Age

Estimates based on the age distribution of AIDS cases suggest that in recent years as many as half of new infections may be among young persons under 25 years of age (CDC, 1997; Hays et al., 1997). Among young men (13 to 24 years) who were becoming infected, 55% of the reported cases in 1995 were among young MSM, 10% were among young men infected through IDU, and 6% were among young men infected heterosexually. Young women in the same age group were infected heterosexually (51%) and through IDU (17%) (CDC, 1997). However, trends in incidence varied greatly by ethnicity. Whereas AIDS incidence fell 16% among young (13 to 25 years) whites between 1990 and 1995, it rose 20% among young Latinos and 65% among young African-Americans (Denning & Fleming, 1997). The decrease in young whites

Table 1–2 ▪ Geographic Distribution of AIDS by Exposure, Age, Gender, and Ethnic Group (in Percent) in Leading Metropolitan Statistical Areas

	United States	New York City	Newark	Washington, DC
EXPOSURE CATEGORY				
Male-male sexual contact	49	32	10	54
Injecting drug use (IDU)	26	45	57	27
Male-male sexual contact/IDU	6	3	4	5
Hemophilia/coagulation disorder	<1	0	<1	0
Male-female sexual contact	9	8	14	9
Transfusion with blood/products	4	1	1	1
Perinatal	1	2	2	1
Undetermined	7	10	12	2
AGE AND GENDER				
*Adults**	98.7	98	98	98
Male	85	78	67	85
Female	15	22	33	15
Children†	1.3	2	2	2
AGE AND ETHNIC GROUP				
Adults				
White	47	31	4	24
African-American	35	38	83	73
Latino	18	29	13	3
Other‡	1	2	0	0
Children				
White	18	7	2	2
African-American	58	56	85	95
Latino	23	37	13	3
Other‡	1	0	0	0

Statistics based on surveillance data provided by the Centers for Disease Control and Prevention and the states and cities listed as of summer 1997.
*Includes all patients 13 years of age and older.
†Inlcudes all patients less than 13 years of age.
‡Includes Asian/Pacific Islander and American Indian/Alaska Native.
Note: Totals may not equal 100% because of rounding.

was due mostly to the decline in cases among young white MSM, whereas the increase in young blacks was due primarily to a 150% rise in heterosexual contacts, which affects women predominantly. Because this rise in incidence among young heterosexual contacts affects women predominantly, there was a 73% increase in HIV incidence in young women (Denning & Fleming, 1997). The HIV epidemic among young persons is spreading fastest among heterosexual contacts, especially African-American women.

Ethnicity

African-Americans account for an increasing proportion of yearly reported cases, from 25% in

1985 to 40% in 1995. Similarly, the proportion of newly reported cases among Latinos has increased steadily from 15% of the annual total in 1985 to 19% in 1995. The proportion of cases among Asian/Pacific Islanders in the United States and American Indian/Alaskan Natives has remained at less than 1% each. The proportion of cases among whites has decreased from 60% in 1985 to 40% in 1995 (CDC, 1997). The disproportionate occurrence of AIDS in ethnic people of color is true in all regions, genders, age groups, and exposure categories. The majority of cases of AIDS among women and children in all regions of the country occur among African-American and Latino women. In Los Angeles African-

	Atlanta	Miami	Philadelphia	Chicago	Houston	Los Angeles	San Francisco
	51	39	46	43	63	74	81
	19	19	35	34	11	7	6
	6	4	6	3	9	6	10
	0	0	0	<1	0	<1	0
	11	12	10	9	9	4	1
	1	1	1	<1	1	1	1
	1	2	1	1	1	<1	0
	10	23	2	9	7	6	1
	99	98	98	99	99	99	99
	86	79	84	80	89	94	97
	14	21	16	20	11	6	3
	1	2	2	1	1	1	1
	40	19	27	20	56	53	76
	58	47	62	64	30	19	11
	2	33	10	13	14	26	10
	0	0	1	1	0	2	3
	21	4	7	9	16	19	41
	77	87	78	69	61	33	34
	20	9	15	21	23	5	15
	0	0	1	1	0	6	10

American women (37%) and children (33%) and Latino women (33%) and children (45%) make up 70% and 78% of AIDS cases, respectively, among women and children (Los Angeles County Department of Health Services, July 15, 1997). In Chicago between 1994 and 1997, 72% of AIDS cases in women occurred in African-American women, 14% occurred in white women, and 14% occurred in Latino women. Among children, 69% of cases occurred in African-American children, 21% in Latino children, and 9% in white children (Chicago Department of Public Health, 1997). In Philadelphia 73% of AIDS cases cumulatively occurred in black women, 13% in white women, and 14% in Latino women (Philadelphia Department of Public Health, June 1997). In New York City in the first 6 months of 1997, 55% of new cases in children occurred in African-American children, 34% in Latino children, and 9.5% in white children (New York State Department of Health, June 30, 1997).

Cumulatively, white men still account for 50.6% of AIDS prevalence in the United States (CDC, December 31, 1996). However, in 1996–1997 in New York City, African-American men made up 38% of the total number of adult males with AIDS, Latino men made up 31%, and white men made up 30% of the total (New York State Department of Health, June 30, 1997). In

Chicago from 1994 to 1997 African-American men made up 57% of the adult male total, white men 27%, and Latino men 15% (Chicago Department of Public Health, 1997). In Los Angeles the percent of new cases of AIDS in men in 1990 among African-Americans (18%) and Latinos (24%) made up 42% of the total new cases, and in 1996 these two groups made up 56% of new cases in men (Los Angeles County Department of Health Services, July 15, 1997).

As noted earlier, in New York City, Los Angeles, and San Francisco, rates of new AIDS diagnoses among MSM decreased between 1989 and 1994 among white men in these cities, with rates declining by 20% in New York City, 16% in Los Angeles, and 3% in San Francisco. In contrast, in these same cities, new AIDS diagnoses among African-American MSM have increased dramatically during this period by 49% in New York City, 48% in Los Angeles, and 53% in San Francisco (CDC, 1997).

From 1989 to 1994 the proportion of young (13 to 25 years) MSM who were white declined from 53% to 38% while the proportion who were African-American increased from 30% to 39%, and the proportion who were Latino increased from 15% to 21%. The proportions who were Asian/Pacific Islander or American Indian/Alaskan Native remained relatively constant at 1% each (Denning et al., 1996). Among injecting drug users, new infections are increasingly concentrated in ethnic people of color, particularly African-Americans. In Chicago between 1994 and 1997, 38% of male IDUs with AIDS were African-American, 11% were white, and 31% were Latino, principally Puerto Rican (Chicago Department of Public Health, 1997). In New York City 46% of the IDUs with new cases of AIDS are African-American, 40% are Latino, and 14% are white (New York State Department of Health, June 30, 1997). In Philadelphia 69% of new cases of AIDS in IDUs, MSM IDUs, and heterosexual IDUs combined occurred in African-Americans, 16% in whites, and 15% in Latinos (Philadelphia Department of Health, June 1997).

The AIDS epidemic in the United States has taken on a new face: In the last 4 years greater concern has arisen regarding young people, women, children, and ethnic people of color. As of this writing, it is clear that AIDS is spreading to the smaller cities and rural areas of the United States. It is also an epidemic out of control among people of color. The epidemiology of AIDS makes it clear that it is virtually impossible to provide health care services in the United States without knowledge of AIDS and the multiple epidemics it spawns in the various regions and human groups that it affects.

The explosion of knowledge about AIDS has been phenomenal. Health care workers need in-depth and up-to-date knowledge of AIDS to practice. Health professionals have close and constant contact with PLWH in a variety of settings and are involved in AIDS education and prevention in the community.

HIV DISEASE

To speak knowledgeably and to understand the disease known as AIDS, one must define the problem in all its complexity. The term *AIDS* is used to indicate only the most severe diseases or clinical conditions (i.e., infections, neoplasms) observed in the continuum of illness related to infection with the retrovirus human immunodeficiency virus type 1 (HIV-1). HIV-1 and AIDS are not synonymous terms. Studies of the natural history of HIV infection have documented a wide spectrum of disease conditions, ranging from asymptomatic infection to life-threatening conditions characterized by severe immunodeficiency, serious opportunistic infections, and cancers (CDC, December 18, 1992). This range of disease conditions has a strong association with the levels of CD4+ T-lymphocytes per microliter of blood and with HIV RNA quantitation (viral load) (Ho et al., 1995; Melroe et al., 1997). In the past, published classification schemes for HIV infection stratified various HIV-related illnesses into separate syndromes, such as AIDS-related complex and lymphadenopathy syndrome. AIDS itself was classified according to various clinical conditions known as AIDS indicator conditions (CDC, May 23, 1986). These different presentations of HIV disease are now considered a continuum of host response to HIV infection and not separate syndromes. In 1993 in the United States, HIV disease was reclassified according to CD4+ T-lymphocyte count and clinical conditions associated with HIV infection (CDC, December 18, 1992; Singleton et al., 1996). The

Table 1–3 ▪ Comparison: 1993 Revised Classification System for HIV Infection (CDCP) and WHO Proposed Staging System for HIV Infection and Disease, 1993

CD4+ T-cell Categories CDC: 1,2,3 WHO: A,B,C	(A) Asymptomatic, HIV-1, PGL (1) Asymptomatic		(B) Symptomatic (2) Early (3) Intermediate		(C) AIDS-indicator (3) Intermediate (4) Late	
	CDCP	WHO	CDCP	WHO	CDCP	WHO
1 or A CD4+ ≥500	A1	1A	B1	2A and 3A	C1	3A and 4A
2 or B CD4+ 200–499	A2	1B	B2	2B and 3B	C2	3B and 4B
3 or C CD4+ <200	A3	1C	B3	2C and 3C	C3	C3 and 4C

Note: HIV RNA quantitation roughly corresponds to CD4 categories.
Category 1 = <10,000 HIV copies per milliliter with low risk of disease progression.
Category 2 = 10,000 to 100,000 HIV copies per milliliter with moderate risk of disease progression.
Category 3 = >10,000 HIV copies per milliliter with high risk of disease progression.

World Health Organization proposed a somewhat different classification scheme based on stages of clinical condition and CD4+ T-lymphocyte count. The WHO system incorporated a performance scale and total lymphocyte count in lieu of CD4+ determinations to be used in countries where these are not available (Global AIDS News, 1993). These two classification schemes are presented in Table 1–3 for comparison purposes.

The expanded AIDS surveillance criteria have improved estimates of the number and characteristics of persons with severe HIV disease and have allowed them access to antiretroviral treatment and insurance coverage of this treatment. The expanded criteria increased the usefulness of AIDS surveillance data in describing HIV-related severe immunosuppression, morbidity, and mortality. However, it also complicated the interpretation of trends by increasing the number of reported AIDS cases in 1993, primarily among persons with severe immunosuppression (CDC, November 18, 1994). The expansion continued to affect reporting in 1994 but diminished in the last quarter of 1994 and stabilized in 1995. Pantaleo et al. (1993) described the typical course of HIV-1 infection as (1) primary or acute infection with HIV-1, followed by (2) a prolonged period of clinical latency (median, 10 years) during which the person is usually free of symptoms, followed by (3) clinically apparent disease with con-

stitutional symptoms, and finally (4) the development of AIDS-indicator disease(s). The hallmarks of HIV-1 disease progression are the functional abnormalities and quantitative depletion of CD4+ T lymphocytes, resulting in profound immunosuppression.

Asymptomatic Stage

For purposes of description here, the CDC and WHO classifications are combined. The asymptomatic stage of HIV disease (category A or 1) includes an acute primary HIV infection, an asymptomatic condition, a persistent generalized lymphadenopathy (PGL), or both (CDC, December 18, 1992). The primary or acute HIV infection phase is the period of time following initial entry of HIV into a person's body. In the acute infection phase, the virus replicates in huge numbers in the blood; there is an initial depression of T cells and a buildup in p24 antigen levels (Anderson, 1996; Ryan, 1997, pp. 268–284). During this phase antibody testing for HIV usually does not yield positive results. Although some persons may be free of symptoms after their initial exposure to HIV, up to 70% of persons have symptoms within 5 to 30 days, with a median duration of symptoms of 14 days (Rosenberg & Cotton, 1997; Tindall & Cooper, 1991). The majority of newly infected persons seek medical attention (Rosenberg & Cotton, 1997). In a review of the literature reporting the observed signs and symptoms manifested during primary HIV infection (N = 365 cases), Katsufrakis and Daar (1997) noted fever (94%), adenopathy (69%), sore throat (66%), rash (54%), myalgia or arthralgia (48%), headache (39%), diarrhea (32%), and nausea or vomiting (29%). Other manifestations of primary HIV infection include aphthous ulcers, leukoplakia, thrombocytopenia, elevated liver enzymes, and neurologic symptoms ranging from aseptic meningitis to encephalitis (Katsufrakis & Daar, 1997). Differential diagnoses include influenza, Epstein-Barr or cytomegalovirus virus infection, toxoplasmosis, rubella, and syphilis (Rosenberg & Cotton, 1997). The initial burst of HIV-1 activity can produce an intense viremia that can result in drastically reduced CD4+ cell counts. A healthy, uninfected person usually has between 500 and 1500 CD4+ cells per cubic millimeter of blood. This initial attack can, in some instances, reduce the CD4+ cell count to less than 100/mm³ (or less than 7.5% of total lymphocytes), leaving the patient vulnerable to the development of an opportunistic infection. In fact, primary infection may produce severe immunosuppression and an illness that requires hospitalization, and both esophageal candidiasis and PCP have been reported to occur in patients with primary HIV-1 infection (Tindall & Cooper, 1991; Vento et al., 1993). After the initial infection, lymph node swelling persists in about one third of the cases. PGL is a phase of HIV infection that is characterized by lymph nodes that are located in at least two extrainguinal sites and that are swollen to more than 1 cm for 3 months or longer.

After the initial infection and during the asymptomatic phase, the viral load in the blood falls and most people have no significant symptoms (Anderson, 1996). Early in this phase (2 to 18 weeks after infection) the HIV antibody test result will become positive. Commonly used tests are the enzyme-linked immunosorbent assay (ELISA) and the enzyme immunoassay (EIA); the Western blot assay and the immunofluorescence assay (IFA) are used to confirm positive results. Other confirmatory tests for HIV infection include direct identification of the virus in host tissues, HIV antigen detection, or a positive result on any other highly specific licensed test for HIV. The asymptomatic stage of infection is matched by the latent phase of virus replication shown in low levels of p24 antigen. In most instances, primary acute HIV infection is followed by a clinically latent period in which the infected person is virtually free of symptoms. Although the person has no symptoms (hence the term *clinical latency*), viral replication continues and cellular destruction takes place in many tissues and organs of the body (Pantaleo et al., 1993). This microbiologically active phase of disease is characterized by an often insidious decline in CD4+ T-cells. There is a steady decrease in CD4+ T-cell levels during this stage, about 40 to 80/μl for each year of infection (Anderson, 1996; CDC, May 8, 1992). With the use of viral load measurement, it has been established that HIV load correlates with CD4+ cell counts and with disease progression (Mellors et al., 1996). CD4+ cell counts greater than 500/ml have been found to be significantly correlated with viral loads of HIV copy counts less than 10,000/ml. Persons with HIV copy counts greater than 10,000/ml were found to have a median time to death of 6.8 years (Mellors et al., 1996). Time to death for persons with HIV copy counts less than 10,000/ml could not be calculated because the majority (70%) were still alive (Mellors et al., 1996; Melroe et al., 1997).

Early Symptomatic Stage

As the years pass, eventually clinically apparent disease manifests itself with conditions that are associated with HIV infection or are indicative of a defect in cell-mediated immunity. The early symptomatic stage (clinical category B or 2 and 3) develops when CD4+ T-cell counts drop to around 500/μl and HIV viral load copy count increases from greater than 10,000/ml up to 100,000/ml (AIDS Clinical Care, 1996). Viral loads in this range indicate moderate risk of disease progression. Examples of clinical conditions in this stage include candidiasis (oropharyngeal and vulvovaginal), cervical dysplasia, herpes zoster, pelvic inflammatory disease, listeriosis, and peripheral neuropathy (CDC, December 18, 1992).

Late Symptomatic Stage

The late symptomatic stage (clinical categories C or 3 and 4) begins when the CD4+ T-cell count drops to less than 200/μl and viral load HIV copy counts increase to more than 100,000/ml (AIDS Clinical Care, 1996; Ryan, 1997, pp. 268–284). Severe symptoms along with life-threatening infections and cancers characterize this stage. At this stage the infection has reached a level where it meets the CDC criteria for AIDS (CDC, December 18, 1992). In addition to the 1986 and 1987 clinical conditions (Kaposi's sarcoma, *Pneumocystis carinii* pneumonia, other opportunistic infections, HIV encephalopathy, HIV wasting syndrome), the CDC has added pulmonary tuberculosis, recurrent bacterial pneumonia, and invasive cervical cancer to the list of AIDS indicator illnesses (Singleton et al., 1996). These conditions are covered in depth in Chapters 3 through 6.

Advanced HIV Disease Stage

When the CD4+ cell count drops to less than 50/µl, the immune system is so impaired that there is an increasing chance of treatment failure. In this stage, severe opportunistic infections and malignant lesions occur. Death becomes likely, usually within 1 year.

EMERGING CLINICAL ISSUES

The last decade of the 20th century has produced significant breakthroughs in the prevention, treatment, and understanding of HIV disease and AIDS. Perhaps one of the most interesting aspects of this devastating pandemic is that HIV poses a challenge to scientists unparalleled in history, given the fact that it can change its genetic makeup so rapidly. Just as scientists begin to unravel one strain of the virus, a new one is discovered.

Research also has revealed that while most people with HIV infection remain free of symptoms for many years, HIV continues to destroy host defenses. The ability to quantify HIV activity with viral load testing has provided clinicians with a more accurate method of prescribing and monitoring antiretroviral therapy. Perhaps the most significant breakthrough in understanding the pathogenesis of HIV-I is research in the role of chemokines and chemokine receptors. The knowledge gained regarding the way these proteins can either attract or repel HIV can lead to more effective therapeutic interventions and vaccine development.

Approaches to treatment have expanded. The most effective treatment strategies have shifted from the use of monotherapeutic to combination drug therapy, especially with nucleoside analogs and protease inhibitors. Our ability to treat HIV as well as to prevent some of the related diseases has resulted in increased survival since the disease was first discovered in 1981. Therapy to enhance immune function is emerging. While vaccine research has not as yet produced an effective HIV vaccine, the knowledge gained thus far has given hope for the future.

HIV Diversity

The hallmark of the HIV is its genetic promiscuity. Currently there are two major strains of HIV, and both cause AIDS: HIV-1, which is distributed worldwide but is most prevalent in the Americas and Europe, and HIV-2, which is prevalent in West African countries, with limited distribution in other geographic locations. Blood screening for both HIV-1 and HIV-2 has detected 62 persons in the United States with HIV-2, among whom 77% were born in, had traveled to, or had a sex partner from Western Africa (CDC, 1995).

The viral subtypes, or clades, of HIV that have caused the worldwide pandemic of AIDS have been designated as either group M viruses or group O viruses. Group M viruses have been assigned to ten distinct genetic subtypes, and are designated as types A, B, C, D, E, F, G, H, I, and J according to phylogenetic analysis of their genes (Barre-Sinoussi, 1996; Kostrikis et al., 1996). These subtypes also vary in their distribution worldwide. Of the 10 genetic subtypes of HIV that exist in the world, subtype B predominates in North America and Europe (Brodine et al., 1995). However, subtypes A, D, and E have been detected in U.S. servicemen who acquired HIV infections while assigned to duty overseas (Brodine et al., 1995). In India, subtypes A, B, C, and E, as well as HIV-2, have been identified (Quinn, 1996).

In addition to the type "M" strain of HIV viruses, a second group that is genetically very different, has been identified and classified as HIV type O. The designation of the letter "O" was deliberate since this particular variant is an outlier of the HIV strain because it is not detectable by enzyme immunoassay (EIA) tests that are commercially available in the United States and Europe.

Group O viruses have been detected in fewer than 100 persons from West and Central Africa (Cameroon, Gabon, Niger, Nigeria, Senegal, and Togo), and in nationals of these countries living in Europe, as well as in one French national. In 1996 the first case of HIV strain O was identified in the United States in a woman who had immigrated from Africa (CDC, 1996). The CDC is currently working with the manufacturers of HIV test kits to ensure that the tests are reconfigured to detect all known HIV variants. The dispersal of HIV subtypes throughout the world may have important implications for the epidemiology of the disease as well as the efficacy of therapeutic interventions and vaccine development.

Adding to the complex nature of the changing makeup of HIV is the fact that researchers have found that approximately 10% of the samples of blood isolated from HIV-infected people do not fall neatly into one clade or another but, instead, are hybrids of two or more clades (Ezzell, 1995). Researchers have noted that in several countries there is evidence of recombinants, such as A/E and B/F (Quinn, 1996).

HIV Pathogenesis

HIV-1 is a retrovirus belonging to the lentivirus family of viruses, which are generally known to result in neurotropic and lymphotropic viremic disease as a result of an indolent infection process characterized by a long period of clinical latency. HIV-1 is one of five retroviruses, along with HIV type 2 (HIV-2) and human T-lymphotropic viruses type I, II, and IV (HTLV-I, HTLV-II, HTLV-IV), associated with human disease. Both HIV-1 and HIV-2 are considered to be causes of AIDS. HTLV-I, which is found predominantly in Southern Japan, the South Pacific, and parts of West Africa, as well as in persons of African descent in the Western Hemisphere, is associated with chronic degenerative neurologic disease and is strongly implicated in T-cell leukemia/lymphoma. Although HTLV-II and HTLV-IV have been found in patients with leukemia and lymphoma, there is no evidence to support the theory that these retroviruses are the direct causes of these illnesses. HIV-1 as a retrovirus has the ability to reverse the usual flow of genetic information with the enzyme reverse transcriptase, using viral RNA as a template for making DNA.

Retroviruses are found in nearly all animal species. Infection can occur through sexual activities, through exposure to blood, and perinatally. The life cycle of HIV-1 includes the following components:

1. Attachment of the virus to the host cell
2. Uncoating, followed by reverse transcription
3. Integration of newly synthesized DNA into the host cell DNA, with transcription and translation of the viral genetic message into viral protein (structural, regulatory, and functional)
4. Assembly, with release of the virus out of the host cell

HIV-1 is composed of a central cylindrical core of diploid RNA surrounded by a spherical lipid envelope. Three structural components make up the viral genome and code for essential protein components. These genes are found on terminal repeat segments. The first, *pol,* encodes the enzymes reverse transcriptase, integrase, and protease located in the viral core. The second, *gag,* encodes for p24, which is also found in the viral core and surrounds the viral RNA, and for protease. It also codes for numerous other core proteins, p7 and p9. The third gene, called *env,* produces two glycoproteins that are part of the viral envelope and appear to be important in the recognition and attachment of HIV-1 to its CD4+ lymphocyte target cell. HIV-1 also possesses genes that code for proteins that have important regulatory functions for the virus. Examples include *tat* (transactivator), *rev* (regulator of expression of virion proteins), *nef* (negative factor), *vif* (virion infectivity factor), *vpu* (required for efficient viral budding), and *vpr* (a weak activator of transcription).

The pathophysiology of HIV-1 relates to this ability to infect human cells that possess CD4 membrane receptors. Clinically apparent disease with its immunodeficiency syndrome is a direct result of depletion of CD4+ lymphocytes and infection of macrophages and monocytes. Other cell types, including epithelial gut cells, uterine cervical cells, and Langerhans cells of the skin, have also been identified as harboring HIV-1 infection.

By the 1990s scientists had established that, for infection to occur, HIV had to bind to the CD4+ molecule on T-helper cells and macrophages; it was known that binding to a cell was insufficient to cause infection and that fusion and entry into the HIV-attached cell was necessary to complete the infecting process. For many years, CD4+ was presumed to be the exclusive cellular receptor for HIV. However, many researchers believed that another receptor or even several other receptors were necessary to mediate this process. Further research has identified that chemokines and chemokine receptors play a significant role in the pathogenesis of HIV.

Chemokines are small proteins that exert their function on target cells by binding to a cell surface without entering it and acting as a messenger, attracting lymphocytes, neutrophils, and macrophages. Chemokines are classified according to the sequencing of the amino acid cysteine (C). Chemokines that contain adjacent copies of C are labeled cysteine-cysteine receptor (CCR), and chemokines that have another amino acid between the cysteines are labeled cysteine-X-cysteine receptor (CXCR). Certain strains of HIV are T-cell-tropic (also called non-syncytium-inducing or NSI) while others are macrophage-tropic (also called syncytium-inducing or SI).

In 1996 Feng and associates discovered a protein receptor, designated as LESTR or "fusion" and now labeled CXCR4, which they found to mediate NSI strains of HIV. CCR3 and CCR5 are additional chemokines that facilitate viral entry in SI strains of HIV (He et al., 1997). However, polymorphism has been noted in CCR5, and some people (more often white persons than people of African or Asian descent) have a homozygous or mutant genetic defect in their CCR5 gene that actually prevents HIV from binding to a cell, explaining a genetic resistance to HIV even in the presence of repeated exposure (Huang et al., 1997; Liu et al., 1996). Other chemokines that may inhibit infection in NSI strains of HIV include regulated-upon-activation, normal T-cell expressed and secreted (RANTES), macrophage inflammatory protein (MIP)-1-alpha, and MIP-1-beta (Cocchi et al., 1996). According to Eron (1997) these discoveries increased the knowledge base of HIV pathogenesis by explaining

1. The ability of HIV to enter cells
2. How HIV switches its tropism from macrophages and T-cells, to T-cells alone over the illness trajectory

3. How some persons remain resistant to HIV infection despite repeated exposure
4. Why there are different rates of HIV disease progression among infected persons

Although much further study is needed regarding the role of chemokine receptors, scientists are developing new therapies based on receptor mimics, receptor ligands, chemokines, and chemokine analogs (McNicholl et al., 1997).

Through the mechanism of binding site capability, HIV-1 fuses with the target cell's membrane, enters the host cell's cytoplasm, sheds its envelope coat, and releases its contents. Reverse transcription then occurs, creating viral DNA that exists in free form or becomes integrated into the cellular DNA as some provirus. Infected cells can remain dormant. Cofactors may be important to their activation. Once activated, the gene products modulate viral progenesis with synthesizing of viral proteins. From these proteins, new virions are assembled and burst from the infected cell and circulate to a new receptor site (CD4) on another target cell.

As many as 10 billion new virions can be produced daily in an HIV-infected person (Feinberg, 1996). Although some types of the host's infected cells die with the budding forth of a new virion, macrophages and monocytes survive and therefore carry the virus in their travels through the lymphoid and blood systems. This serves to protect the virus and enhance the opportunity for further infections to occur, leading to a compromised immune response. The functions of the macrophage and monocyte are compromised as well, leading to further immunosuppression. The virus gains access to the central nervous system by way of these infected macrophages, which cross the blood-brain barrier and cause damage.

Long-term Nonprogressors

Long-term nonprogressors (LTNPs) are persons who (1) have documented evidence of HIV-1 infection for more than 10 years, (2) have remained asymptomatic, (3) have normal and stable immune profiles, and (4) have not required or received any antiretroviral therapy for HIV-1. LTNPs should not be confused with long-term survivors. Long-term survivors are persons who, despite having a definitive diagnosis of an AIDS-indicator disease, have survived for several years.

They have all the clinical manifestations of HIV-1 disease and have required AIDS-related treatment. LTNPs are persons infected with HIV who never became ill.

Researchers have found that although HIV-1 continues to replicate in LTNPs, these persons produce vigorous serum antibody responses, resulting in extremely low viral burden, and their lymph tissue and immune function remains intact (Montefiori et al., 1996). Studies of the role of chemokines in disease progression have found that although nonprogressors who possess at least one copy of the mutant CCR5 gene are more likely to become a LTNP, neither the presence of CCR5 nor serum levels of RANTES, MIP-1 alpha, and MIP-1 beta can explain the natural history of HIV in this population (Cohen et al., 1997; McKenzie et al., 1996). Researchers continue to study LTNPs with great interest with the hope that they may gain insight into potential therapies for HIV-1 as well as vaccine development.

Monitoring Disease Progression

Until 1990, the backbone of most clinical evaluations of HIV-1 disease progression, as well as research studies, has been the absolute CD4+ cell count. However, problems with the absolute CD4+ cell count included the fact that interlaboratory variability, diurnal variations, and intercurrent variations produced laboratory results with cell count changes between 50 and 300/mm^3 between reports. Clinicians soon learned that a more consistent surrogate marker was the percentage of lymphocytes that were CD4+ cells (e.g., a CD4+ cell count of 200/mm^3 corresponded to a CD4+ percentage of 14). Although these tests provided indirect information on disease progression, they did not directly measure HIV-1 activity.

As noted earlier, a more direct method of measuring HIV-1 activity that has been developed measures viral load, also referred to as viral burden. By measuring the amount of HIV-1 RNA in plasma, clinicians can more accurately assess the amount of HIV-1 activity that is taking place in the body and can treat the patient appropriately. The test results are reported in the number of copies per milliliter: Fewer than 10,000/ml indicate a low risk of advancing disease. Test results showing 10,000 to 100,000/ml indicate a medium risk of advancing disease, and those

showing more than 100,000/ml indicate a high risk of advancing disease (Sax, 1996).

Testing is usually performed as part of the initial workup, when CD4+ cell counts indicate a clinical problem, and 3 to 4 weeks after starting or changing antiretroviral therapy. Illnesses such as influenza, herpes, or pneumonia, as well as vaccines, can cause a temporary increase in test results. Although high viral loads are generally correlated with a low CD4+ cell count and low levels with a high count, the correlation is weak and inconsistent. Some patients with low CD4+ cell counts have low viral loads and vice versa (Mellors et al., 1996). Therefore CD4+ cell counts are not reliable substitutes for viral load tests when one is trying to determine the degree of HIV-1 disease activity or evaluating the efficacy of treatment. Chapters 5 and 6 contain additional information on the clinical use of HIV RNA tests, and Appendix III contains information on test interpretation.

Chemotherapeutic Interventions

Research and drug development have focused on antiretroviral agents to inhibit disease progression, prophylactic therapy to prevent opportunistic infections associated with the diagnosis of AIDS, immunomodulator therapy to restore the depleted immune system, and vaccine development. Among these four approaches in managing HIV disease, the greatest accomplishments have been achieved in the development of antiretroviral therapy to suppress the destructive forces of HIV activity.

Development of antiretroviral therapy has focused on the knowledge that two single strands of viral RNA and the viral enzymes reverse transcriptase, RNAse, polymerase, integrase, and protease are essential for HIV replication. Until 1995, the mainstay of antiretroviral therapy was the use of nucleoside analog reverse transcriptase inhibitors (NRTIs), commonly referred to as nucleoside analogs. When incorporated into the DNA of HIV during viral replication, the NRTI terminates the DNA chain, preventing viral replication, and results in viral stasis. These agents will prevent the spread of HIV to new cells, but they do not interfere with viral replication in cells that are already infected. Examples of NRTIs include zidovudine, didanosine, zalcitabine, stavudine, and lamivudine.

In 1995 a second group of drugs for treatment of HIV, known as proteinase or, more commonly, protease inhibitors (PIs), was approved. PIs inhibit viral replication by blocking protease activity and acting on chronically infected cells to render viral particles noninfectious. Examples of PIs include saquinavir, indinavir, ritonavir, and nelfinavir.

A third type or class of antiretroviral drugs known as nonnucleoside reverse transcriptase inhibitors (NNRTIs) was introduced in 1996. Although NNRTIs do not actually terminate the DNA chain, they are similar to NRTIs and act by stopping the process of reverse transcription. Examples of NNRTIs include delavirdine and nevirapine.

Over the past few years, scientists have learned that a major factor decreasing the durability and efficacy of antiretroviral therapy is the use of one drug at a time (monotherapy). Combination therapy produces a more sustained antiviral effect in a person with HIV infection, decreases the emergence of drug resistance, and has more effect on a wider range of cell and tissue reservoirs of HIV. Combination therapy using NRTIs with either a PI or an NNRTI has reduced viral load below detectable levels and dramatically improved the overall health and well-being of HIV-infected persons. Chapters 3 and 5 contain a detailed discussion of antiretroviral therapy in care management.

Chemoprophylactic therapy to prevent AIDS-defining opportunistic infections (OIs) has led to significant decreases in certain diseases, such as *Pneumocystis carinii* pneumonia and *Mycobacterium avium-intracelluare* disease, in both adults and children. Continuing research in this area has recently shown that other OIs such as cytomegalovirus can also be prevented. Details of current recommendations for preventing both primary and secondary AIDS-related infections are contained in Chapters 3 through 6.

In addition to developing successful strategies that interfere with HIV activity, researchers have also spent considerable energy in developing agents that restore normal host immunity. However, the development of drugs for immune reconstitution therapy has been limited by the fact that knowledge of the interactions between HIV, immune cells, and various cytokines is just emerging. One such therapy that shows promise is interleukin-2 (IL-2). IL-2, formerly known as T-cell growth factor, is produced in the body and has significant effects on the proliferation and differentiation of several types of immune cells, including T cells, B cells, and natural killer cells. Recombinant IL-2 administered parenterally on an intermittent basis to HIV-infected patients with CD4+ T-cell counts greater than 500/mm^3, and in combination with oral antiretroviral agents has resulted in resulted in sustained increases in CD4+ T-cell counts to normal levels and delayed the progression of HIV disease (Davey et al., 1997; Jacobson et al., 1996; Kovacs et al., 1996). However, the use of IL-2 to treat advanced disease may be limited since the therapeutic response was more favorable in patients with higher baseline CD4+ T-cell counts (Davey et al., 1997). Another form of immune therapy, which actually replaces cells rather than stimulating host immune cell function, is the administration of intravenous immune globulin (IVIG). IVIG, derived from pooled immunoglobulin G, provides significant passive antibody protection against a wide range of bacterial and viral infections. The results of this therapy, although short-lived, have been more successful in children than in adults. See Chapter 3 for an in-depth discussion of IVIG therapy in children.

On a global basis, the major obstacle to the development of a universally effective HIV-preventive vaccine is the genetic variability that exists in the occurrence of the numerous subtypes of HIV in different parts of the world. Basic research is still needed to determine whether a vaccine based on one HIV subtype will provide protection against some, all, or none of the other subtypes. Since 1987, approximately 15 HIV-1 experimental vaccines have been tested in the United States, in 25 trials involving more than 1900 healthy, noninfected adults (NIAID News, 1996). These trials have been conducted by the National Institutes of Health's National Institute of Allergy and Infectious Diseases (NIAID) AIDS Vaccine Evaluation Group (AVEG).

Several types of preventive vaccines have been tested in humans, including

1. A recombinant subunit vaccine, genetically engineered to simulate the outer surface or other part of HIV
2. A peptide vaccine, synthetically producing proteins that simulate HIV proteins

3. A particle or pseudo-virion vaccine, a noninfectious particle resembling HIV and its proteins
4. A live vector vaccine, a live bacteria or virus that is harmless to humans and is used to transport a gene to make HIV proteins
5. DNA immunization, direct inoculation of genetic material that produces HIV proteins (Heyward et al., 1997)

Two other types that have been tested in animal models include a whole-killed or inactivated vaccine, live HIV that has been treated chemically or by other means and rendered noninfectious, and a live-attenuated vaccine derived from live HIV that has had genes responsible for viral replication deleted. According to Heyward and associates the candidate vaccines tested in humans thus far have been found to be safe and well tolerated, and almost all of them have produced some type of HIV-specific immune response with varying degrees of success. However, only two recombinant subunit preventive vaccines have made it to phase II trials because of a lack of economic incentives for pharmaceutical companies, along with such other deterring concerns as a lack of adequate resources, legal and liability concerns, and the social and political issues involved in vaccine development (Heyward et al., 1997).

Most of the vaccines developed thus far are composed of recombinant proteins, such as the envelope glycoprotein gp160 and gp120. The results of the trials have shown that (1) gp120 vaccines induce more neutralizing antibodies than gp160 vaccines, although the gp160 vaccines induce more vigorous proliferation of lymphocytes, and (2) vaccines developed in mammalian cells perform better, and more antigen stimulates better immune responses than smaller quantities of antigen (Doepel, 1996).

Plans have been made for prevention trials to study phase III vaccine efficacy. The objectives of the study include

1. Enrolling and retaining volunteers at high risk of HIV-1 infection
2. Monitoring risk behavior and detecting early infection
3. Evaluating strategies for informed consent
4. Engaging target communities in planning the trials
5. Evaluating behavioral interventions that could augment future trials

A total of 4884 persons have been recruited in Boston, Chicago, Denver, New York, Philadelphia, San Francisco, and Seattle (Doepel, 1996).

The use of HIV vaccines as a therapeutic strategy for HIV-infected persons to stimulate host immune responses is also under study. Both recombinant gp160 and gp120 have shown favorable results in stimulating both cellular and humoral responses (Levine et al., 1996; Valentine et al., 1996). See Chapter 14 for a review of policy regarding HIV vaccine development.

RESEARCH IN HIV HEALTH CARE

HIV research is addressed specifically in some chapters in this text. The content of each chapter is based on up-to-date research on the pathogenesis of AIDS, immunology, pharmacology, treatment, community care, health promotion, behavior change, quality of life, psychosocial interventions, and so forth. Some chapters also make recommendations for future research and point out areas of particular research need.

Here an overview is given of general research needs in HIV/AIDS care:

1. Developing and testing community-based models of care. The care of persons with HIV disease is given increasingly in the community. The range of care and services needed by persons with HIV disease and their families makes this population particularly appropriate for the development and testing of community-based models. Every aspect of health care, from health promotion to treatment and palliation, from physiologic to psychosocial, from acute to long-term, and from cost-effective home care to referral for care, could be studied in a community-based health care network for persons with HIV. Community-based care in a climate of managed care is especially worthy of investigation. Results of these studies might be generalized to the community care and service needs of other populations as well. A summary of research in this area and recommendations for future research are addressed in more depth in Chapter 10.

2. Assessing the effectiveness of health care interventions in HIV/AIDS. Both physiologic health care interventions and psychosocial interventions could be identified and tested with the use of experimental designs. Research in the area of physiologic care especially is needed to test the effects of symptom management in HIV care: fatigue, nausea, weight loss, dry skin, diarrhea, shortness of breath, cough, fever, pain, and so forth. The use of viral load (HIV RNA quantitation) as a marker of symptom onset and management is a significant area of study. Interventions specific to adults and children, men and women, and various cultural groups should be identified and tested. Studies on symptom management might be generalizable to other illness conditions as well. A summary of research specific to these areas and recommendations for HIV research are addressed particularly in Chapters 4 and 6 but also in Chapter 8.

3. Developing and testing approaches to remediating cognitive impairment. For persons with HIV disease, cognitive dysfunction occurs because of HIV dementia and because of various other fungal, parasitic, and viral infections. In addition to treatment with drugs, persons with cognitive dysfunction can be retrained in memory and concentration and in self-care skills (activities of daily living). Interventions could be designed and tested to determine the outcomes for persons with HIV in self-care skills and the reduction of stress in caregivers. Results might be generalizable to other cognitively impaired persons, such as those with Alzheimer's disease, and their caregivers. A summary of research specific to this area and recommendations for future research are addressed in more depth in Chapter 7.

4. Testing interventions for coping with chronic illness. Increasingly, HIV disease has come to be a chronic illness. From the early infection stage to advanced HIV disease, PLWH need a range of health and human services and therapeutic interventions. Special importance should be given to client adherence to medical regimens, especially since the advent of protease inhibitors. Study results may be generalized to persons with other chronic, life-threatening diseases such as cancer. A research summary and recommendations in this area are addressed in greater depth in Chapter 10.

5. Identifying biologic-behavioral factors and testing interventions to promote immunocompetence. The effects of nutrition, exercise, rest, stress reduction, changes in lifestyle factors such as smoking and the use of recreational drugs, preventive and therapeutic health care, and so forth all suggest interventions that may enhance immunocompetence. The synergy between HIV infection and other STDs and between TB and HIV disease progression suggests a special research emphasis. Programs instituting these biobehavioral factors need to be designed and tested with PLWH. Study results may be generalizable to persons with other immunodeficiency diseases as well. Research to date and research needed in this area are addressed in more depth in Chapter 2.

Finally, some investigators have encouraged collaborative research between clinicians and researchers. The benefits of such research are obvious in terms of applicability to HIV health care. Multidisciplinary research efforts also would lead to a more comprehensive understanding of HIV disease and its effects on physiologic and psychologic processes.

SUMMARY

Many changes in HIV disease and the AIDS epidemic have occurred in the past 4 years. This chapter provides an overview of those changes and refers the reader to subsequent chapters in which current information is presented in depth. Two areas not addressed elsewhere are covered here: the pathogenesis of HIV and the changing regional epidemiology of HIV infection. Finally, suggestions are made for HIV research based on general areas of need and current changes in the epidemic.

Information about HIV disease is changing so rapidly that it is impossible to publish anything that is completely up to date. For this reason, it is especially important for health professionals to remain aware of new developments and changes in information about HIV. Close attention to AIDS- and HIV-related research, conferences, and information in the professional and popular media can help health care workers keep up with issues and information about HIV disease and the AIDS epidemic.

REFERENCES

Abrams, D.I. (1986). AIDS: Battling a retroviral enemy. *California Nursing Review, 8*(6), 36–37, 44.

AIDS Clinical Care. (April, 1996). For your information. *AIDS Clinical Care.*

Anderson, R.M. (1996). The spread of HIV and sexual mixing patterns. In J. Mann, D. Tarantola (Eds.),

AIDS in the world II (pp. 71–86). New York: Oxford University Press.

Asch, S.M., London, A.S., Barnes, P.F., et al. (1997). Testing for human immunodeficiency virus infection among tuberculosis patients in Los Angeles. *American Journal of Respiratory and Critical Care Medicine, 155,* 378–381.

Bacchetti, P., Osmond, D., Chaisson, R., et al. (1988). Survival patterns of the first 500 patients with AIDS in San Francisco. *Journal of Infectious Diseases, 157*(5), 1044–1047.

Barre-Sinoussi, F. (1996). HIV-1 as the cause of AIDS. *Lancet, 348*(9019), 31–35.

Barre-Sinoussi, F., Chermann, J.C., Rey, F., et al. (1983). Isolation of a T-lymphotropic retrovirus from a patient at risk for acquired immune deficiency syndrome (AIDS). *Science, 220*(4599), 868–871.

Bennett, C.L., Adams, J., Gertler, P., et al. (1992). Relation between hospital experience and in-hospital mortality for patients with AIDS-related *Pneumocystis carinii* pneumonia: Experience from 3,126 cases in New York City in 1987. *Journal of Acquired Immune Deficiency Syndromes, 5*(9), 856–864.

Brown, L.S., Siddiqui, N.S., Chu, A.F. (1996). Natural history of HIV infection and predictors of survival in a cohort of HIV seropositive injecting drug users. *Journal of the National Medical Association, 88*(1), 37–42.

Brodine, S.K., Mascola, J.R., Weiss, P.J., et al. (1995). Detection of diverse HIV-1 genetic subtypes in the USA. *Lancet, 346*(8984), 1198–1199.

Caliendo, A.M., Hirsch, M.S. (1994). Combination therapy for infection due to human immunodeficiency virus type 1. *Clinical Infectious Diseases, 18*(4), 516–524.

Carpenter, C.C.J., Fischl, M.A., Hammer, S.M., et al. (1997). Antiretroviral thrapy for HIV infection in 1997. *Journal of the American Medical Association, 277*(24), 1962–1968.

Cegielski, J.P., Goetz, M.B., Jacobson, J.M., et al. (1997). Gender differences in early suspicion of tuberculosis in hospitalized, high-risk patients during 4 epidemic years, 1987–1990. *Infection Control and Hospital Epidemiology, 18*(4), 237–243.

Center for Studying Health System Change. (1997). The trajectory of managed care. *Issue Brief, 9,* 1–4.

Centers for Disease Control. (June 5, 1981). Pneumocystis pneumonia—Los Angeles. *Morbidity and Mortality Weekly Report, 30*(21), 250–252.

Centers for Disease Control. (September 24, 1982). Update on acquired immune deficiency syndrome (AIDS): United States. *Morbidity and Mortality Weekly Report, 31*(37), 507–514.

Centers for Disease Control. (July 9, 1982). Opportunistic infections and Kaposi's sarcoma among Haitians in the United States. *Morbidity and Mortality Weekly Report, 31*(26), 353–354, 360–361.

Centers for Disease Control. (July 16, 1982). *Pneumocystis carinii* pneumonia among persons with hemophilia A. *Morbidity and Mortality Weekly Report, 31*(27), 365–367.

Centers for Disease Control. (May 23, 1986). Classification system for human T-lymphotropic virus III/lymphadenopathy-associated virus infection. *Morbidity and Mortality Weekly Report, 35*(20), 334–339.

Centers for Disease Control. (May 8, 1992). Guidelines for the performance of CD4+ T-cell determinations in persons with human immunodeficiency virus infections. *Morbidity and Mortality Weekly Report, 41*(RR-8), 1–12.

Centers for Disease Control. (December 18, 1992). 1993 revised classification system for HIV infection: An expanded surveillance case definition for AIDS among adolescents and adults. *Morbidity and Mortality Weekly Report, 41*(RR-17), 1–19.

Centers for Disease Control and Prevention. (November 18, 1994). Update: Trends in AIDS diagnosis and reporting under the expanded surveillance definition for adolescents and adults—United States, 1993. *Morbidity and Mortality Weekly Report, 43*(45), 826–836.

Centers for Disease Control and Prevention. (1995). Update: HIV-2 infection among blood and plasma donors—United States, June 1992–June 1995. *Morbidity and Mortality Weekly Report, 44*(32), 603–606.

Centers for Disease Control and Prevention. (August 18, 1995). Update: HIV-2 infection among blood and plasma donors—United States. June 1992–June 1995. *Morbidity and Mortality Weekly Report, 44*(32), 603–606.

Centers for Disease Control and Prevention. (1996). Identification of HIV group O infection—Los Angeles County, California, 1996. *Morbidity and Mortality Weekly Report, 45*(26), 561–565.

Centers for Disease Control and Prevention. (January 19, 1996). Surveillance of tuberculosis and AIDS co-morbidity—Florida, 1981–1993. *Morbidity and Mortality Weekly Report, 45*(2), 38–40.

Centers for Disease Control and Prevention. (June 7, 1996). Update: Provisional public health service recommendations for chemoprophylaxis after occupational exposure to HIV. *Morbidity and Mortality Weekly Report, 45*(22), 468–478.

Centers for Disease Control and Prevention. (1997). HIV and AIDS trends: The changing landscape of the epidemic: A closer look. *Centers for Disease Control and Prevention (www.cdcnac.org//hivtrend.html).*

Centers for Disease Control and Prevention. (December 31, 1997). *HIV/AIDS Surveillance Report, 9*(2), 1–39, Atlanta, GA: The Center.

Centers for Disease and Control and Prevention. (July 1997). Female adult/adolescent AIDS rates per 100,000 population, for cases reported in 1996, United States. *HIV/AIDS Prevention,* p. 13.

Centers for Disease Control and Prevention. (September 5, 1997). Anergy skin testing and preventive therapy for HIV-infected persons: Revised recommendations. *Morbidity and Mortality Weekly Report, 46*(RR-15), 1–10.

Centers for Disease Control and Prevention. (September 19, 1997). Update: Trends in AIDS incidence—United States, 1996. *Morbidity and Mortality Weekly Report, 46*(37), 861–866.

Centers for Disease Control and Prevention. (September 26, 1997). Gonorrhea among men who have sex with men—Selected sexually transmitted diseases clinics, 1993–1996. *Morbidity and Mortality Weekly Report, 46*(38), 889–894.

Chaisson, R.E., Keruly, J.C., Moore, R.D. (1995). Race, sex, drug use, and progression of human immunodeficiency virus disease. *New England Journal of Medicine, 333*(12), 751–756.

Chicago Department of Public Health. (Second Quarter, 1997). *AIDS Chicago.* Chicago Department of Public Health, HIV/AIDS Surveillance Program.

Cocchi, F., DeVico, A.L., Garzino-Demo, A., et al. (1995). Identification of RANTES, MIP-1 alpha, and MIP-1 beta as the major HIV-suppressive factors produced by CD8+ T cells. *Science, 270*(5343), 1811–1815.

Cohen, O.J., Fauci, A., Vaccarezza, M., et al. (1997). Heterozygosity for a defective gene for CC chemokine receptor 5 is not the sole determinant for the immunologic and virologic phenotype of HIV-infected long-term nonprogressors. *Journal of Clinical Investigation, 100*(7), 1581–1589.

Crespo-Fierro, M. (1997). Compliance/adherence and care management in HIV disease. *Journal of the Association of Nurses in AIDS Care, 8*(4), 7–25.

Currier, J., Fliesler, N. (1995). Demographics of HIV survival revisited. *AIDS Clinical Care, 7*(11), 94.

Dade County Health Department. (August 30, 1997). Monthly Surveillance Report. Dade County Health Department; Office of Epidemiology and Disease Control.

Dallas County Heath and Human Services Department. (September 2, 1997). Acquired Immunodeficiency Syndrome (AIDS) HIV/AIDS Reporting System Surveillance Report.

Davey, R.T., Chaitt, D.G., Piscitelli, S.C., et al. (1997). Subcutaneous administration of interleukin-2 in human immunodeficiecy virus type 1-infected persons. *Journal of Infectious Diseases, 175*(4), 781–789.

DeCock, K.M., Brun-Vezinet, F. (1996). HIV-2 infection: Current knowledge and uncertainties. In J. Mann, D. Tarantola (Eds.), *AIDS in the world II* (pp. 171–176). New York: Oxford University Press.

Denning, P., Fleming, P. (1997). *Estimating recent patterns of HIV infection among adolescents and young adults* (abstract 375). Presented at 4th Conference on Retroviruses and Opportunistic Infections, Washington, DC.

Denning, P., Ward, J., Chu, S., et al. (1996). *Current trends in AIDS incidence among young men who have sex with men, United States* (abstract TuC2405). Presented at XIth International Conference on AIDS, Vancouver, British Columbia.

Department of Health and Human Services. (August 31, 1997). *AIDS: Cumulative summary of Houston MSA cases.* Houston Department of Health and Human Services.

Doepel, L.K. (March, 1996). Fauci presents NIAID strategy HIV vaccine development. *NIAID AIDS Agenda.* National Institute of Allergy and Infectious Diseases.

Enger, C., Graham, N., Peng, Y., et al. (1996). Survival from early, intermediate, and late stages of HIV infection. *Journal of the American Medical Association, 275*(17), 1329–1334.

Eron, J. (1997). *Crucial co-receptor discoveries.* Presented at 4th Conference on Retroviruses and Opportunistic Infections, Washington DC: available: http://www.healthcg.com/hiv/4thconf/

Ezzell, C. (1996). Recombination between HIV clades not so rare. *Journal of NIH Research, 7*(6), 24–26.

Feinberg, M.B. (1996). Changing the natural history of HIV disease. *Lancet, 348,* 239–246.

Feng, Y., Broder, C.C., Kennedy, P.E., Berger, E.A. (1996). HIV-1 entry cofactor: Functional cDNA cloning of a seven-transmembrane, G protein-coupled receptor. *Science, 272,* 872–877.

Gelberg, L., Panarites, C.J., Morgenstern, H., et al. (1997). Tuberculosis skin testing among homeless adults. *Journal of General Internal Medicine, 12,* 2–33.

Global AIDS News. (1993). New CDC definition will cause surge in reported U.S. AIDS cases. *Global AIDS News, 1,* 4.

Gorman, C. (June, 1997). If the condom breaks. *TIME,* p. 48.

Graham, H.M.H., Jacobson, L.P., Kuo, V., et al. (1994). Access to therapy in the multicenter AIDS cohort study, 1989–1992. *Journal of Clinical Epidemiology, 47*(9), 1003–1012.

Hays, R.B., Paul, J., Ekstrand, M., et al. (1997). Actual versus perceived HIV status, sexual behaviors and predictors of unprotected sex among young gay and bisexual men who identify as HIV-negative, HIV-positive and untested. *AIDS, 11,* 1495–1502.

He, J., Chen, Y., Farzan, M., et al. (1997). CCR3 and CCR5 co-receptors in HIV microglia. *Nature, 385*(6617), 645–649.

Heyward, W.L., MacQueen, K.M., Jaffe, H.W. (1997). Obstacles and progress toward development of a preventive HIV vaccine. *Journal of the International Association of Physicians in AIDS Care, 3*(8), 28–34.

Hirsch, M.S., D'Aquila, R.T. (1993). Therapy for human immunodeficiency virus infection. *New England Journal of Medicine, 328*(23), 1686–1695.

Ho, D.D., Neumann, A.U., Perelson, A.S., et al. (1995). Rapid turnover of plasma virions and CD4 lymphocytes in HIV-1 infection. *Nature, 373,* 123–126.

Hogg, R.S., Strathdee, S.A., Craib, K.J., et al. (1994). Lower socioeconomic status and shorter survival following HIV infection. *Lancet, 344*(8930), 1120–1124.

Huang, Y., Paxton, W.A., Wolinsky, S.M., et al. (1996). The role of a mutant CCR5 allele in HIV transmission and disease progression. *Nature Medicine, 2*(11), 1240–1243.

Huebscher, R. (1997). Overdrugging and undertreatment in primary health care. *Nursing Outlook, 45*(4), 161–166.

Jacobson, E.L., Pilaro, F., Smith, K.A. (1996). Rational interleukin-2 therapy for HIV positive indiviuals: Daily low doses enhance immune function without toxicity. *Proceedings of the National Academy of Science USA, 93*(19), 10405–10410.

Katsufrakis, P.J., Daar, E.S. (1997). HIV/AIDS assessment, testing, and natural history. *Primary Care Clinics in Office Practice, 24*(3), 479–496.

Katz, M.H., Gerberding, J.L. (1997). Postexposure treatment of people exposed to the human immunodeficiency virus through sexual contact or injection-drug use. *New England Journal of Medicine, 336*(15), 1097–1100.

Kitahata, M.M., Koepsell, T.D., Deyo, R.A., et al. (1996). Physicians' experience with the acquired immunodeficiency syndrome as a factor in patients' survival. *New England Journal of Medicine, 334*(11), 701–706.

Kostrikis, L.G., Cao, Y., Ngai, H., et al. (1996). Quantitative analysis of serum neutralization of human immunodeficiency virus type 1 from subtypes A, B, C, D, E, F, and I: Lack of direct correlation between neutralization serotypes and genetic subtypes and evidence for serum-dependence. *Journal of Virology, 70*(1), 445–458.

Kovacs, J.A., Vogel, S., Albert, J.M., et al. (1996). Controlled trial of interleukin-2 infusions in patients infected with the human immunodeficiency virus. *New England Journal of Medicine, 335*(18), 1350–1356.

Lai, D., Tsai, S.P., Hardy, R.J. (1997). Impact of HIV/AIDS on life expectancy in the United States. *AIDS, 11,* 203–207.

Laraque, F., Greene, A., Triano-Davis, J.W. (1996). Effect of comprehensive intervention program on survival of patients with human immunodeficiency virus infection. *Archives of Internal Medicine, 156*(2), 169–176.

Levine, A.M., Groshen, S., Allen, J., et al. (1996). Initial studies on active immunization of HIV-infected subjects using a gp120-depleted HIV-1 immunogen: Long-term follow-up. *Journal of Acquired Immune De-ficiency Syndromes and Human Retrovirology, 11*(4), 351–364.

Levy, J.A., Hoffman, A.D., Kramer, S.M., et al. (1984). Isolation of lymphocytopathic retroviruses from San Francisco patients with AIDS. *Science, 225*(4664), 840–842.

Liu, R., Paxton, W.A., Choe, S., et al. (1996). Homozygous defect in HIV-1 coreceptor accounts for resistance of some multiply-exposed individuals to HIV-1 infection. *Cell, 86*(3), 367–377.

Los Angeles County Department of Health Services. (July 15, 1997). Advanced HIV disease (AIDS) surveillance summary. Los Angeles County Department of Health Services; HIV Epidemiology Program.

Mann, J., Tarantola, D. (Eds). (1996). *AIDS in the world II: Global dimensions, social roots, and responses.* New York: Oxford University Press.

Mascolini, M. (1996). The rolling uncertainties of antiprotease prescribing. *Journal of the International Association of Physicians in AIDS Care, 2*(2), 6–10.

Mastro, T.D., Kunanuson, C., Dondero, T.J., et al. (1997). Why do HIV-1 subtypes segregate among persons with different risk behaviors in South Africa and Thailand? *AIDS, 11,* 113–116.

McKenzie, S.W., Dallio, G., North, M., et al. (1996). Serum chemokine levels in patients with non-progressing HIV infection. *AIDS, 10*(9), F29–F33.

McNicholl, J.M., Smith, D.K., Qari, S.H., Hodge, T. (1997). *Emerging Infectious Diseases, 3*(3), 261–267.

Medicaid Access Study Group. (1994). Access of Medicaid recipients to outpatient care. *New England Journal of Medicine, 330*(20), 1426–1430.

Mellors, J.W., Rinaldo, C.R., Jr., Gupta, P., et al. (1996). Prognosis in HIV-1 infection predicted by the quantity of virus in plasma. *Science, 272,* 1167–1170.

Melroe, N.H., Stawarz, K.E., Simpson, J., et al. (1997). HIV RNA quantitation: Marker of HIV infection. *Journal of the Association of Nurses in AIDS Care, 8*(5), 31–38.

Melnick, S.L., Sherer, R., Louis, T.A. (1994). Survival and disease progression according to gender of patients with HIV infection. *Journal of the American Medical Association, 272*(24), 1915–1921.

Mocroft, A., Johnson, M.A., Phillips, A.N. (1996). Factors affecting survival in patients with the acquired immunodeficiency syndrome. *AIDS, 10*(10), 1057–1065.

Montefiori, D.C., Pantaleo, G., Fink, L.M., et al. (1996). Neutralizing and infection-enhancing antibody responses to human immunodeficiency virus type 1 in long-term non-progressors. *Journal of Infectious Diseases, 173*(1), 60–67.

Moore, R.D., Stanton, D., Gopalan, R., Chaisson, R.E. (1994). Racial differences in the use of drug therapy for HIV disease in an urban community. *New England Journal of Medicine, 330*(11), 763–768.

Mukhopadhyay, A. (1996). HIV/AIDS: An overview of national demographics (comment). *ABNF Journal, 7*(2), 35–36.

Mulder, D. (1996). Disease progression and mortality following HIV-1 infection. In J. Mann, D. Tarantola (Eds.), *AIDS in the world II* (pp. 15–17). New York: Oxford University Press.

Najera, R., Herrera, M.I., de Andres, R. (1987). Human immunodeficiency virus and related retroviruses. *Western Journal of Medicine, 147*, 694–696.

New York State Department of Health. (June 30, 1997). HIV/AIDS quarterly updates. New York State Department of Health.

Osmond, D., Charlesbois, E., Lang, W., et al. (1994). Changes in AIDS survival time in two San Francisco cohorts of homosexual men, 1983–1993. *Journal of the American Medical Association, 271*(14), 1083–1087.

Paauw, D.S., Wenrich, M.D., Curtis, J.R., et al. (1995). Ability of primary care physicians to recognize physical findings associated with HIV infection. *Journal of the American Medical Association, 274*(17), 1380–1382.

Pantaleo, G., Graziosi, C., Fauci, A.S. (1993). The immunopathogenesis of human immunodeficiency virus infection. *New England Journal of Medicine, 328*(5), 327–335.

Philadelphia Department of Public Health. (June 1997). AIDS Surveillance Quarterly Update. Philadelphia, PA: Department of Public Health.

Phillips, J.D. (1996). Protease inhibitors: A new weapon and a new strategy against HIV. *Journal of the Association of Nurses in AIDS Care, 7*(5), 57–64.

Popovic, M., Sarngodharan, M.G., Reed, E., et al. (1984). Detection, isolation, and continuous production of cytopathic retrovirus (HTLV-III) from patients with AIDS and pre-AIDS. *Science, 224*(46480), 497–500.

Quinn, T.C. (1996). Global burden of the HIV pandemic. *Lancet, 348*(9020), 99–106.

Randolph, L.B. (April, 1997). The magic "miracle." "The Lord has healed Earvin." *Ebony,* 73–76.

Rosenberg, E., Cotton, D. (1997). Primary HIV infection and the acute retroviral syndrome: The urgent need for recognition. *AIDS Clinical Care, 9*(3), 19, 23–25.

Ryan, F. (1997). *Virus X: Tracking the new killer plagues.* Boston: Little, Brown & Company.

Sax, P. (1996). Viral load testing. *AIDS Clinical Care, 8*(4), 31–32.

Shernoff, M., Ball, S. (1997). Sex secrets and lies. *OUT,* 105–147.

Singleton, J.A., Tabnak, F., Kuan, J., et al. (1996). Human immunodeficiency virus disease in California—Effects of the 1993 expanded case definition of the acquired immunodeficiency syndrome. *Western Journal of Medicine, 164*, 122–129.

Stone, V.E., Seage, G.R., Hertz, T., Epstein, A.M. (1992). The relation between hospital experience and mortality for patients with AIDS. *Journal of the American Medical Association, 268*(19), 2655–2661.

Strathdee, S.A., Veugelers, P.J., Page-Shafer, A., et al. (1996). Lack of consistency between five definitions of nonprogressors in cohorts of HIV-infected seroconverters. *AIDS, 10*(9), 959–965.

Tindall, B., Cooper, D.A. (1991). Primary infection: Host responses and intervention strategies. *AIDS, 5*(1), 1–14.

Torian, L.V., Weisfuse, I.B., Makki, H.A., et al. (1996). Trends in HIV seroprevalence in men who have sex with men: New York City Department of Health sexually transmitted disease clinics, 1988–1993. *AIDS, 10*, 187–192.

Tu, X.M., Meng, X.M. (1993). Survival differences and trends in patients with AIDS in the United States. *Journal of Acquired Immune Deficiency Syndromes, 6*(10), 1150–1156.

Turner, B.J., Ball, J.K. (1992). Variations in inpatient mortality for AIDS in a national sample of hospitals. *Journal of Acquired Immune Deficiency Syndromes, 5*(10), 978–987.

Valentine, F.T., Kundu, S., Haslett, P.A., et al. (1996). A randomized, placebo-controlled study of the immunogenicity of human immunodeficiency virus (HIV) rgp160 vaccine in HIV-infected subjects with > or = 400/mm³ CD4 T lymphocytes (AIDS Clinical Trials Group Protocol 137). *Journal of Infectious Diseases, 173*(6), 1336–1346.

van Harmelen, J., Wood, R., Lambrick, M., et al. (1997). An association between HIV-1 subtypes and mode of transmission in Cape Town, South Africa. *AIDS, 11*, 81–87.

Vento, S., DiPerri, G., Garofano, T., et al. (1993). *Pneumocystis carinii* pneumonia during primary HIV-1 infection. *Lancet, 342*(8862), 24–25.

Volberding, P.A. (1996). Medicine and HIV. *Lancet, 348,* 1007–1008.

von Reyn, C.F., Mann, J.M. (1987). AIDS: A global perspective: Global epidemiology. *Western Journal of Medicine, 147*(6), 694–701.

Weniger, B.G., Brown, T. (1996). The march of AIDS through Asia. *New England Journal of Medicine, 335*(5), 343–345.

Williams, A.B. (1997). New horizons: Antiretroviral therapy in 1997. *Journal of the Association of Nurses in AIDS Care, 8*(4), 26–38.

2

Health Promotion and Maintenance

Jacquelyn Haak Flaskerud

Health promotion in the case of HIV disease means promoting a lifestyle and behaviors that will prevent or decrease the chances of infection with HIV as well as promoting a healthy lifestyle and behaviors in persons who are already infected. Similarly, disease prevention means not only decreasing or preventing the behaviors that cause initial infection with the virus but also decreasing or preventing behaviors and conditions that foster disease expression, prolonging the asymptomatic stage of HIV infection, and postponing the occurrence of AIDS-indicator diseases. Finally, disease prevention in AIDS means prophylactic and therapeutic treatment of the AIDS-indicator conditions, rehabilitation, and palliation. From this perspective, the public health model of primary prevention, early intervention, and rehabilitative and palliative efforts is exceptionally applicable to the spectrum of HIV disease.

Some constructs that have received added emphasis in public health prevention since the advent of HIV disease are harm reduction and stages of change (Fitzgerald et al., 1996; McKirnan et al., 1996; Prochaska et al., 1994). Harm reduction focuses on persons moving toward goals of safer behavior on a continuum that includes absence of the behavior as one of the poles among many other options along the continuum. It does not focus on the morality of the behavior (Fitzgerald et al., 1996; McKirnan et al., 1996). Harm reduction is a collaborative approach to decision making that includes the client and a multidisciplinary health care team. Members of the community are mobilized as peer educators (Zevin, 1997). The Stages of Change model accepts that behavior change is a long-term and dy-

namic process that includes both progression and relapse in the behavior change process and among the stages of change (Prochaska et al., 1994). This model suggests that people move along a continuum of five stages of change from precontemplation to maintenance of behavior change. The model proposes interventions congruent with and appropriate to each stage of change. From a community perspective also, the health promotion–harm reduction–stages of change framework is uniquely suited to decreasing and preventing the incidence and prevalence of HIV (Hamburg, 1996; Wardrop, 1993).

VARIABLE PATHOGENESIS OF HIV

Ever since HIV/AIDS was first recognized, it has been apparent that the rate at which persons become infected with HIV and immunodeficient or contract complicating diseases when infected varies considerably. Within groups of infected persons, it is still uncertain in whom and when AIDS will develop. This variable expression of pathogenic properties is true of all but a few microorganisms infecting humans (Cole & Kemeny, 1997; Royce et al., 1997). The proportion of people who are exposed to HIV and become infected or who are infected and will develop AIDS cannot be absolutely determined on the basis of observed data. On a population level, host-related factors (e.g., susceptibility, infectiousness), environmental factors (e.g., social, cultural, and political milieu), and agent factors (e.g., HIV type) determine HIV infectivity (Lewin, 1996; Royce et al., 1997). More and more frequently the factors that contribute to infection and disease progression are being identified for persons in all exposure categories. Knowledge of these factors makes targeted health promotion and disease prevention a more practical reality. Recent developments have encouraged health care workers to implement health-promoting and harm-reducing behaviors and lifestyles in persons who are infected. Clinical and research findings have provided health professionals with knowledge to give concrete direction and advice to their clients in specific situations. In February 1992 the National Institutes of Health (NIH) identified three groups of resistant "rule breakers":

1. Those exposed to HIV but not infected
2. Those who are infected but do not show immunologic progression (CD4+ T-cell counts stabilize at above 200)
3. Those who show progression (CD4+ T-cell counts fall to less than 200) but do not develop AIDS—advanced HIV disease (Rowe, 1993).

Several reports of long-term survivors of HIV disease have prompted investigators to study healthy persons to learn about resistance to HIV. Persons exposed to HIV but not infected may share some of the same immune system characteristics of long-term nonprogressors to HIV disease (Clerici et al., 1992; Detels et al., 1994, 1996).

Immune Response

The presence of a cellular immune response characterized by high levels of CD8+ cells may explain the lack of infection in persons exposed to HIV as well as those infected now for 20 years whose immune systems look very much like those of uninfected exposed persons (Giorgi & Majchrowica, 1996). HIV suppressor factors known as chemokines may be at work in blocking HIV infection of CD4+ cells (Ferbas, 1996; Royce et al., 1997). As an example, among prostitutes in Kenya, 60 of 424 women (14%) remained persistently seronegative despite repeated exposure to infection (Fowke et al., 1996). Investigators postulated that the women have an HIV-1 specific cellular immune response that protects them from infection, probably a CD8-mediated suppression of HIV-1 replication.

About 5% of HIV-1 infected people appear to experience nonprogressing infection (Staprans & Feinberg, 1997). Long-term survivors have several immunologic characteristics in common. They have lower levels of plasma HIV-1 RNA

and maintain strong cytotoxic lymphocyte activity many years after HIV infection. They maintain strong suppressor T-cell activity, and they have higher levels of antibodies directed against several HIV proteins and subregions of proteins (Staprans & Feinberg, 1997; Ferbas, 1996). Various reasons for the delay in the progression to AIDS have been postulated: for example, variation in pathogenic strain of HIV, viral replication rate, and genetic protection through a stronger human leukocyte antigen (HLA) type (Ezzell, 1996; Levy, 1993; Pelletier & Wain-Hobson, 1996; Staprans & Feinberg, 1997; Tingley, 1996).

An intensive psychoimmunologic study of long-term survivors who are alive and well after an AIDS diagnosis was begun in 1987 by investigators in California (Ironson et al., 1995; Leiphart, 1997; Solomon et al., 1987). They are studying psychosocial and immunologic variables associated with survival. These variables include hardiness, the use of problem-solving help, altered lifestyle, hopeful psychological mood, an emotionally expressive personality type, a "fighting spirit," and several immunologic markers. Another study identified attitudinal dimensions associated with long-term survival. These dimensions included a positive attitude, planning for the future, and focusing one's energies (Barroso, 1996). In addition to such psychosocial characteristics, clinicians and researchers recommend healthy lifestyle practices and safer sexual practices to prevent reexposure to additional strains of HIV or to pathogens that cause other STDs.

Immune Status

Whether a person becomes infected with HIV is related also to the immune status of the infected person who is transmitting the virus. In perinatal transmission, male-male sexual contact, and male-female sexual contact, the rate of HIV transmission is consistently related to the immunologic status of the infected person (mother or partner). Infected sexual partners and pregnant women with low CD4+ cell counts (400 and below) or percentages (0.50), higher viral loads, and detectable p24 antigen had higher rates of transmission to partners and the fetus than did those who had high CD4+ counts, lower viral load, and no antigenemia (Bulterys & Goedert, 1996; CDC, April 29, 1994; Gallagher & Klima, 1996; Staprans & Feinberg, 1997). Exposure to a person with a primary infection also was associated with increased infectiousness (Royce et al., 1997). In pregnant women the risk of infection to the fetus increased tenfold with decreased immunologic status of the mother (Royce et al., 1997). In a study of heterosexual exposure, the risk of infection to the female partner increased fivefold with lower immunologic status of the male partner (Downs & de Vincenzi, 1996; Royce et al., 1997).

Disease Course

Currently, HIV disease is understood as a chronic disease with a recognizable course. Several prospective studies and estimates have shown that the asymptomatic incubation period of HIV disease is long (10 or more years) (Levy, 1993; Zeller et al., 1996). Considerable variation exists in the time it takes for clinical disease to develop, with a minority of persons getting ill in 2 years and, at the other end of the spectrum, long-term survivors who have been free of symptoms for more than 15 years (Staprans & Feinberg, 1997). These figures are estimates and a way of looking at all persons with AIDS. If clinical findings, immunologic findings, and environmental factors are combined, it is possible to make a more specific estimate about the rate of progression to AIDS. Persons who are considered at higher risk of having a more rapid progression of disease and mortality can be recognized by the clinical presentation of symptomatic primary HIV infection with fever and skin rash, the presence of HIV p24 antigenemia, the absence of a serologic response to HIV core protein, decreased cytotoxic function, and reduced access to health care (Brennan & Porche, 1997; Easterbrook et al., 1996; Keet et al., 1993). It may be assumed that for persons without these clinical, laboratory, and environmental characteristics the prognosis would be for a longer asymptomatic incubation period and perhaps for long-term survival. Survival is enhanced also by the use of prophylactic treatment of conditions such as *Pneumocystis carinii* pneumonia and cytomegalovirus (Frost, 1996; Munoz et al., 1993).

The trend in increased survival time also varies considerably on the basis of geographic region, ethnicity, gender, and exposure category (Montoya & Atkinson, 1996). Despite the scientific advances made in understanding HIV infection and disease progression, some studies have found that survival time comparable to that of white men who have sex with men (MSM) has not occurred in Latinos/Hispanics, in African-Americans, in IDUs, and in MSM who are also IDUs (Easterbrook et al., 1996; Montoya & Atkinson, 1996; Prins & Veugelers, 1997). The opposite findings have been reported also, with no differences in disease progression or mortality between male MSM and IDUs and no differences based on ethnicity (Easterbrook et al., 1996; Gordon et al., 1996; Poole et al., 1996; Prins & Veugelers, 1997). However, women who were IDUs had decreased survival time (Poole et al., 1996), and IDUs in general tended to have a pre-AIDS mortality rate that was much higher than that of homosexual men (Prins & Veugelers, 1997). Another study comparing men and women with HIV also found decreased survival time in the HIV-infected women, regardless of whether they were IDUs (Melnick et al., 1994). Some of the reasons for the conflicting findings among these groups have been related to environmental factors, such as poverty, differential access to health care and standard treatments, discrimination, and less social support for women than for men.

Other reasons for these findings are related to behaviors and are modifiable if the client agrees. For instance, among IDUs, concurrent infection with sexually transmitted disease (STD), current injecting drug use, abscess at the injection site, and multiple, concurrent sexual partners are predictive in estimating the transmission rate (CDC, July 1997). Such findings raise three important questions:

1. Why do some people become infected but others do not?
2. Why do some who are infected not become immunodeficient or contract disease?
3. What is there about some persons that makes them susceptible to infection and disease progression?

Something in addition to HIV exposure seems to be required both to acquire the virus and to become ill from it. Knowledge of these conditions and the various human groups most affected by them will assist health care workers in developing health promotion and disease prevention programs.

FACTORS RELATED TO HIV TRANSMISSION AND DISEASE PROGRESSION

Several factors appear to be involved in determining the pathogenesis of HIV disease (Levy, 1993; Royce et al., 1997). These factors might be viewed as occurring in two categories: conditions of exposure and trigger mechanisms (see Box). Conditions of exposure are those that might affect or facilitate acquisition of HIV infection. Trigger mechanisms are those that either increase

a person's likelihood of being infected during exposure to HIV or contribute to HIV disease progression in those who have been infected.

Conditions of Exposure

Numerous studies in the United States and Europe have documented the relationship between specific life events, sexual and lifestyle practices, and exposure to HIV infection (Brennan & Porche, 1997; Bulterys & Goedert, 1996; Choi et al., 1996; Fowke et al., 1996; Gresenguet et al., 1997; Levy, 1993; Norris et al., 1996; Royce et al., 1997; Tabet et al., 1996; Torian et al., 1995). Receptive anal intercourse, multiple, concurrent sexual partners, vaginal and rectal douching or rectal enemas in conjunction with receptive anal intercourse, sexual intercourse during menstruation and pregnancy, sexual intercourse with sex workers, the presence of genital ulcers, and not being circumcised are all factors associated with the acquisition of HIV infection (Brennan & Porche, 1997; CDC, March 1, 1997; Morris & Kretzschmar, 1997; Torian et al., 1995; Warszawski et al., 1996). These conditions expose a person to HIV by increasing the probability of sexual contact with an infectious partner, providing a route for transmission, causing trauma to the local mucosa, exposing a larger mucosal surface, or producing membrane disruption that permits access of the viral agent to the bloodstream. It should be noted that evidence suggests that the virus probably can pass through an intact mucous membrane as well (Levy, 1993; Staprans & Feinberg, 1997).

Other conditions that may facilitate acquisition of HIV infection have been associated with various aspects of drug and alcohol use (Caetano & Hines, 1995; Montoya & Atkinson, 1996; Ostrow et al., 1995; Turner & Solomon, 1996). The disinhibiting effects on behavior caused by alcohol and other drugs, such as crack cocaine, are well known and possibly allow more frequent or anonymous sexual exposure to the virus (CDC, March 1, 1996; Turner & Solomon, 1996). Some drugs also blunt the sensation of pain, permitting or extending sexual practices that might not ordinarily be tolerated. The most obvious association of drugs and HIV infection is the direct transmission of the virus through the sharing of hypodermic needles, syringes, and other paraphernalia among IDUs. The risk of seropositivity increases

---

▪ HOST-RELATED FACTORS AFFECTING TRANSMISSION OF HIV ▪

Exposure Factors
Anal receptive sex
Rectal douching
Multiple sexual partners
Needle and syringe sharing
Use of "shooting galleries"
Frequency of injection
Use of recreational drugs
Receipt of factor VIII concentrate
Receipt of blood, blood products, tissue
In utero and intrapartal exposure
Needlestick, occupational exposure

Trigger Mechanisms
Noninfectious
Malnutrition
Substance use
Allergic conditions
Genetics (HLA type, mutation of chemokine receptor gene)
Emotional stress
Age
Gender
Pregnancy
Menstruation
Intrauterine devices
Hormonal contraceptives
Cervical ectopy
Presence of foreskin
Genital tract trauma

Infectious
Immune activation—coincident viral infection
Local infection (ulcer of rectal, genital, oral mucosa)
STDs
Stage of HIV infection of vector (primary, late)

with increasing numbers of persons with whom needles are regularly shared and with more frequent injections. In addition, a consistent relationship has been shown between the use of "shooting galleries" or injection in semipublic places and seropositivity (Jewett & Hecht, 1993; Latkin et al., 1996; Montoya & Atkinson, 1996). These conditions produce exposure by increasing the probability of contact with the virus.

Other exposure factors exist for persons with hemophilia and for recipients of blood, blood products, and tissue (CDC, May 20, 1994; CDC, April 12, 1996; Gilmore, 1996; Lee et al., 1996; Levy, 1993). The risk of seropositivity associated with hemophilia increases as the number of exposures to factor VIII concentrate, pooled blood components, and multiple strains of HIV increases. Similarly, among recipients of blood and blood products, the exposure to plasma-rich pooled blood components and multiple strains of HIV and the volume of blood received are significant risk factors for HIV seropositivity (Balfour, 1993; Gilmore, 1996; Levy, 1993; Mellors et al., 1996; Royce et al., 1997). Transfusion of HIV-infected blood is the most efficient mode of HIV transmission and is associated with a 90% probability that the recipient will become infected.

The probability of being infected through in utero or intrapartal exposure or postnatally through breast-feeding has been estimated downward and varies considerably throughout the world (Brennan & Porche, 1997). The probability varies from 14% in Europe, to 31% in New York City and San Francisco, to 45% in Kenya (Staprans & Feinberg, 1997; Wara, 1993). Since introduction of the use of zidovudine in HIV-infected women in the United States, mother-to-child HIV transmission has decreased by two thirds (NIH, March 26, 1997). The addition of HIV immune globubulin to the zidovudine protocol further reduced transmission to 4.8% (NIH, March 26 1997). Poor clinical health, depressed immunologic status of the mother, and the method of delivery (vaginal vs. cesarean section) are exposure factors related to an increased risk of perinatal transmission (Tovo et al., 1996). Without treatment, the overall transmission rate in the United States is approximately 23% (NIH, March 26, 1997). There is also a possibility of infant infection through breast milk.

Trigger Mechanisms

Trigger mechanisms exert an effect on the expression of disease that is independent of any role in producing exposure to HIV. These mechanisms augment or accelerate immunodeficiency. They increase the likelihood of being infected during exposure or contribute to the expression of active disease in those with HIV positivity. Trigger mechanisms may have additive, deterministic, synergistic, or facilitative roles in the cytopathic effects of HIV on the immune system. Trigger mechanisms are postulated to contribute to T-cell immunodeficiency and immunologic abnormality through a variety of mechanisms.

NONINFECTIOUS FACTORS. Both noninfectious and infectious factors are involved in the cause of and susceptibility to HIV infection and symptomatic AIDS. Noninfectious factors include nutrition and diet; use of injection, recreational, or prescribed drugs; genetic predisposition; allergic disorders; stress; age; gender; pregnancy; and so forth (see Box, p. 29). The most common cause of T-cell immunodeficiency worldwide is protein-calorie malnutrition. Malnutrition reduces the total number of T-lymphocytes and helper and suppressor cells, impairs cell-mediated immunity and secretory immunity, reduces complement secretion, alters phagocytic function, and decreases natural killer cell activity (Casey, 1997). In addition, malnourishment leads to significant mineral, trace element, and vitamin deficiencies that affect overall immune function (Burns et al., 1995; Elion, 1997). Malnutrition may be related to a lack of food supplies, to non-nutritional food choices, to the use of drugs to control appetite, and to loss of appetite related to injection or recreational drug use.

Alcohol, nitrites (poppers), amphetamines, marijuana, tobacco (cigarettes), and injection drugs (heroin, cocaine, and morphine) have all been suggested as possible factors in immunosuppression (Casey, 1997; Cronk & Sarvela, 1997; Ostrow et al., 1995; Poole et al., 1996; Prins & Veugelers, 1997; Schoenbaum, 1997). Cohort studies of persons living with HIV (PLWH) have sometimes supported the association of substance use and decreased immune function and other times have not (Caetano & Hines, 1995; Casey, 1997; Colebunders, 1996; Park et al., 1993). In a study of HIV-infected pregnant women who did not take antiretroviral drugs, women who smoked during pregnancy had a 31% risk of transmitting the virus to the fetus compared with 22% who did not smoke (Turner, 1997). In addition, smoking tobacco or marijuana and nitrite inhalation might predispose the lungs to opportunistic infections, especially PCP.

Exposure to allogeneic semen and sperm has been suggested as a possible mechanism in HIV disease (Levy, 1993). Immunosuppression could result from exposure to allogeneic cells in passive partners during anogenital or vaginal sex if sperm and semen can reach the lymphatic and vascular systems. This could occur by way of genital, rectal, or lower bowel lesions resulting from trauma caused by sexual practices or from other infections.

A relationship between psychobiologic factors and decreased immune function has been proposed frequently (Cole, 1997; Cole & Kemeny, 1997; Leiphart, 1997). In the case of HIV disease, this relationship has been hypothesized to be related to disease progression as measured by decline in CD4+ levels and lymphocyte function. Findings have been mixed. In an extensive review of more than 50 studies, Cole and Kemeny (1997) summarized the literature that relates immune function and HIV morbidity and mortality to stressful life events, coping, bereavement, response to bereavement, hardiness, depression, social support, and personality characteristics. Although several studies reported an effect on immune function (usually CD4+ levels), very few measured progression to HIV morbidity and mortality. In those studies in which clinical outcomes were measured, HIV morbidity and mortality frequently did not correspond to immune function.

Only 12 studies were methodologically sound and measured clinical outcomes. In these studies, negative expectations about future health were related to significant increases in symptom onset and HIV mortality (Reed et al., 1994; in press). Repeated bereavement and self-reproach in response to bereavement were significantly related to decreased CD4+ levels but not to clinical outcomes (Kemeny & Dean, 1995). Active coping was related to significant *increase* in symptom onset (Keet et al., 1993). Depression in one study was not related to CD4+ level, AIDS onset, or HIV mortality (Lyketsos et al., 1993), and in another study it was related to a decrease in CD4+ level but not to morbidity or mortality (Burack et al., 1993). Social support was significantly related to an *increase* in symptom onset in one study (Patterson et al., 1996) and to a *decrease* in CD4+ level in another (Miller et al., 1997) but not to clinical outcomes. Finally, psychological inhibition was significantly related to a decrease in CD4+ level and an increase in AIDS onset and HIV mortality (Cole et al., 1996). In summary, it is not clear how much influence psychosocial factors have on the physical health of seropositive persons.

Age is related to immunologic status. Infants have undeveloped natural resistance systems, which makes them susceptible to multiple infections, including HIV infection. Younger infants (6 months of age) with HIV infection also have the poorest prognosis (Colebunder, 1996). In addition, the more premature that infants are, the more immunologically abnormal they are and the more likely they are to be infected with HIV (Wara & Dorenbaum, 1997). Recently it has been reported that adolescents and young adults (13 to 25 years of age) have a shorter incubation period, that is, a shorter time from HIV infection to AIDS (Denning & Fleming, 1997). Older adults (over 45 to 50 years of age) have an age-related loss of natural resistance, which might make them more susceptible to HIV and other infections (Prins & Veugelers, 1997). Among persons with hemophilia and other recipients of blood transfusions, older age is strongly related to disease progression (Colebunder, 1996).

Pregnancy represents a relatively immunosuppressed state to protect the fetus from immune rejection. Gestational immunosuppression occurs naturally in the second and third trimesters and can be measured by depressed CD4-bearing lymphocytes, which return to normal 1 month postpartum (Landers & Shannon, 1997). A relationship between pregnancy and disease progression in seropositive women has been hypothesized. Currently, the evidence is not clear as to whether pregnancy exerts an influence on the course of HIV disease (Landers & Shannon, 1997). Trends toward earlier manifestation of HIV-related symptoms in pregnant women and toward a higher maternal mortality rate in seropositive women than in seronegative women have been found, but other factors such as nutritional status may have been involved (Burns et al., 1995).

Gender differences in response to survival and disease progression have been noted among persons in community programs in 13 U.S. cities (Melnick et al., 1994). Women were at increased risk of death but not of disease progression. Risks of most OIs were similar for men and women; however, women were at an increased risk of bacterial pneumonia. In another study of 1171 subjects from clinical centers in Chicago, Detroit, Los Angeles, Newark, New York, and San Francisco, women IDUs had the worst survival rates (Poole et al., 1996). Women had an increased risk of bacterial pneumonia and bacterial sepsis than men. In both of these studies the difference was attributed to different socioeconomic and lifestyle factors, differential access to health care and standard treatments, general poor health, and less social support for women (e.g., lower income, less education, more depression, more symptoms, more use of tobacco, and less use of medicine). A review of U.S. adult AIDS cases diagnosed between January 1988 and June 1991 showed that the prevalence of certain AIDS-defining conditions was reported significantly more frequently in women than in men: infection with herpes simplex virus (HSV), infection with cytomegalovirus (CMV), and esophageal candidiasis (Fleming et al., 1993; Newman & Wofsy, 1997). These conditions commonly are associated with CD4+ cell counts in a more advanced stage of disease progression.

Genetics may also play a role in HIV disease progression and the likelihood that specific disease manifestations will develop. HLA type (e.g., HLA B37 and B49) has been associated with clinical disease progression (Colebunder, 1996; Ezzell, 1996); HLA type may also protect HIV-infected persons from disease progression (for example, HLA B27, B57, B51) (Ezzell, 1996). In addition, persons who are homozygous for a chemokine receptor gene (CKR5) mutation appear to be resistant to HIV infection and those who are heterozygous have a slower progression to disease (Royce et al., 1997).

Finally, of the possible noninfectious conditions that facilitate HIV disease, allogeneic blood and blood products, especially plasma-rich blood components such as fresh frozen plasma, whole blood, and platelets, may be immunosuppressive. The transfer of allogeneic blood and blood products might compromise the immune system of recipients (Levy, 1993; Vamvakas & Kaplan, 1993). In persons with hemophilia, immunosuppression may result from infusion of factor VIII as replacement therapy. The transfusion of stored anticoagulated plasma has been suggested as one factor that may affect host immune defenses and facilitate expression of clinical HIV disease.

INFECTIOUS FACTORS. Infectious processes are involved also in the cause of and susceptibility to AIDS. Inflammation and immune activation can facilitate infection as well as accelerate the course of HIV disease (Royce et al., 1997; Whalen et al., 1995). If the immune system is continually stimulated by a high antigenic load in association with various chronic infections, this overstimulation may interfere with the host's capacity to eliminate infectious agents. A history of multiple infectious diseases, among them tuberculosis, syphilis, giardiasis, gonorrhea, chancroid, and parasitic diseases, has been suggested as a factor in the acquisition of HIV infection (Boland, 1997; CDC March 1, 1996; Hopewell, 1997; Mostad & Kreiss, 1996; Royce et al., 1997; Torian et al., 1995). Soft tissue infections, such as injection site abscesses, as well as such infections as viral hepatitis and bacterial endocarditis, may result from the injection of drugs dissolved in nonsterile water, mixed with contaminated diluents and impure narcotics, and self-administered through needles and syringes contaminated by blood and dirt (Alcabes et al., 1993; Newman & Wofsy, 1997; Poole et al., 1996; Solomon et al., 1993). These infections are thought to produce sufficient insult to the immune system to enhance the pathologic effects of HIV on the host.

Another infectious factor that might be operative in the progression from asymptomatic infection to overt disease is immune activation caused by viruses other than HIV. Chief among those suggested as playing an additive or synergistic role in potentiating the cytopathic effects of HIV are chronic infections with CMV, Epstein-Barr virus (EBV), hepatitis B and C viruses (HBV and HCV), herpesviruses, and human papillomavirus (HPV) (Drew et al., 1997; Rochon, 1997; Royce et al., 1997). These viruses significantly impair the immune system and may facilitate the progression of HIV infection. The effect of infection with other viruses might be simply immunosuppressive, providing opportunities for reactivation of HIV, or the viruses may activate cells that carry HIV, resulting in the full expression of cyto-pathologic effects (Drew et al., 1997).

Finally, reinfection with HIV, stage of HIV infectivity, and type of HIV strain may be interacting factors in the acquisition of HIV infection and in progression to clinical disease (Royce et al., 1997). The stage of infectivity determines the amounts of circulating virus and antibody. Transmission of the virus to others may vary, depending on the amount of circulating virus or stage of infection in an HIV-infected person (Downs & de Vincenzi, 1996; Staprans & Feinberg, 1997). Infectivity is increased during primary HIV infection and late-stage HIV infection. Furthermore, HIV-1 strain types differ between persons and between population groups (Downs & de Vincenzi, 1996; Mastro et al., 1994). Strains of HIV vary in their virulence. Strain type is correlated with primary HIV infection, disease course, and clinical outcome. Because HIV strain types differ, a more virulent strain of HIV may infect a person who has thus far avoided infection even though exposed and may alter the course of disease progression in a person who has remained free of symptoms.

The various factors discussed here play a role in exposure to the virus, transmission of the virus, immunosuppression of the host, and activation or facilitation of the virus. Depending on their virulence and combination, they can increase or decrease the susceptibility to HIV infection and the potentiating effect on expression of HIV disease.

PERSONAL AND SOCIAL GROUP EFFORTS TO PREVENT HIV INFECTION

A comprehensive public health approach to cause, prevention, and cure is needed to control the spread of HIV infection. A comprehensive approach to combating disease considers changes in the host, the agent, and the environment. Host-related changes are behaviors that individuals, partners, and families can engage in or modify to prevent exposure to HIV or progression to disease. Agent-related efforts include identifying the virus, finding antiviral treatments, and developing a vaccine against the virus. Environmental efforts involve HIV infection control in the community through changing access to care and the social, cultural, and political milieu. This section

begins with health promotion and changes in disease prevention needed in host behavior. A later section in this chapter addresses environmental (community) efforts to promote health and prevent disease.

Health Promotion

Knowledge of exposure to HIV disease and the factors that potentiate disease expression can assist health professionals in planning health care activities that individuals and their partners, families, and friends can implement on their own behalf or with the assistance of health care workers. These take the form of health promotion, disease prevention, and harm reduction activities. Health promotion strategies pose few risks, have a positive effect on well-being, and may contribute to slowing disease progression (Jewett & Hecht, 1993).

Health promotion behaviors and activities are applicable to all persons, regardless of HIV status. Behaviors and activities discussed here are those related to a healthy lifestyle and those believed to enhance immunocompetence. These behaviors apply also to persons who are infected with HIV and to those in all stages of HIV disease.

DIET. As noted earlier, malnutrition is the major cause of immunosuppression worldwide. The impact of specific nutrients on immune status has been documented: deficiencies in calorie-protein intake have consistent and profound effects on cell-mediated immunity, lymphocyte subsets, complement secretion, phagocyte function, secretory antibody response, and antibody affinity (Casey, 1997; Coodley et al., 1994; Nerad & Gorbach, 1994).

Currently, a health-promoting diet that promotes optimal immune functioning consists of a variety of foods from each of the seven food groups and is composed of 50% to 55% calories from carbohydrates, 15% to 20% calories from protein, and 30% or fewer calories from fat (Aron, 1994; Wong, 1993). Two or three servings of food from each of the protein and dairy groups are recommended for each day, seven to twelve servings from the starch-grain group, two servings of vitamin C–rich fruits and vegetables, one serving of vitamin A–rich fruits and vegetables, and three servings of other fruits and vegetables.

MICRONUTRIENTS. Vitamins and minerals are essential for optimal immune functioning (Coodley et al., 1994; Elion, 1997). A diet rich in micronutrients should supply the vitamins and minerals essential for immune functioning. The addition of a multivitamin-mineral supplement to the diet provides sufficient essential nutrients (Coodley et al., 1994; Wong, 1993). Recent reports have suggested that enhanced immune response may be related to adequate amounts of vitamins A and E, beta-carotene, zinc, and selenium (Abrams, 1997; Elion, 1997). Researchers at Johns Hopkins Medical Center have been studying the use of vitamins A, B_1, C, and niacin in doses larger than the recommended amount with 28 HIV-positive men for up to 6 to 8 years. In an interim report these investigators found that micronutrient intake for at least 2 years, started early in the course of HIV infection, seemed to slow the onset of AIDS (*HIV Frontline Update*, 1994). According to the researchers, these results need to be confirmed by additional studies. However, it should be noted carefully that megadoses of vitamins and minerals may be dangerous. Megadoses can create nutrient-nutrient or nutrient-medication competitive environments, cause toxic effects and neurologic damage, and result in a weakening of the immune system (Abrams, 1997).

Information on nutrition and meal planning is an important aspect of health promotion education for all groups (Abrams, 1997; Flaskerud, 1994; Jewett & Hecht, 1993; Sowell et al., 1997). Special attention may be required for some groups. Some homosexual men and heterosexual women may have eating disorders or may diet excessively in an effort to be exceptionally thin to enhance their physical attractiveness (Gold, 1995). Information on the dangers of this kind of dieting and on what constitutes adequate nutrition may be needed.

Another group that may need nutrition information consists of the urban poor. Even when diets are adequate in calories in this group, they are often deficient in protein, vitamins, vegetables, and fruit and high in fat (Sowell et al., 1997). Among the urban poor are the IDUs and other substance abusers, who often are poorly nourished because of the appetite-suppressant effects of drugs, toxic effects of alcohol on the gastrointestinal tract, and inadequate assimilation of

vitamins and amino acids as a result of damaged liver cells (Casey, 1997). Chapter 11 contains additional information on nutrition and HIV.

REGULAR EXERCISE. Physical exercise is recommended as a health-promoting activity because it increases lung capacity, muscle-to-fat ratio, endurance, energy, and flexibility, and improves circulation (Centers for Disease Control and Prevention [CDC], September 10, 1993, July 11, 1996). It also improves sleeping, appetite, and regular bowel activity and decreases stress. Solomon and colleagues (1993) have proposed a relationship between psychosocial factors, exercise, and immunity based on studies of athletes, elderly persons, and PLWH. Currently, an exercise program of 30 to 45 minutes, 4 or more days per week, is recommended. Exercise should use muscle groups in both the arms and legs, should be fitted to personal endurance, and should not be painful or boring.

Acceptable and feasible exercise programs must be designed specifically for individual interests, physical capabilities, financial restrictions, and other personal characteristics. Walking is an exercise available to all that is not overly taxing and may be done in the company of children or other adults (Sowell et al., 1997). The benefits of exercise are not readily apparent to some people, such as the urban poor or mothers with young children, who may believe that it is too expensive and will make them more tired and pressured for time.

Balancing the need for regular exercise is the need for adequate, regular rest and sleep. For some persons, sleep programs must be designed that will allow them to fall asleep and stay asleep (McEnany et al., 1996). Others need education on the negative effects of sleep deprivation. Sleep deprivation is associated with fatigue and clinical depression. Taken together, these represent added strains, which may facilitate symptom expression (McEnany et al., 1996).

STRESS AND EMOTIONS. Reduction and control of stress is the goal of stress management programs. Stress may be associated with immunosuppression and may increase a person's vulnerability to disease. Sympathetic nervous system response may influence immune system function and viral replication through alterations in cytokine production (Cole, 1997). Adequate sleep and rest and regular exercise are important stress-reduction activities (McEnany et al. 1996; Solomon et al., 1993). Mental exercises, such as meditation, visualization, and biofeedback, are all types of relaxation techniques that may reduce stress (Eller, 1995; Taylor, 1995).

An adequate coping response has been suggested as a means of moderating stress. Active or involved coping is believed to have beneficial health effects (Folkman et al., 1993). Active coping includes problem-solving activity, increased expression of emotions, seeking advice and information, altering one's lifestyle, taking control of one's health and well-being, and having a sense of purpose and commitment to life. Active coping seems to work best in situations of specific, highly stressful personal events, such as at the time of notification of HIV infection, the occurrence of AIDS onset, or bereavement, rather than being related to a general state of mind and behavior (Keet et al., 1993; Kemeny & Dean, 1995; Patterson et al., 1996). Studies of active coping as a general state of behavior have found associations with *poorer* rather than better health status (Keet et al., 1993). To date, the relationship of most of these behaviors, attitudes, and values is in a hypothetical stage of research and should not be promoted with clients as preferable to other forms of coping. Rather, a repertoire of coping behaviors seems to offer the most useful approach to life events and stresses.

Other stress-reduction techniques involve social group relationships. These include being involved in altruistic ways with other persons and groups, providing and receiving social support, involvement in spiritual and religious activities, taking part in recreational activities and play, taking breaks at work and vacations, and being involved in committed relationships (Cole & Kemeny, 1997; Gaskins & Brown, 1997; Sowell et al., 1997). Avoidance of stress-producing situations has also been recommended. However, it should be noted that avoidance of stress is almost impossible in today's world, and using it as a health promotion strategy may produce guilt (Segerstrom et al., 1996).

Special attention should be given to the benefit of emotional expression. In several studies, strong sympathetic nervous system reactivity to the expression of basic emotions (fear, anger, surprise, disgust, happiness, and sadness) was related to increased immune function and enhanced mental and physical health (Cole et al., 1996; Gross & Levenson, 1993; Petrie et al., 1995). Some people may believe mistakenly that suppression of emotion is one method of stress reduction and think that by suppressing emotions they will reduce stress and promote immune function. The studies cited here found the opposite. There were complex interactions among emotional expression, strong autonomic reactivity, and increased immune response. Helping persons find avenues for emotional expression through family, friends, partners, social groups, clergy and religious groups, and professional counseling may enhance both physical and mental health (Cole & Kemeny, 1997).

Recommending stress-reduction programs as a health promotion activity on the basis of current evidence may seem premature, but there are probably at least three reasons for doing so. These programs pose few risks, they may have a positive effect on well-being, and they increase participation of people in their own health care (Cole & Kemeny, 1997; Jewett & Hecht, 1993). Such programs also provide more general information about health promotion, stress, and immune function that may be applicable to HIV disease as well. Finally, if there is a possibility that health promotion and stress reduction may affect immune status and, consequently, HIV disease status, it would be unthinkable not to offer these programs, especially since they rarely involve adverse side effects and have a psychologic benefit.

RECREATIONAL DRUG USE. The overuse of chemical stimulants, alcohol, and recreational drugs such as tobacco, marijuana, and "speed" may have an immunosuppressant effect (Casey, 1997; Klein, 1996; Ostrow et al., 1995). These substances are associated with a variety of physical and mental health problems. Avoiding or limiting their use should be part of health promotion activities. Several self-help programs, as well as professional programs, exist to assist persons who wish to modify their substance use behaviors. These substances, in addition to their possible immunosuppressant characteristics, limit or interfere with the health promotion activities and behaviors described earlier in this section. These substances suppress appetite, irritate the gastrointestinal tract, lead to impaired absorption of food, and damage liver cells. All these consequences reduce the health-promoting benefits of nutrition. They also interfere with regular exercise, sleep, and rest and may therefore exacerbate distress indirectly; direct exacerbation of distress may come from their effect on personal and social relationships.

Prevention of Primary Infection With HIV

Epidemiologic studies indicate that semen, cervical and vaginal secretions, breast milk, and blood products are the predominant, if not exclusive, vehicles of viral transmission (Brennan & Porche, 1997). HIV-1 is transmitted through unprotected anal and vaginal intercourse, the sharing of injection drug equipment, transfusions of blood and blood products, and tissue transplants and between mother and infant in utero, intrapartally, and postnatally through breast-feeding. Transmission can occur also in health care settings through needle-stick injuries and exposures to cuts or mucous membranes. Each of these forms of exposure can be prevented or reduced.

SEXUAL EXPOSURE. No risk of sexual transmission exists for those who practice sexual abstinence. Likewise, there is no risk of infection if neither partner is infected. This would be true of couples who have been mutually monogamous since the introduction of HIV in the United States (mid-1970s) and of mutually monogamous couples who have been shown by serologic testing to have HIV antibody negativity.

For persons outside these situations, the risk can be reduced by limiting the number of concurrent sexual partners and by practicing protective sex. Protective sex is sexual activity in which no semen, vaginal secretions, or blood is exchanged between partners. Protective sex practices involve kissing, hugging, caressing, and genital manipulation (all in the absence of an open lesion). Receptive anal penetrative sex is the most risky sexual practice for men and women. Unprotected vaginal intercourse is the next level of risk, with women more frequently infected (Erhardt, 1996). There is disagreement between health educators in Europe and the United States about whether fellatio with ejaculation poses a risk of HIV infection and should be protected against with condoms (Coxon, 1996; Ostrow et al.,

1995). Risks can be reduced in vaginal and anal intercourse, provided a condom is worn consistently or even occasionally (CDC, August 6, 1993; Pinkerton & Abramson, 1996; Royce et al., 1997). It is important to note here that the use of spermicides with condoms was recommended in the past. It is now thought that spermicides may increase transmission through irritation of rectal mucosa or vaginal lining cells (Feldblum et al., 1995; Royce et al., 1997). The relative risk of sexual transmission in various practices is provided in Table 2–1.

The risk of infection can be reduced by avoiding specific sexual behaviors and practices. These include anal receptive intercourse, vaginal and rectal douching, and multiple, concurrent sexual partners. In combination, these behaviors and practices produce the highest risk of HIV infection in the United States. Genital sores also increase the risk of infection (Torian et al., 1995; Warszawski et al., 1996). Avoidance of unprotected anal intercourse is the principal focus of efforts to reduce risk in male-to-male sexual contact and should also be a major focus of prevention efforts in male-to-female sexual contact.

Vaginal intercourse has lower risks than anal but has become a more frequent route of exposure (Erhardt, 1996). Women are infected at a higher rate than men through this means of exposure. The risk of transmission is higher if there are preexisting sores in the genital area, such as herpes lesions (Brennan & Porche, 1997; Mostad & Kreiss, 1996; Royce et al., 1997).

For those engaging in vaginal intercourse, reducing the number of concurrent, sexual partners and practicing protective sex, preferably at all times but even on occasional times, can reduce the risk of infection and is consistent with a harm-reduction model (Pinkerton & Abramson, 1996). In an effort to assist its health care workers in an area that many find difficult and uncomfortable, Kaiser Permanente has been teaching its health care workers to use a 60-second sexual history interview. This interview is presented in the Box on page 38.

Oral sex, especially fellatio with ejaculation, may play a possible a role in transmission through exposure of the oral mucosa to semen or vaginal fluid (Ostrow et al., 1995). It has been established that HIV-1 shedding occurs in the genital tract of both men and women (Mostad & Kreiss, 1996).

Table 2–1 ■ Risk of Exposure to HIV Related to Behaviors and Practice

Risk/Levels of Safety	Sexual Contact	Injecting Drug Use	Perinatal Exposure
Absolutely safe	Abstinence Mutually monogamous with noninfected partner	Not using injection drugs	Abstinence Sterilization
Safe	Noninsertive sexual practices Dry kissing Masturbation on intact skin Oral sex with a condom External "water sports" Touching Fantasy	Exchanging needles and syringes for sterile supplies Using sterilized injection paraphernalia	Abortion
Possibly safe	Insertive sexual practices with the use of condoms	Not sharing equipment Cleaning injection paraphernalia with full-strength bleach	Use of hormonal contraceptives, intrauterine devices Use of condoms
Risky	Wet kissing Fellatio, cunnilingus without a latex barrier Masturbation on broken skin	Cleaning equipment with other disinfectants, water	Pregnancy
Dangerous	Intercourse without a condom Internal "water sports" Fisting Rimming	Sharing equipment Use of "shooting galleries" Sex under the influence of drugs or alcohol	Pregnancy Breast-feeding

Sores around or in the mouth could theoretically provide an exposure route. Condoms can also help reduce risk in oral sex (Coxon, 1996). Deep kissing with an exchange of saliva has theoretical but not much practical risk. In one reported case a woman possibly became infected through deep kissing when she had inflamed gingival mucosa and her partner had bleeding gums and exudative oral lesions (CDC, July 11, 1997). There also have been rare bite-related instances of HIV transmission (Vidmar et al., 1996).

Other conditions also may modify sexual behaviors. The use of alcohol may lead to risky sexual activities by reducing inhibitions and affecting judgment. The use of crack cocaine has been consistently implicated in these behaviors (Caetano & Hines, 1995; CDC, March 1, 1996; Montoya & Atkinson, 1996; Turner & Solomon, 1996).

INJECTING DRUG USE. Injecting drug use is the second most frequently reported risk for AIDS in the United States (CDC, June 30, 1997). The risk of HIV infection from injecting drug use differs by geographic region, social setting of injec-

tion (e.g., shooting galleries), and frequency of injection (Montoya & Atkinson, 1996). A history of STDs, pyogenic bacterial infections, and soft tissue infection at the injection site increases the risk of infection for IDUs (CDC, July 1997). IDUs can reduce their chances of exposure to HIV infection by stopping the use of injection drugs. For this to occur, addicted persons need referrals to rehabilitation programs. Currently, the number of rehabilitation programs available is inadequate to meet the need if the goal is to stop drug use or if all drug users wish to enroll in such a program. A massive infusion of government and public support is necessary for a major rehabilitation effort (Mann & Tarantola, 1996, pp. 414–426). Because epidemiologic evidence suggests that HIV infection affects African-American and Latino IDUs disproportionately (CDC, November 18, 1994), much of this effort and money will have to be concentrated in communities of color.

If injecting drug use cannot be stopped, exposure to HIV infection can be prevented or reduced by ending the sharing of unsterilized injec-

---

▨ A 60-SECOND SEXUAL HISTORY SCREENING INTERVIEW ▨

1. Are you sexually active? (Do you have sex on a regular basis?)
   a. If YES: "Are you . . .?" (GO TO QUESTION 2)
   b. If NO: "How long since you've been sexually active?"
   c. If > 10 years: STOP
   d. If < 10 years:
      (1) "How long has it been since you had sexual relations on a regular basis?"
      (2) "When you were sexually active, were you . . .?" (GO TO QUESTION 2)
2. ". . . sexually active with men, women, or both?"
   a. If response indicates only one partner (man or woman), ask:
      "How long have you had just one partner?"
   b. If > 10 years: (GO TO QUESTION 4)
   c. If < 10 years: "And before that?" (GO TO QUESTION 3)
3. "How many partners do you (did you) have over the last two years (of activity)?"
   If more than one:
   a. "How many men?"
      "How many women?"
   b. "How long have you been or were you active with each?"
4. "How likely is it that your partner(s) had sexual contacts with an intravenous drug user?"
   "Several other persons?"
   a. If monogamous, partner is not bisexual, and has no-risk contacts: (GO TO QUESTION 5)
   b. If multiple partners, regardless of sex, ask:
      (1) "How often do you have sex with each?"
      (2) "What kind of sexual practices do you engage in, that is, oral, anal, or vaginal sex?"
      (3) If anal, ask: "receptive or insertive?"
5. "Do you have any problems with sexual functioning that you would like to talk about?" Give examples depending on gender of patient.
6. If relevant, based on answers to questions 1 through 4:
   "Have you ever had a sexually transmitted disease, such as gonorrhea or syphilis?"
7. If relevant (multiple partners/partner at risk), ask:
   "Do you use condoms?"

From Southern California Kaiser Permanente Medical Group, Physicians AIDS, Symposium, February 1992, with permission.

tion paraphernalia. Commonly shared injection paraphernalia in which HIV-1 has been detected includes cookers, cotton filters, and drug solutions in addition to needles and syringes (Koester et al., 1996). Risk to female IDUs may be greater than to male IDUs because some investigators have found that females are more likely to share equipment, especially with partners (Neaigus et al., 1994). At a minimum, persons who use injection drugs should clean their equipment with bleach and not share drug solution, cookers, or cotton filters (Koester et al., 1996). Recently the CDC (June 4, 1993) recommended the use of full-strength bleach to clean disposable needles and syringes because they are not intended for reuse and are very difficult to clean. Another possibility is to provide sterile needles and syringes

for IDUs (CDC, September 22, 1995; Gostin et al., 1997). Needle and syringe exchange programs have been effective in decreasing the spread of HIV and have not encouraged drug use in the process (Des Jarlais et al., 1996; Gostin et al., 1997). To decrease their risk of seropositivity through parenteral and injecting drug use, drug users should also stop using semipublic places and/or shooting galleries for injection and decrease the frequency of injection (see Table 2–2) (Montoya & Atkinson, 1996).

Outside the addicted population, there is a substantial number of persons who experiment with drugs. Educational programs for teenagers, for communities in which drug use is high, and for the staffs of drug clinics must emphasize the danger of sharing needles and equipment. The use of drugs in conjunction with sexual practices dramatically increases the risk of exposure to HIV.

PERINATAL EXPOSURE. Perinatal transmission of HIV can be avoided if infected women do not become pregnant. Pregnancy is associated with a moderate risk of infection to infants in untreated mothers (NIH, March 26, 1997). It is unclear whether pregnancy accelerates the development of AIDS in HIV-infected mothers (Brennan & Porche, 1997; Burns et al., 1995; Landers & Shannon, 1997). The risk of perinatal transmission of HIV is higher in women with clinical symptoms of AIDS, with viremia and viral replication, with p24 antigenemia, and with CD4+ cell counts less than 400 (Wara, 1993; Wara & Dorenbaum, 1997). Women at greater risk of exposure (IDUs, prostitutes, women with multiple, concurrent sexual partners, with STDs, or with sexual partners at high risk of exposure) should be encouraged to undergo testing for HIV infection. Those who are infected may be encouraged to postpone pregnancy until more is known about the risks to themselves and their infants. Infected women should be counseled about the risk of transmission on the basis of their immunologic and clinical status and their risk behaviors (Landers & Shannon, 1997). Women should be counseled about the advantages of perinatal zidovudine therapy and of enrolling in clinical trials of zidovudine.

The most recent evidence of the perinatal use of zidovudine demonstrated a 67.5% reduction in the risk of vertical HIV transmission in 364 women participating in ongoing clinical trials (Brennan & Porche, 1997; CDC, April 29, 1994; Landers & Shannon, 1997). Zidovudine is given to the mother during pregnancy and delivery and to the newborn for the first 6 weeks of life. The addition of HIV immunoglobulin to the zidovudine protocol further reduced transmission to 4.8% (NIH, March 26, 1997). Mothers who take zidovudine are given monthly infusions of hyperimmune HIV immunoglobulin (HIVIG) or intravenous immunoglobulin (IVIG) during the pregnancy. Their infants receive a single infusion of HIVIG or IVIG and the 6 weeks of oral zidovudine (Landers & Shannon, 1997). Women who are infected with HIV and become pregnant also should be given family-planning and abortion counseling in the first trimester (Landers & Shannon, 1997).

Women in developing countries where antiretrovirals and immunoglobulin are not available have been treated with microbicide vaginal douching before giving birth, but this treatment has not proved effective (Biggar et al., 1996). All women who are infected with HIV should be told not to breast-feed their babies because the infants may be exposed to HIV through this route as well. HIV-1 has been detected in breast milk and colostrum and increases the risk of infection by 14% (La Coeur & Lallemant, 1996; Wara & Dorenbaum, 1997).

BLOOD AND BLOOD PRODUCT TRANSFUSION AND TISSUE TRANSPLANTATION. Infection through the use of donated blood, blood products, and tissue can be prevented by donor exclusion, serologic testing for HIV antibodies, and heat inactivation of products such as factor VIII concentrate (Brennan & Porche, 1997; Gilmore, 1996). Because processing semen from HIV-infected persons has not been shown to prevent transmission of HIV, semen implantation should be avoided (Edlin & Holmberg, 1993). Donor exclusion can be facilitated by education of donors, interviews at blood banks, and confidential postdonation self-exclusion (CDC, March 1, 1996; Gilmore, 1996). Serologic testing of donors for HIV antibody uses both the enzyme-linked immunosorbent assay (ELISA) or enzyme immunoassay (EIA) technique and the confirmatory Western blot assay. The indirect immunofluorescence assay (IFA) has provided an external standard against which ELISA performance can be judged. Current laboratory screening for HIV-1 will also detect HIV-2, although this infection is extremely rare in the United States (CDC, August 18, 1995). Early hopes that the testing for p24 antigen could "close the window" of false-negative results have not been met because p24 antigenemia is present during only a portion of the window period (Busch & Alter, 1995; CDC March 1, 1996).

The recent addition of HBV antibody core testing of blood donors might further eliminate donors at risk of acquiring HIV infection, because a substantial proportion of those at risk of acquiring HIV infection are also at risk of acquiring HBV infection (Gilmore, 1996). Heat inactivation of factor VIII concentrate suggests that this approach can protect persons with hemophilia who receive factor VIII from acquiring HIV infection almost 100%. Another recommendation is that cryoprecipitate be used instead of concentrated products, because a product from only one person should be safer than pooled blood products. These precautions in combination would virtually eliminate the risk of HIV infection from transfusion of blood and blood products. Currently, in the United States the risk of acquiring HIV from screened blood is estimated at 1 in 450,000 to 660,000 donations (Lackritz et al., 1995).

Several practices can further reduce the risk of exposure through blood and blood products. One of these is participation in autologous blood donation programs for persons who are seronegative. Autologous blood programs are also important for persons who are seropositive, to prevent reinfection with other HIV strains and to prevent transfusion-related lowering of CD4+ cell counts (Vamvakas & Kaplan, 1993). Another practice that has been found to be effective in reducing transfusion transmission is to encourage donations from volunteers while discouraging donations from paid donors (Gilmore, 1996). Finally, a practice that will reduce transfusion transmission is the institution of appropriate transfusion protocols (Ghali et al., 1994; Gilmore, 1996; Weiskopf, 1997). Single-unit transfusions and transfusions of blood as a prophylactic measure are almost never necessary (Ghali et al., 1994; Weiskopf, 1997). In 1984 the World Health Organization estimated that 20% to 25% of blood transfusions and 90% of albumin transfusions were not necessary. In industrialized countries such as the United States, excessive and inappropriate use of transfusions may be common because they are available and affordable.

Asymptomatic HIV Disease: Health Education and Maintenance

Primary health education begins at the time of HIV antibody testing and counseling. A program of HIV testing and counseling must be concerned with complex social and psychologic issues. Testing has both benefits and harms, and pretest and posttest counseling guidelines must be followed to ensure a safe and beneficial program (AAHCPR, January 1994; CDC, January 15, 1993a; CDC,

May 20, 1994; CDC, July 7, 1995). At least 50% of persons receive HIV testing at a private site (physician's office, HMO, clinic); publicly funded sites commonly used include health departments, STD or TB clinics, and drug treatment programs (CDC, March 10, 1995). Hospitals and clinics, drug treatment centers, mental health facilities, and independent practitioners should consider the provision of voluntary HIV counseling for their clients. These settings can offer ready access, appropriate client referral, evaluation, and therapy. Counseling should occur also in blood-bank settings when blood and plasma donors have positive or indeterminate HIV tests (CDC, March 1, 1996). Knowledge of HIV status allows individuals and their partners to seek treatment and prolong their lives and to change high-risk behaviors and prevent transmission. Routine, voluntary HIV testing services may result not only in benefits to clients but in societal and economic benefits as well. Despite these benefits, before embarking on an HIV testing and counseling program, health care facilities and professionals should consider carefully the social issues involved and the wide-ranging responsibilities engendered by such a service.

ISSUES IN HIV TESTING. The assurance of confidentiality is of the highest importance among the issues associated with testing. Disclosure of confidential information can result in discrimination in health care, insurance, employment, and housing. In addition, the impact on interpersonal relationships can be devastating. To protect themselves and their clients, agencies must have clearly written and enforced policies regarding disclosure of test results and maintenance of confidentiality throughout the system. Chapters 12 and 13 provide detailed information related to HIV testing and legal and ethical issues.

A second concern is the presence of a comprehensive standard of care or a teaching program within which HIV antibody testing is conducted. Among persons receiving testing at a public site, 61% received counseling with their test results. In comparison, 28% received counseling at private sites (CDC, March 10, 1995). Severe psychologic trauma to persons being tested has occurred because of the way in which seropositive test results were revealed to them. This trauma is compounded by lack of counseling, failure to make referrals, disclosure of inaccurate test results, or institution of inappropriate procedures (e.g., isolation) based on test results. The standard of care for HIV testing and counseling is mandated by law in some states and is recommended in guidelines by the CDC and the U.S. Public Health Service AHCPR (AHCPR, January 1994, pp. 15–21; CDC, January 15, 1993a; CDC, July 7, 1995; CDC, 1997).

The standard of care involves pretest and posttest counseling and may be characterized by emphasis on completeness and consistency. A personalized client risk assessment is the foundation of pretest counseling. Chapter 5 contains detailed information on taking a comprehensive health history. All relevant information must be provided to persons considering testing. The information provided must be consistent from one person to the next and in accord with standards of practice (CDC guidelines) and the current understanding of HIV disease. Problems arise when clients are provided with more or less information or with conflicting information. For this reason, the CDC recommends adequate training for HIV counselors with ongoing periodic observation, monitoring of counseling sessions, and subsequent feedback for quality assurance. Finally, as part of any comprehensive standard of care, appropriate referral sources for continued counseling, education, medical care, and psychiatric emergencies must be in place before HIV testing begins. HIV counseling should result in a personalized plan of risk reduction, health promotion, and health maintenance negotiated with the client.

Another issue is the predictive value of HIV antibody testing. Like all laboratory tests, HIV antibody tests are imperfect. Both false-positive and false-negative results can occur. Because false-positive results may have tragic psychologic and legal consequences, additional testing of a second specimen by means of the Western blot test should be required before test results are communicated. Testing for p24 antigen can detect HIV infection earlier (6 days on average) than antibody tests but is not useful after antibodies to HIV become detectable because of antigen-antibody complexing and viral clearance (CDC, March 1, 1996). In persons with no high-risk behaviors, positive results should be repeated on two new serum specimens in a reference labora-

tory. For instance, false-positive results have been reported among blood donors after influenza vaccination (CDC, March 12, 1993). False-negative antibody results also may occur. After infection, there is a window period in which antibody cannot be detected. A negative result may be misleading and falsely reassuring to a tested person. Seroconversion may take up to 3 months or, in rare cases, longer. Continued high-risk behaviors may lead to infection of the person and of his or her sexual or needle-sharing partners. Before HIV testing is conducted, persons considering testing must be carefully instructed about the occurrence of false-positive and false-negative test results. They must also be informed in detail about what an HIV antibody test result does and does not mean.

Several additional issues that must be considered in HIV testing have been raised recently. There is a strong association between tuberculosis (TB) and HIV infection (Asch et al., 1997; CDC, January 19, 1996). HIV seroprevalence in persons with TB ranges from 66% in Uganda to 5.2% in Brazil (Raviglione et al., 1996). In the United States estimates vary from 2% to 14%, depending on the population group studied (Hopewell, 1997). In Los Angeles nearly half of the urban patients with TB are also infected with HIV; yet physicians tested only one third of TB patients for HIV. The failure to test was due to provider choice rather than patient refusal (Asch et al., 1997). Clearly, it is necessary that persons with TB be tested routinely for HIV and that TB screening be a routine part of management of patients with HIV infection (Hopewell, 1997; Raviglione et al., 1996). An integral part of HIV test counseling should include counseling and referral for TB screening.

A second issue that has gained recent attention is the failure of persons who are tested for HIV antibody to return for test results. The published failure-to-return rate ranges from 24% to 58% (Bell et al., 1997). Among some populations, this rate may be even higher. The major reasons for failure to return involve fears about the results, issues surrounding confidentiality of results, a perceived lack of risk, and lifestyle or life circumstances that do not permit return (e.g., drug use, transportation problems) (Bell et al., 1997; Irwin et al., 1996; Solomon et al., 1996; Sowell et al., 1996; Stall et al., 1996; Valdiserri et al., 1993).

Clearly, an extremely important aspect of pretest counseling should focus on the personal, medical, and social benefits of returning to receive the test results (Irwin et al., 1996).

Finally, home testing for HIV antibody is a recent development that deserves discussion. Home testing in the United States is available through a fingerstick blood test and a test of saliva (Schopper & Vercauteren, 1996). Home testing involves collecting a blood or saliva sample at home and mailing it to a laboratory for antibody testing. After about a week, negative results are given to the person by telephone or voice mail and positive results are given person-to-person. The issues surrounding home testing concern the absence of pre- and post-HIV test counseling. The home collection kit contains a pretest counseling booklet. Persons whose test results are positive are advised or take it upon themselves to contact appropriate health services.

Proponents of home testing argue that it increases considerably the number of persons who have access to and may use an HIV antibody test (Schopper & Vercauteren, 1996). Persons who preferred a home test to a clinic test in a national survey in the United States had less education and lower income, did not know where to go for a test, and were nonwhite (Phillips et al., 1995). This would be a population that has been less involved in testing, and getting this population involved is seen as a benefit of home testing (Irwin et al., 1996; Solomon et al., 1996; Valdiserri et al., 1993). Proponents cite other benefits, such as earlier treatment, avoidance of perinatal transmission, decreased sexual transmission, and decreased cost. Proponent arguments are based on assumptions that persons with positive test results will change their risk behaviors and will become involved in treatment. There is little evidence that HIV testing, even with counseling, results in enough behavior change to have a public health impact on HIV transmission (Schopper & Vercauteren, 1996; Sowell et al., 1996).

Opponents of home testing point to the lack of counseling as a risk to mental health and include in their argument the lack of information about false-positive or false-negative tests. More worrisome is the potential for abuse in coercive situations by employers, insurance companies, police, and border controls and by men against women. Negative effects of home testing are more likely in situations where people are powerless, poor, and of unequal status and where health services are not readily available.

There is as yet little direct evidence about the issues surrounding home testing or its effectiveness. Until August 1997, there were two home testing kits available: Home Access, Health Corporation and Johnson & Johnson Direct Access. Johnson & Johnson took their Confide home test off the market in August, citing poor sales. However, the Food and Drug Administration (FDA) warned Johnson & Johnson about its quality-control procedures and noted that they had not submitted mandatory reports to the FDA after consumer complaints that the wrong test results were given to some persons (*HIV News Briefs,* 1997). The benefits and risks of home testing are yet to be determined.

BENEFITS AND RISKS OF TESTING. More than most clinical laboratory tests, HIV antibody testing has benefits, risks, and responsibilities that must be weighed before health facilities and professionals offer a program of testing and before an individual decides on whether to be tested (Irwin et al., 1996; Schopper & Vercauteren, 1996). The benefits to individuals and to society follow. For persons with seronegative test results, the benefits include the following:

- Reassurance and reduction of anxiety
- Motivation for behavior change to prevent infection
- Information on which to base decisions about marriage, sexual relationships, childbearing, breast-feeding, and immunizations for infants
- Support for an alternative medical diagnosis for unexplained symptoms when HIV disease is under consideration

Symptom-free persons with seropositive test results may receive the following benefits:

- Closer medical follow-up
- Laboratory measurement of disease prognostic markers
- Opportunity for involvement in experimental protocols, early intervention programs, and alternative therapies
- Treatment or prophylaxis for other infectious diseases

- Protection of sexual partners
- Information as a basis for decisions about marriage, sexual relationships, childbearing, breast-feeding, and immunizations for infants
- Information for use in future plans for employment, insurance, housing, legal affairs, and so forth

Society receives the following benefits from testing:

- Prevention of new HIV infections through sexual exposure, injecting drug use, blood supply and organ donations, and perinatal exposure
- Assistance to scientists and researchers through enrollment in experimental protocols, through tracking of the natural history of HIV infection and disease, and through establishment of the incidence and prevalence of infection
- Assistance to health providers and planners in designing programs to meet the HIV-related needs of the community and to provide treatment and services
- Decrease of the economic costs to society of HIV disease

There are also risks and harm associated with HIV antibody testing programs. Persons with seronegative test results may have had a false-negative result, fostering a false sense of security, high-risk behaviors, and infection of others. Symptom-free persons with seropositive test results may have the following problems:

- Possibility of false-positive test results accompanied by psychologic trauma
- Discrimination and ostracism by health care professionals, resulting in medically inappropriate procedures
- Severe psychologic reactions, including anxiety, depression, sleep disturbances, and suicidal behavior
- Disrupted interpersonal relationships
- Sexual dysfunction
- Preoccupation with physical symptoms
- Stigmatization and ostracism by society
- Discrimination in housing and employment
- Loss of insurance
- Exposure to hatred and violence

The potential harm of HIV testing far exceeds that of any other laboratory clinical test. Therefore in any HIV antibody testing program every effort must be made to maximize the benefits and minimize the harm to persons tested. These goals can be achieved best through a comprehensive pretest and posttest counseling program.

PRETEST COUNSELING. A comprehensive pretest counseling program that meets standards of care in both completeness and consistency has several essential elements (AHCPR, January 1994; CDC, January 15, 1993a; CDC, March 10, 1995; CDC, July 7, 1995). The pretest counseling program should be extremely comprehensive, both to maximize its benefits and because posttest counseling often occurs in a situation of such relief or anxiety that concentration is compromised. HIV counseling should be culturally competent, sensitive to issues of sexual identity, developmentally appropriate, and linguistically relevant (CDC, January 15, 1993a; Irwin et al., 1996; Valdiserri et al., 1993). The essential elements of a comprehensive pretest counseling program include the following:

- A personalized client risk assessment
- Analysis of reasons for seeking testing and assessment of risk behaviors
- Review of test procedures
- Review of what both positive and negative test results mean and do not mean
- Review of possibility of false-negative and false-positive results
- Review of agency's policy for protecting confidentiality
- General information on the virus and AIDS
- A personalized risk-reduction plan that will include the following as necessary:
  - Advice on safer sexual practices, abstinence, and safer drug use
  - Information on drug treatment programs
  - Provision of condoms and bleach
  - Information on pregnancy, breast-feeding, and immunizations for infants
  - General health information on diet, rest, exercise, alcohol and tobacco use, and avoidance of infections (e.g., TB, STDs, and soft tissue infections)
  - Review of potential psychologic and emotional reactions to test results

– Review of potential interpersonal and societal reactions to test results
– Information on alternative testing sites for partners
– Information on medical, social, and psychiatric resources and follow-up counseling
– Review of the risks and benefits of testing
– Emphasis on the personal benefits of returning to obtain test results

When the pretest counseling session is completed, the counselor should obtain a written informed consent for testing.

POSTTEST COUNSELING. As noted earlier, often when the HIV antibody test results are disclosed, the person may be distracted by feelings of relief or anxiety. Therefore a comprehensive approach should be taken during pretest counseling. However, some elements of posttest counseling are essential. These should be both discussed with the person and given in a written format so that he or she can review them later. For persons with seronegative test results, posttest counseling includes the following:

• Interpretation of the test results
• Advice on HIV retesting after 3 months if the person engages in high-risk behaviors
• Information on safer sex and drug use practices
• Provision of condoms and bleach if desired
• Information on needle-exchange programs where available
• Information on how to maintain a negative status
• General information on healthy lifestyle practices
• Information on alternative test sites or home testing for partners
• Referral for psychologic, social, medical, and psychiatric services and drug rehabilitation programs as needed
• Follow-up for retesting of persons engaging in high-risk behaviors
• An assessment of whether further posttest counseling is needed

For symptom-free persons with seropositive test results, posttest counseling includes the following:

• Reconfirmation of test results on a second serum specimen in a reference laboratory
• Interpretation of the results (including the information that the person does not have AIDS)
• Evaluation of suicide potential
• Crisis intervention counseling as needed
• Information on alternative test sites or home testing for partners
• Discussion of follow-up for partners and children
• Referral to a partner-notification program if needed
• Information on transmission, safer sex and drug use practices, and reinfection
• Information on pregnancy and perinatal transmission
• Information on tuberculosis and TB screening
• Information on symptoms associated with the spectrum of HIV disease
• Referral to an early-intervention program that includes attention to lifestyle practices that may suppress the immune system and activate the disease
• Referral to the appropriate support group(s)
• Referral for medical follow-up, including TB screening
• Referral to drug rehabilitation program(s) as needed
• Referral to clinical trials or experimental protocols and information on the personal benefits of these programs
• Referral for psychologic, social, and psychiatric services as needed
• Discussion of potential discrimination and effects on housing, employment, insurance, and so forth
• Assessment of whether further posttest counseling is needed

Symptom-free infected persons will benefit from a full range of health and human services during the course of their HIV disease. At the time of immediate posttest counseling, they may be extremely anxious and unable to absorb the information presented. They should be given written information as well and encouraged to return for additional counseling. Such persons need continual reassurance and support and access to consistent health care. That health care should promote clients' concern for their condition and encourage monitoring and prevention, but it should avoid an excessive approach that can lead to undue anxiety. One of the most useful forms of support is an ongoing involvement with groups or individuals who share the person's situation and concerns. The overall goals of a comprehensive program for HIV-infected persons with no symptoms are to assist them to (1) manage their psychologic reactions, (2) manage information and resources, and (3) develop a personal health and medical care plan.

The same guidelines and procedures may be used for pretest and posttest counseling for HIV-2 and human T-lymphotropic viruses I and II (CDC, June 25, 1993; Levy, 1996). Transmission of these viruses is similar, although perhaps not as efficient (Mann & Tarantola, 1996, p. 10). Health maintenance and monitoring guidelines are likewise very similar.

Health Education and Maintenance

Primary health maintenance involves taking a comprehensive health history and making a physical and psychosocial assessment. Taking of a health history and physical assessment are covered in depth in Chapter 5 and Appendix I. Psychosocial, psychiatric, and neuropsychologic assessment are discussed in Chapter 7. Secondary health education and maintenance begins when HIV seropositivity has been established and the client enters the longest period of HIV disease, known as the asymptomatic stage. This stage may last for 10 or more years and is thought to be enhanced and possibly extended by health promotion activities and behaviors that increase immunocompetence. Persons who have HIV antibody and are free of symptoms can engage in a number of activities that may slow or prevent progression to clinical disease. These activities center on minimizing or eliminating the effects of both infectious processes and noninfectious conditions and may be broadly categorized as health education and health maintenance activities.

HEALTH EDUCATION. All persons who are infected with HIV need information on the meaning of infection. Secondary health education should include the person's sexual partner and family whenever possible. Persons with HIV infection should not assume that they will or will not develop clinical disease and should take all precautions possible to extend life. However, they should be informed that they are probably infected for life and probably contagious for life. This information means that they should not engage in unsafe sexual practices or needle sharing; nor should they donate blood, plasma, body organs, or other tissue. In addition, they should be told that anything that may be contaminated by their blood, semen, or vaginal fluid may constitute a risk of infection. For example, toothbrushes and razors should not be shared. Tampons and other blood-contaminated articles should be double bagged in plastic bags and marked as contaminated, and any needles or sharp objects used in treatment should be disposed of in a rigid container. Persons with HIV can thus help to prevent the spread of HIV to noninfected persons. On the other hand, sharing food and toilet facilities, sneezing and coughing, and expressing affection in a casual manner will not transmit HIV.

It is important that persons with HIV not engage in unsafe sexual practices or share needles with other seropositive persons. Repeated exposures to the virus may involve more virulent strains and may increase the likelihood of progression to AIDS (Leiphart, 1997; Levy, 1996; Royce et al., 1997). Unsafe (unprotected) anal sexual practices also expose the person to allogeneic sperm and semen. Repeated exposure to sperm and semen through the rectum can have immunosuppressant effects that HIV-infected persons need to avoid.

Health education must be directed also at prevention of infections other than HIV. Many of the infectious diseases that facilitate HIV disease can be prevented by the same changes in sexual practices that could prevent HIV infection: avoidance of anal intercourse and multiple, concurrent sexual partners. These practices are associated not only with HIV infection but also with other STDs that present a health threat: HBV, CMV, HPV, and HSV infections, amebiasis, syphilis, and gonorrhea (CDC, July 1997; Rochon, 1997). Whether through the ability of immunosuppression to provide opportunity for activation of HIV, or through actual activation of cells carrying HIV, coincident chronic infections have significant effects on the immune system and on the progression of HIV infection. Avoiding concurrent STDs should be a principal focus of any health education program (CDC, July 1997). Short of abstinence, condoms should be used, at a minimum, for all insertive sexual practices to reduce the risk of infection.

Injecting drug users can eliminate or significantly reduce the risks of concurrent infections by stopping the use of intravenous drugs, using disinfected needles and syringes, stopping needle and equipment sharing, decreasing the number of injections, and avoiding the use of shooting galleries for injection. All of these practices, uncorrected, result not only in HIV infection but also in other infections among IDUs. Chief among these infections are frequent and chronic soft tissue infections (cellulitis, abscesses), bacterial endocarditis, and the viral hepatitides. In addition, injecting drug users may be infected with all the STDs described previously. These chronic multiple infections can play a role as facilitators in the progression of disease in HIV-infected persons (CDC, July 1997). The focus of health education for drug users should be on stopping the use of drugs, stopping the sharing of dirty needles and syringes, and encouraging safer sex (use of condoms, cessation of anal receptive intercourse, and reduction in number of sexual partners).

Other strategies for prevention of infection revolve around controlling exposure to pathogens that naturally exist in such things as soil, pets, other humans, and food. Food safety may be maintained by keeping foods at the proper temperature (cold or hot); cooking them properly; washing foods, food preparation areas, and utensils thoroughly; and avoiding contamination of foods with one another (Meer, 1994). Finally, good hygiene practices and maintenance of skin integrity are barriers to infection. These strategies are addressed also in Chapter 6.

HEALTH MAINTENANCE. A health maintenance program involves symptom surveillance, treatment, hygiene, nutrition, stress reduction, and involvement in supportive interpersonal relationships, in work, in spiritual activities, and in volunteerism (Baigis-Smith et al., 1995; Leiphart, 1997; Mota, 1996; Sowell et al., 1997). Through lifestyle changes, persons with HIV infection can also minimize or eliminate immunosuppressive factors and emphasize factors that promote immune function. First, regular medical and psychiatric evaluations and follow-up are advised for HIV-infected persons. (Monitoring of health status requires an initial evaluation to establish baseline findings.) Secondary health maintenance involves prophylaxis and treatments to prevent disease progression (addressed in depth in Chapters 5 and 6). Finally, health maintenance efforts include proper nutrition, elimination of recreational drug and alcohol use, stress management, and careful consideration of future pregnancy, all of which may be influential in affecting the rate of disease progression (Leiphart, 1997). Secondary health maintenance should be directed at lifestyle changes in these areas.

Nutrition was discussed earlier in this chapter in the section on health promotion. In addition to the health-promoting activities described there, persons in the asymptomatic stage of HIV disease should focus on maintaining their weight and increasing calorie and protein intake as necessary. High-calorie, high-protein foods are from the protein, dairy, starch and grain, and fat food groups. Using food supplements and eating between meals are strategies for increasing intake. Evidence that nutrition plays a role in enhancing immunocompetence in persons with HIV comes from a prospective study of dietary intake in HIV seropositive homosexual men (Abrams, 1997). In this study, dietary intake affected CD4+ cell count and HIV symptom variables. Furthermore, the use of micronutrients (vitamin A, B_1, C, and niacin) may slow the onset of AIDS (Aron, 1994; Casey, 1997; Coodley et al., 1994; Elion, 1997; Semba et al., 1995).

Assisting persons with HIV to limit or give up the use of alcohol, recreational drugs, and tobacco is also part of secondary health maintenance. These substances reduce immunocompetence (Caetano & Hines, 1995; Casey, 1997). Limiting or removing their use may slow or prevent disease progression in HIV-infected persons. Programs such as Alcoholics Anonymous, smoking cessation, and drug rehabilitation may be indicated.

Women who are infected with HIV must be informed of the effects of pregnancy on the progression of disease. Pregnancy itself has a small immunosuppressant effect. There is conflicting evidence about whether pregnancy accelerates the pace of disease expression. However, seropositive women should be cautioned about the risks of pregnancy. Other information that women need to know about pregnancy and AIDS is that more than 90% of pediatric AIDS is attributed to maternal transmission, that they do not need to be sick to pass HIV to the fetus, that there are ways to reduce the risk of the fetus's becoming infected if the mother is infected, and that the virus may be contracted through breast milk. Women also need information on the use of zidovudine and HIV immunoglobulin during pregnancy. Counseling on birth control, pregnancy, enrolling in clinical trials, abortion, and breast-feeding should be part of any health maintenance program for women.

Stress reduction programs may be useful also in secondary health maintenance. They contribute to quality of life and may also contribute to immunocompetence. Information on stress reduction was given in the section on health promotion. In addition to regular exercise, rest, and sleep, personal use of relaxation techniques may be of help to some persons. Avenues for expression of emotion can be obtained through friends and family, social support groups, and professional counseling. Involvement in work, spiritual activities, and volunteerism all have been found to enhance quality of life (Gaskins & Brown, 1997; Mota, 1996; Sowell et al., 1997).

Two current ongoing programs that have been developed to boost immunity serve as examples (Leiphart, 1997). A look at each of these programs summarizes the health maintenance activities described in this section. In San Diego, California, the L.I.F.E. Program (Learning Immune Function Enhancement) teaches seropositive participants over a 1-year period of self-management of 19 immune factors. These are fatalism, impatience, survival-related stress, grief and loss, depression, life purpose and goals, self-assertiveness, trust and support, crisis management, breathing patterns, water, diet and nutrition, sleep, substance use, exercise, hygiene, exposure to infection, reexposure to HIV, health knowledge, and medical care. Each participant receives peer support and individualized immune factor counseling. Persons completing the program improve their quality of life and decrease the number of HIV symptoms (Leiphart, 1997).

At the Harvard Medical School, the Mind/Body/Spirit Program for HIV/AIDS is a 10-week program for seropositive persons designed to boost their immunity. Activities focused on are stress reduction; commitment, control, life goals and volunteerism; cognitive restructuring; physical exercise with yoga; nutrition; emotional expression via writing; exploring spirituality and hope; and humor and laughter. Clients completing the program experience reduction in psychologic and physical symptoms (Leiphart, 1997). Finally, Lands (1996) summarizes similar activities in her 10 commandments of living with HIV, which emphasize diet, nutrition, micronutrients, disease management, avoiding infections, taking antiviral medication, exercise, and mental attitude.

Symptomatic HIV Disease

During the symptomatic stage of HIV disease, the person has various kinds of opportunistic infections and malignancies. They may also experience weakness, fatigue, pain, weight loss, and wasting. Chronic diarrhea may be a particular problem, causing a deterioration in social activity, work, daily living, energy, and cognition (Jones, 1997). Clinical manifestations of HIV and AIDS are discussed comprehensively in Chapters 5 and 6. The primary care management of the symptomatic stage of HIV disease is discussed in Chapter 6 and focuses on symptoms and human responses to HIV illness. At this stage, infections generally respond to medical treatment. Symptom control is a major goal of primary health care.

Secondary health maintenance behaviors and activities discussed in the previous section are also applicable here. Enhancing immunocompetence to prevent infections is still the focus of care for the person with HIV, whether provided by self and family or by health care providers. In addition to the information already provided, further information on nutrition is given here. Common problems related to nutrition in symptomatic-stage HIV infection may be lack of appetite; mouth sores and problems in swallowing; taste changes; bloating, fullness, and heartburn; nausea and diarrhea; and weight loss (Casey, 1997).

The latter course of HIV disease is most frequently influenced by malnutrition and wasting (2nd International Conference on Nutrition and HIV, 1997; Jones, 1997). Wasting syndrome, cachexia, loss of lean body mass, and decrease in body cell mass are associated with inadequate nutrition, altered metabolism, opportunistic infections, and poor patient outcomes. Several therapies are in use to reverse or alter the progressive weight loss associated with AIDS. These include many complementary medicine approaches and alternative therapies (Abrams, 1997; Elion, 1997; Nemechek et al., 1997). Several that are being tested are anabolic steroids, and human growth hormone to maintain or build body mass (Abrams, 1997; Mascolini, 1996; Nemechek et al., 1997). Use of these therapies with concomitant antiretroviral therapy and dietary evaluation and supplementation has allowed persons with AIDS to reestablish nutritional stores. Appetite stimulants have been used also, including marijuana and dronabinol. Because of FDA regulation, clinical trials comparing the two have not been conducted (Abrams, 1997; Corless & Miramontes, 1997). Dronabinol as a treatment for anorexia has been tested, with an increase in appetite and a decrease in nausea over a control group receiving placebos (Beal et al., 1995).

When diarrhea is a problem, replacement therapy, antidiarrheal agents, diet modification, or bowel rest may be indicated (Jones, 1997). If oral intake is limited, tube feeding may provide nutrients if the gastrointestinal system is functioning. If the person has severely compromised bowel function and if oral or gastrointestinal tube feedings are inadequate or contraindicated, a short course of either peripheral parenteral nutrition or total parenteral nutrition might be considered (Jones, 1997; Thomson, 1994). Recent evidence, however, suggests that the use of parenteral feedings should be reserved for persons who meet objective criteria for protein-calorie malnutrition and that the use of lipid emulsions (e.g., soybean oil) may increase the risk of infectious complications and have a negative effect on immunity (Phinney et al., 1996).

Chapters 5, 6, and 11 address in detail the health care needs of persons with HIV disease. These chapters include complete information on nutrition as well as on alternative therapies.

Late HIV Disease

In the late stage of HIV disease, immune functioning is severely compromised and pharmacologic treatments have little effect. Palliation and quality of life become the major goals of care. Management of pain, skin care, mouth care, provision of fluids and oxygen, and positioning take precedence in making clients comfortable. Spiri-

tual care and psychosocial care are important for clients, partners, and family. These aspects of care are addressed in depth in Chapter 7. They are considered the final stage of a health promotion and disease-prevention approach on an individual and family level.

COMMUNITY EFFORTS

Health promotion and disease prevention also occur at the community level. Community interventions are discussed next, with an emphasis on environmental factors that facilitate HIV disease, various human groups affected by HIV, strategies for successful community programs, and existing community resources.

Environmental factors that facilitate HIV transmission tend to cluster in different human groups, producing social groups more or less at risk of acquiring infection. The social, economic and political milieu places some groups at greater risk than others for HIV infection and accelerated disease progression (Fahs et al, 1994; Hamburg, 1996; Hu et al., 1995; Royce et al., 1997). Poverty is probably the best environmental predictor of infection and disease progression (Fahs et al., 1994; Hamburg, 1996). As the AIDS epidemic matures, it becomes compellingly clear that HIV affects populations that are denied human rights—those that are marginalized, stigmatized, and discriminated against (Mann & Tarantola, 1996, pp. 463-476). In the United States the epidemic has turned toward populations at risk or vulnerable populations. Vulnerable populations include women, children, people of color, men who have sex with men, sex workers, IDUs, and others denied human rights (Merson, 1996). Community-based programs have emerged to reduce HIV transmission, and some of these are targeted to the vulnerable populations noted here. These programs are discussed under the exposure categories of sexual practices and injecting drug use.

Changes in Sexual Practices

For more than a decade public health resources and services and community-based programs have been involved in educating the public about HIV disease and how to prevent its transmission. These programmatic efforts are necessary and impressive. They are, however, focused on changing individual behavior within a societal context that has not changed. The long-term effect on behavior change has been disappointing. Epidemiologic reports from various geographic areas in the United States provide evidence of the effectiveness of these efforts. Changes in sexual practices appear to be greatest in white men who have sex with men (MSM) and identify themselves as homosexuals (CDC, June 2, 1995). African-American and Latino MSM and those who do not identify themselves as homosexual have not experienced the same changes (Denning et al., 1996). Less change in sexual behavior is observed in adolescents, heterosexual men, and women (Choi & Catania, 1996; Denning & Fleming, 1997). Finally, among ethnic groups, African-Americans and Latinos have experienced less change (CDC, November 18, 1994, Singleton et al., 1996; Torian et al., 1996). A study in California and another in New York City illustrate the trends in sexual behavior (Singleton et al., 1996; Torian et al., 1996), as do the results of two national surveys (Choi & Catania, 1996).

The AIDS epidemic in California plateaued in 1992. Cases declined in Los Angeles and San Francisco counties and increased in the rest of the state. The decline was the result of a decrease in cases among white MSM. Women, African-Americans, and Latinos (male-to-male, male-to-female, and female-to-male contact) all experienced an increase in AIDS incidence (CDC, November 18, 1994). In addition, cases of AIDS increased in the group aged 13 to 19 years (Singleton et al., 1996). A study of MSM in New York City showed that AIDS case rates have flattened in white MSM but that case rates continue to rise in African-American and Latino MSM (Torian et al., 1996). In two national surveys, heterosexual risk behaviors through sexual exposure were assessed (Choi & Catania, 1996). The overall HIV risk levels of U.S. heterosexuals remained unchanged over time, with similar proportions of persons reporting multiple sexual partners and a risky partner. There was also no change in HIV testing behavior. There was an increase in condom use among persons with less than a high school education who reported sex with a risky partner. However, there was a substantial increase in the number of risky sexual partners in these groups (Choi & Catania, 1996).

Despite the population-based changes noted

in white MSM, risk behaviors in MSM as an aggregate have not changed substantially. Among young gay men there has been an increase in risky sexual behaviors (Denning & Fleming, 1997; Hays et al., 1997; Hickson et al., 1996; *Los Angeles Times,* September 3, 1995). Risk behaviors associated with anal penetrative sex, multiple partners, and lack of condom use have remained constant (Hickson et al., 1996). The high number of newly infected homosexual and bisexual men has led to a call for additional intervention initiatives (*Los Angeles Times,* September 3, 1995). Among MSM who do not self-identify as homosexual or who do not disclose their homosexuality or bisexuality, unprotected anal intercourse continues at high rates and the use of condoms is infrequent and inconsistent (CDC, January 15, 1993b; Heckman et al., 1995; *Los Angeles Times,* September 3, 1995). Ethnic identity is associated with increased risk of HIV infection among MSM, with the highest rates among African-American and Latino men (CDC, 1997; Denning et al., 1996). African-American MSM also had a substantially higher prevalence of unprotected anal intercourse than white MSM in San Francisco (Peterson et al., 1996).

Changes in sexual practices among heterosexuals have not been observed. Even among heterosexual couples who were aware of a partner's seropositive status, use of condoms was not consistent (Wells & Mayer, 1997). The lack of safer sexual practices is particularly notable in young and adolescent heterosexuals, among whom sexual activity has been steadily increasing since the 1970s (CDC, September 27, 1996a; Denning & Fleming, 1997; Hein, 1993). Among heterosexuals, women are more likely than men to continue unsafe sexual practices (CDC, May 28, 1993; Sikkema et al., 1996; Wells & Mayer, 1997). This behavior may be due to women not knowing the risk behaviors of their partners. In two studies, however, personal perception of risk, involvement with multiple sexual partners, and infection with an STD did not motivate women to adopt low-risk behaviors (Erickson, 1997; CDC, September 27, 1996b). In some studies, unsafe sexual practices were greater among ethnic women of color than among white women (CDC, September 27, 1996a; Turner & Solomon, 1996).

Among persons who identified multiple, concurrent sexual partners as a major risk factor, men, regardless of sexual orientation, were more likely to use condoms than women (CDC, May 28, 1993; CDC, September 27, 1996b). Furthermore, among persons whose sexual contacts were both paying and nonpaying partners, the use of condoms was more frequent with paying partners (McKirnan et al., 1995; Montoya & Atkinson, 1996). Although there have been some positive changes overall in sexual behavior, it is apparent that for many groups risk practices have not decreased in response to public health campaigns and programs and that there are many and varying subepidemics of HIV regionally.

Changes in Injecting Drug Use Practices

For IDUs also, there has been a barrage of information on prevention, the use of bleach, distribution of condoms, and free needle and syringe exchange programs. Despite these efforts, there has been a continued rise in the number of HIV-seroprevalent persons whose risk behavior is injecting drug use (CDC, June 30, 1997; Gostin et al., 1997). Sharing of needles is associated with use of shooting galleries and injection in semipublic places, reported as high-risk behaviors for HIV exposure (Latkin et al., 1996; Montoya & Atkinson, 1996). Several studies have found that IDUs have modified their needle use behaviors in response to programs for needle and syringe exchange and for use of bleach and condoms. However, sharing of needles has been reported as more prevalent among women than among men (Neaigus et al., 1994). Women inject drugs more frequently with a partner than do men, and sharing tends to go on in this situation and role relationship and in social networks to which the woman belongs (Amaro, 1995; Latkin et al., 1996; Neiagus et al., 1994).

Complicating injecting drug use practices are the sexual behaviors of IDUs. It is frequently impossible to know whether exposure to HIV is occurring because of injecting drug use or because of sexual practices (Rietmeijer et al., 1996). For example, the severity of heroin dependence was found to be related to unprotected sexual activity with multiple partners, often for money or drugs (Turner & Solomon, 1996). Crack cocaine use also has been related to high-risk sexual activities (Montoya & Atkinson, 1996). Finally, intravenous drug use was significantly associated with sexual risk taking, with women more likely than men to have an IDU as a sexual partner (Turner

& Solomon, 1996). There is evidence that changing the sexual behavior of IDUs is much more difficult than changing drug-injection risk behaviors (CDC, February 23, 1996; Des Jarlais & Friedman, 1996). It becomes apparent from these reports that it is extremely difficult to separate the risks of exposure because of drug use from those of drug-related sex practices.

Needle and syringe exchange programs and needle-disinfection programs have been supported and implemented to decrease the risk of transmission among IDUs. It seems clear that these programs have caused a change in needle and syringe use behavior, with increased use of sterile needles and syringes and of bleach to clean needles and syringes (Des Jarlais et al., 1996; Rietmeijer et al., 1996). It is far from certain that changing needle and syringe use will decrease transmission of HIV in IDUs. Changes in sexual behavior may be a more overriding concern (CDC, February 23, 1996; Des Jarlais & Friedman, 1996).

Components of Successful Community Intervention

Several community-based intervention models and strategies for change in sexual and drug use behavior have been implemented and evaluated. Some of these have been successful and have identified common and unique characteristics that may provide guidelines for future community prevention efforts. The Centers for Disease Control and Prevention (May 10, 1996) implemented the AIDS Community Demonstration Projects in Dallas, Denver, Long Beach, California, New York City, and Seattle. These projects were based on risk reduction incorporating elements of three social-behavioral models and the Transtheoretical Model of Change. A comprehensive community-level intervention was designed and implemented. On the basis of experience with this intervention, the CDC made six recommendations for community-level prevention programs:

1. Before implementing an intervention, health departments and other agencies should develop a thorough understanding of the target population.
2. Concepts from social-behavioral theories and models should be used to develop and guide prevention and risk-reduction activities.

3. An intervention protocol should be designed to allow for adaptation to different populations and communities.
4. Ongoing qualitative research should be used to ensure that the intervention responds to changes in the community.
5. Persons within the communities to be served should be recruited to deliver intervention messages.
6. Community-level HIV prevention interventions should be used to reach less accessible populations at risk of HIV infection.

In all the city sites there were changes in behavior on four outcomes measures: in condom use for vaginal intercourse with a primary and nonprimary partner, in condom use for anal intercourse with nonprimary partner, and in consistent use of bleach to clean injection equipment (CDC, May 10, 1996). In a separate report the CDC (May 2, 1997) discussed changes among low-income men in five cities in condom use to prevent HIV and other STDs while maintaining their contraceptive methods to protect against pregnancy.

The CDC has recommended also HIV-prevention case management to prevent transmission of HIV when one partner is infected (CDC, June 18, 1993). On the basis of the experiences of community health centers in Miami, New York City, and Newark, New Jersey, the CDC reported changes in risk behaviors related to case-managed care. The essential features of this care were a one-on-one client service associated with ongoing medical preventive care for an extended period. Case-managed care was designed around HIV testing and counseling, risk-reduction counseling, and a care plan for medical and psychosocial services. Although the study employed no comparison group, the participants reported reduced sexual risk behaviors (CDC, June 18, 1993). In a study on syringe-exchange programs (SEP) in the United States, the CDC reported that SEP use improved threefold in the United States since the programs were implemented and were effective in reducing viral infections among IDUs in selected study site cities. Included in the syringe-exchange programs were provision of alcohol swabs, latex condoms, counseling services, and assistance in obtaining health and social services (CDC, September 22, 1995). Finally, in a community-based HIV-prevention program in Colorado with homeless, chemically dependent, and mentally ill participants, the CDC reported that high proportions were involved in HIV high-risk behaviors and in previous HIV testing and were willing to use outreach services. Community organizations that provided medical and social services were in closest contact with these persons (CDC, February 21, 1997).

The San Francisco model for changing high-risk sexual behavior among chiefly white gay and bisexual men was expanded in 1994 to other ethnic, gender, age, language, and drug-use groups. Several reports of program success have been attributed to the design and implementation of this multifaceted community program (Dearing et al., 1996; Meyer & Dearing, 1996; Rogers et al., 1995). These programs were built on the same principles of community-level intervention derived from cardiovascular disease risk-reduction programs, smoking-cessation programs, and family-planning interventions to reduce adolescent pregnancy. These programs incorporated information, motivation, skills training, existing community structures and social networks, attention to normative behaviors, and methods of diffusing information. These programs used peer educators; they were approached as long-term efforts with multiple and repeated strategies to initiate and sustain ongoing change; they incorporated a comprehensive range of services (medical, psychosocial, and so forth); and they used a field experimental design to evaluate their effectiveness. The most effective aspect of these programs was the use of community peer educators in the design, implementation, and evaluation of the programs. An added benefit in San Francisco was a dramatically altered sense of community.

In a call for action for effective AIDS education for adolescents, Hein (1993) emphasized some of these same principles: peer education, realistic behavior change expectations, normative and explicit risk-reduction messages, joining of HIV prevention with HIV services, and joining of HIV programs with existing community agencies serving youth. Intervention for HIV prevention with inner-city adolescent and young adult women in Boston compared a peer educator–delivered intervention with a provider-delivered intervention (Quirk et al., 1993). The study took place in a community family health center. Both interventions significantly affected knowledge, attitudes, and sexual behaviors (reduced vaginal intercourse, increased skills in discussing sexual behavior with a partner). Peer education achieved greater knowledge of injecting drug use, and provider education achieved greater knowledge of sexual risks. In a nationwide survey of high school students, 86.3% had been taught about HIV in school and, as a consequence, two thirds had talked with parents about HIV/AIDS (CDC, September 27, 1996a). Female students were more likely than male students to talk with a parent, and black students were more likely than white or Latino students to talk with a parent.

An already existing community agency to which women were attracted for food coupons was used to deliver an HIV prevention intervention for low-income Latina (Mexican and Central American) women in Los Angeles (Flaskerud et al., 1997). Women attending the Public Health Foundation's Nutrition Program for Women, Infants, and Children (WIC) in an inner-city neighborhood were given free HIV antibody testing and counseling and 1 year of follow-up care. The program consisted of counseling before and after HIV testing, counseling in risk reduction and health promotion, skill development in condom use and in negotiating with a partner, free condoms as often as desired, and referral and advocacy for medical, psychosocial, financial, legal, and social services. The intervention was based on a conceptual model of illness, prevention, and treatment that was specific to the cultural beliefs of the subjects (Flaskerud & Calvillo, 1991a). A one-on-one intervention was delivered by peer educators who shared the ethnicity, language, and gender of the participants. Snacks and child care were provided during visits. Three visits during the 1-year period were required. Additional visits for condoms and additional counseling were encouraged. The program employed a study group and a comparison group who did not receive the intervention. Significant changes occurred in knowledge of HIV transmission, in sexual behavior, and in condom use. These changes did not occur in the comparison group. No HIV seroconversions occurred during the follow-up period. Eighty-five percent of the women came for more than the required three visits to obtain additional condoms and medical and human services referral and advocacy. However, there were

problems associated with the intervention protocol that did not facilitate the transfer of information to use of needles for home medication (Flaskerud & Nyamathi, 1996). In addition, the main reason for using condoms was to prevent pregnancy (Flaskerud et al., 1996).

In addition to community-based organizations (CBOs) that are formed within and are accountable to specific communities, many other groups outside government are involved in responding to HIV/AIDS and are referred to collectively as NGOs (nongovernmental organizations). There are examples of NGO involvement in every sector and country (O'Malley et al., 1996). Among the greatest strengths of NGOs are their roots in communities and their responses based on assessed needs, priorities, and the dynamics of local people. Most of the NGOs now involved in AIDS work are not AIDS-specific organizations but are oriented to broader and more comprehensive goals of health and development (O'Malley et al., 1996). Common approaches to AIDS prevention and health goals include peer education, involvement of the community to be served, use of existing social networks and community agencies, ability to speak the language of the community served and use of images common to its culture, provision of HIV prevention within a comprehensive program of primary and public health care, provision of long-term ongoing services, and use of the mass media to reinforce messages and create behavioral norms. NGOs also typically are involved in contextual (societal) factors that increase suspectibility to HIV, such as gender inequality, discrimination, and racism (O'Malley et al., 1996).

All successful intervention programs reviewed in this section have incorporated many and sometimes most of the common principles and components identified by these various groups and organizations and considered essential to behavior change and maintenance strategies. The cultural norms or beliefs of the community must frame the message. Finally, motivation through peer role models and others such as the participants who have been successful will encourage belief in personal capability and community-level change (Holtgrave et al., 1995).

Community Settings for HIV Prevention

Several existing community resources lend themselves to the prevention of HIV. Their relationship to known exposure routes of HIV, to factors facilitating HIV infection and disease expression, and to particular human groups recommends them for special consideration in community efforts to control HIV disease. Targeted interventions in conjunction with these existing resources may make a major difference where some others have so far failed. In designing community intervention programs in these settings, public health educators may take direction from the success of programs described in the preceding section.

SEXUALLY TRANSMITTED DISEASE CLINICS. The relationship between HIV and other STDs is highly dynamic and synergistic (AHCPR, January 1994; CDC, May 21, 1997). Persons who have a history of STDs are at increased risk of acquiring HIV, and HIV-infected persons have an increased susceptibility to infection with other STDs. In persons with HIV who are coinfected with other STDs, these infections usually have severe and protracted courses. In addition, the STD may facilitate disease expression (AIDS) in persons with HIV (CDC, July 1997). Transmission is similar, and issues for STD prevention and control are applicable to the full range of infections, including HIV.

Locating education programs for HIV prevention in STD or STI (sexually transmitted infection) clinics makes use of the concept of *core groups* for preventive interventions. Core groups are defined as segments of the population who are (in this case) more likely than others to transmit infections sexually. The public health importance of this concept rests in its potential to permit targeting of limited resources to groups that are most susceptible to transmission. The concept of the core group suggests a focus for behavioral interventions in persons with risky sexual or drug use practices (CDC, July 1997; Katz & Gerberding, 1997; McKirnan et al., 1996). Comprehensive and well-integrated preventive services that address both HIV infection and other STDs may have a greater chance of success than separate programs. STD programs have a long history of control measures, treatment, follow-up and partner notification, and professional experience and expertise. The programs are an existing community resource, and they are used by sexually active persons who are engaged in risky sexual practices

(CDC, March 1, 1996; May 2, 1997). For many persons, such sexual practices are inextricably intermixed with drug use practices.

FAMILY PLANNING AND PERINATAL CLINICS. There is a dynamic interaction between HIV and various activities related to reproduction. Women of reproductive age and their infants may constitute another core group for programs of HIV infection prevention. Reproductive clinics provide opportunities to educate women about sexual transmission, in utero and intrapartal transmission, and breast-feeding. Furthermore, pregnancy itself may enhance disease expression (AIDS) in women who are infected with HIV. In addition to contraceptive services, prenatal and postnatal care, and infant care, family planning and perinatal clinics also might offer voluntary HIV testing and counseling, prevention education, health promotion teaching, and follow-up (AHCPR, January 1994; CDC, May 2, 1997; September 27, 1996b; Kelly et al., 1994; Lauver et al., 1995). These clinics constitute an existing community resource. The established history of such clinics, the professional experience and expertise that they embody, and their frequent use by women of reproductive age all recommend them for well-integrated preventive services that address both HIV infection and pregnancy. Family planning clinics also treat substantial numbers of women who are infected with STDs (CDC, September 27, 1996b; May 2, 1997). Another possible setting for reaching women of reproductive age is the abortion clinic. Prevention interventions for women differ substantially from those for men. Locating these interventions in clinics associated with reproduction will ensure that these programs are specific to women and teach prevention methods unique to women (Landers & Shannon, 1997; Lauver et al., 1995; Newman & Wofsy, 1997). Because reproductive clinics are often community based, it would be possible to design programs specific to the unique concerns of the population(s) served, such as teenagers and ethnic and cultural groups. As with the core groups who use STD clinics, women who use reproductive health clinics might be susceptible not only to sexual exposure but also to drug-use exposure or drug-related sexual exposure.

PROGRAMS RELATED TO DRUG (AND NEEDLE) USE. Injecting drug use and HIV infection have an obvious link because the injection provides a parenteral route for infection. The interaction between HIV infection and the use of noninjectable drugs may also have an effect on sexual transmission. Combining HIV prevention and education in conjunction with various programs related to drug use may provide another opportunity for reaching a core group of susceptible persons (Caetano & Hines, 1995; CDC, February, 23, 1996; Erickson, 1997; McKirnan et al., 1996; Swan, 1995). Drug and alcohol rehabilitation programs provide one such existing community resource that may be used for HIV prevention. Once again, professional experience and expertise and a history of working with drug users on a continuous, long-term basis recommend these programs for combination preventive strategies. Methadone programs provide the potential for reaching heroin IDUs. Oral opiate substitution programs can also be effective in reducing the risk of acquiring HIV infection. Needle and syringe exchange centers or pharmacies also offer the opportunity for education on HIV prevention and transmission. In all these existing community facilities, the risk of transmission through sexual practices needs equal emphasis with the risk of transmission through injection or the parenteral route (CDC, February 23, 1996; Des Jarlais & Friedman, 1996).

Despite the potential represented by these existing community resources, a tremendous amount of information must still be learned about addiction itself, needle-sharing practices, gender-specific risks, and sexual behavior of drug users. With this gap in understanding, prevention efforts currently focus on reduction of risk and reduction of harm (i.e., through the use of clean needles). Harm-reduction messages have had success, but more must be done about the social roots of drug use to stop the spread of HIV in drug users through injection or sexual exposure.

IN-SCHOOL PROGRAMS. Children and adolescents who attend school can be targeted for health education and disease-prevention programs that include prevention of HIV infection. To meet the needs of students and their communities, HIV-prevention programs in schools should be integrated into a comprehensive health promotion approach that begins in elementary school (CDC, September 27, 1996a). The CDC has initiated youth risk behavior surveys to help monitor and evaluate changes in behavior related to comprehensive school health programs. Among children and adolescents, health promotion and counseling must focus on the prevalence of behaviors that lead to intentional and unintentional injuries, tobacco use, alcohol and other drug use, sexual behaviors, dietary behaviors, and physical activity (CDC, September 27, 1996a).

For students who are engaged already in unsafe behaviors, schools may plan and implement HIV-prevention programs that meet local standards. These programs are usually designed to help students stop risky behaviors or teach them methods to reduce risk. In some instances, local areas have permitted the distribution of condoms and bleach. According to one leading clinician-researcher-educator who works with adolescents, HIV education in schools must be joined with on-site condom availability (Hein, 1993). A national survey by the CDC in 1995 showed that 53% of U.S. teenagers engaged in sexual intercourse, 18% of them with four or more partners. Among sexually active students, 54.4% used condoms (CDC, September 27, 1996a). Overall, black students (73.4%) were more likely to have had sexual intercourse than white (48.9%) and Hispanic (57.6%) students. This was true for both males and females. An alarming report issued by the CDC (August 13, 1993) noted that during the period from 1981 through 1991, 24% to 30% of the reported morbidity from gonorrhea and 10% to 12% of the reported morbidity from syphilis in the United States were in adolescent age groups. Prevalence was higher in the South and in African-American youth.

According to the Youth Risk Behavior Surveillance survey (CDC, September 27, 1996a), drug use among students in grades 9 to 12 varied widely, depending on the substance used. Nationwide, 71% of students had tried cigarettes, 11% smokeless tobacco, 80% alcohol, 42% marijuana, 7% cocaine, 3.7% steroids, 2% injectable drugs, 16% other illegal drugs, and 20% inhalants (CDC, September 27, 1996a).

Other aspects of in-school programs related to HIV specifically and to healthy attitudes and behaviors in general (e.g., dietary behaviors, physical activity) are coordination of in-school programs with a variety of community health services and health professionals. In-school programs should also help teachers, parents, and students understand HIV disease and deal compassionately with students who are infected.

OTHER COMMUNITY SETTINGS. Selection of community settings for HIV education, prevention, and treatment that already are in existence and are providing health and human services makes sense for several reasons. These settings are known to the community and are being used by community members. Recruitment of core group members is not a problem. Professionals working in these settings have experience and expertise in specific areas that involve the behaviors of their core group. The structure for administering and delivering services is in place. If these existing agencies would incorporate the new strategies gained in field experiments of community HIV-prevention programs, they would offer advantages over other settings in the battle to prevent HIV infection.

Several in-place community settings come to mind other than those described here: WIC programs, Job Corps programs, and college campuses, to name a few. Community health workers are aware of many others that would be similarly well suited. However, a note of warning is necessary. The dramatic increase in the incidence and prevalence of HIV and its dynamic synergy with TB should alert health care workers who provide services to a variety of populations to test for both TB and HIV (Asch et al., 1997; CDC, January 19, 1996; Gelberg et al., 1997; Hopewell, 1997). These populations include immigrants, migrant workers, homeless, and institutionalized persons (e.g., elderly, prisoners, incarcerated youth, orphans, mentally ill). It is imperative that all community-based organizations begin testing for TB and HIV in their clients. Education for community health workers on the relationship between TB and HIV is needed as well as a strong commitment to infectious disease control. In-place community settings are the logical sites for providing both HIV and TB testing and treatment. These two diseases exemplify the concept of providing comprehensive care within a health setting that people are already using (McKirnan et al., 1996).

HIV RESEARCH IN HEALTH PROMOTION AND DISEASE PREVENTION

Summary of Research

For the purposes of this chapter, research on health promotion and disease prevention and harm reduction is considered behavioral (host-related) and environmental (social, political milieu) in that it focuses on behaviors of people and communities and on societal conditions that promote health, prevent disease, and enhance immunocompetence. Although biologic research (agent-related) may also include health promotion through the discovery of a vaccine or the roles of chemicals, micronutrients, and genetics and their effects on the virus or immune function, the area of research emphasized here focuses on behaviors involved with biologic processes, such as drinking, smoking, eating, and reproducing, and societal conditions that foster or impede such behaviors. To date, for example, behavioral research has explored the role of nutrition in the immunocompetence of persons with HIV, the role of stress management in the quality of life of PLWH, correlates of psychological inhibition and of stress in HIV disease, and the coping responses used by persons at risk of acquiring HIV infection (see, for instance, Burns et al., 1995; Cole & Kemeny, 1997; Elion, 1997; Keet et al., 1993; Kemeny & Dean, 1995). These areas of research lend themselves to health promotion questions and interventions and are being pursued all over the country. Several studies of health promotion, disease prevention, and harm reduction have direct applicability to HIV: predicting the health-promoting behaviors of gay men; changing codependent and health-promoting behaviors in families of substance abusers; reducing sexual transmission of STDs; and identifying condom-use control variables for women and their partners (see, for instance, Amaro, 1995; Erickson, 1997; Latkin et al., 1996; Neaigus et al., 1994; Peterson et al, 1996; Torian et al., 1996).

Environmental research has focused also on health promotion and health maintenance activities by and for persons with HIV infection, as they are affected by poverty, lack of health insurance, accessibility of health care, and use of health care services (see, for instance, Fahs et al., 1994; Fleishman et al., 1994; Gordon et al., 1996; Hu et al., 1995). Especially in the AIDS epicenters in the United States, these areas of research are of interest to health professionals because of their direct effects on and applicability to community health care. Furthermore, community-based HIV research has been involved with screening programs and designing and testing the effects of community-based AIDS-prevention programs on changes in knowledge and behaviors (see, for instance, CDC, May 10, 1996; Dearing et al.,

1996; Flaskerud et al., 1997; Meyer & Dearing, 1996) and with evaluating community-based case management of symptoms in PLWH. The research reviewed in this chapter has involved a wide range of subjects. Homosexual and bisexual men, women, children, and adolescents, ethnic people of color, homeless persons, low-income persons, injecting drug users and their partners, and others exemplify a range of study participants. The results of this research have made meaningful contributions to a science of health promotion and disease prevention for health-related disciplines.

Research Needed

Health promotion, disease prevention, and harm reduction are fruitful areas of research for health professionals because of the long-standing interest and support among community health care workers for preventive practice. Research that continues to be needed may be divided into four categories: (1) behavioral and environmental factors to prevent or reduce exposure, (2) behavioral and environmental factors to promote health, (3) behavioral and environmental factors to maintain health, and (4) community-based interventions to change knowledge, attitudes, and behaviors. On a societal level, health professionals can be involved in social and political change to reform health care in the United States and to decrease poverty, discrimination, and racism. Each of these areas may be further subdivided on the basis of the population(s) served. A summary of the research that is needed follows.

1. Research that describes, explains, and predicts behavioral conditions that facilitate exposure:
   a. Preventing or limiting risky sexual practices
   b. Preventing or decreasing risky drug use practices
   c. Preventing or reducing behaviors resulting from an interaction of drug use and sexual practices
   d. Preventing or limiting pregnancy, intrapartal infection, and transmission through breast-feeding
   e. Preventing inappropriate use of transfusions, tissue transplants, and unsafe donations
2. Research that describes, explains, and predicts factors related to health promotion:

   a. Effects of nutrition
   b. Effects of physical exercise, rest, and sleep
   c. Effects of stress management
3. Research that describes, explains, and predicts factors related to health maintenance in HIV-infected persons:
   a. Prevention of infections
   b. Effects of health promotion behaviors (listed above)
   c. Effects of treatment: physiologic, psychosocial, and neuropsychiatric
   d. Effects of comfort measures
   e. Effects of palliation
   f. Accessibility, availability, and responsiveness of health care services
   g. Promotion and maintenance of self-care activities
4. Research that describes, explains, and predicts successful community-level interventions:
   a. Essential elements of successful programs
   b. Strategies of successful programs with a wide variety of populations
   c. Effect of the use of in-place community settings for HIV prevention programs
   d. Field experiments testing the effectiveness of specific community programs on behavior change with particular populations

Community-based health professionals have a special interest in all these areas of research. They also are uniquely qualified because of their community practice to conduct research in these areas. Finally, research in these areas will help develop a science of health promotion, disease prevention, and harm reduction that will guide efforts at limiting the HIV epidemic and will be useful and generalizeable to future public health programs.

SUMMARY

Host, environmental, and agent-related factors all play a major role not only in exposure to HIV infection but also in disease expression and progression. Identifying the behavioral and environmental factors and making them a focus of public health education programs have been emphasized in this chapter and are crucial to HIV disease control. Health promotion, health education, harm reduction, and health maintenance programs can be designed to take into account host and environmental factors related to immunocompetence and immunosuppression. Changes in behaviors and in the social and political milieu have been demonstrated to improve health for everyone and at all stages of HIV infection.

Community health promotion and prevention programs have identified the essential components of successful intervention programs. However, these need further testing and evaluation. When validated, these components can be incorporated into the design of future programs. Placing these programs in community settings that are already providing services for similar behaviors may enhance their effect and appeal. Research in all areas of health promotion, disease prevention, and harm reduction should inform health care practices and develop the base for interventions.

REFERENCES

Abrams, D.I. (1997). Alternative therapies for HIV. In M.A. Sande, P.A. Volberding (Eds.), *The medical management of AIDS* (ed. 5, pp. 143–158). Philadelphia: Saunders.

Agency for Health Care Policy and Research (AHCPR), Public Health Service, USDHHS. (January 1994). Evaluation and management of early HIV infection. *Clinical Practice Guideline,* No. 7, AHCPR publication No. 94-0572, Rockville, MD.

Alcabes, P., Schoenbaum, E.E., Klein, R.S. (1993). Correlates of the rate of decline of CD4+ lymphocytes among injection drug users infected with the human immunodeficiency virus. *American Journal of Epidemiology, 137*(9), 989–991.

Amaro, H. (1995). Love, sex, and power. *American Psychologist, 50*(6), 437–447.

Aron, J.M. (1994). Optimization of nutritional support in HIV disease. In R.R. Watson (Ed.), *Nutrition and AIDS* (pp. 215–233). Boca Raton, FL: CRC Press.

Asch, S.M., London, A.S., Barnes, P.F., et al. (1997). Testing for human immunodeficiency virus infection among tuberculosis patients in Los Angeles. *American Journal of Respiratory and Critical Care, 155*(1), 378–381.

Baigis-Smith, J., Gordon, D., McGuire, D.B., et al. (1995). Healthcare needs of HIV-infected persons in hospital, outpatient, home, and long-term care settings. *Journal of the Association of Nurses in AIDS Care, 6*(6), 21–36.

Balfour, H.H., Jr. (1993). Transfusion and the human immunodeficiency virus. *Transfusion, 33*(2), 101–102.

Barroso, J. (1996). Focusing on living: Attitudinal approaches of long-term survivors of AIDS. *Issues in Mental Health Nursing, 17,* 395–407.

Beal, J.E., Olson, R., Laubenstein, L., et al. (1995). Dronabinol as a treatment for anorexia associated with weight loss in patients with AIDS. *Journal of Pain and Symptom Management, 10,* 89–97.

Bell, R.A., Molitor, F., Flynn, N. (1997). On returning for one's HIV test result: Demographic, behavioral and psychological predictors. *AIDS, 11*(2), 263–264.

Biggar, R., Miotti, P., Taha, T., et al. (1996). *Perinatal HIV-1 transmission in Africa and the effect of birth canal cleansing* (abstract 27). Presented at the 3rd Conference on Retroviruses and Opportunistic Infections, Washington, D.C.

Boland, G. (1997). Management of syphilis in HIV-infected persons. In M.A. Sande, P.A. Volberding (Eds.), *The medical management of AIDS* (5th ed., pp. 399–409). Philadelphia: Saunders.

Brennan, C., Porche, D.J. (1997). HIV immune pathogenesis. *Journal of the Association of Nurses in AIDS Care, 8*(4), 7–22.

Bulterys, M., Goedert, J.J. (1996). From biology to sexual behaviour—towards the prevention of mother-to-child transmission of HIV. *AIDS, 10,* 1287–1289.

Burack, J.H., Barrett, D.C., Stall, R.D., et al. (1993). Depressive symptoms and CD4 lymphocyte decline among HIV-infected men. *Journal of the American Medical Association, 270,* 2568–2573.

Burns, D., et al. (1995). *Changes in CD4 and CD8 cell levels cohort of HIV-1 seronegative and seropositive women* (abstract 14). Presented at 35th Annual Interscience Conference on Antimicrobial Agents and Chemotherapy, San Francisco, California.

Busch, M.P., Alter, H.J. (1995). Will human immunodeficiency virus p24 antigen screening increase the safety of the blood supply, and, if so, at what cost? *Transfusion, 35,* 536–539.

Caetano, R., Hines, A.M. (1995). Alcohol, sexual practices, and risk of AIDS among blacks, Hispanics, and whites. *Journal of Acquired Immune Deficiency Syndromes Human Retrovirology, 10*(5), 554–561.

Casey, K. (1997). Malnutrition associated with HIV/AIDS. Part one: Definition and scope, epidemiology, and pathophysiology. *Journal of the Association of Nurses in AIDS Care, 8*(3), 24–34.

Centers for Disease Control and Prevention. (January 15, 1993a). Recommendations for HIV testing services for inpatients and outpatients in acute-care hospital settings and technical guidance on HIV counseling. *Morbidity and Mortality Weekly Report, 42*(RR-2), 1–5, 11–16.

Centers for Disease Control and Prevention. (January 15, 1993b). Condom use and sexual identity among men who have sex with men: Dallas, 1991. *Morbidity and Mortality Weekly Report, 42*(9), 7–14.

Centers for Disease Control and Prevention. (March 12, 1993). False-positive serologic tests for human T-cell lymphotropic virus type 1 among blood donors following influenza vaccination, 1992. *Morbidity and Mortality Weekly Report, 42*(9), 173.

Centers for Disease Control and Prevention. (May 28, 1993). Sexual behavior and condom use—District of Columbia, January–February 1992. *Morbidity and Mortality Weekly Report, 42*(20), 390–397.

Centers for Disease Control and Prevention. (June 4, 1993). Use of bleach for disinfection of drug injection equipment. *Morbidity and Mortality Weekly Report, 42*(2), 418–419.

Centers for Disease Control and Prevention. (June 18, 1993). HIV prevention through case management for HIV-infected persons: Selected sites. *Morbidity and Mortality Weekly Report, 42*(23), 448–456.

Centers for Disease Control and Prevention. (August 6, 1993). Update: Barrier protection against HIV infection and other sexually transmitted diseases. *Morbidity and Mortality Weekly Report, 42*(30), 589–597.

Centers for Disease Control and Prevention. (September 10, 1993). Physical activity and the prevention of coronary heart disease. *Morbidity and Mortality Weekly Report, 42*(35), 669–672.

Centers for Disease Control and Prevention. (May 20, 1994). Guidelines for preventing transmission of human immunodeficiency virus through transplantation of human tissue and organs. *Morbidity and Mortality Weekly Report, 43*(RR-8), 1–17.

Centers for Disease Control and Prevention. (April 29, 1994). Zidovudine for the prevention of HIV transmission from mother to infant. *Morbidity and Mortality Weekly Report, 43*(16), 285–287.

Centers for Disease Control and Prevention. (November 18, 1994). Update: Trends in AIDS diagnosis and reporting under the expanded surveillance definition for adolescents and adults—United States, 1993. *Morbidity and Mortality Weekly Report, 43*(45), 826–831.

Centers for Disease Control and Prevention. (June 2, 1995). Update: Trends in AIDS among men who have sex with men—United States, 1989–1994. *Morbidity and Mortality Weekly Report, 44*, 401–404.

Centers for Disease Control and Prevention. (July 7, 1995). U.S. Public Health Service recommendations for human immunodeficiency virus counseling and voluntary testing for pregnant women. *Morbidity and Mortality Weekly Report, 44*(RR-7), 1–15.

Centers for Disease Control and Prevention. (March 10, 1995). HIV Counseling and testing—United States, 1993. *Morbidity and Mortality Weekly Report, 44*(9), 169–175.

Centers for Disease Control and Prevention. (August 18, 1995). Update: HIV-2 infection among blood and plasma donors—United States, June 1992–June 1995. *Morbidity and Mortality Weekly Report, 44*(32), 603–606.

Centers for Disease Control and Prevention. (September 22, 1995). Syringe Exchange Programs-United States, 1994–95. *Morbidity and Mortality Weekly Report, 44*(37), 684–692.

Centers for Disease Control and Prevention. (January 19, 1996). Surveillance of tuberculosis and AIDS comorbidity—Florida, 1981–93. *Morbidity and Mortality Weekly Report, 45*(2), 38–40.

Centers for Disease Control and Prevention. (February 23, 1996). Continued sexual risk behavior among HIV-seropositive, drug-using men—Atlanta; Washington, D.C., and San Juan, Puerto Rico, 1993. *Morbidity and Mortality Weekly Report, 45*(7), 151–159.

Centers for Disease Control and Prevention. (March 1, 1996). Outbreak of primary and secondary syphilis—Baltimore City, Maryland, 1995. *Morbidity and Mortality Weekly Report, 45*(8), 165–169.

Centers for Disease Control and Prevention. (April 12, 1996). Hepatitis B virus infection among hemodialysis patients. *Morbidity and Mortality Weekly Report, 45*(14), 285–288.

Centers for Disease Control and Prevention. (May 10, 1996). Community-level prevention of human immunodeficiency virus infection among high-risk populations: The AIDS Community Demonstration Projects. *Morbidity and Mortality Weekly Report, 45*(RR-6), 1–24.

Centers for Disease Control and Prevention. (July 11, 1996). Physical activity and health: A report of the Surgeon General. *Morbidity and Mortality Weekly Report, 45*, 591–592.

Centers for Disease Control and Prevention. (1997). HIV and AIDS trends: The changing landscape of the epidemic: A closer look. Centers for Disease Control and Prevention (www.cdcnac.org//hivtrend.html).

Centers for Disease Control and Prevention. (September 27, 1996a). Youth risk behavior surveillance—United States, 1995. *Morbidity and Mortality Weekly Report, 45*(SS-4), 1–81.

Centers for Disease Control and Prevention. (September 27, 1996b). Contraceptive method and condom use among women at risk for HIV infection and other sexually transmitted diseases. *Morbidity and Mortality Weekly Report, 45*(38), 820–831.

Centers for Disease Control and Prevention. (February 21, 1997). Community-based HIV prevention in presumably underserved populations—Colorado Springs, Colorado, July–September 1995. *Morbidity and Mortality Weekly Report, 46*(7), 152–154.

Centers for Disease Control and Prevention. (March 1, 1997). Outbreak of primary and secondary syphilis—Baltimore City, Maryland, 1995. *Morbidity and Mortality Weekly Report, 45*(8), 166–169.

Centers for Disease Control and Prevention. (May 2, 1997). Contraceptive practices among women—selected U.S. sites, 1993–1995. *Morbidity and Mortality Weekly Report, 46*(17), 373–379.

Centers for Disease Control and Prevention. (June 30,

1997). *HIV/AIDS Surveillance Report, 5*(3), 1–39, Atlanta, GA: The Center.

Centers for Disease Control and Prevention. (July 1997). Female adult/adolescent AIDS annual rates per 100,000 population, for cases reported in 1996, U.S. *HIV/AIDS Prevention,* 13.

Centers for Disease Control and Prevention. (July 11, 1997). Transmission of HIV possibly associated with exposure of mucous membrane to contaminated blood. *Morbidity and Mortality Weekly Report, 46*(27), 620–623.

Choi, K., Catania, J.A. (1996). Changes in multiple sexual partnerships, HIV testing, and condom use among US heterosexuals 18 to 49 years of age, 1990–1992. *American Journal of Public Health, 86*(4), 554–556.

Choi, K., Lew, S., Vittinghoff, E., et al. (1996). The efficacy of brief group counseling in HIV risk reduction among homosexual Asian and Pacific Islander men. *AIDS, 10,* 81–87.

Clerici, M., Giorgi, J.V., Chou, C.C., et al. (1992). Cell-mediated immune response to immunodeficiency virus (HIV) type 1 in seronegative homosexual men with recent sexual exposure to HIV-1. *Journal of Infectious Disease, 165,* 1012–1019.

Cole, S.W. (1997). The biological basis for psychoneuroimmunology. *Focus, 12*(3), 5–6.

Cole, S.W., Kemeny M.E. (1997). Psychobiology of HIV Infection. *Critical Reviews in Neurobiology, 11*(4), 289–321.

Cole, S.W., Kemeny, M.E., Taylor, S.E., et al. (1996). Accelerated course of HIV progression in gay men who conceal their homosexual identity. *Psychosomatic Medicine, 58,* 219–231.

Colebunders, R. (1996). Long-time survivors: What can we learn from them? In J. Mann, D. Tarantola (Eds.), *AIDS in the world II* (pp. 165–170). New York: Oxford University Press.

Coodley , G.O., Loveless, M.O., Merrill, T.M. (1994). The HIV wasting syndrome: A review. *Journal of Acquired Immune Deficiency Syndrome, 7,* 681–694.

Corless, I.B., Miramontes, H.M. (1997). Is it better to inhale? An examination of the medical use of marijuana controversy in the United States. *Journal of the Association of Nurses in AIDS Care, 8*(3), 17–20.

Coxon, A.P.M. (1996). Male homosexuality and HIV. In J. Mann, D. Tarantola (Eds.), *AIDS in the world II* (pp. 252–258). New York: Oxford University Press.

Cronk, C.E., Sarvela, P.D. (1997). Alcohol, tobacco, and other drug use among rural/small town and urban youth: A secondary analysis of the monitoring the future data set. *American Journal of Public Health, 87*(5), 760–769.

Dearing, J.W., Rogers, E.M., Meyer, G., et al. (1996). Social marketing and diffusion-based strategies for communicating with unique populations: HIV prevention in San Francisco. *Journal of Health Communication, 1,* 343–363.

Denning, P., Fleming, P. (1997). *Estimating recent patterns of HIV infection among adolescents and young adults* (abstract 375). Presented at 4th Conference on Retroviruses and Opportunistic Infections, Washington, D.C.

Denning, P., Ward, J., Chu, S., et al. (1996). *Current trends in AIDS incidence among young men who have sex with men, United States* (abstract Tu.C. 2405). Presented at XI International Conference on AIDS, Vancouver, British Columbia.

Des Jarlais, D.C., Friedman, S.R. (1996). Risk reduction among injecting drug users. In J. Mann, D. Tarantola (Eds.), *AIDS in the world II* (pp. 264–265). New York: Oxford University Press.

Des Jarlais, D.C., Marmor, M., Paone, D., et al. (1996). HIV incidence among injecting drug users in New York City syringe-exchange programs. *Lancet, 348,* 987–991.

Detels, R., Liu, A., Hennessey, K. (1994). Resistance to HIV-1 infection. Multicenter AIDS cohort study. *Journal of Acquired Immune Deficiency Syndromes and Human Retrovirology, 7*(2), 1263–1269.

Detels, R.I., Mann, D., Carrington, M., et al. (1996). Resistance to HIV infection may be genetically mediated [Letter]. *AIDS, 10,* 102–104.

Downs, A.M., de Vincenzi, I. (1996). Probability of heterosexual transmission of HIV: Relationship to the number of unprotected sexual contacts. *Journal of Acquired Immune Deficiency Syndrome Human Retrovirology, 11,* 388–395.

Drew, W.L., Stempien, M.J., Erlich, K. (1997). Management of herpesvirus infections (CMV, HSV, VZV). In M.A. Sande, P.A. Volberding (Eds.), *The medical management of AIDS* (5th ed., pp. 381–398). Philadelphia: Saunders.

Easterbrook, P.J., Farzadegan, H., Hoover, D.R., et al. (1996). Racial differences in rate of CD4 decline in HIV-1 infected homosexual men. *AIDS, 10,* 1147–1155, 1157.

Edlin, B.R., Holmberg, S.D. (1993). Insemination of HIV-negative women with processed semen of HIV-positive partners. *Lancet, 341*(8844), 570–571.

Elion, R.A. (May 1997). Complementary medicine and HIV infection. *HIV Hotline, 7*(3), 2.

Eller, L.S. (1995). Effects of two cognitive-behavioral interventions on immunity and symptoms in persons with HIV. *Annals of Behavior Medicine, 17,* 339.

Erhardt, A.A. (1996). Sexual behavior among heterosexuals. In J. Mann, D. Tarantola (Eds.), *AIDS in the world II* (pp. 259–265). New York: Oxford University Press.

Erickson, J.R. (1997). Human immunodeficiency virus infection risk among female sex partners of intravenous drug users in Southern Arizona. *Holistic Nursing Practice, 11*(2), 9–17.

Ezzell, C. (1996). Tissue type may determine AIDS progression. *Journal of NIH Research, 8*(5), 42.

Fahs, M.C., Waite, D., Sesholtz, M., et al. (1994). Results of the ACSUS for pediatric AIDS patients: Utilization of services, functional status, and social severity. *Health Services Research, 29*(5), 549–568.

Feldblum, P., Morrison, C., Cates, W. (1995). The effectiveness of barrier methods of contraception in preventing the spread of HIV. *AIDS, 9,* S85–S93.

Ferbas, J. (1996). Naturally produced factors that regulate viral infections: Are there more than one? *UCLA AIDS Institute Perspectives, 4*(2), 10.

Fitzgerald, B., Aranda-Naranjo, B., Ferri, R., et al. (1996). Applying the transtheoretical and harm reduction models. *Journal of the Association of Nurses in AIDS Care, 7*(Suppl. 1), 33–40.

Flaskerud, J.H. (1994). AIDS and traditional food therapies. In R.R. Watson (Ed.), *Nutrition and AIDS* (pp. 235–237). Boca Raton, FL: CRC Press.

Flaskerud, J.H., Calvillo, E.R. (1991a). Beliefs about AIDS health, and illness among low income Latina women. *Reseach in Nursing and Health, 14,* 431–438.

Flaskerud, J.H., Nyamathi, A. (1996). Home medication injection among Latina women in Los Angeles: Implications for health education and prevention. *AIDS Care, 8*(1), 95–102.

Flaskerud, J.H., Nyamathi, A.M., Uman, G. (1997). Longitudinal effects of an HIV testing and counseling program for low income Latina women. *Ethnicity and Health, 2*(1/2), 89–103.

Flaskerud, J.H., Uman, G., Lara, R., et al. (1996). Sexual practices, attitudes, and knowledge related to HIV transmission among low income Los Angeles Hispanic women. *Journal of Sex Research, 33*(6), 1–11.

Fleishman, J.A., Hsia, D.C., Helliger, F.J. (1994). Correlates of medical service utilization among people with HIV infection. *HSR: Health Services Research, 29*(5), 527–548.

Fleming, P.L., Ciesielski, C.A., Byers, R.H., et al. (1993). Gender differences in reported AIDS-indicative diagnoses. *Journal of Infectious Diseases, 68*(1), 61–67.

Folkman, S., Chesney, M., Pollack, L., et al. (1993). Stress, control, coping, and depressive mood in human immunodeficiency virus-positive and negative gay men in San Francisco. *Journal of Nervous and Mental Disease, 181*(7), 409–416.

Fowke, K.R., Negelkerke, N.J.D., Kimani, J., et al. (1996). Resistance to HIV-1 infection among persistently seronegative prostitutes in Nairobi, Kenya. *Lancet, 348,* 1347–1351.

Frost, K.R. (1996). Cytomegalovirus resistance. *AmFAR Report,* pp. 1–5.

Gallagher, M.A., Klima, C. (1996). The challenge of maternal-infant transmission of HIV. *Journal of the Association of Nurses in AIDS Care, 7*(1), 47–54.

Gaskins, S., Brown, K. (1997). Helping others: A response to HIV disease. *Journal of the Association of Nurses in AIDS Care, 8*(3), 35–57.

Gelberg, L., Panarites, C.J., Morgenstern, H., et al. (1997). Tuberculosis skin testing among homeless adults. *Journal of General Internal Medicine, 12,* 2–33.

Ghali, W.A., Palepu, A., Paterson, W.G. (1994). Evaluation of red blood cell transfusion practices with the use of preset criteria. *Canadian Medical Association Journal, 150,* 1449–1454.

Gilmore, N. (1996). Blood and blood product safety. In J. Mann, D. Tarantola (Eds.), *AIDS in the world II* (pp. 287–292). New York: Oxford University Press.

Giorgi, J.V., Majchrowica, M.A. (1996). Mechanisms of HIV resistance. *UCLA AIDS Institute Perspectives, 4*(2), 1–2.

Gold, R.S. (1995). Why we need to rethink AIDS education for young men. *AIDS Care, 7*(Suppl.), S11–S19.

Gordon, H.S., Harper, D.L., Rosenthal, G.E. (1996). Racial variation in predicted and observed in-hospital death. *JAMA, 276*(20), 1639–1644.

Gostin, L.O., Lazzarini, Z., Jones, S., et al. (1997). Prevention of HIV/AIDS and other blood-borne diseases among injection drug users. *JAMA, 277*(1), 53–62.

Gresenguet, G., Kreiss, J.K., Chapko, M.K., et al. (1997). HIV infection and vaginal douching in Central Africa. *AIDS, 11,* 101–106.

Gross, J.J., Levenson, R.W. (1993). Emotional suppression: Physiology, self-report, and expressive behavior. *Journal of Personality and Social Psychology, 64,* 970.

Hamburg, M.A. (1996). Public health and urban medicine. *Lancet, 348,* 1008–1010.

Hays, R.B., Paul, J., Ekstrand, M., et al. (1997). Actual versus perceived HIV status, sexual behaviors and predictors of unprotected sex among young gay and bisexual men who identify as HIV-negative, HIV-positive and untested. *AIDS, 11,* 1495–1502.

Heckman, T.G., Kelly, J.A., Sikkema, K.J., et al. (1995). Differences in HIV risk characteristics between bisexual and exclusively gay men. *AIDS Education and Prevention, 7,* 504–517.

Hein, K. (1993). "Getting real" about HIV in adolescents. *American Journal of Public Health, 83*(4), 492–494.

Hickson, F.C.I., Reid, D.S., Davies, P.M., et al. (1996). No aggregate change in homosexual HIV risk behaviour among gay men attending the Gay Pride festivals, United Kingdom, 1993–1995. *AIDS, 10,* 771–774.

HIV Frontline Update. (March–April 1994). Vitamins could slow AIDS onset. *HIV Frontline, 17,* 3.

HIV News Briefs. (July/August 1997). Home HIV test taken off market. *HIV Frontline, 29,* 7.

Holtgrave, D.R., Qualls, N.L., Curran, J.W., et al. (1995). An overview of the effectiveness and efficiency of HIV prevention programs. *Public Health Reports, 110*(2), 134–146.

Hopewell, P.C. (1997). Tuberculosis in persons with human immunodeficiency virus infection. In M.A.

Sande, P.A. Volberding (Eds.), *The medical management of AIDS* (pp. 311–325). Philadelphia: Saunders.

Hu, D.J., Fleming, P.L., Castro, K.G., et al. (1995). How important is race/ethnicity as an indicator of risk for specific AIDS-defining conditions? *Journal of Acquired Immune Deficiency Syndromes and Human Retrovirology, 10*(3), 374–380.

Ironson, G., Solomon, G., Cruess, D., et al. (1995). Psychosocial factors related to long-term survival with HIV/AIDS. *Clinical Psychology and Psychotherapy, 2,* 249–266.

Irwin, K.L., Valdiserri, R.O., Holmberg, S.D. (1996). The acceptability of voluntary HIV antibody testing in the United States: A decade of lessons learned. *AIDS, 10,* 1707–1717.

Jewett, J.F., Hecht, F.M. (1993). Preventive health care for adults with HIV infection. *Journal of the American Medical Association, 269*(9), 1144–1153.

Jones, S.G. (1997). Implementing a multidisciplinary HIV diarrhea critical pathway in the acute care setting. *Journal of the Association of Nurses in AIDS Care, 8*(3), 59–68.

Katz, M.H., Gerberding, J.L. (1997). Postexposure treatment of people exposed to the human immunodeficiency virus through sexual contact or injection-drug use. *New England Journal of Medicine, 336*(15), 1097–1100.

Keet, I.P.M., Krijnen, P., Koot, M., et al. (1993). Predictors of rapid progression to AIDS in HIV-1 seroconverters. *AIDS, 7*(10), 51–57.

Kelly, J.A., Murphy, D.A., Washington, C.D., et al. (1994). The effects of HIV/AIDS intervention groups for high-risk women in urban clinics. *American Journal of Public Health, 84,* 1918–1922.

Kemeny, M.E., Dean, L. (1995). Effects of AIDS-related bereavement on HIV progression among New York City gay men. *AIDS Education and Prevention, 7*(Suppl. 5), 36–47.

Klein, T.W. (1996). Cannabinoids and immunity to *Legionella pneumophila* infection. Presented at the PsychoNeuro Immunology Research Society, April 17–20, 1996. *Research Perspectives in Psychoneuroimmunology,* Abstract S.5.

Koester, S., Booth, R.E., Zhang, Y. (1996). The prevalence of additional injection-related HIV risk behaviors among injection drug users. *Journal of Acquired Immune Deficiency Syndromes and Human Retrovirology, 12,* 202–207.

La Coeur, S., Lallemant, M. (1996). Pediatric HIV/AIDS. In J. Mann, D. Tarantola (Eds.), *AIDS in the world II* (pp. 273–277). New York: Oxford University Press.

Lackritz, E.M., Satten, A., Aberle-Grasse, J., et al. (1995). Estimated risk of transmission of the human immunodeficiency virus by screened blood in the United States. *New England Journal of Medicine, 333,* 1721–1725.

Landers, D.V., Shannon, M.T. (1997). Management of pregnant women with HIV infection. In M.A. Sande, P.A. Volberding (Eds.), *The medical management of AIDS* (5th ed., pp. 459–467). Philadelphia: Saunders.

Lands, L. (Ed.). (1996). *Positively well: Living with HIV as a chronic, manageable, survivable disease.* New York: Irvington.

Latkin, C., Mandell, W., Vlahov, D., et al. (1996). People and places: Behavioral settings and personal network characteristics as correlates of needle sharing. *Journal of Acquired Immune Deficiency Syndromes and Human Retrovirology, 13,* 273–280.

Lauver, D., Armstron, K., Marks, S., et al. (1995). HIV risk status and preventive behaviors among 17,619 women. *Journal of Obstetric, Gynecologic, and Neonatal Nursing, 24*(1), 33–39.

Lee, T.H., Sakahara, N., Fiebig, E., et al. (1996). Correlation of HIV-1 RNA levels in plasma and heterosexual transmission of HIV-1 from infected transfusion recipients. *Journal of Acquired Immune Deficiency Syndromes and Human Retrovirology, 12,* 427–428.

Leiphart, J.M. (1997). Psychoneuroimmunology: A basis for HIV treatment. *Focus: A Guide to AIDS Research and Counseling, 12*(3), 1–4.

Levy, J.A. (1993). The transmission of HIV and factors influencing progression of AIDS. *American Journal of Medicine, 95,* 86–98.

Levy, J.A. (1996). HIV heterogeneity in transmission and pathogenesis. In J. Mann, D. Tarantola (Eds.), *AIDS in the world II* (pp. 177–183). New York: Oxford University Press.

Lewin, D.I. (1996). Cell cofactors give HIV its specificity. *Journal of NIH Research, 8,* 27–28.

Los Angeles Times. (September 3, 1995). Young gays stray from safe sex, new data shows. *Los Angeles Times,* pp. A1, A28.

Lyketsos, C.G., Hoover, D.R., Guccione, M., et al. (1993). Depressive symptoms as predictors of medical outcomes in HIV infection. *Journal of the American Medical Association, 270,* 2563–2567.

Mann, J., Tarantola, D. (Eds). (1996). *AIDS in the world II: Global dimensions, social roots, and responses.* New York: Oxford University Press.

Mascolini, M. (1996). HIV and the mind. *AIDS Care, 2*(6), 18–26.

Mastro, T.D., Satten, G.A., Nopkesorn, T., et al. (1994). Probability of female-to-male transmission of HIV-1 in Thailand. *Lancet, 343,* 204–207.

McEnany, G.W., Hughes, A.M., Lee, K.A. (1996). Depression and HIV. *Nursing Clinics of North America, 31*(1), 57–80.

McKirnan, D.J., Ostrow, D.G., Hope, B. (1996). Sex, drugs and escape: A psychological model of HIV-risk sexual behaviours. *AIDS Care, 8*(6), 655–659.

McKirnan, D., Stokes, J.P. (1995). Bisexually active men: Social characteristics and sexual behavior. *Journal of Sex Research, 32*(1), 66–75.

Meer, R. (1994). AIDS and food safety. In R.R. Watson (Ed.), *Nutrition and AIDS* (pp. 189–199). Boca Raton, FL: CRC Press.

Mellors, J., Rinaldo, C.R., Guta, P., et al. (1996). Prognosis in HIV-1 infection predicted by the quantity of virus in plasma. *Science, 272,* 1167–1170.

Melnick, S.L., Sherer, R., Louis, T.A., et al. (1994). Survival and disease progression according to gender of patients with HIV infection. *JAMA, 272*(24), 1915–1921.

Merson, M.H. (1996). Returning home: Reflections on the USA's response to the HIV/AIDS epidemic. *Lancet, 347,* 1673–1676.

Meyer, G., Dearing, D. (1996). Respecifying the social marketing model for unique populations. *Social Marketing Quarterly,* 44–52.

Miller, G.E., Kemeny, M.E., Taylor, S.E., et al. (1997). Social relationships and immune processes in HIV seropositive gay men. *Annals of Behavioral Medicine, 9,* 139–151.

Montoya, I.D., Atkinson, J.S. (1996). Determinants of HIV seroprevalence rates among sites participating in a community-based study of drug users. *Journal of Acquired Immune Deficiency Syndromes and Human Retrovirology, 13,* 169–176.

Morris, M., Kretzschmar, M. (1997). Concurrent partnerships and the spread of HIV. *AIDS, 11,* 641–648.

Mostad, S.B., Kreiss, J.K. (1996). Shedding of HIV-1 in the genital tract. *AIDS, 10,* 1305–1315.

Mota, R.G. (1996). Personal care strategies of people living with HIV/AIDS. In J. Mann, D. Tarantola (Eds.), *AIDS in the world II* (pp. 398–403). New York: Oxford University Press.

Munoz, A., Schrager, L.K., Bacellar, H., et al. (1993). Trends in the incidence of outcomes defining acquired immunodeficiency syndrome (AIDS) in multicenter AIDS cohort study: 1985–1991. *American Journal of Epidemiology, 137*(4), 423–438.

National Institutes of Health. (March 26, 1997). *NIH Press Release, 3,* 1.

Neaigus, A., Friedman, S.R., Curtis, R., et al. (1994). The relevance of drug injectors' social and risk networks for understanding and preventing HIV infection. *Social Science and Medicine, 38*(1), 67–78.

Nemechek, P.M., Sackuvich, L., Zakovich, P., et al. (May 1997). Maintenance of body cell mass and phase angle after discontinuation of human growth hormone. *HIV Hotline, 7*(3), 11–15.

Nerad, J.L., Gorbach, S.L. (1994). Nutrition aspects of HIV infection. *Infectious Disease Clinics of North America, 8,* 499–515.

Newman, M.D., Wofsy, C.B. (1997). Gender-specific issues in HIV disease. In M.A. Sande, P.A. Volberding (Eds.), *The medical management of AIDS* (5th ed., pp. 475–502). Philadelphia: Saunders.

Norris, A.E., Ford, K., Shyr, K., et al. (1996). Heterosexual experiences and partnerships of urban, low income African and Hispanic youth. *Journal of AIDS and Human Retrovirology, 11,* 288–300.

O'Malley, J., Nguyen, V.K., Lee, S. (1996). Nongovernmental organizations. In J. Mann, D. Tarantola (Eds.), *AIDS in the world II* (pp. 341–342). New York: Oxford University Press.

Ostrow, D.G., DiFranceisco, W.J., Chmiel, J.S., et al. (1995). A case-control study of human immunodeficiency virus type 1 seroconversion and risk-related behaviors in the Chicago MACS/CCD Cohort, 1984–1992. *American Journal of Epidemiology, 142*(8), 875–883.

Park, L.P., Margolick, J.B., Georgi, J.V., et al. (1993). Influence of HIV-1 infection and cigarette smoking on leukocyte profile in homosexual men. *Annals of New York Academy Science, 667*(March), 433–436.

Patterson, T.L., Shaw, W.S., Semple, S.J., et al. (1996). Relationship of psychosocial factors to HIV disease progression. *Annals of Behavioral Medicine, 18,* 30.

Pelletier, E., Wain-Hobson, S. (1996). Research commentary: AIDS is not caused by the extreme genetic variability. *Journal of NIH Research, 8,* 45–48.

Peterson, J.L., Coates, T.J., Catania, J., et al. (1996). Evaluation of an HIV risk reduction intervention among African-American homosexual and bisexual men. *AIDS, 10,* 319–325.

Petrie, K.J., Booth, R.J., Pennebaker, J.W., et al. (1995). Disclosure of trauma and immune response to a hepatitis B vaccination program. *Journal of Consulting and Clinical Psychology, 63,* 787.

Phillips, K.A., Flatt, S.J., Morrison, K.R., et al. (1995). Potential use of home HIV testing. *New England Journal of Medicine, 332,* 1308–1310.

Phinney, S.D., Siepler, J., Bach, H.T. (1996). Is there a role for parenteral feeding in clinical medicine? *Western Journal of Medicine, 164*(2), 130–136.

Pinkerton, S.D., Abramson, P.R. (1996). Occasional condom use and HIV risk reduction. *Journal of Acquired Immune Deficiency Syndromes and Human Retrovirology, 13,* 456–460.

Poole, W.K., Fulkerson, W., Lou, Y., et al. (1996). Overall and cause-specific mortality in a cohort of homo-/bisexual men, injecting drug users, and female partners of HIV-infected men. *AIDS, 10,* 1257–1264.

Prins, M., Veugelers, P.J. (1997). Comparison of progression and non-progression in injecting drug users and homosexual men with documented dates of HIV-1 seroconversion. *AIDS, 11,* 621–631.

Prochaska, J., Harlow, R.L., Rossi, J., et al. (1994). The transtheoretical model of change and HIV prevention: A review. *Health Education Quarterly, 21*(4), 471–486.

Quirk, M.E., Godkin, M.A., Schwenzfeier, E. (1993). Evaluation of two AIDS prevention interventions for inner-city adolescent and young adult women. *American Journal of Preventive Medicine, 9*(1), 21–26.

Raviglione, M., Nunn, P.P., Kochi, A., et al. (1996). The pandemic of HIV-associated turberculosis. In J. Mann, D. Tarantola (Eds.), *AIDS in the world II* (pp. 87–92). New York: Oxford University Press.

Reed, G.M., Kemeny, M.E., Taylor, S.E., et al. (1994). Realistic acceptance as a predictor of decreased survival time in gay men with AIDS. *Health Psychology, 13,* 299.

Reed, G.M., Kemeny, M.E., Taylor, S.E., et al. (In press). Negative HIV-specific expectancies and AIDS-related bereavement as predictors of symptom onset in asymptomatic HIV seropositive gay men. *Health Psychology.*

Rietmeijer, C.A., Kane, M.S., Simons, P.Z., et al. (1996). Increasing the use of bleach and condoms among injecting drug users in Denver: Outcome of a targeted, community-level HIV prevention program. *AIDS, 10,* 291–298.

Rochon, D. (July/August 1997). Opportunistic infections and neoplasms: Focus on cervical cancer. *HIV Frontline, 29,* 6.

Rogers, E.M., Dearing, D., Rao, N., et al. (1995). Communication and community in a city under siege: The AIDS epidemic in San Francisco. *Communication Research, 22*(6), 664–678.

Rowe, P.M. (1993). Resistance to HIV infection. *Lancet, 341*(8845), 624.

Royce, R.A., Sena, A., Cates, W., et al. (1997). Sexual transmission of HIV. *New England Journal of Medicine, 336*(15), 1072–1078.

Sande, M.A., Volberding, P.A. (Eds.). (1997). *The medical management of AIDS* (5th ed.). Philadelphia: Saunders.

Schoenbaum, M. (1997). Do smokers understand the mortality effects of smoking? Evidence from the Health and Retirement Survey. *American Journal of Public Health, 87*(5), 755–759.

Schopper, D., Vercauteren, G. (1996). Testing for HIV at home: What are the issues? *AIDS, 10,* 1455–1465.

Segerstrom, S., Taylor, S.E., Kemeny, M.E., et al. (1996). Causal attributions of immune decline in HIV seroprevalence in gay men. *Health Psychology, 15,* 485.

Semba, R.D., Caiaffa, W.T., Graham, N.M., et al. (1995). Vitamin A deficiency and wasting as predictors of mortality in human immunodeficiency virus-infection drug users. *Journal of Infectious Disease, 171,* 1196–1202.

Sikkema, K.J., Heckman, T.G., Kelly, J.A., et al. (1996). HIV risk behaviors among women living in low-income, inner-city housing developments. *American Journal of Public Health, 86*(8), 1123–1128.

Singleton, J.A., Tabnak, F., Kuan, J., et al. (1996). Human immunodeficiency virus disease in California. *Western Journal of Medicine, 164,* 122–129.

Solomon, G.F., Temoshok, L., O'Leary, A., et al. (1987). An intensive psychoimmunologic study of long-surviving patients with AIDS. *Annals of New York Academy of Sciences, 496,* 647–655.

Solomon, G.F., Benton, D., Harker, B.D., et al. (1993). Prolonged asymptomatic states in HIV-seropositive persons with 50 CD4+ T-cells/mm^3: Preliminary psychoimmunologic findings (letter). *Journal of Acquired Immune Deficiency Syndromes and Human Retrovirology, 6*(10), 1172–1173.

Solomon, L., Moore, J., Gleghorn, A., et al. (1996). HIV testing behaviors in a population of inner-city women at high risk for HIV infection. *Journal of Acquired Immune Deficiency Syndromes and Human Retrovirology, 13,* 267–272.

Sowell, R.L., Moneyham, L., Guillory, J., et al. (1997). Self-care activities of women infected with human immunodeficiency virus. *Holistic Nursing Practice, 11*(2), 18–26.

Sowell, R.L., Seals, B.F., Phillips, K.D. (1996). Knowledge of risk behaviors of people seeking HIV antibody testing at a community site. *Journal of the Association of Nurses in AIDS Care, 7*(3), 33–42.

Stall, R., Hoff, C., Coates, T.C., et al. (1996). Decisions to get HIV tested and to accept antiretroviral therapies among gay/bisexual men: Implications for secondary prevention efforts. *Journal of Acquired Immune Deficiency Syndromes and Human Retrovirology, 11,* 151–160.

Staprans, S.I., Feinberg, M.B. (1997). Natural history and immunopathogenesis of HIV-1 disease. In M.A. Sande, P.A. Volberding (Eds.), *The medical management of AIDS* (5th ed., pp. 29–55). Philadelphia: Saunders.

Swan, N. (1995). Drug abuse links to AIDS prompt highly targeted responses. *NIDA Notes, 10*(6), 94–95.

Tabet, S.R., de Moya, A., Holmes, K.K., et al. (1996). Sexual behaviors and risk factors for HIV infection among men who have sex with men in the Dominican Republic. *AIDS, 10,* 201–206.

Taylor, D.N. (1995). Effects of a behavioral stress-management program on anxiety, mood, self-esteem, and T-cell count in HIV-positive men. *Psychological Report, 76,* 451.

Thomson, C. (1994). Specialized nutrition support. In R.R. Watson (Ed.), *Nutrition and AIDS* (pp. 201–213). Boca Raton, FL: CRC Press.

Tingley, D.W. (1996). Disarming the immune system: HIV-1 uses multiple strategies. *Journal of NIH Research, 8*(2), 33–37.

Torian, L.V., Weisfuse, I.B., Makki, H.A., et al. (1995). Increasing HIV-1 seroprevalence associated with genital ulcer disease, New York City, 1990–1992. *AIDS, 9,* 177–181.

Torian, L.V., Weisfuse, I.B., Makki, H.A., et al. (1996). Trends in HIV seroprevalence in men who have sex with men: New York City Department of Health sexually transmitted disease clinics, 1988–1993. *AIDS, 10,* 187–192.

Tovo, P.A., de Martino, M., Gabiano, C., et al. (1996). Mode of delivery and gestational age influence perinatal HIV-1 transmission. *Journal of Acquired Immune Deficiency Syndromes and Human Retrovirology, 11,* 88–94.

Turner, B. (1997). Pregnancy, smoking, and HIV. *Journal of Acquired Immune Deficiency Syndromes and Human Retrovirology, 14*(4), 327–337.

Turner, N.H., Solomon, D.J. (1996). HIV risks and risk reduction readiness in hard-to-reach, drug-using Africa American women: An exploratory study. *AIDS Education and Prevention, 8*(3), 236–246.

Valdiserri, R.O., Moore, M., Gerber, R., et al. (1993). A study of clients returning for counseling after HIV testing: Implications for improving rates of return. *Public Health Reports, 108*(1), 12–18.

Vamvakas, E.H., Kaplan, H.S. (1993). Early transfusion and length of survival in acquired immunodeficiency syndrome: Experience with a population receiving medical care at a public hospital. *Transfusion, 33*(2), 111–118.

Vidmar, L., Poljak, M., Tomazic, J., et al. (1996). Transmission of HIV-1 by human bite. *Lancet, 347,* 1762–1763.

Wara, D. (1993). Pediatric AIDS. II. Perinatal transmission and early diagnosis. *AIDS Clinical Care, 5*(3), 21–22.

Wara, D.W., Dorenbaum, A. (1997). Pediatric AIDS: Perinatal transmission and early diagnosis. In M.A. Sande, P.A. Volberding (Eds.), *The medical management of AIDS* (5th ed., pp. 469–473). Philadelphia: Saunders.

Wardrop, K. (1993). A framework for health promotion: A framework for AIDS. *Canadian Journal of Public Health, 84*(Suppl. 1), S9–S13.

Warszawski, J., Meyer, L., Bajos, N. (1996). Is genital mycosis associated with HIV risk behaviors among heterosexuals? *American Journal of Public Health, 86*(8), 1108–1111.

Weiskopf, R.B. (1997). Practice guidelines for blood component therapy summarized. *Western Journal of Medicine, 166*(3), 204–205.

Wells, E.K., Mayer, R.R. (July/August 1997). HIV-negative women in serodiscordant couples. *HIV Frontline, 29,* 4.

Whalen, C., Horsburgh, C.R., Hom, D., et al. (1995). Accelerated course of human immunodeficiency virus infection after tuberculosis. *American Journal of Respiratory Critical Care Medicine, 151,* 129–135.

Wong, G. (1993). *HIV disease nutrition guidelines.* Chicago: Physicians Association for AIDS Care.

Zeller, J.M., McCain, N.L., Swanson, B. (1996). Immunological and virological markers of HIV disease progression. *Journal of the Association of Nurses in AIDS Care, 7*(1), 15–28.

Zevin, B. (1997). Harm reduction and HIV treatment. *HIV Frontline, 28,* 3–4.

3

Infants and Children
HIV DISEASE CARE MANAGEMENT

Mary Boland ■ Pamela Rothpletz-Puglia ■ James Oleske

By 1997, 7629 cases of AIDS in children under the age of 13 years were reported in the United States (CDC, 1996a). Perinatal transmission not only accounts for 90% of all cases of AIDS in this age group but also is the cause of virtually all new cases of HIV infection in infants. In addition, 1507 cases involving infants and children have been reported from the 21 states where HIV infection is a reportable condition. According to the results of anonymous newborn seroprevalence data, it is estimated that around 7000 infants are born to HIV-infected women in the United States each year. On the basis of an estimated average perinatal transmission rate without treatment intervention of 24.5%, more than 5000 HIV-infected infants were born in the United States during the 3 years 1995 through 1997. AIDS has become the ninth leading cause of death in the United States among children between the ages of 1 and 4 years (CDC, 1996b).

HIV TRANSMISSION IN INFANTS AND CHILDREN

Perinatal Transmission

Perinatal transmission of HIV accounts for virtually all new HIV infections in children (CDC, 1997a). Transmission from mother to infant (vertical transmission) can occur prenatally and at the time of delivery. Studies examining fetal tissue suggest that prenatal transmission of HIV can occur as early as the eighth week of gestation (Lewis et al., 1990). HIV has been cultured as early as the twelfth week of gestation from fetal brain, thymus, liver, spleen, and lung and has been identified, with the use of other techniques, in fetal brain tissue as early as the fourteenth week of gestation (Falloon et al., 1989; Lyman, et al., 1988). Although the placenta prevents the actual mixing of maternal and fetal circulation, cellular elements and soluble factors can cross the placenta. CD4+ positive cells have been demonstrated in the lining of the stroma of the chorionic villi, which is in close contact with maternal blood (Maury et al., 1989). HIV-specific IgA-containing immune complexes have been documented in amniotic fluid. The fact that up to one third of infants have AIDS-defining symptoms in the first 2 years of life is consistent with early prenatal infection in these infants (Duliege et al., 1992).

There is now ample evidence that HIV transmission also occurs, perhaps in the majority of perinatally infected infants, during the peripartum period. Serial serologic evaluations of infants have provided strong evidence of HIV transmission around the time of delivery (Pyun et al., 1987). Only 24% to 50% of infected infants test positive by culture or polymerase chain reaction (PCR) within the first week of life, and fewer than one in four have a positive p24 antigen capture assay (Rouzioux, et al., 1993). A meta-analysis of data from 271 HIV-infected children revealed that only 38% of HIV-infected children had a positive DNA PCR test result within the first 48 hours of life. By 14 days of age 93% of infected children had positive PCR findings (Dunn et al., 1995).

HIV transmission at the time of delivery is most likely associated with exposure to maternal body fluids, including blood and vaginal secretions. This is supported by recent studies evaluating the impact of the mode of delivery on transmission rates. Data from the European Collaborative Study (1994; Dunn et al., 1994) of 1254 maternal-infant pairs reveals that the odds of transmission via cesarean section relative to vaginal delivery are about 0.5; this refutes the findings of an earlier study that did not support a lower rate of transmission with cesarean sections (Maury et al., 1989). A UCLA-based study of 68 mother-infant pairs indicated that there is an increased risk of transmission with increased peripartum exposure to maternal blood, such as occurs with fetal scalp monitoring, episiotomy, or severe lacerations (Boyer et al., 1994). In one study rupture of membranes more than 4 hours before delivery was associated with a perinatal transmission rate of 25%, compared with 14% in cases with rupture of membrane less than 4 hours before delivery (Landsman et al., 1996).

A study of HIV transmission to twins reported an increased transmission rate to the firstborn of twins, implying that significant peripartum transmission to the firstborn might be related to increased exposure to maternal secretions at the time of delivery (Goedert et al., 1991). This finding is similar to studies of other bloodborne viruses transmitted during the peripartum period, such as hepatitis B virus. Studies evaluating the rate of perinatal transmission of HIV from mother to infant have yielded estimates ranging between 13% and 58% (CDC, 1996b). Transmission rates vary by geographic location, with lower transmission rates reported from industrialized countries than from developing countries.

Why some infants become infected and others do not is a subject of ongoing research. Studies evaluating the impact of maternal antibody against gp120 on transmission rates have been inconsistent. A study of the ability of maternal antibodies to neutralize autologous virus showed that neutralizing antibodies are more frequently found in mothers who do not transmit HIV perinatally than in transmitting mothers (Scarlatti et al., 1993). Women who are more immunocompromised (lower CD4+ count), have increased viral load (HIV RNA PCR counts), or who have symptoms of HIV-related disease at the time of delivery are more likely to transmit infection to their infants. In one study, none of 63 women with HIV RNA copy counts less than 20,000/ml transmitted HIV perinatally, compared with 13 of 13 women with HIV RNA PCR counts greater than 80,000/ml (Dickover et al., 1996). This is consistent with the belief that the main determinant of transmission is the level of maternal viral burden at the time of pregnancy and delivery (Levy, 1993). The risk of perinatal transmission appears to be greatest at the time of initial maternal infection, before the development of HIV-specific immunity and coincident with high levels of viremia, and at the later stages of disease when viremia increases and HIV-specific immunity wanes (Cao et al., 1997; Shearer et al., 1997).

Interrupting Perinatal Transmission

Zidovudine administered in the dose and on the schedule employed in AIDS Clinical Trials Group (ACTG) protocol 076 has been shown to reduce dramatically the likelihood of perinatally acquired HIV infection (see Table 3–1) (Connor & Mofenson, 1995; Connor et al., 1994). Updates of data from the study continue to show a reduction in transmission from 22.6% to 7.6%. Numerous organizations, including the U.S. Public Health Service, now recommend this regimen to prevent transmission from mother to infant. Subsequent published reports continue to show a decrease in transmission rate in communities where this regimen has been implemented (Englund et al., 1997; Kline et al., 1997; Luzuriaga et al., 1997). From 1984 through 1992, the estimated number of children with perinatally acquired AIDS diagnosed each year increased; then it declined by 43% during 1992 and 1996 (CDC, 1997a).

A CDC-supported study conducted in Thailand, which sparked a public ethics debate over the use of placebo in the United States, found that the short-course zidovudine (ZDV) regimen was effective in decreasing transmission by half (CDC, 1998). The short-course regimen—ZDV for 3 to 4 weeks prior to delivery, an oral dose at delivery, and no infant dose—is a more realistic regimen for countries where the cost of ZDV has been the major barrier to its use.

Worldwide, approximately 500,000 infants are infected with HIV perinatally each year. Most of these children are born in developing countries

Table 3–1 ▪ Clinical Situations and Recommendations for Use of Zidovudine (ZDV) to Reduce Perinatal Transmission

Clinical Situation	Recommendations
I. Pregnant HIV-infected women with CD4+ lymphocyte counts >200/μl who are at 14–34 wk of gestation and who have • No clinical indications for ZDV • No history of extensive (>6 mo) prior antiretroviral therapy	I. Infants who are born to HIV-infected women who have received no intrapartum ZDV therapy • Full ACTG Protocol 076 regimen* – During gestation: ZDV 100 mg PO 5/d – During labor: loading dose of ZDV, 2 mg/kg IV, then 1 mg/kg/h by continuous IV infusion until umbilical cord is clamped – In newborn infants: ZDV syrup 2 mg/kg PO q6h for 6 wk
II. Pregnant HIV-infected women who are at >34 wk of gestation, who • Have no history of extensive (>6 mo) prior antiretroviral therapy • Do not require ZDV for their own health	II. Full ACTG Protocol 076 regimen
III. Pregnant HIV-infected women with CD4 lymphocyte counts <200/μl who are at 14–34 wk of gestation, who have • No other clinical indications for ZDV • No history of extensive (>6 mo) prior antiretroviral therapy	III. • Antenatal ZDV therapy to the woman for her own health benefit • Intrapartum and neonatal components of the ACTG Protocol 076 regimen
IV. Pregnant HIV-infected women who have a history of extensive (>6 mo) ZDV therapy or other antiretroviral therapy before pregnancy	IV. Consider recommending the ACTG Protocol 076 regimen on a case-by-case basis
V. Pregnant HIV-infected women who have not received antepartum antiretroviral therapy and who are in labor	V. Discuss the benefits and potential risks of the intrapartum and neonatal components of the ACTG Protocol 076 regimen

*Zidovudine regimens used in the ACTG 076 study from Reduction of maternal-infant transmission of human immunodeficiency virus type 1 with zidovudine treatment, by E. Connor, R. Sperling, T. Gelber, P. Kiselev, G. Scott, M. O'Sullivan, et al., 1994. *New England Journal of Medicine, 331,* 1173–1180.
Adapted from Centers for Disease Control and Prevention. (1994). Zidovudine for the prevention of HIV transmission from mother to infant. *Morbidity and Mortality Weekly Review, 43,* 285–287.

(WHO, 1997). Governments in these countries, donor agencies, and other interested groups are now addressing implementation issues. CDC estimates that the $50 cost for the short-course regimen is dramatically less than the cost of the longer version. Subsequently, Glaxo, the manufacturer of ZDV, with prodding from UNAIDS, has agreed to negotiate a price with each country.

The long-term consequences of zidovudine (ZDV) when it is used solely to reduce perinatal transmission are unknown, but concerns include potential mutagenic and carcinogenic effects, possible teratogenicity, and possible effects on neurodevelopment and on the reproductive system. A National Institute of Allergy and Infectious Diseases panel (1997) convened to review studies of

transplacental toxicity of ZDV concluded that the known benefits of ZDV in preventing perinatal transmission outweigh the hypothetical concerns of transplacental carcinogenesis raised by animal studies. Nonetheless, the panel recognized the potential for long-term consequences and strongly emphasized the need for long-term follow-up of all children exposed in utero to antiviral therapy, particularly those who are not infected.

The expanding number of antiviral agents available to women complicates decision making regarding treatment for both patient and clinician. Pregnant women should be the beneficiaries of any clinical advantage offered by the new regimens and should not be restricted to single-drug therapy. (Minkoff & Augenbraun, 1997). Both maternal indications and perinatal prevention of HIV transmission must be considered by clinicians providing care to pregnant women.

Early Identification of At-Risk and HIV-Infected Infants

Although there is currently no cure for HIV infection, there are several interventions that can reduce morbidity, delay progression of disease, and reduce perinatal transmission. New treatments directed at both HIV and the opportunistic infections secondary to HIV are increasingly being investigated. For these reasons, adults are encouraged to undergo confidential and voluntary HIV testing with informed consent.

Knowledge of the HIV status of pregnant women or voluntary testing of newborns is reasonable from a medical standpoint. Effective antiretroviral agents are available both for treating the mother's illness and for preventing mother-to-infant transmission. Infants who are at risk can be identified for (1) early initiation of antiretroviral therapy when appropriate of both mother and infant, (2) change in immunization schedule from the use of oral poliovirus vaccine (OPV) to inactivated poliovirus vaccine (IPV) and the inclusion of pneumococcal and influenza vaccines, (3) access to social service benefits to assure health care, and (4) avoidance of breast-feeding in the United States and other areas where formula substitutes are available. Along with voluntary testing of infants and women, there must be assurance of confidentiality, protection against discrimination, and access to state-of-the-art health care.

Transmission Through Breast-Feeding

Postpartum transmission of HIV infection from mother to newborn through breast-feeding has been reported and documented in women who acquired HIV infection after delivery through sexual relations and blood transfusion (Ziegler et al., 1985). A meta-analysis of studies with varying perinatal transmission rates from different parts of the world suggests that breast-feeding increases the rate of perinatal transmission of HIV by 14% (Dunn et al., 1992). Although the timing of HIV transmission by breast milk during the course of lactation remains unknown, HIV-1 DNA can be detected in more than 50% of breast milk samples, and its presence correlates with CD4+ depletion and vitamin A deficiency (Kreiss, 1997).

The risk/benefit ratio for breast-feeding in HIV-infected women is influenced by the infant mortality rate associated with infectious disease or malnutrition in conjunction with the relative risk for bottle-fed infants (American Academy of Pediatrics, 1995). Where sterile formula is readily available, this ratio is clearly in favor of bottle-feeding, and HIV-infected women should bottle-feed rather than breast-feed their infants. However, for parts of Africa and many other developing nations, the situation is much less clear and favors breast-feeding in areas where the infant mortality attributable to bottle-feeding is greater than one in seven infants. Recognizing that failure to breast-feed has health and social consequences for women throughout the world, Kuhn and Stein (1997) modeled the frequency of adverse outcomes associated with different infant feeding practices in the context of the HIV epidemic. Noting that complete avoidance of breast-feeding by the entire population in developing nations will never be a reasonable option, they concluded that early cessation of breast-feeding may be a more realistic or desirable alternative for many women.

Global and national recommendations regarding breast-feeding can be viewed as extreme since they are based on population rather than individual risk. Individual maternal and infant factors related to HIV transmission are complex and interrelated; for example, disease state and viral load will vary among women, and within a woman over time, and maternal nutrition influences immune system function and may modulate the response of lactating women to HIV infection. Therefore generalizations on which to base global recommendations may be impossible. Such recommendations are necessary and should always be based on scientific data. At present, however, it appears that insufficient data are available to develop recommendations regarding breast-feeding. Instead, experienced clinicians will need to consider the individual situation, the desires of the woman, and the social context of breast-feeding before providing advice to the patient.

Sexual Abuse

Sexual abuse has been reported as a mode of transmission of HIV infection in infants, children, and adolescents (Gellert et al., 1993). It is estimated that approximately 200,000 children are sexually abused each year in the United States (Krugman, 1991). Identifying these children is difficult, however, since sexual transmission of HIV is not a reportable category of HIV exposure for children, and there are many barriers to identification of children infected with HIV through sexual abuse (Gutman et al., 1993). Gutman and colleagues (1991) from Duke University reported that 14.6% of the HIV-infected children (N = 96) who tested positive for HIV had been sexually abused. All of these children did not necessarily become HIV infected as a result of sexual abuse, and in some instances the perpetrators knew that the child was already infected and did not use barrier precautions. This is noteworthy, since child abuse within the home may also involve siblings.

DIAGNOSTIC EVALUATION OF THE HIV-EXPOSED INFANT

All infants born to HIV-infected women should be evaluated on a regular basis until a definitive determination is made regarding their HIV status. The preferred method for diagnosing HIV infection in infants is by HIV culture or PCR testing (see Fig. 3–1). Assays should be performed at least twice: (1) once at ≥1 month of age and (2) once at ≥4 months of age. If any test result is positive, testing should be repeated to confirm the diagnosis of HIV infection.

Viral culture is performed on peripheral blood mononuclear cells that are co-cultured with uninfected mononuclear cells to promote HIV growth and detect latent HIV-infected cells by stimulating viral replication. Evidence of p24 antigen, reverse transcriptase activity, or syncytial formation indicates the presence of HIV in such samples. The sensitivity of this test is dependent on age. Results of studies indicate a sensitivity of 24% during the first week of life, 85% at 1 month, greater than 90% in infants by 2 to 3 months of age, and nearly 100% by 6 months of age (McIntosh et al., 1994).

The HIV DNA polymerase chain reaction assay facilitates the detection of minute amounts of HIV proviral DNA that have become incorporated into the DNA of infected cells. The sensi-

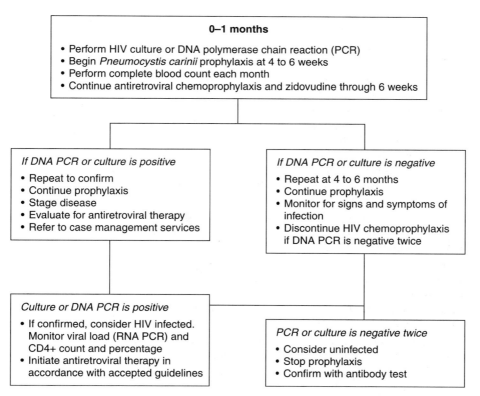

Figure 3–1 ▪ Diagnosis and evaluation of the HIV-exposed infant. (Adapted from Burr, C., O'Hara, M.J. [1996]. Clinical management of pediatric HIV patients [p. 378]. In K.M. Casey, F. Cohen, A. Hughes [Eds.], *ANAC's core curriculum for HIV/AIDS nursing*. Philadelphia: Nursecom.)

tivity and specificity of PCR as a diagnostic tool are similar to those of HIV culture. A meta-analysis of data from 271 infants revealed that 38% of HIV-infected infants had a positive PCR assay within the first 48 hours of life and that 93% of infected infants had a positive reaction by 14 days of age (Dunn et al., 1995). The use of these assays for diagnostic purposes has been recommended after 1 month of age for infants born to HIV-infected women (El-Sadr et al., 1994).

A presumptive diagnosis of HIV infection can be made with one positive HIV culture or PCR assay on noncord blood, and a definitive diagnosis can be made with a confirmatory test on a different blood sample. HIV infection can be reasonably excluded with two negative HIV culture or PCR results, one obtained at ≥1 month of age and the other at ≥4 months of age (Grubman et al., 1995). Some experienced clinicians feel reasonably comfortable with the exclusion of HIV infection by means of these assays at earlier ages. The current standard of care requires a negative HIV enzyme immunoassay (EIA) and Western blot at 18 months of age to rule out HIV infection definitively.

Whereas the EIA tests for anti-HIV antibody, the antigen capture assay tests directly for the HIV p24 antigen levels in serum. Isolated false-positive antigen capture assay results have been reported in infancy, and the question remains whether it is possible that viral particles can be transferred from mother to infant without actual infection ensuing. After the first few weeks of life, though, this test is very specific and, if positive, can be used to help establish the diagnosis. Antigen capture is not at all sensitive, with fewer than 50% of infected infants having positive reactions in the first year of life. Thus antigen capture cannot be used to rule out HIV infection and, although it is readily available and relatively easy to perform, it is not the assay of choice in diagnosing disease in infants. The reason for the low sensitivity of the standard p24 antigen capture assay is that maternal HIV-specific IgG antibody can result in antibody excess immune complexes' producing a negative result. Through a modification in the assay that involves immune complex dissociation (ICD), the sensitivity of this assay has been greatly enhanced while maintaining its specificity. There is, however, a lack of published data on age-specific sensitivity, and therefore the

ICD p24 antigen capture assay cannot be used to rule out HIV infection at this time. The recommended virologic diagnosis assays are the HIV DNA PCR and culture, with the HIV DNA PCR preferred by most clinicians because of its availability and quick turnaround time.

In children and infants older than 18 months, definitive diagnosis of HIV infection is made in the same way as it is in adults, by means of the EIA and confirmatory Western blot assays. These provide serologic evidence of a humoral immune response to HIV by detecting HIV-specific IgG antibodies. However, since maternal IgG antibody is transferred to infants across the placenta, all infants born to HIV-infected women have a positive EIA at birth. An IgG antibody response cannot be used to diagnose HIV infection definitively in infants until they are 18 months of age, when maternal antibody is no longer present and the infant's own humoral immune response should have been mounted.

In some developing countries virologic diagnostic assays are not universally available to many practitioners, and a presumptive diagnosis frequently requires correlation of clinical symptoms with surrogate laboratory parameters in HIV-exposed infants. The most frequently used laboratory parameter of immune function is the CD4+ T-cell count, and a depressed CD4+ T-cell count or a reversed CD4+/CD8 ratio is indicative of immunocompromise. However, healthy infants and children normally have much higher counts than healthy adults, and this varies with age (see Table 3–2). Although the absolute number of CD4+ T-cells is higher in infants and children, the percentage of CD4+ T-cells is relatively stable from infancy to adulthood, with a normal median value of approximately 50%. It is important to be familiar with the normal age-specific lymphocyte counts when evaluating the immune status of infants and children.

The CD4+ count and percentage are used not only to monitor the immune system in children with HIV infection but also to guide treatment decisions. The clinician making a treatment decision based on this count must be sure that the pediatric, and not the adult, value is used. These counts are subject to variation, such as intercurrent illness or immunization that produces a transient decrease in CD4+ numbers and percentages, so counts are best measured when the infant or

Table 3–2 ■ Immunologic Categories Based on Age-Specific CD4+ Lymphocyte Count and Percentage

	Age of Child		
Immune Category	<12 mo	1–5 y	6–12 y
Category 1: No suppression	>1500 mm^3 (≥25%)	≥1000 mm^3 (≥25%)	≥500 mm^3 (≥25%)
Category 2: Moderate suppression	750–1499 mm^3 (15–24%)	500–999 mm^3 (15–24%)	200–499 mm^3 (15–24%)
Category 3: Severe suppression	<750 mm^3 (<15%)	<500 mm^3 (<15%)	<200 mm^3 (<15%)

Data from Centers for Disease Control and Prevention. (1994). 1994 Revised classification system for human immunodeficiency virus infection in children less than 13 years of age. *Morbidity and Mortality Weekly Report, 34*(RR-12), 1–18.

child is clinically well. No changes in therapy should be made on the basis of a change in CD4+ number until the count has been measured twice, with at least 1 week between measurements. CD4+ counts and percentages should be measured in all HIV-exposed infants at 1 and 3 months of age. CD4+ monitoring is not required once HIV infection has been reasonably excluded. For those infants with a diagnosis of HIV, CD4+ values should be monitored at 6, 9, and 12 months of age.

Not only is the immune status monitored with CD4+ T-cell counts, but HIV activity is quantified with viral load testing. Relatively high viral burden may persist in infants during the first year of life, with 98% having greater than 100,000 copies per milliliter. Viral load is measured by HIV RNA PCR as opposed to HIV DNA PCR , which is used to diagnose HIV infection. Typically, viral burden decreases slowly, reflecting the influence of an immature immune system or a greater number of HIV-susceptible HIV cells in the infant (Palumbo et al., 1995). Preliminary data indicate that high RNA levels in infants less than 12 months of age may be correlated with disease progression and survival. Very high RNA levels (above 100,000/ml) in children more than 2 years of age have been associated with increased mortality risk. The risk for disease progression is age independent; that is, it is driven by RNA value (viral load) and not age.

Recent published data from a cohort of infants and children showed that plasma RNA and CD4+ lymphocyte count are independent predictors of clinical course (Palumbo et al., 1998). This study showed CD4+ lymphocyte count had strong, independent predicative ability for disease progression, as is true for adults. Further, the study documented a linear relationship between plasma log$_{10}$ RNA and relative risk for disease progression in children. The clinical implication is obvious: control and suppression of viral load through agressive antiretroviral treatment should be the goal of therapy. For the first time, clinicians have targeted laboratory values that can be used to monitor therapy and risk of disease progression.

Most infants and children with HIV infection have polyclonal hypergammaglobulinemia, very high levels of all immunoglobulins—IgG, IgM, and IgA (Joshi et al., 1990). Normal immunoglobulin levels in infants and children are also age-specific and need to be considered when a child is being evaluated for hypergammaglobulinemia. Elevated beta-2 microglobulin and neopterin levels have been reported in HIV-infected children. Other laboratory abnormalities seen in pediatric HIV infection include (1) hypogammaglobulinemia, seen in 3% to 5% of cases, (2) anemia, which is usually secondary to chronic disease and has been associated with disease progression (other causes such as iron deficiency, sickle cells, and lead toxicity must be ruled out), (3) thrombocytopenia, seen in about 10% to 20% of HIV-infected children and documented to be associated with antiplatelet antibody in 80% of these, and (4) leukopenia.

PRESENTATION AND PROGNOSIS IN INFANTS AND CHILDREN

There are two general patterns of presentation of HIV infection in children. The first pattern, representing about one third of all perinatally acquired infections, is a fulminant course of illness represented by early onset of severe disease with rapid progression and poor prognosis (Duliege et al., 1992). Rapid progressors are infants with early onset of disease manifestations who die by the age of 4 years. Infants in this group usually have severe opportunistic infections (most often *Pneumocystis carinii* pneumonia [PCP]), encephalopathy, or both, within the first 2 years of life. Many of these children become identified as being infected with HIV because of severe illnesses that arise abruptly. PCP in this group is seldom insidious; the primary care provider may see an infant with some mild general symptoms, and then 1 week later the child may manifest fulminant, life-threatening PCP. Because these infants are prone to rapid-onset PCP, early primary chemoprophylaxis is required.

The second pattern of pediatric HIV infection involves later onset of disease symptoms and is associated with a better prognosis. These children generally are seen after the first year of life with a more indolent disease course, consisting of a variety of the more general clinical manifestations. Compared with children in whom AIDS is diagnosed in the first year of life, these children more often have a diagnosis of lymphoid interstitial pneumonitis (LIP) and manifest other signs of lymphoproliferation, such as generalized lymphadenopathy and parotitis. In some instances, the child is school-age before LIP develops and a diagnosis of perinatal HIV infection is established; in other cases the diagnosis of AIDS or HIV infection is not made until the child is 10 or 11 years of age. One study has reported a median incubation period of more than 6 years in this group, which is comparable to the adult experience (Auger et al., 1988). In a cohort of perinatally infected children between the ages of 9 and 16 years followed at the Children's Hospital AIDS Program in Newark, New Jersey, the mean age at diagnosis of HIV infection was 7.3 years (88 months). Although most of the children in this cohort had HIV-related symptoms or significant disease, almost one fourth of them remained free of symptoms with relatively intact immune systems at a mean age of 11.3 years (Grubman et al., 1995).

Children whose symptoms appear later in life may be clinically similar to asymptomatic adults or may show only subtle HIV-related signs and symptoms before demonstrating more obvious conditions, such as oral candidiasis. Recurrent bacterial infections are likely to occur as AIDS-defining conditions in both early- and late-onset presentation of HIV. Frequently, renal and cardiac involvement occurs later in the illness after other significant HIV-related disease has been diagnosed (see Chapter 4).

A number of factors may contribute to a more fulminant course of HIV disease in some children than in others. Rapid progressors are more likely to have been infected during the early prenatal period or to have been born to women with more advanced disease. Blanche and colleagues (1994) studied 162 HIV-infected infants and noted that the risk of opportunistic infection or encephalopathy in the first 18 months of life correlated directly with the degree of maternal HIV-related symptoms as well the p24 antigen level and was inversely related to maternal CD4+ T-cell count at the time of delivery. In this study, 50% of infants born to mothers with AIDS had OIs or encephalopathy by the age of 18 months, compared with 14% of infants born to mothers who were either free of symptoms or had generalized lymphadenopathy. Mayaux and associates (1996) observed that infants who have positive virologic test results within the first week of life are more likely to progress rapidly to AIDS within the first year. Unpublished data presented at the Eleventh International Conference on AIDS in July 1996 indicate that infants with rapidly progressing disease have higher plasma HIV RNA copy counts during the first 12 months of life and are more likely to have positive HIV cultures within the first 2 days of life.

Two major clinical factors that appear to affect the prognosis in children with HIV infection are the specific HIV-related diseases that they develop and their age at presentation of disease. Scott and colleagues (1990) studied 172 perinatally infected children and found a median survival rate from diagnosis of:

- 1 month for those with PCP
- 5 months for those with nephropathy
- 11 months for those with encephalopathy
- 12 months for those with *Candida* esophagitis
- 50 months for those with recurrent bacterial infection
- 72 months for those with LIP

A study at the Children's Hospital of New Jersey showed a median survival of 2 months after PCP (Connor et al., 1991). PCP continues to be a leading AIDS indicator disease in infants less than 1 year of age and carries a grave prognosis in this group. On the basis of these data, it appears that both delayed clinical presentation and infectious disease are associated with longer survival.

It is important to note that the prognosis is related to the specific AIDS-indicator disease and not to the general nonspecific diagnosis of AIDS. For example, opportunistic infections and encephalopathy are associated with significantly higher morbidity and mortality rates than either LIP or recurrent bacterial infections. Although an AIDS diagnosis may be of epidemiologic interest and can be important in accessing public entitlement programs such as Social Security Insurance (SSI), without specifying the AIDS-indicator diseases, it is of limited value in predicting survival time. This is an extremely important issue for primary care providers, since many parents and caregivers assume that a diagnosis of AIDS means that a child will die within a very short period of time. It is important for health care workers to discuss the prognosis for a child in the context of the specific diseases that the child has developed.

CLINICAL MANIFESTATIONS

HIV infection in infants and children is a chronic disease with multiorgan system involvement. As in adults, HIV disease appears in infants and children with a broad spectrum of manifestations, some of which are unique to children. The present CDC classification system considers both immunologic and clinical criteria (see Table 3–3). The scheme divides children into four clinical categories according to clinical presentation. Most of the symptomatic clinical manifestations of pediatric HIV disease are related to either the direct cytopathic effect of HIV infection or the consequences of immunosuppression. Clinical symptoms vary widely and range from common, nonspecific findings to severe manifestations of common childhood illnesses, AIDS-defining conditions, or end-organ dysfunction (see Box, p. 74). Immunologic categories are based on age-specific CD4+ T- lymphocyte counts and percentages (see Table 3–2).

Common clinical findings in children with HIV that are not AIDS-defining include lymphadenopathy, hepatomegaly, splenomegaly, parotis, recurrent diarrhea, failure to thrive, and recurrent fevers. It is important to evaluate children for specific infectious etiologic factors for these conditions, although HIV or the ensuing immunodeficiency may be the sole cause. Common oropharyngeal signs include persistent candidiasis, severe painful gingivitis, HIV-specific periodontal disease, recurrent aphthous stomatitis, and recurrent herpetic gingivostomatitis. Some of these conditions are extremely common, and, as commonly seen in adults, lymphoproliferation

---

Table 3–3 ■ Pediatric HIV Classification System*

Immunologic Categories	Clinical Categories			
	N: No Signs or Symptoms[†]	A: Mild Signs or Symptoms[‡]	B: Moderate Signs or Symptoms[§]	C: Severe Signs or Symptoms[‖]
(1) No evidence of immune suppression	N1	A1	B1	C1
(2) Evidence of moderate immune suppression	N2	A2	B2	C2
(3) Severe immune suppression	N3	A3	B3	C3

*Children whose HIV infection is not confirmed are classified by the above system with a letter *E* (perinatally exposed) before the classification (e.g., E/N2).
[†]No signs or symptoms or only one of those in category A.
[‡]Two or more of the following: lymphadenopathy, hepatomegaly, splenomegaly, dermatitis, parotitis, recurrent or persistent upper respiratory infection or sinusitis, recurrent or persistent otitis media.
[§]Symptomatic conditions not listed in category A or C (including LIP).
[‖]Any of the conditions in the 1987 surveillance case definition of AIDS with the exception of LIP that is in category B.
Data from Centers for Disease Control and Prevention. (1994). 1994 Revised classification system for human immunodeficiency virus infection in children less than 13 years of age. *Morbidity and Mortality Weekly Report, 43*(RR-12), 1–19.

▨ CLINICAL CATEGORIES FOR CHILDREN WITH HIV INFECTION ▨

Category N: Not Symptomatic
Children who have no signs or symptoms considered to be the result of HIV infection or who have only *one* of the conditions listed in Category A

Category A: Mildly Symptomatic
Children with *two* or more of the following conditions but none of the conditions listed in Category B or C:

Lymphadenopathy	Dermatitis
Hepatomegaly	Parotitis
Splenomegaly	Recurrent or persistent upper respiratory infection, sinusitis, or otitis media

Category B: Moderately Symptomatic
Children who have symptomatic conditions other than those listed for Category A or C that are attributed to HIV infection. Examples of conditions in Category B include but are not limited to:

Anemia (<8 g/dl, neutropenia (<1000/mm^3), or thrombocytopenia (<100,000/mm^3) persisting ≥30 days
Bacterial meningitis, pneumonia, or sepsis (single episode)
Candidiasis, oropharyngeal (thrush), persisting >2 months in children >6 months of age
Cardiomyopathy
Cytomegalovirus infection, with onset before 1 month of age
Diarrhea, recurrent or chronic
Hepatitis
Herpes simplex virus (HSV) stomatitis, recurrent (more than two episodes within 1 year)

HSV bronchitis, pneumonitis, or esophagitis with onset before 1 month of age
Herpes zoster (shingles) involving at least two distinct episodes or more than one dermatome
Leiomyosarcoma
Lymphoid interstitial pneumonia (LIP) or pulmonary lymphoid hyperplasia complex
Nephropathy
Nocardiosis
Persistent fever (lasting >1 month)
Toxoplasmosis, onset before 1 month of age
Varicella, disseminated (complicated chickenpox)

Category C: Severly Symptomatic
Children who have any condition listed in the 1987 surveillance case definition for acquired immunodeficiency syndrome, with the exception of LIP (which is a Category B condition)

Data from Centers for Disease Control and Prevention. (1994). 1994 revised classification system for human immunodeficiency virus infection in children less than 13 years of age. *Morbidity and Mortality Weekly Report, 43*(RR-12), 1–19.

---

manifesting as lymphadenopathy may be the first objective sign of disease.

There is a broad clinical spectrum of neurologic abnormalities seen in pediatric HIV infection. Most children have some degree of developmental delay, whether subtle or obvious, that affects both motor and cognitive milestones. The presentation of developmental delay is variable. There may be a relatively normal development period suddenly followed by either a loss of milestones or a failure to attain new milestones. Periods of relative stability in neurologic function (static encephalopathy) or a course of rapid neurodevelopmental deterioration (progressive encephalopathy) may follow the onset of develop-

mental delay. Pyramidal tract involvement may be seen, with resulting spastic paresis. Hypertonicity and hyperreflexia are common manifestations of motor involvement.

Static encephalopathy is seen in about one fourth of children with HIV and is characterized by developmental delay of varying severity without loss of previously attained milestones. Children in this group can have improvement in neurologic function with continued acquisition of developmental skills, but usually in a delayed manner. Progressive encephalopathy, characterized by progressive deterioration in cognitive, motor, or language skills and a loss of previously attained developmental milestones is often seen in patients who also have OI. Progressive encephalopathy, which is associated with a very poor prognosis, can be characterized by a plateau course without continued loss of milestones, by a subacute progressive course associated with slow continued losses in motor and nonmotor developmental milestones, or by a rapidly progressive course. Neuroimaging studies of HIV infection in children include findings of ventricular enlargement, cerebral atrophy, attenuation of white matter, and calcification of cerebral and basal ganglia (DeCarli et al., 1993). The possibility of a central nervous system (CNS) lymphoma must always be considered in the child in whom new neurologic signs and symptoms develop.

Antiretroviral therapy with zidovudine has been shown to improve the neurodevelopmental functioning of infants and children with HIV. With therapy, children can regain lost motor and developmental milestones, and in some the response is dramatic, with the reversal of incontinence, gait abnormalities, or lost cognitive milestones.

HIV-associated malignant neoplasms are reported in approximately 3% of children, including non-Hodgkin's lymphoma, Burkitt's lymphoma, immunoblastic lymphoma, and CNS lymphoma (Mueller et al., 1994). Other reported cancers such as leiomyoma and leiomyosarcoma are believed to be associated with Epstein-Barr virus infection. Kaposi's sarcoma is unusual in children in the United States. Diagnosis and management of these malignant conditions are similar to those in other children, and referral to an experienced pediatric oncology center, a tertiary care setting, or both is appropriate.

TREATMENT OF HIV INFECTION AND RELATED CONDITIONS

The medical management of children with HIV includes (1) regular immunologic monitoring with CD4+ T-cell counts and percentages, (2) regular virologic monitoring with HIV RNA determinations, (3) HIV-specific antiretroviral treatment, (4) prevention and treatment of infections, both bacterial and opportunistic, and (5) general supportive management.

General supportive management includes psychosocial support, symptom management, nutritional supplementation, developmental intervention, patient education, and advocacy. Education of parents or other caregivers about supportive care is basic and important. Topics covered should include hand washing; bathing the child regularly (daily or every other day); keeping the child's skin clean and dry, especially in the diaper area; moisturizing the skin in other areas to prevent cracking and itching and thus prevent fungal infections and impetigo; changing diapers; and cleaning bottles. Providers need to educate caregivers concerning the signs and symptoms that require medical attention.

Medical management should encompass general well-child care, including childhood immunizations. Because HIV-infected children are particularly susceptible to disease, all at-risk children should be immunized against childhood diseases (see Fig. 3–2). Immunizations represent the cornerstone of preventive medicine for children. The childhood immunization schedule recommended by the Advisory Committee on Immunization Practices and the American Academy of Pediatrics (1997) should be used in HIV-infected children with some modifications. Paralytic poliomyelitis is a potential complication of the oral polio vaccine (OPV) for both the immunocompromised patient and immunocompromised family members because of virus excreted in the patient's stool. The use of inactivated polio vaccine (IPV) instead of OPV is recommended for HIV-infected infants and children as well as for uninfected infants and children living in households with infected adults.

There is also a potential for serious complications from other attenuated viral vaccines, such as measles vaccine. Although the use of measles-mumps-rubella (MMR) vaccine is recommended for most HIV-infected children, the CDC (1996c) currently recommends consideration of withholding MMR vaccine from severely immunocompromised HIV-infected children. HIV-infected children who have been exposed to such diseases as measles should be immunized within 72 hours of exposure, even if they have not yet reached the normal age for immunization. Any HIV-infected child who is exposed to measles should receive intramuscular serum immune globulin as prophylaxis. The increased mortality and morbidity rates for measles have led to the recommendation that children in high-prevalence measles areas, who fail to develop protective anti-

Age → / Vaccine ↓	Birth	1 mo	2 mo	4 mo	6 mo	12 mo	15 mo	18 mo	24 mo	4–6 y	11–12 y	14–16 y
↓	Recommendations for these vaccines are the same as those for immunocompetent children											↓
Hepatitis B†	Hep B-1											
		Hep B-2			Hep B-3						Hep B	
Diphtheria, Tetanus, Pertussis‡		DTaP or DTP	DTaP or DTP	DTaP or DTP		DTaP or DTP				DTaP or DTP	Td	
Haemophilus§ *influenzae* type b		Hib	Hib	Hib		Hib						
↓	Recommendations for these vaccines differ from those for immunocompetent children											↓
Polio‖			IPV	IPV		IPV				IPV		
Measles, Mumps, Rubella¶						MMR	MMR					
Influenza#						Influenza (a dose is required every year)						
*Streptococcus pneumoniae***									Pneumo-coccal			
Varicella						CONTRAINDICATED in *all* HIV-infected persons						

NOTE: Modified from the immunization schedule for immunocompetent children. This schedule also applies to children born to HIV-infected mothers whose HIV infection status has not been determined. Once a child is known not to be HIV-infected, the schedule for immunocompetent children applies. This schedule indicates the recommended age for routine administration of currently licensed childhood vaccines. Some combination vaccines are available and may be used whenever administration of all components of the vaccine is indicated. Providers should consult the manufacturers' package inserts for detailed recommendations.

*Vaccines are listed under the routinely recommended ages. Bars indicate range of acceptable ages for vaccination. Shaded bars indicate catch-up vaccination: at 11 to 12 years of age, hepatitis B vaccine should be administered to children not previously vaccinated.

†**Infants born to HBsAg-negative mothers** should receive 2.5 μg of Merck vaccine (Recombivax HB) or 10 μg of SmithKline Beecham (SB) vaccine (Engerix-B). The second dose should be administered more than1 month after the first dose. **Infants born to HBsAg-positive mothers** should receive 0.5 ml of hepatitis B immune globulin (HBIG) within 12 hours of birth and either 5 μg of Merck vaccine (Recombivax HB) or 10 μg of SB vaccine (Engerix-B) at a separate site. The second dose is recommended at 1 to 2 months of age and the third dose at 6 months of age. **Infants born to mothers whose HBsAg status is unknown** should receive either 5 μg of Merck vaccine (Recombivax HB) or 10 μg or SB vaccine (Engerix-B) within 12 hours of birth. The second dose of vaccine is recommended at 1 month of age, and the third dose at 6 months of age. Blood should be drawn at the time of delivery to determine the mother's HBsAg status; if it is positive,the infant should receive HBIG as soon as possible (no later than 1 week of age). The dosage and timing of subsequent vaccine doses should be based on the mother's HBsAg status. **Children and adolescents who have not been vaccinated against hepatitis B in infancy** may begin the series during any childhood visit. Those who have not previously received three doses of hepatitis B vaccine should initiate or complete the series during the 11- to 12-year-old visit. The second dose should be administered at least 1 month after the first dose, and the third dose should be administered at least 4 months after the first dose and at least 2 months after the second dose.

‡DTaP (diphtheria and tetanus toxoids and acellular pertussis vaccine) is the preferred vaccine for all doses in the vaccination series, including completion of the series in children who have received more than one dose of whole-cell DTP vaccine. Whole-cell DTP is an acceptable alternative to DTaP. The fourth dose of DTaP may be administered as early as 12 months of age, provided 6 months have elapsed since the third dose and provided the child is considered unlikely to return at 15 to 18 months of age. Td (tetanus and diphtheria toxoids, absorbed, for adult use) is recommended at 11 to 12 years of age if at least 5 years have elapsed since the last dose of DTP, DTaP, or DT. Subsequent routine Td boosters are recommended every 10 years.

§Three *Haemophilus influenzae* type b (Hib) conjugate vaccines are licensed for infant use. If PRP-OMP (PedvaxHIB [Merck]) is administered at 2 and 4 months of age, a dose at 6 months is not required. After the primary series has been completed, any Hib conjugate vaccine may be used as a booster.

‖Inactivated poliovirus vaccine (IPV) is the only polio vaccine recommended for HIV-infected persons and their household contacts. Although the third dose of IPV is generally administered at 12 to 18 months of age, the third dose of IPV has been approved to be administered as early as 6 months of age. Oral poliovirus vaccine (OPV) should *not* be administered to HIV-infected persons or their household contacts.

¶Measles, Mumps, Rubella (MMR) should not be administered to severely immunocompromised children. HIV-infected children without severe immunosuppression should routinely receive their first dose of MMR as soon as possible on reaching the first birthday. Consideration should be given to administering the second dose of MMR vaccine as soon as 1 month (i.e., a minimum of 28 days) after the first dose, rather than waiting until school entry.

#Influenze virus vaccine should be administered to all HIV-infected children >6 months of age each year. Children 6 months to 8 years of age who are receiving influenza vaccine for the first time should receive two doses of split-virus vaccine separated by at least 1 month. In subsequent years a single dose of vaccine (split virus for persons ≤12 years of age, whole or split for persons >12 years of age) should be administered each year. The dose of vaccine for children 6–35 months of age is 0.25 ml; the dose for children ≥3 years of age is 0.5 ml (page •••).

**The 23-valent pneumococcal vaccine should be administered to HIV-infected children at 24 months of age. Revaccination should generally be offered to HIV-infected children vaccinated when 3–5 years (children aged ≤10 years of age) or >5 years (children aged >10 years of age) earlier.

Figure 3–2 ▪ Recommended immunization schedule for HIV-infected children. (From Centers for Disease Control and Prevention. [1997]. USPHS/IDSA guidelines for the prevention of opportunistic infections in persons with human immunodeficiency virus. *Morbidity and Mortality Weekly Report, 46*[RR-12], 34.)

bodies after two MMR immunizations, should receive regular intravenous infusions of immune globulin (IVIG). Children already receiving IVIG therapy may be protected but should receive an additional dose if the exposure occurs more than 2 weeks after the last infusion. Some children with life-threatening manifestations of measles, such as pneumonitis, have been also treated with intravenous ribavirin on a compassionate use basis.

The recently approved varicella vaccine is a live attenuated vaccine and should not be used in HIV-infected children. Parents should report varicella (chickenpox) exposure immediately, and HIV-infected children should receive varicella-zoster immune globulin (VZIG) within 96 hours of exposure to prevent or modify infection. Providers must be aware that VZIG prolongs the incubation period to 10 to 28 days.

Normally, varicella virus is controlled by cell-mediated immune mechanisms and is a self-limited illness. In children with immune system impairment, however, it can cause prolonged and disseminated morbidity, with such complications as neurologic encephalitis and pneumonia. Symptoms include a pruritic vesicular rash on the face, scalp, and trunk, preceded by systemic symptoms, including fever, chills, myalgia, and arthralgia. The treatment of choice is intravenous administration of acyclovir until lesions dry to decrease pain and hasten healing. Immunocompromised children who have had varicella are at risk of its reactivation as herpes zoster (shingles), which can be severe and disseminated.

A yearly injection of influenza vaccine is recommended, and the pneumococcal vaccine should be administered to infected children at 2 years of age. Ramilo and associates (1996) reported that the administration of influenza vaccine was associated with a significant increase in viral load in 5 of 16 children who did not receive antiretroviral therapy. Although the HIV viral load returned to its baseline level by 6 to 8 weeks after immunization, it is not clear what impact, if any, these repeated immunizations have on the course of the disease; however, influenza vaccine is still recommended.

Symptom-free, immunocompetent children would be expected to produce protective antibodies in response to immunization. Information on the antibody response after immunization can be obtained by performing postvaccination serum titers. Children with symptomatic infection, documented humoral or antibody deficiencies, or both, may have a poor immunologic response, resulting in lack of protective antibodies. Such children, when exposed to a vaccine-preventable disease such as measles, should be considered susceptible regardless of the history of vaccination. Even with appropriate immunization, many HIV-infected children, especially those with low CD4+ T-cell counts, do not mount protective antibody responses against measles and continue to be susceptible because of their impaired humoral immune response (Palumbo et al., 1992).

As the CD4+ T-cell count declines and immunodeficiency increases, HIV-infected children with documented antibodies in response to exposure to or immunization against an infectious agent can lose this protection. Therefore it is extremely important for primary care providers to review immunization status regularly, particularly at those times of the year when measles and chickenpox are reported in the community.

Antiretroviral Therapy

The majority of data from trials of antiretroviral therapy, including those with clinical end points and those with surrogate marker end points, have been obtained in the HIV-infected adult population. This is especially true regarding data on the more recently approved reverse transcriptase inhibitors (lamivudine and stavudine) and protease inhibitors. Of the eleven antiretroviral agents currently approved for use in adults and adolescents in the United States, only five (zidovudine, didanosine, and lamivudine, nelfinavir, and indinavir) are approved for use in infants and children under the age of 13 years. The approval of lamivudine was based almost entirely on adult data.

The Working Group on Antiretroviral Therapy and Medical Management of HIV Infected Children (1997) has outlined the indications for the initiation of antiretroviral therapy in HIV-1–infected children, including (1) clinical symptoms related to HIV-1 infection (clinical category A, B, or C), (2) evidence of immune suppression, as indicated by CD4+ lymphocyte absolute number or percentage in CDC immune category 2 or 3, (3) all HIV-1–infected infants under 12 months of age regardless of clinical, immunologic, or virologic status, and (4) asymptomatic HIV-1–infected children over 1 year of age with normal immune status who have a rapidly declining CD4+ lymphocyte number or percentage to values approaching the moderate immune status level (CDC immune category 2) or have a high or increasing HIV RNA viral load.

Zidovudine was approved by the FDA for use in children 3 years after it was approved for use in adults. Its approval for children was based on the results of efficacy trials in adults, pharmacokinetic and toxicity trials in children, and some efficacy data that were deduced from phase I and phase II studies in children. It is important that drug development for use in children proceed in parallel with development for use in adults and not after that development. This situation does not seem to be improving, as three new protease inhibitors have been approved for use in adults without adequate pharmacokinetic data being available on their use in infants and children.

INITIATION OF ANTIRETROVIRAL THERAPY. The first consensus guidelines for antiretroviral treatment in children, published in 1993, recommended therapy only for the infected child with evidence of significant immunodeficiency (based on age-related CD4+ count) or with HIV-associated symptoms. ZDV monotherapy was recommended as the standard of care. In the years since these recommendations were made, dramatic advances in basic and clinical research have occurred. It is now recognized that the rapidity and magnitude of HIV-1 replication during all stages of infection are much greater than previously thought and account for the emergence of drug-resistant variants when antiretroviral therapy is not adequate to suppress replication. Therapeutic strategies now focus on early institution of regimens capable of suppressing viral replication to reduce the development of resistance and to preserve immunologic function.

Perinatal HIV infection occurs in immunologically naive and developing persons, leading to differences in HIV manifestations, rate of disease progression, and response to available interventions. In addition, there are well-documented changes in drug pharmacokinetics during the transition from the newborn period to adulthood that require specific evaluation of drug dosing and toxicity in infants and children. Finally, treatment of perinatally transmitted HIV infection will happen in the context of exposure to antiretroviral drugs given during pregnancy, delivery, and the neonatal period to treat mothers, to prevent perinatal transmission, or both.

There are many issues that a care provider must grapple with in deciding when to initiate antiretroviral therapy and determining which agents are most appropriate as initial therapy for HIV-infected infants and children. It is reasonable to assume that the underlying virologic character of HIV infection is similar in the adult and pediatric populations. The fact that such infections generally progress more rapidly in infants and children than in adults is consistent with the current understanding of the prognostic value of viral load in the adult population and emerging data of higher HIV RNA copy numbers in infants and children as compared with adults. It is safe, therefore, to assume that in infants and children, as in adults, a high viral load indicates a poor prognosis and a low viral load indicates a good one. Unfortunately, there are insufficient data regarding the absolute numbers of viral loads in infants and children to provide concrete guidelines for antiretroviral therapy. In addition, providers must decide how appropriate it is to extrapolate from adult clinical and surrogate marker data (discussed in Chapter 5) for their patients. Management of infants and children infected with HIV is increasingly complex and rapidly evolving. Such management requires the direction of care by a specialist in pediatric HIV or consultation when such a specialist is not available in the geographic area.

Other important questions are (1) whether it is appropriate to initiate therapy with the one agent or a combination of agents with the strongest documented antiretroviral activity (based on adult viral load data) or (2) whether it is best to reserve this therapy for patients with progressing disease and adding drugs to the initial therapy. These questions are difficult to answer because available antiretroviral agents are virustatic and not virucidal (effecting a cure) and because of the plethora of data showing limited efficacy due to the emergence of antiretroviral drug resistance in patients receiving combination therapy. Although both approaches can be defended and may be considered appropriate, there is little controversy regarding some issues.

Antiretroviral therapy has been shown to provide significant clinical benefit to children with clinical or immunologic symptoms of HIV infection. More recently, pediatric trials in antiretroviral-naive children with symptoms have demonstrated that combination therapy with either zidovudine, lamivudine, or zidovudine and didanosine are clinically, immunologically, and virologically superior to initial monotherapy with zidovudine or didanosine (Englund et al., 1997; Kline et al., 1997; Luzuriaga et al., 1997).

Results of clinical trials of antiretroviral therapy in asymptomatic infants and children with normal immune function are not yet available. The theoretical benefits of early therapy must be weighed with the potential risks such as short- and long-term drug toxicity, antiretroviral resistance, and limitation of future treatment options. Published recommendations from the Working Group on Antiretroviral Therapy and Medical Management of HIV Infected Children (1997) convened by the National Pediatric and Family HIV Resource Center support early combination treatment for certain groups of children (see Box below). Treatment is now recommended for all infants under 12 months of age as soon as a confirmed diagnosis is established, regardless of clinical status, immunologic status, or viral load. Antiretroviral dosing in neonates is extremely complex, and data are lacking on drugs other than zidovudine. There are currently no data available regarding drug dosage, safety, or tolerance of any of the protease inhibitors in neonates. Therefore newborn infants should be treated only by providers who are experienced in perinatal HIV infection.

Clinicians who are uncomfortable with such an aggressive approach could consider careful monitoring of the infant's clinical, immunologic, and viral status and could delay therapy in situations where the risk of clinically significant disease progression is low (e.g., low viral load) and other factors favor deferring treatment. In such situations, therapy should be initiated when clinical symptoms appear, when there is a rapid decline in CD4+ T-cell count or percentage of CD+ T-cells indicating moderate immune suppression, and when there is a high or increasing HIV RNA level.

CHANGING THE ANTIRETROVIRAL REGIMEN. A change in the initial antiretroviral regimen should

---

■ INDICATIONS FOR INITIATION OF ANTIRETROVIRAL THERAPY IN HIV-INFECTED CHILDREN* ■

1. Clinical symptoms related to HIV infection (clinical category A, B, or C, see Box, p. 74).
2. Evidence of immune suppression, as indicated by CD4+ lymphocyte absolute number or percentage in immunologic category 2 or 3 (Table 3–2).
3. All HIV-infected infants under 12 months of age regardless of clinical, immunologic, or virologic status.
4. For asymptomatic HIV-infected children over 1 year of age with normal immune status:
   a. Most Working Group members recommend initiating therapy in all HIV-infected children regardless of age or symptomatic, immunologic, or virologic status.
   b. Some Working Group members would recommend considering deferral of treatment in situations in which the risk of clinically significant disease progression is low (see text) and other factors (e.g., concern for the durability of response, safety, adherence) favor deferring treatment. In such cases, clinical, immunologic, and virologic status should be closely monitored. Factors that should be considered in deciding to initiate therapy include
      (1) Development of clinical symptoms
      (2) Rapidly declining CD4+ lymphocyte number or percentage to values approaching the moderate immune suppression (CDC immune category 2) level
      (3) High or rising HIV RNA copy count (see text for further discussion of HIV RNA levels)

*Indications for initiation of antiretroviral therapy in HIV-infected adolescents should follow the Adult Guidelines (PanelRec 97).
Data from Working Group on Antiretroviral Therapy and Medical Management of HIV-infected Children (1997).

be considered in any patient with clinical, immunologic, or virologic disease progression or demonstrated drug intolerance. When a child, while undergoing therapy, progresses from one CDC-defined immunologic category to another or demonstrates a rapid or persistent decline in CD4+, a change should be considered. Any observed change should be validated with at least one repeated measurement obtained at least 1 week after the initial test. Which agent(s) should be used as second- and third-line therapy depends on which agent(s) the patient had been given initially, whether there had been drug intolerance, and the toxicity profile of other available agents. A physician who is experienced in pediatric HIV disease should be consulted when these decisions are made.

The goal of antiretroviral therapy is to obtain suppression of viral replication below levels capable of detection with current HIV-1 RNA assays. Because HIV-1 RNA levels in perinatal infection are extremely high, it may take as much as 8 to 12 weeks to see a response to treatment, and complete suppression to undetectable levels may not be achieved in some children despite combination therapy. Therefore virologic indications for changing therapy differ from those of adults. Adult guidelines should be followed for adolescents (see Chapter 5, Box, p. 151). Failure to maximally suppress replication is thought to be associated with viral mutation and emergence of resistance. Clinicians need to recognize that changing a regimen may limit future options for therapy. The choice of a new regimen is dictated by the clinical, immunologic, and virologic situation as well as by the drug options available.

The antiretroviral agents used to treat HIV infection in children have demonstrated individual as well as drug class toxicities that limit both the dosages and combinations that can be used. When drug toxicities do occur in children, the frequency and severity may differ significantly from toxicities observed in adults. All efforts should be made to continue therapy in the presence of non-life-threatening toxicities. This should include liberal use of adjunctive measures such as granulocyte colony-stimulating factor for treatment of neutropenia and erythropoietin, transfusions for treatment of anemia, and symptom management for side effects.

Intravenous Immune Globulin Therapy

Intravenous immune globulin (IVIG) is standard therapy for children and adults with primary humoral immunodeficiency disorders such as Bruton's agammaglobulinemia. Passive immunotherapy in the form of IVIG provides protection against a wide range of bacterial and viral pathogens. Children with HIV infection often have functional abnormalities of the B-cell–mediated immune system that place them at risk of infections that require an intact humoral immune response. Although most children with HIV infection have elevated immunoglobulin levels, this is believed to represent nonspecific polyclonal B-cell activation. Many children fail to mount an antibody response to routine childhood immunization, indicating a functional immunodeficiency.

Pediatric immunologists have been using IVIG in HIV-infected children with B-cell immunodeficiency since early in the epidemic, resulting in (1) a reduced frequency of sepsis and other clinical symptoms, (2) improvements in mitogen-induced lymphoproliferative responses, and (3) in some cases, a decrease in the concentration of circulating immune complexes. Mofenson and colleagues (1993), in a placebo-controlled trial, studied the efficacy of IVIG therapy for HIV-infected children and found that IVIG prolonged the time the children were free from serious or minor bacterial and viral infections and was also associated with a slowing of CD4+ T-cell count decline. The study did not separately evaluate the efficacy in those children with documented B-cell defects but looked only at groups based on CD4+ counts. Other studies have not shown any additional protection against bacterial infections in children receiving IVIG and trimethoprim-sulfamethoxazole. Increases in survival related to IVIG have not been reported.

On the basis of available research and clinical experience in treating children with humoral immunodeficiency and HIV infection, many pediatric HIV specialists have agreed that IVIG (400 mg/kg every 28 days) should be considered for use in HIV-infected children with the following conditions: (1) evidence of humoral immunodeficiency (hypo- or hypergammaglobulinemia) as defined by severe recurrent bacterial infections despite appropriate antimicrobial prophylaxis and therapy, (2) residence in a community with a high prevalence of measles, without detectable antibody to measles despite two measles immunizations, (3) thrombocytopenia, and (4) chronic bronchiectasis with failure to respond to antibiotics and pulmonary care (Working Group on Antretroviral Therapy and Medical Management of HIV Infected Children, 1997).

Prophylaxis for Opportunistic Diseases

A comprehensive approach to prevention of opportunistic and recurrent serious infection requires integration of monitoring of immunologic function, administration of immunizations, prophylactic antimicrobials, and use of immunoglobulin. For those conditions in which prophylaxis is known to be safe and effective, primary prophylaxis can reduce the likelihood of infection. With the exception of PCP and *Mycobacterium avium-intracellulare* complex, opportunistic diseases common in adults occur infrequently in children. Therefore, primary prophylaxis for

Table 3–4 ▪ Prophylaxis for First Episode of Opportunistic Disease in HIV-infected Infants and Children

Pathogen	Indication	First Choice	Alternatives
I. STRONGLY RECOMMENDED AS STANDARD OF CARE			
*Pneumocystis carinii**	HIV-infected or HIV-indeterminate infants aged 1–12 mo HIV-infected children aged 1–5 y with CD4+ count <500/µl or CD4+ percentage <15% HIV-infected children aged 6–12 y with CD4+ count <200/µl or CD4+ percentage <15%	Trimethoprim-sulfamethoxazole (TMP-SMZ)	Aerosolized pentamidine (children aged ≥5 y) via Respirgard II nebulizer; dapsone (children aged ≥1 mo); IV pentamidine
Mycobacterium tuberculosis Isoniazid-sensitive	TST reaction ≥5 mm or prior positive TST result without treatment or contact with case of active tuberculosis	Isoniazid	Rifampin
Isoniazid-resistant	Same as above; high probability of exposure to isoniazid-resistant tuberculosis	Rifampin	Uncertain
Multidrug (isoniazid and rifampin)-resistant	Same as above; high probability of exposure to multidrug-resistant tuberculosis	Choice of drug requires consultation with public health authorities	None
Mycobacterium avium complex	For children aged ≥6 y, CD4+ count <50/µl; aged 2–6 y, CD4+ count <75/µl; aged 1–2 y, CD4+ count <500/µl; aged <1 y, CD4+ count <750/µl	Clarithromycin or azithromycin	Children aged ≥6 y, rifabutin; children aged <6 y, 5 mg/kg PO qd when suspension becomes available; azithromycin
Varicella zoster virus[†]	Significant exposure to varicella with no history of chickenpox or shingles	Varicella zoster immune globulin (VZIG)	None
Vaccine-preventable pathogens	HIV exposure/infection	Routine immunizations (see text and Fig. 3–2)	None

*The efficacy of parenteral pentamidine (e.g., 4 mg/kg/mo) is controversial. TMP-SMZ, dapsone-pyrimethamine, and possibly dapsone alone appear to protect against toxoplasmosis, although data have not been prospectively collected. Daily TMP-SMZ reduces the frequency of some bacterial infections. Patients receiving therapy for toxoplasmosis with sulfadiazine-pyrimethamine are protected against *Pneumocystis carinii* pneumonia (PCP) and do not need TMP-SMZ.

[†]Children routinely being given intravenous immune globulin (IVIG) should receive VZIG if the last dose of IVIG was administered >21 days before exposure. *Table continued on following page*

Table 3–4 ▪ Prophylaxis for First Episode of Opportunistic Disease in HIV-infected Infants and Children *Continued*

Pathogen	Indication	First Choice	Alternatives
II. GENERALLY RECOMMENDED			
Toxoplasma gondii[‡]	IgG antibody to *Toxoplasma* and severe immunosuppression	TMP-SMZ	Dapsone (children aged ≥1 mo), plus pyrimethamine plus leucovorin
III. NOT RECOMMENDED FOR MOST PATIENTS; INDICATED FOR USE ONLY IN UNUSUAL CIRCUMSTANCES			
Invasive bacterial infections[§]	Hypogammaglobulinemia	IVIG	None
Candida species	Severe immunosuppression	Nystatin or topical clotrimazole	None
Cryptococcus neoformans	Severe immunosuppression	Fluconazole	Itraconazole
Histoplasma capsulatum	Severe immunosuppression, endemic geographic area	Itraconazole	None
Cytomegalovirus (CMV)[‖]	CMV antibody positivity and severe immunosuppression	Children aged 6–12 y (oral ganciclovir under investigation)	None

[‡]Protection against *Toxoplasma* is provided by the preferred anti-*Pneumocystis* regimens. Pyrimethamine alone probably provides little, if any, protection. For definition of severe immunosuppression, see Table 3–1.
[§]Respiratory syncytial virus (RSV) IVIG may be substituted for IVIG during the RSV season.
[‖]Data on oral ganciclovir are still being evaluated; durability of effect is unclear. Acyclovir is not protective against CMV.
From Working Group on Antiretroviral Therapy and Medical Management of HIV Infected Children. (1997). *Guidelines for the use of antiretroviral agents in pediatric HIV infection.* Rockville, MD: Health Resources Services Administration, Public Health Service, U.S. Department of Health and Human Services.

such conditions as cryptosporidiosis and toxoplasmosis is not recommended (CDC, 1997b). Table 3–4 outlines the current recommendations for primary prophylaxis for opportunistic infection (OI) in infants and children with HIV infection.

Acute episodes of OI are frequently life-threatening. With the exception of bacterial infections, none of the OIs complicating HIV are curable with currently available treatments. Once an initial episode occurs, suppressive treatment, secondary prophylaxis, or both is essential.

PCP occurred in 34% of perinatally infected children reported to the CDC through 1996 and is associated with a high rate of morbidity and mortality (Working Group on Antiretroviral Therapy and Medical Management of HIV Infected Children, 1997). Many HIV-exposed children are not identified early enough to receive prophylaxis before the period of highest risk of PCP. In children, PCP is a primary illness and not a reactivation of previously acquired infection, as it is in adults. It presents acutely with a peak incidence in the first 12 months of life. PCP prophylaxis guidelines are contained in Table 3–4. PCP prophylaxis can be stopped when HIV has been reasonably excluded on the basis of two or more negative PCR or HIV cultures, one obtained after 1 month of age and one obtained after 4 months of age. Prophylaxis can be discontinued for children with HIV infection at 1 year of age if the CD4+ T-cell count is above the age-adjusted parameters on serial measurements.

Adherence to a prophylaxis regimen is difficult for parents. It is a particular challenge for the parents of a young, healthy-appearing infant. It can help to involve the parents early in the decision-making process by having them make decisions regarding days or times of administration. One should review the prophylaxis regimen at all visits and keep a record of prescription refills. Most HIV care programs have seen acute PCP develop in an infant receiving prophylaxis only to find that the parent had stopped the drug. Reasons given vary with each situation. Nonetheless, it is up to the health care provider to work with the parents to minimize treatment nonadherence. When the clinician acknowledges the difficulty of compliance, parents can volunteer what is really happening regarding drug administration.

NUTRITIONAL CONCERNS IN CHILDREN WITH HIV INFECTION

Pediatric HIV infection frequently results in nutritional deficiencies and growth failure. Failure to gain weight or weight loss can occur as early as the first 4 months of life or in later years when the child becomes symptomatic (McKinney & Robertson, 1993). The reasons for growth failure are multifactorial and are primarily related to the underlying pathologic disease processes. In addition, psychosocial, behavioral, and environmental problems can also influence growth patterns and nutritional status.

Researchers have established that nutrition and immunology are inextricably correlated. Studies of the immunologic consequences of single-nutrient deficiencies and generalized malnutrition have identified that poor nutrition alone can have a negative impact on the host's immunologic responses (Beisel, 1995; Chandra, 1991; Raiten, 1992). Malnutrition has also been proposed as a cofactor of immune dysfunction in HIV infection and has been recognized as a cause of increased morbidity and mortality in HIV infection (Chlebowski et al., 1989; Ikeogu et al., 1997; Kotler et al., 1989).

A number of vitamin and mineral deficiencies can complicate the clinical course of HIV infection. Specific deficiencies that affect the immune response are inadequate amounts of selenium, iron, zinc, vitamin B_6, vitamin A, vitamin E, iron, and vitamin C (Cunningham-Rundles et al., 1996; Semba et al., 1995). In young infants who are dependent on proper nutrition for CNS development, nutritional deficiencies may result in neurologic impairments. Therefore proactive and aggressive nutritional interventions are necessary not only to improve the overall nutritional status of an HIV-infected child but also to improve the child's immune status, decrease morbidity, and improve the quality of life.

Reasons for Growth Failure

HIV causes morbidity in two equally destructive ways that directly affect the child's growth and development: (1) the virus directly infects cells, resulting in destruction of the immune system and making the child vulnerable to opportunistic infections, and (2) the virus can also infect virtually every body organ, causing system dysfunction. In general, linear growth and weight gain in HIV-infected children are significantly reduced early in life (McKinney & Robertson, 1993; Miller et al., 1993; Moye et al., 1996). Cachexia or preferential loss of lean body mass associated with HIV infection has been described in both children and adults (Kotler et al., 1985; Miller, 1996). Micronutrient deficiencies have also been identified as a possible explanation for growth failure in pediatric HIV infection (Cunningham-Rundles et al., 1996; Omene et al., 1996).

Hirschfeld (1996) has proposed that dysregulation of growth and development, seen in children with HIV infection, is related to either normal metabolism but inadequate energy for growth or abnormal metabolism leading to inappropriate or inadequate substrate use. Normal metabolism but energy that is inadequate for growth may be related to (1) inadequate intake associated with anatomic complications, infectious complications, pain, behavioral factors, or pharmacologic interventions or (2) growth disorders despite apparently adequate intake associated with an inappropriate diet lacking in essential nutrients, malabsorption due to a metabolic or structural defect in the small intestine that does not allow proper digestion or absorption of nutrients, or inadequate absorption due to a defect in ion or fluid resorption, bacterial overgrowth, or structural abnormality that results in excess losses in the large intestine. Abnormal metabolism leading to inappropriate or inadequate substrate use may be related to (1) an intrinsic defect in intermediary metabolism, (2) dysregulation of metabolic pathways, (3) cellular signaling defects due to (4) endocrine abnormalities (e.g., thyroid, adrenal, or hypothalamic dysfunction), (5) global organ dysfunction, (6) chronic infections, or (7) tumors.

Nutritional Assessment

Nutritional assessment begins with taking a thorough nutritional history from the parent or caregiver and when age appropriate, the child. The interview involves investigation of the child's feeding skill abilities, food availability, social history, behavioral problems, cultural practices, dental health, appetite, symptoms, vitamins and supplements taken, activity level, and a diet history. Equally important are the nutrition patterns of the family (e.g., the number of meals they eat together, snacking habits, composition of each meal prepared).

Since there are multiple problems that may develop throughout the course of HIV disease, it is important to establish a regular nutrition surveillance program for the child that includes anthropometric monitoring. In the United States, weight-for-height percentiles are typically used to assess acute undernutrition. Some HIV-infected children have abnormalities in height velocity; thus their weight-for-height level will be near normal. Therefore, weight-for-age and weight-growth velocities are more sensitive markers of a decline in nutritional status. The Waterlow and Gomez classification system for malnutrition, wasting, and stunting is also useful for assessing the nutritional status of children (Waterlow, 1972). Growth velocities and z scores are also helpful in monitoring the growth of children who fall below the fifth percentiles for both height and weight.

In addition, measurements of body composition may reflect nutrition status more accurately than standard weights, especially in the presence of conditions such as inadequate hydration. Skinfold measurements are an accessible and inexpensive tool for measuring body composition as long as the practitioner is trained to accurately and consistently perform the procedure (Miller, 1996). Miller and colleagues (1993) found that HIV-infected children had significantly less lean body mass by 2 years of age as measured by arm muscle circumference. Bioimpedance analysis (BIA) in the prediction of total body water and free fat mass in HIV-infected children has been found to be efficacious with the use of BIA equations developed specifically for HIV-infected children (Arpadi et al., 1996). However, clinicians should be aware of the fact that the BIA may not be totally accurate because of the variability in body water during the course of HIV disease (Miller, 1996). To determine the accuracy of findings, clinicians may consider using the dual x-ray absorptiometry (DEXA) as the standard with which to compare other body composition analyses.

Evaluation of laboratory data as part of the nutritional assessment includes regular monitoring of the hemoglobin and hematocrit along with red blood cell indices, albumin (prealbumin and serum retinol-binding protein levels), and serum ferritin and retinol-binding protein if anemia is present. Other indices of nutritional status should be monitored as indicated (e.g., liver enzymes, if the child is receiving hyperalimentation, and fecal fat, D-xylose, hydrogen breath tests) when a child has suspected malabsorption. Micronutrient deficiencies that have a direct effect on the integrity of the immune system such as A, D, E, C, B_6, folate, selenium, copper, iron, and zinc may also be evaluated (Beach et al., 1989; Cunningham-Rundles et al., 1996).

Ongoing nutritional evaluation includes a review of the current medications that have been prescribed for the child. Medications ordered to treat HIV infection and the related conditions can provide a plethora of problems that affect the nutritional status of the child, including but not limited to liver and kidney problems, hypersensitivity reactions, and nausea and vomiting. Protease inhibitors often cause diarrhea and are known to cause hyperglycemia and diabetes. Additional problems to look for are drug-nutrient interactions and the effect of food on the bioavailabilty of certain drugs. Evaluation of the effects of drugs is no easy task, since some children may be taking as many as 10 to 15 different medications at a time.

Finally, as part of the assessment, the clinician should be aware of the child's disease classification and current diagnoses since nutritional interventions vary according to diagnoses. Table 3–5 was designed to reflect the CDC classification scheme and can serve as a general guide to nutrition interventions particular to disease classification.

Nutrition Intervention

Nutrition intervention should begin as early as possible in the disease process (Oleske et al., 1996). Strategies should be proactive, and the focus should be on prevention rather than intervention only when a problem occurs; the goals are to enhance immune function and improve the quality of life. The primary objective of preventive nutrition counseling is to increase the nutrient density of the child's diet. Teaching of the parent or caregiver should be based on cultural preferences and food likes and dislikes and should include

Table 3-5 ■ CDC Clinical Categories and Nutritional Interventions

Nutrition Assessment	N: No Signs/Symptoms Interventions	A: Mild Signs/Symptoms Interventions	B: Moderate Signs/Symptoms Interventions	C: Severe Signs/Symptoms Interventions
Anthropometrics Laboratory data Nutritionally significant medications Developmental age Activity level Food access Social history Disease classification 24-Hour recall Food frequency Dental health Cultural practices Calorie counts Food allergies Appetite	Calories and protein 1.5–2 × RDA if growth velocity is not appropriate for age Nutrient-dense diet Multivitamin with minerals Increase food access Reduce caffeine intake Promote feeding development Meal psychology Dental health Plus food safety with moderate and severe immune suppression (to avoid food poisoning)	Calories and protein 1.5–2 × RDA if growth velocity is not appropriate for age Nutrient-dense diet Multivitamin with minerals Increase food access Reduce caffeine intake Promote feeding development Meal psychology Dental health Plus food safety with moderate and severe immune suppression	All of the interventions listed in A plus; with • Increase calories with weight loss • Evaluation for oral supplements, may have to use elemental product and or products containing MCT **Iron Deficiency Anemia** High-iron foods with vitamin C source Dietary folic acid and B_{12} Iron supplementation **Diarrhea** Determine origin Check for disaccharide intolerance, usually lactose Malabsorption evaluation Evaluate fiber sources Prevent osmotic diarrhea Reinforce food poisoning prevention *Lactobacillus acidophilus* via yogurt **Cardiomyopathy** Increase selenium-containing foods such as beef, tuna fish, and liver **Oral candidiasis** Lukewarm, nonspicy, nonacidic foods **Fever** Increase calories (7% increase in BEE for every degree F increase) **Nephropathy** Occasional sodium and protein restrictions	All of the interventions listed in A and B plus; with **Encephalopathy** Monitor feeding skills, may have to change texture and consistency of food with developmental deterioration Modified eating techniques and utensils Occupational and physical therapy including feeding therapy **Wasting Syndrome** High-calorie, high-protein diet Malabsorption evaluation Enteral or parenteral nutrition Appetite stimulants or agents that increase lean body mass **MAC** Small, frequent meals Prevent osmotic diarrhea Appetite stimulants with anorexia

From Rothpletz-Puglia, P. (1997). Case reports of nutrition intervention strategies for children with HIV infection. *Topics in Clinical Nutrition, 12*(4), 69–77.

1. Proper hand washing and food and water safety (see Appendix I)
2. Increasing the variety of foods in the diet, especially foods rich in antioxidants, vitamins, and minerals
3. Adapting food-preparation techniques to maintain optimum nutrient content
4. Recommending a variety of textures and consistencies to achieve a diverse, more nutritious diet
5. Planning meals so that the children will be able to participate in food-related activities with their peers

Increasing food availability, which is extremely important, may be a problem for some families and caregivers. Health care providers should assess whether families and caregivers need help with applying for food assistance programs, food budgeting, and consumer purchasing power. In addition, education on how to minimize food waste can help the family and caregiver get the most out of the food budget.

When a child fails to meet growth standards, oral supplements should be instituted. The findings of the nutrition assessment and the child's current diagnoses will determine what type of supplement is appropriate. Formula composition should be prescribed according to the extent of malabsorption and the age of the child. Although these clinically obvious parameters are extremely important, the bottom line in including a nutritional supplement in the plan of care is whether or not the child will drink it. Health care providers often recommend a supplement, go to great lengths to help the family obtain a supply, have a large quantity delivered to the home, and then find that the child will not drink the supplement. Providing the family with a sample, or encouraging the parent or caregiver to purchase a small amount (e.g., one can) will avoid a lot of unnecessary work and frustration. Sometimes it is not the taste but the consistency that the child dislikes. Supplements are available in a variety of compositions (e.g., liquids, powders to be reconstituted or added to foods, and puddings). The initial phase of introducing a nutritional supplement as an intervention includes having the child taste the supplement to assure acceptance. For economic reasons or because of the individual child's, the family's, or the caregiver's preference,

natural, food-based alternatives should be recommended when feasible.

Enteral nutritional support with the use of a feeding tube should be considered when a child fails to grow even after attempts have been made to increase oral consumption. Miller and colleagues (1995) noted that HIV-infected children who received gastrostomy tube feedings gained weight, had fewer hospital admissions, and had a 2.8-fold reduction in the risk of dying. The least traumatic method of tube feeding should be tried first, beginning with a nasogastric enteral tube feeding and evaluating the child's tolerance to the procedure as well as weight gain.

In selected instances, children who fail to gain weight with aggressive enteral nutrition support should be provided with total parenteral nutrition support (TPN). Such therapy is indicated, for example in children with severe symptoms, such as intractable diarrhea and continuing weight loss. Available data on the appropriateness and efficacy of TPN for adults and children with severe HIV-related nutritional problems have demonstrated significant increases in body weight and improved quality of life (Giacomet et al., 1996; Singer et al., 1992). Although TPN may produce weight gain and increased body fat, increases in body cell mass are not likely to occur in the presence of systemic diseases (Kotler et al., 1990).

Other nutritional interventions include the use of appetite stimulants, growth hormone, anticytokine therapies, single-nutrient supplementation of vitamins and minerals, and herbal therapies. Megestrol acetate, an appetite stimulant given to HIV-infected children with failure to grow, has been associated with weight gain but did not affect linear growth (Clarick et al., 1997). The therapy appeared to be well tolerated and was not associated with adverse effects. No data evaluating the effect of megestrol on body cell mass in children are available. Other agents used to treat weight loss and wasting in HIV-infected adults, such as dronabinol, growth hormone, cytokine inhibitors, and thalidomide, have not been evaluated in children. Although the efficacy therapies, such as micronutrient replacement or herbal remedies, have not been formally studied in children, clinicians should be aware that some parents and caregivers do choose to supplement their child's diet with these agents. By understanding the health beliefs and cultural practices of the specific client populations they serve, health care providers can appreciate their importance and anticipate that such complementary therapies will be used (see Chapter 9, Culture and Ethnicity, and Chapter 12, Alternative and Complementary Therapies).

Nutritional interventions vary depending on the child's disease classification, symptoms, and social situation. The following case studies illustrate examples of nutritional interventions for the HIV-infected child.

CASE STUDIES

▪ INFANT WITHOUT SYMPTOMS OF HIV

Medical History   Asymptomatic HIV disease

Summary   T. is a 3-month-old girl with perinatally acquired asymptomatic HIV infection and a high viral load. The infant was born at 28 weeks' gestation and has bronchopulmonary dysplasia (BPD) with reactive airway disease. This infant has spent the first 2½ months of life in the hospital because of prematurity. Since discharge, she has not been growing at an appropriate velocity. She gets extremely irritable and tired when being fed, especially when in respiratory distress.

Nutrition Interventions Provided
by the Health Care Team
1. Monitor growth and development and correct weight and height measurements for prematurity
2. Evaluate current dietary intake
3. Evaluate laboratory data, medications, and vitamins/mineral/herbs taken
4. Assess infant-caretaker bonding since the child has been hospitalized for so long
5. Assess if the caretakers have the time and patience necessary for feeding this infant and explore the family's support network
6. Provide a calorically dense formula and follow-up by assessing that the total caloric intake exceeds that of a regular formula of 20 kcal/oz
7. Provide recommendations for helping the infant relax while being fed (e.g., avoid an overstimulating environment)
8. Provide recommendations for reflux management if necessary
9. Provide recommendations for feeding position, facilitating suckle patterns, nipple size, etc.
10. Evaluate the home environment for such things as incense, which may exacerbate respiratory problems

Outcome   T. began to gain weight at an appropriate rate. Her nutrition status was monitored monthly.

▪ TODDLER WITH MILD SYMPTOMS

Medical History   Mildly symptomatic HIV disease manifested by hepatomegaly and splenomegaly

Summary   P. is a well-nourished 3-year-old boy with perinatally acquired HIV-infection. He had never been hospitalized and was clinically stable. He and his mother lived in a transitional housing program, and his mother was in a substance-abuse rehabilitation program. He was still dependent on the bottle, and his diet consisted of a pediatric supplement (PediaSure) and limited pureed food.

Nutrition Interventions Provided
by the Health Care Team
1. Assess the transitional housing program's meal program and the child's individual intake
2. Evaluate laboratory data, medication, vitamins/minerals/herbs taken
3. Assess whether the mother has made long-term plans for food and housing and make appropriate referrals
4. Provide recommendations for transitioning this toddler to a cup and age-appropriate food textures
5. Strategize with the mother about cooking and meal preparation
6. Strategize with the mother about how to increase food variety and nutrient density and discuss the importance of adequate nutrition to enhance immune function
7. Discuss food and water safety issues (see Appendix I, food and water safety)
8. Evaluate whether dental caries is interfering with dietary intake and make appropriate referrals
9. Assess whether the child's day care provider can reinforce the nutrition plan

Outcome   P.'s nutrition status remained stable.

▪ CHILD WITH MODERATE SYMPTOMS

Medical History   Moderately symptomatic HIV disease manifested by recurrent otitis media, hepatomegaly, oral candidiasis, cardiomyopathy, and diarrhea with weight loss

Summary   M. is a 9-year-old boy with perinatally acquired HIV infection. His CD4+ T-cell count was decreasing and his viral load was increasing. His chief complaint was odynophagia. His father is his primary caretaker and works during the night. At night M. is left with a neighbor, and during the day he attends school.

Nutrition Interventions Provided
by the Health Care Team

1. Evaluate growth velocity
2. Evaluate dietary intake
3. Evaluate laboratory data, medications, vitamins/minerals/herbs taken
4. Assess the underlying cause of the diarrhea
5. Recommend a lactose-reduced diet if lactose intolerance is diagnosed or suspected
6. Recommend low-fat diet with MCT (medium-chain triglyceride) oil if fat malabsorption is suspected or confirmed
7. Recommend an elemental oral supplement if protein malabsorption is suspected or confirmed
8. Make recommendations for preventing osmotic diarrhea
9. Recommend increasing soluble fiber and decreasing insoluble fiber
10. Recommend soft, bland, and cool foods for better tolerance with oral candidiasis
11. Recommend increasing the calorie and protein requirements and nutrient density of the child's diet
12. Recommend a multivitamin
13. Assess the father's ability to prepare meals and strategize about fast, easy-to-prepare, nutritious meals
14. Discuss and reinforce food safety issues
15. Monitor the child's growth
16. Assess what meals the child is eating in school

Outcome   M.'s nutrition status remained stable.

PSYCHOSOCIAL ISSUES

The epidemiologic data on pediatric HIV disease make it clear that in the United States there has been a disproportionate impact on traditionally underserved populations, primarily people of color and the poor. In addition, contact with intrusive public agencies may dispose these populations toward distrust of health care providers and discourage them from seeking timely medical care (Boyd-Franklin & Aleman, 1990; Boyd-Franklin et al., 1995). Often one of the first relationships that HIV-affected families must develop is with the health care providers who treat their children. Health care professionals should attempt to establish a partnership with the family rather than reinforcing the more traditional role of passivity and dependence.

The conditions of poverty, including inadequate housing, may interfere with the delivery of optimal health care. Mothers are typically the strongest advocates for their children, but this advocacy may be hindered by the fact that the mothers of HIV-infected children are often single parents and poor. In some cases, symptomatic HIV infection or drug use may interfere with a mother's ability to properly care for her child, although more often mothers are assertive in seeking care for their children while neglecting their own care needs. There is a significant shortage of treatment programs for drug-dependent persons in the United States. However, the availability is most limited when it comes to programs willing to treat HIV-infected women who are pregnant or have children. These systemic problems must be addressed when one is designing effective health care systems for families with HIV infection.

Families need psychosocial support in dealing with the HIV diagnosis in a child. The diagnosis of HIV infection in the child may be the first evidence that a parent is infected and may evoke feelings of guilt or anger, leading to further disruption in family dynamics. Even apparently resolved emotional issues may require periodic reexamination (e.g., when parents are confronted repeatedly with the differences between a child who is developmentally delayed and healthy peers) (Jessop & Stein, 1989).

Decisions about the disclosure of an HIV diagnosis may have to be made on multiple occasions as different audiences are encountered, such as family, friends, siblings of the infected child, the child himself, day care workers, school nurses, and teachers. Many parents choose to disclose the diagnosis on a "need-to-know" basis. However, children and their siblings often find it less stressful to know the diagnosis and the reality of the situation than to be left in the dark about something that is not discussed but is very apparent to them. Counseling may help parents to decide whether and how to disclose the diagnosis in a developmentally appropriate way. There is evidence that children, parents, and health care providers are unable to deal directly with the breadth of concerns related to HIV infection. In a cohort of 42 perinatally infected children, 9 to 16 years old of age, followed at Children's Hospital AIDS Program in Newark, New Jersey, fewer than 60% were specifically told their diagnosis (Grubman et al., 1995). Clinical experience suggests that it is beneficial for children with normal cognitive development to have the opportunity to discuss aspects of their illness with trusted adults (Lipson, 1994). The issue of disclosure of diagnosis is particularly important, since perinatally infected children live into middle and late adolescence.

The hidden population in the HIV epidemic consists of the uninfected children in families with HIV/AIDS. In a study of 172 consecutive admissions to the Visiting Nurse Service of New York Home Care, there were 26 HIV-infected parents caring for a total of 49 uninfected children under the age of 18 years (Ungvarski, 1996). Uninfected siblings have mental health needs as well, particularly related to the disruptions in family life that result from HIV-related illness in multiple family members as well as feelings of fear, shame, grief, and bereavement. Although much has been written about "AIDS orphans," very little is truly understood regarding effective programming to assist them (Michaels & Levine, 1992). The implications for care management include (1) planning for child care if the parent should require hospitalization, (2) obtaining help in the home if the parent is too ill to provide child care, (3) assessing the need for legal assistance with guardianship, (4) ascertaining the HIV serostatus of all family members, and (5) preventing transmissible infections such tuberculosis, cryptosporidiosis, and viral skin lesions such as herpes simplex and shingles (Ungvarski, 1996).

Challenges of Community-Based Care

The ideal locus for the management of chronic childhood illnesses is the home. The parent or caregiver of a chronically ill child is the only consistent link in the health care system and the person who knows the most about the child's symptoms, treatments, and responses. Even in the best of circumstances, however, managing a chronic illness introduces stresses into the family since it must reorient its existence around the child's constant need for care and deal with the concomitant financial, social, and emotional strains. In addition, in the case of HIV-infected children, drug addiction, poverty, substandard housing, inadequate support networks, and poor access to community resources, including medical care, may already have compromised family stability. Moreover, HIV infections in parents frequently are diagnosed only when HIV symptoms are diagnosed in their newborn child. This discovery, which may be the first concrete ev-

idence of one partner's drug use or bisexuality, invariably transforms the relationship, often further destabilizing family life. The first reaction may be a denial of the child's diagnosis.

HIV-infected children and their families require services from many professionals, including nurses, physicians, social workers, psychologists, dietitians, teachers, clergy, and occupational, physical, speech, and recreational therapists. The more service providers involved in care, the greater the need for case management to prevent one of two extremes—failure to meet needs or duplication of services—from occurring (see Chapter 10, Case Management).

Primary health care is most accessible and effective if it is offered in special clinics that provide comprehensive care for both children and adults (family care). In all care settings the special needs of children, such as the need to play, should be acknowledged and accommodated. In addition, health care professionals must be culturally sensitive, supportive, and nonjudgmental so as to promote positive attitudes in families who bear the burden of care.

The need for preventive therapy should be reviewed early in the course of a child's illness and should include consideration of prophylaxis against PCP, the potential benefits of intravenous administration of gamma globulin, and the timing of antiretroviral therapy. For school-age children, the development of treatment protocols and drug regimens should take into account school schedules, late afternoon or evening clinic visits, and the need for adjusted medication schedules. HIV-infected parents should be encouraged to obtain regular health care, and primary care providers should look for signs of parental compromise that could affect the care of the child, such as fatigue, weight loss, forgetfulness, or an inability to follow through with prescribed treatments.

A formal assessment of the family is important to determine not only their willingness but also their ability to provide care for the HIV-infected child. If home care services are requested, the home care staff should be apprised of the family's understanding of HIV infection and the illness trajectory, as well as who in the family is aware of the diagnosis. Families may also have a general suspicion of authorities, including health care providers, if injection drug use was the route of infection. Even without these complicating factors, caretakers often do not understand the complexities of HIV disease or they may be overwhelmed by the amount of information provided to them, and many have difficulty remembering what was said. In addition, competing priorities may exist at the time of client-provider contact (e.g., the dietitian is worried about and focusing on weight loss, and the mother is worried about paying for the new prescription the doctor just handed her). Health care providers should attempt to assess clients' immediate needs and priorities rather than assume that a problem that is obvious to them is of immediate concern to the client. Client teaching should be provided on the many occasions in which clients encounter health professionals, and it should be reinforced with printed and audiovisual materials when available. Some parental concerns can be addressed in the context of support groups, although many parents of infected children shy away from formal support group meetings. An alternative is organized group social activities, which can also provide an opportunity for informal support, as such group activities often spawn informal support systems.

Surrogate Caregivers

In some circumstances, surrogate caregivers are needed for infected children. Often they can be found within the extended family (e.g., in many black or Hispanic families the pattern of care often involves grandmothers or aunts). However, these caregivers may be impeded by struggles related to the lifestyles, illnesses, or the deaths of their own children. If they are advanced in age, they may lack the physical strength and stamina to provide care for young children at a time in their lives when they themselves might reasonably expect to receive care. Although extended family members in some places are reimbursed for the foster care of a relative, services available to other caregivers, such as respite care, may not be available to them.

Early in the pediatric HIV epidemic there were periodic horror stories in the press about infected children who lived their entire lives as "boarder babies" in acute-care hospitals. By 1990 the situation had changed markedly. Most states had improved their resources for recruiting and training foster care families, and transitional care facilities for children awaiting foster care placement had been developed in many localities. Although foster parents of HIV-infected children have some of the same fears of rejection and isolation as do natural parents, they face some additional challenges. They may lack the legal authority to participate in decision making about a child's medical treatment, or they may be unrealistic in their expectations about what will be involved in caregiving. Their involvement may grow out of spiritual beliefs, a sense of higher calling, a strong sense of advocacy, or a belief that love will heal. Proper training of foster parents, conducted in hospitals and transitional care facilities, can help prepare them for the realities of caring for chronically ill children (Groth, 1993).

Dealing With Stress

The manner in which a biologic, extended, or foster family copes with an HIV diagnosis in a child is related to its previously established ways of dealing with crises and stresses. A diagnosis of HIV infection can magnify feelings of hopelessness and precipitate suicidal ideation in some adults, and in some cultural contexts adults may view illnesses as a moral judgment or punishment for past behavior. Similar feelings are involved when a child has HIV infection. A parent's guilt may manifest itself in overprotective or permissive behavior toward the child, possibly interfering with the child's development. If family members fear the stigma often attached to an HIV diagnosis, they may be secretive and may isolate themselves. This may confuse older siblings, who frequently become involved in caring for an ailing child and parents. These children may face the prospect of requiring a new home without understanding the illness that is the cause of their relocation. Because of difficulty in adjusting to the diagnosis, the family may have only intermittent contact with clinics at crisis or decision points and may otherwise be unavailable. This intermittent contact may also be an outgrowth of a family's perception of outside agencies as intrusive, which may be more common in families with multiple socioeconomic problems that are most in need of help.

Families with HIV-infected children may have to deal with the illness for many years and are likely to encounter practical problems that have no easy solutions. Most families with infected children are totally dependent on public health care programs, such as Medicaid, that are often inadequately funded. Even adequately insured families may have difficulty in getting complete coverage for HIV-related conditions in children. Other financial stressors include the loss of work time when a child must be supervised constantly, lost opportunities for career advancement, and the expenses involved in transporting the child to the clinic and other social service appointments. Chronic illnesses such as HIV infection can also be more draining emotionally than acute illnesses. Parents of chronically ill children often experience a variety of reactions, including shock, denial, sadness, and anger, that fluctuate between periods of relative acceptance and equilibrium. Their feelings of guilt or inadequacy are brought to the surface repeatedly when they are confronted by the child's difference from healthy peers, especially at such critical developmental stages as starting day care or school or approaching adolescence. Most of the literature on chronic illness has focused on children in middle-class families, so there is little understanding of how poor, disenfranchised families may deal with a chronic illness such as HIV infection over a long period of time. In addition, families with an HIV-infected child typically have more than one chronically ill member. In fact, in some inner-city neighborhoods three generations of HIV-infected persons can reside in the same household. Early results from one study of biologic, extended, and foster parents of children indicate similarities in coping styles of the three types of family units (Sherwen & Boland, 1993).

Once AIDS is diagnosed, the prognosis is often poor. Depending on the AIDS-indicator disease, most children die within 2 years of diagnosis. Frequently the AIDS diagnosis is complicated by the comorbidities seen at the later stages of illness, such as failure to thrive, encephalopathy, or difficult-to-treat opportunistic infection. High levels of service and intervention are required, and these greatly increase the potential for parent-provider conflict as the involved parties grapple with the risks and benefits of aggressive, intrusive, and sometimes investigational therapies.

An AIDS diagnosis is frequently accompanied by an immediate family crisis, manifested in guilt, shock, shame, and confusion. Families often need assistance in clarifying issues and getting support for decision making. Some families may assume that the physician is always right and may not realize that they can actively participate in making decisions. The family should be encouraged to discuss feelings about the child's prognosis, including the desire for pain management, use of life support mechanisms, and confidentiality. Often at a time when the medical staff has come to accept the child's impending death, parents favor heroic lifesaving measures. Conversely, some parents perceive and accept impending death before the medical team does. The different expectations of parent and provider must be recognized and addressed openly. The health care provider can initiate discussion and facilitate recognition of differing perceptions. Sometimes a facilitator, a mental health professional not directly involved in the child's care, can assist both the family and the primary care provider in reaching a decision.

Maintaining Family Autonomy

Health care professionals treating a child with a chronic illness should try to prevent both the illness and the treatment regimen from disrupting the child's development and the family's life. Quite often, health care professionals assume a paternalistic attitude that encourages passivity and dependence in the parents' behavior. Forcing parents into a dependent role is counterproductive in families that are determined to maintain control over the child, and enforced dependence makes the adults, as well as the child, feel out of control. Health care providers should attempt to establish a partnership with the family.

Establishing a partner relationship with the family may be a challenge, especially in the case of families unaccustomed to dealing with the health care system. To them, monthly appointments may appear time-consuming, cost-prohibitive, and unnecessary if they do not result in a prescription, procedure, or treatment. In addition, where case management and coordinated care systems have not been developed, the variety of sources and providers with whom the family must deal may include multidisciplinary providers who make conflicting demands. This situation sets the stage for clashes between the values of middle-class professionals who provide services and those of poor families struggling to survive. Because responsibility for day-to-day supervision falls to family members, it is important to respect their autonomy and provide a flexible system of care.

The family of the HIV-infected child should be able to maintain its independence, autonomy, and self-determination without undue supervision and paternalism. Health care providers must convince families that the services they offer are necessary if they expect parents to make use of them. It is also important to point out that members of the health care team sometimes have to deal with their own feelings of anger and blame toward parents, if fantasies of rescuing children from "evil" parents are to be avoided.

There is a complex interaction among chronic illness, the family's response, and the child's developmental status. Changes in all three occur simultaneously and as the child develops, the chronic condition continues or changes in its course, and the family behaviors change to accommodate the needs of the HIV-infected child. The care of most HIV-infected children requires lifelong treatment involving multiple drug regimens with oral and intravenous treatments and complex medical interventions.

Disclosure of the Diagnosis to the Child

Parents and caregivers of chronically ill older children and adolescents often struggle over (1) whether to tell the children the nature of their illness, (2) exactly what should be told, (3) when to tell them, and (4) who should actually participate in the discussion. The truth is less threatening to children than fear of the unknown, but the information given to a child has to be provided in a way appropriate for his or her developmental level. Psychologists can provide invaluable assistance in the decision-making process, by helping to frame the information given to the child and helping the child to survive the aftermath of the disclosure. Before a disclosure is made, the child's and parents' understanding of illness causality should be assessed. Awareness of the family's level of health knowledge as well as their beliefs about health and illness is also important in determining how to help them integrate and process the necessary medical information. Often families need assistance in finding words that they can say comfortably and that the child will understand. Because an HIV-infected child with neurologic involvement may not be functioning at a normal age level, developmental evaluation may be helpful in determining how to communicate information. It is good practice to repeat the in-formation more than once. Developmentally appropriate language is needed when medical procedures and treatments are explained to children, and follow-up discussion and play therapy may be helpful. The stigma and shame that often accompany an HIV diagnosis must be addressed therapeutically as well. Disclosure should be considered an ongoing process, especially as the survival of children increases.

Overcoming Isolation

Some families of infected children isolate themselves in an attempt to maintain control over the children and the situation, and in some instances their isolation may be the result of disapproval or fear of contagion on the part of family members and friends. Isolated caregivers may believe that they and their children are contaminated, they may be angry with the medical profession, or they may be depressed over the many actual and potential losses they face. Counseling and psychological support may be indicated to help family members and caregivers deal with denial and feelings of shame or fear. Families that have dealt with racism, poverty, and the intrusive scrutiny of entitlement programs may have strict rules about the privacy of family-related matters that have to be overcome. In dealing with isolation, it is important for parents and providers to remember the child's need to have contact with his or her peers, particularly in school settings.

SUMMARY

Both psychosocial issues and the progressive nature of HIV disease complicate the management of HIV infection as a chronic childhood illness. Nevertheless, it is critical for the child that the care management begin early so that appropriate interventions are implemented to reduce disease morbidity and improve the quality of life of the child and family. The expanded use of HIV testing and greater awareness of early signs of pediatric HIV infection by health care workers can potentially result in more diagnoses before the appearance of symptoms indicative of advanced disease. Early diagnosis will require that pediatric health professionals deal with issues that were not typically encountered in pediatric practice in the past, including substance abuse, sexuality, reproductive rights, early death, and bereavement.

In general, persons who provide care for the chronically ill child should strive to minimize the disruptive nature of the disease process and associated treatment regimens in order to maintain family functioning and to enhance the development of the child. In recent years the focus of pediatric health care has shifted from an exclusive concern with medical care toward a recognition of the complex dynamics of child-family care, with a focus on psychosocial problem solving and an awareness of the positive contributions that the interdisciplinary team can make to ongoing health care. This shift has contributed to the development of care models that promote a normal life for the chronically ill child. In the case of HIV-infected children, their health care and psychosocial needs, along with systemic social problems that exist in their families, are particularly complex and demand careful coordination. Community-based providers can meet most of these needs, but regional tertiary care centers should be available to treat the children for severe infection or illness and to provide periodic evaluation and antiretroviral treatment.

Twenty years ago 95% of all children with leukemia died, whereas today up to 85% are cured. The intensity of effort put into controlling childhood leukemia should serve as a template for our efforts to treat HIV-infected children. Efforts to improve quality of life while working toward a cure for HIV will require a multidisciplinary approach, calling on the skills of physicians, nurses, social workers, nutritionists, pharmacists, dentists, developmental specialists, therapists, and case managers. This effort must take the child's entire family into consideration, whether it is the family of birth, an extended family, or a foster family.

REFERENCES

American Academy of Pediatrics, Committee on Pediatric AIDS. (1995). Human milk, breast-feeding and transmission of human immunodeficiency virus in the United States. *Pediatrics, 96,* 977–979.

American Academy of Pediatrics. (1997). HIV infection. In G. Peter (Ed.), *1997 Redbook Report of the committee on infectious diseases* (24th ed., p. 294). Elk Grove Village, IL: American Academy of Pediatrics.

Arpadi, S.M., Wang, J., Cuff, P.A., et al. (1996). Application of bioimpedance analysis for estimating body composition in prepubertal children infected with human immunodeficiency virus type 1. *Journal of Pediatrics, 129*(5), 755–757.

Auger, I., Thomas, P., DeGruttola, V., et al. (1988). Incubation periods for pediatric AIDS patients. *Nature, 336,* 575–577.

Beach, R.S., Mantero-Atienza, E., Van Riel, F., Fordyce-Baum, M. (1989). Potential implications of nutritional deficiencies in early HIV-1 infected patients. *Archives of AIDS Research, 3,* 225.

Beisel, W.R. (1995). Nutrition and immune function: Overview. *Journal of Nutrition, 126,* 2611S–2615S.

Blanche, S., Mayaux, M.J., Rouszioux, C., et al. (1994). Relation of the course of HIV infection in children to the severity of the disease in their mothers at delivery. *New England Journal of Medicine, 330,* 308–312.

Blanche, S., Tardieu, M., Duliege, A.M., et al. (1990). Longitudinal study of 94 symptomatic infants with perinatally acquired human immunodeficiency virus infection; evidence for a bimodal expression of clinical and biological symptoms. *American Journal of Diseases of Children, 144,* 1210–1215.

Boyd-Franklin, N., Aleman, J. (1990). Black, inner-city families and multigenerational issues: The impact of AIDS. *Psychologist, 40*(3), 14–17.

Boyd-Franklin, N., Steiner, G., Boland, M. (Eds.). (1995). *Children, families, and HIV/AIDS: Psychosocial and therapeutic issues.* New York: Guilford Press.

Boyer, P.J., Dillon, M., Navaie, M., et al. (1994). Factors predictive of maternal fetal transmission of HIV-1: Preliminary analysis of zidovudine given during pregnancy and/or delivery. *Journal of the American Medical Association, 271,* 1925–1930.

Cao, Y., Krogstad, P., Korber, B.T., et al. (1997). Maternal HIV-1 viral load and vertical transmission of infection. *Nature Medicine, 3,* 549–552.

Centers for Disease Control. (1988). Measles in HIV infected children. *Morbidity and Mortality Week Review, 37,* 183–186.

Centers for Disease Control and Prevention. (1994a). Recommendation of the U.S. Public Health Service Task Force on the use of zidovudine to reduce perinatal transmission of human immunodeficiency virus. *Morbidity and Mortality Weekly Review, 43*(RR-11).

Centers for Disease Control and Prevention. (1994b). 1994 Revised classification system for human immunodeficiency virus infection in children under 13 years of age. *Morbidity and Mortality Weekly Review, 43*(RR-12), 1–19.

Centers for Disease Control and Prevention. (1994c). Zidovudine for the prevention of HIV transmission from mother to infant. *Morbidity and Mortality Weekly Review, 43,* 285–287.

Centers for Disease Control and Prevention. (1995a). 1995 Revised guidelines for prophylaxis against *Pneumocystis carinii* pneumonia for children infected with or perinatally exposed to human immunodeficiency virus. *Morbidity and Mortality Weekly Review, 44*(RR-4), 1–11.

Centers for Disease Control and Prevention. (1995b). U.S. Public Health Service recommendations for human immunodeficiency virus counseling and voluntary testing for pregnant women. *Morbidity and Mortality Weekly Review, 44*(RR-7), 1–14.

Centers for Disease Control and Prevention. (1996a). *HIV/AIDS Surveillance Report, 8*(2), 1–39.

Centers for Disease Control and Prevention. (1996b). AIDS among children in the United States. *Morbidity and Mortality Weekly Review, 45*(46), 1005–1010.

Centers for Disease Control and Prevention. (1996c). Measles pneumonitis following measles-mumps-rubella vaccination of a patient with HIV infection. *Morbidity and Mortality Weekly Review, 45*(28), 603–606.

Centers for Disease Control and Prevention. (1997a). Update: Perinatally acquired HIV/AIDS—United States, 1997. *Morbidity and Mortality Weekly Report, 46*(46), 1087–1092.

Centers for Disease Control and Prevention. (1997b). 1997 USPHS/IDSA guidelines for the prevention of opportunistic infections in persons infected with human immunodeficiency virus. *Morbidity and Mortality Weekly Report, 46*(RR-12), 1–46.

Centers for Disease Control and Prevention. (1998). Administration of zidovudine during late pregnancy and delivery to prevent perinatal HIV transmission—Thailand, 1996–1998. *Morbidity and Mortality Weekly Report, 47*(RR-02), 151–154.

Chandra, R.K. (1991). Nutrition and immunity: Lessons from the past; new insights into the future. *American Journal of Clinical Nutrition, 53,* 1087–1101.

Chlebowski, R.T., Grovesnor, M.B., Berhard, N.H., et al. (1989). Nutritional status, gastrointestinal dysfunction, and survival in patients with AIDS. *American Journal of Gastroenterology, 84,* 1288–1293.

Clarick, R.H., Hanekom, W.A., Yogev, R., Chadwick, E.G. (1997). Megestrol acetate treatment of growth failure in children infected with human immunodeficiency virus. *Pediatrics, 99*(3), 354–357.

Connor, E., Bagarazzi, M., McSherry, G., et al. (1991). Clinical and laboratory correlates of *Pneumocystis carinii* pneumonia in children infected with HIV. *Journal of the American Medical Association, 265,* 1693–1697.

Connor, E.M., Mofenson, L.M. (1995). Zidovudine for the reduction of perinatal human immunodeficiency virus transmission: Pediatric AIDS clinical trial group protocol 076: Results and treatment recommendations. *Pediatric Infectious Disease Journal, 14*(6), 536–541.

Connor, E.M., Sperling, R.S., Gelber, R., et al. (1994). Reduction of maternal-infant transmission of human immunodeficiency virus type 1 with zidovudine treatment. *New England Journal of Medicine, 331,* 1173–1180.

Cunningham-Rundles, S., Kim, S.H., Dnistrian, A., et al. (1996). Micronutrient and cytokine interaction in congenital pediatric HIV infection. *Journal of Nutrition, 126,* 2674S–2679S.

DeCarli, C., Civitello, A., Brouwers, P., Pizzo, P.A. (1993). The prevalence of computed tomographic abnormalities of the cerebrum in 100 consecutive children symptomatic with human immune deficiency virus. *Annals of Neurology, 34,* 198–205.

Dickover, R.E., Garratty, E.M., Herman, S., et al. (1996). Identification of levels of maternal HIV-1 RNA associated with risk of perinatal transmission: Effect of maternal zidovudine treatment on viral load. *Journal of the American Medical Association, 275,* 599–605.

Duliege, A.M., Messiah, A., Blanche, S., et al. (1992). Natural history of human immunodeficiency virus type 1 infection in children: Prognostic value of laboratory tests on the bimodal progression of the disease. *Pediatric Infectious Disease Journal, 11,* 630–635.

Dunn, D.T., Brandt, C.D., Krivine, A., et al. (1995). The sensitivity of HIV-1 DNA polymerase chain reaction in the neonatal period and the relative contributions of intrauterine and intrapartum transmission. *AIDS, 9,* F7–F11.

Dunn, D.T., Newell, M.L., Ades, A.E., et al. (1992). Risk of human immunodeficiency virus type 1 transmission through breast-feeding. *Lancet, 340,* 585–588.

Dunn, D.T., Newell, M.L., Mayaux, M.J., et al. (1994). Mode of delivery and vertical transmission of HIV-1: A review of prospective studies. Perinatal AIDS Collaborative Transmission Studies. *Journal of Acquired Immune Deficiency Syndromes, 7*(10), 1064–1066.

El-Sadr, W., Oleske, J.M., Agins, B.D., et al. (1994). *Evaluation and management of early HIV infection* (AHCPR Publication No. 94-0572). Rockville, MD: Agency for Health Care Policy and Research, Public Health Service, U.S. Department of Health and Human Services.

Englund, J.A., Baker, C.J., Raskino, C., et al. (1997). Zidovudine, didaosine or both as the initial treatment for symptomatic HIV-infected children. *New England Journal of Medicine, 336,* 1704–1712.

European Collaborative Study. (1994). Caesarean section and the risk of vertical transmission of HIV-1 infection. *Lancet, 343,* 1464–1467.

Falloon, J., Eddy, J., Weiner, L., Pizzo, P.A. (1989). Human immunodeficiency virus infection in children. *Journal of Pediatrics, 114,* 1–30.

Ferguson, F., Berentsen, B., Nachman, S. (1995). Experiences of a pediatric dental program for HIV positive children. In J.S. Greenspan, D. Greenspan (Eds.), *Oral manifestations of HIV infection: Proceedings of the Sec-*

ond *International Workshop on the Oral Manifestations of HIV Infection, January 31–February 3, 1993, San Francisco, California.* Chicago: Quintessense.

Gellert, B., Dufree, M., Berkowitz, C., et al. (1993). Situation and sociodemographic characteristics of children infected with human immunodeficiency virus for pediatric sexual abuse. *Pediatrics, 91,* 39–44.

Giacomet, V., Ruga, E., Rampon, O., et al. (1996). Central venous catheter in HIV-infected children receiving total parenteral nutrition for severe failure to thrive. *International Conference on AIDS, 11(2),* 293. Abstract no. THB-4242.

Goedert, J.J., Duliege, A.M., Amos, C., et al. (1991). High risk of HIV-1 infection for the firstborn of twins. *Lancet, 338,* 1471–1475.

Groth, B. (1993). Resource availability versus need: Perceptions of foster parents of HIV positive children. *Pediatric AIDS & HIV Infection: Fetus to Adolescent, 4,* 367–372.

Grubman, S., Gross, E., Lerner-Weiss, N., et al. (1995). Older children and adolescents living with perinatally acquired HIV infection. *Pediatrics, 95,* 657–663.

Gutman, L.T., Herman-Giddens, M.E., McKinney, R.E. (1993). Pediatric acquired immunodeficiency syndrome: Barriers to recognizing the role of child sexual abuse. *American Journal of Diseases of Children, 147,* 775–780.

Gutman, L.T., St. Claire, K.K., Weedy, C., et al. (1991). Human immunodeficiency virus transmission by child sexual abuse. *American Journal of Diseases of Children, 145,* 137–141.

Hirschfeld, S. (1996). Dysregulation of growth and development in HIV-infected children. *Journal of Nutrition, 126,* 2641S–2650S.

Ikeogu, M.O., Wolf, B., Mathe, S. (1997). Pulmonary manifestations in HIV seropositivity and malnutrition in Zimbabwe. *Archives of Diseases of Children, 76(2),* 124–128.

Jessop, D.J., Stein, R.E. (1989). Meeting the needs of individuals and families. In R. Stein (Ed.), *Caring for children with chronic illness* (pp. 63–74). New York: Springer Publishing Co.

Joshi, V.V., Oleske, J.M., Connor, E.M. (1990). Morphologic findings in children with acquired immune deficiency syndrome: Pathogenesis and clinical implications. *Pediatric Pathology, 10(1–2),* 155–165.

Kline, M.W., Lindsey, J.C., Culnane, M., et al. (1997). A randomized comparative trial of zidovudine (ZDV) versus stavudine (d4T) in children with HIV infection [Abstract 724]. *Abstracts of the 4th Conference on Retroviruses and Opportunistic Infections, Washington, DC, January 22–26, 1997.*

Kotler, D.P., Tierney, A.R., Culpepper-Morgan, J.A., et al. (1990). Effect of home total parenteral nutrition on body composition in patients with acquired immuno-deficiency syndrome. *Jounal of Parenteral and Enteral Nutrition, 14(5),* 454–458.

Kotler, D.P., Tierney, A.R., Francisco, A., et al. (1989). The magnitude of body cell mass depletion determines the timing of death from wasting in AIDS. *American Journal of Clinical Nutrition, 50,* 444–447.

Kotler, D.P., Wang, J., Pierson, R.N. (1985). Body composition studies in patients with the acquired immuno-deficiency syndrome. *American Journal of Clinical Nutrition, 42,* 1255–1265.

Kreiss, J. (1997). Breastfeeding and vertical transmission of HIV-1. *Acta Paediatrica Supplement, 421,* 113–117.

Krugman, R.D. (1991). Child abuse and neglect: Critical first steps in response to a national emergency. The report of the U.S. Advisory Board on Child Abuse and Neglect. *American Journal of Diseases of Children, 145(5),* 513–515.

Kuhn, L., Stein, Z. (1997). Infant survival, HIV infection, and feeding alternatives in less developed countries. *American Journal of Public Health, 87(6),* 926–931.

Landsman, S.H., Kalish, L.A., Burns, D.N., et al. (1996). Obstetrical factors and the transmission of human immunodeficiency virus type 1 from mother to child. *New England Journal of Medicine, 334,* 1617–1623.

Levy, J. (1993). Pathogenesis of human immunodeficiency virus infection. *Microbiology Review, 57,* 183–289.

Lewis, S.H., Reynolds-Kohler, C., Fox, H.E., Nelson, J.A. (1990). HIV-1 in trophoblastic and villous Hofbauer cells and haematological precursors in eight-week fetuses. *Lancet, 1,* 565–568.

Lipson, M. (1994). Disclosure of diagnosis to children with human immunodeficiency syndrome. *Developmental and Behavioral Pediatrics, 15,* S61–S65.

Luzuriaga, K., Bryson, Y., Krogstad, P., et al. (1997). Combination treatment with zidovudine, didanosine and nevirapine in infants with human immunodeficiency virus type 1 infection. *New England Journal of Medicine, 336,* 1343–1349.

Lyman, W.D., Kress, Y., Rashbaum, W.K., et al. (1988). An AIDS virus-associated antigen localized in human fetal brain. *Annals of the New York Academy of Science, 540,* 628–629.

Maury, W., Potts, B.J., Rabson, A.B. (1989). HIV-1 infection of first trimester and term human placental tissue: A possible mode of maternal-fetal transmission. *Journal of Infectious Diseases, 160,* 583–588.

Mayaux, M.J., Burgard, M., Teglas, J.P., et al. (1996). Neonatal characteristics in rapidly progressive perinatally acquired HIV-1 disease. *Journal of the American Medical Association, 275,* 606–610.

McIntosh, K., Pitt, J., Brambilla, D., et al. (1994). Blood culture in the first 6 months of life for the diagnosis of vertically transmitted human immunodeficiency virus infection. *Journal of Infectious Diseases, 170,* 996–1000.

McKinney, R.E., Robertson, W.R. (1993). Effect of human immunodeficiency virus on the growth of young children. *Journal of Pediatrics, 123,* 579–582.

Michaels, D., Levine, C. (1992). Estimates of the number of motherless youth orphaned by AIDS in the United States. *Journal of the American Medical Association, 268*(24), 3456–3461.

Miller, T.L. (1996). Nutrition assessment and its clinical application in children infected with the human immunodeficiency virus. *Journal of Pediatrics, 129*(5), 633–636.

Miller, T.L., Awnetwant, E.L., Evans, S., et al. (1995). Gastrostomy tube supplementation for HIV-infected children. *Pediatrics, 96*(4), 696–702.

Miller, T.L., Evans, S., McIntosh, K., Winter, H.S. (1993). Growth and body composition in children with human immunodeficiency virus-1 infection. *American Journal of Clinical Nutrition, 57,* 588–592.

Minkoff, H., Augenbraun, M. (1997). Antiretroviral therapy for pregnant women. *American Journal of Obstetrics & Gynecology, 176*(2), 478–489.

Mofenson, L.M., Bethel, J., Moye, J., et al. (1993). Effect of intravenous immunoglobulin (IVIG) on CD4+ lymphocyte decline in HIV-infected children in a clinical trial of IVIG infection prophylaxis. *Journal of Acquired Immune Deficiency Syndrome, 6,* 1103–1113.

Moye, J., Rich, K.C., Kalish, L.A., et al. (1996). Natural history of somatic growth in infants born to women infected by human immunodeficiency virus. Women and Infants Transmission Study Group. *Journal of Pediatrics, 128*(1), 58–69.

Mueller, B., Shad, A.T., Magrath, I.T., Horowitz, M.E. (1994). Malignancies in children with HIV infection. In P. Pizzo, C. Wilfert (Eds.), *Pediatric AIDS: The challenge of HIV infection in infants, children and adolescents* (pp. 603–622). Baltimore: Williams & Wilkins.

National Institute of Allergy and Infectious Diseases. (1997). *Summary of the meeting of a panel to review studies of transplacental toxicity of AZT, January 14, 1997.* Bethesda, MD: National Institute of Allergy and Infectious Diseases, Office of Communications.

Oleske, J.M., Rothpletz-Puglia, P.M., Winter, H. (1996). Historical perspectives on the evolution in understanding the importance of nutritional care in pediatric HIV. *Journal of Nutrition, 126,* 2616S–2619S.

Omene, J.A., Easington, C.R., Glew, R.H., et al. (1996). Serum beta carotene deficiency in HIV infected children. *Journal of the National Medical Association, 88,* 789–793.

Palumbo, P., Hoyt, L., Demasio, K., et al. (1992). Population-based study of measles and measles immunization in human immunodeficiency virus-infected children. *Pediatric Infectious Disease Journal, 11,* 1108–1114.

Palumbo, P.E., Kwok, S.H., Waters, S., et al. (1995). Viral measurement by polymerase chain reaction-based assays in human immunodeficiency virus-infected infants. *Journal of Pediatrics, 126,* 582–585.

Palumbo, P., Raskino, C., Fiscus, S., et al. (1998). Predicative value of quantitative plasma HIV RNA and CD4+ lymphocyte count in HIV-infected infants and children. *Journal of the American Medical Association, 279,* 756–761.

Pyun, K.H., Ochs, H.D., Dufford, M., Wedgewood, R.J. (1987). Perinatal infection with human immunodeficiency virus: Specific antibody responses by the neonate. *New England Journal of Medicine, 317,* 611–614.

Raiten, D.J. (1992). Nutritional correlates of human immunodeficiency virus infection. *European Journal of Gastroenterology & Hepatology, 4,* 428–442.

Ramilo, O., Hicks, P., Borvak, J., et al. (1996). T cell activation and human immunodeficiency virus replication after influenza immunization of infected child. *Pediatric Infectious Disease Journal, 15,* 197–203.

Rouzioux, C., Constagliola, D., Burgard, M., et al. (1993). Timing of mother-to-child HIV-1 transmission depends on maternal status. *AIDS, 7*(Suppl. 2), 249–252.

Scarlatti, G., Letiner, T., Hodara, V., et al. (1993). Neutralizing antibodies and viral characteristics in mother-to-child transmission of HIV-1. *AIDS, 7*(Suppl. 2), S45–S48.

Scott, G.B., Hutto, C., Makuch, R.W., et al. (1990). Survival in children with perinatally acquired HIV-1 infection. *New England Journal of Medicine, 321,* 1791–1796.

Semba, R.D., Caiffa, V.T., Graham, N., et al. (1995). Vitamin A deficiency and wasting as predictors of mortality in human immunodeficiency virus-infected injection drug users. *Journal of Infectious Diseases, 171,* 1196–1202.

Shearer, W.T., Quinn, T.C., LaRussa, P., et al. (1997). Viral load and disease progression in infants infected with human immunodeficiency virus type 1. *New England Journal of Medicine, 336,* 1337.

Sherwen, L., Boland, M. (1993). Stress, coping and perception of child vulnerability in female caretakers of HIV-infected children: A preliminary report. *Pediatric AIDS & HIV Infection: Fetus to Adolescent, 4,* 358–366.

Singer, P., Rubinstein, A., Askanzi, J., et al. (1992). Clinical effects of lipid-based parenteral nutrition in AIDS. *Journal of Parenteral & Enteral Nutrition, 16,* 165–167.

Ungvarski, P.J. (1996). Challenges for the urban home health care provider: The New York City experience. *Nursing Clinics of North America, 31*(1), 81–95.

Waldholz, M. (March 5, 1998). AZT price cut for Third-World mothers-to-be. *Wall Street Journal,* p. 81.

Waterlow, J.C. (1972). Classification and definition of protein calorie malnutrition. *British Medical Journal, 3,* 565–558.

Working Group on Antiretroviral Therapy and Medical Management of HIV Infected Children. (1997). *Guidelines for the use of antiretroviral agents in pediatric HIV infection.* Rockville, MD: Health Resources Services Administration, Public Health Service, U.S. Department of Health and Human Services.

World Health Organization. (1997). Global AIDS surveillance—part I. *Weekly Epidemiology Record, 72,* 357–360.

Ziegler, J.B., Cooper, D.A., Johnson, R.O., Gold, J. (1985). Post-natal transmission of AIDS-associated retrovirus from mother to infant. *Lancet, 1,* 896–898.

4

Infants and Children
AIDS CARE MANAGEMENT

LYNN CZARNIECKI ■ PAMELA ROTHPLETZ-PUGLIA ■ JAMES OLESKE

HIV infection in children less than 13 years of age continues to progress to advanced disease or AIDS over varying lengths of time. Rapid progressors develop symptoms of advanced disease early in life and live only 3 to 5 years (Delfraissy et al., 1992). In long-term survivors advanced disease may not develop until their school years or adolescence (Grubman et al., 1995).

Advanced HIV disease in children is usually a multisystem disease marked by frequent infections, multiple hospitalizations for acute complications, and many stressful symptoms. The care of the children with advanced HIV disease is challenging, not only for the child and the family or caregivers but also for the health care providers. It requires a comprehensive, multidisciplinary approach to meet all the needs of the child and the family or caregivers. Multiple medical specialists are needed to help manage the various organ complications that develop. Psychosocial professionals are essential to meet the host of psychological, emotional, and financial difficulties that arise. Nurses play a pivotal role as coordinators of care, case managers, and client educators. Nutritionists and dietitians are needed to continually assess the nutritional needs of the child and family or caregivers and to provide proactive nutritional interventions. For the child with AIDS to live in the home, multiple community-based services must be accessed and coordinated.

Infectious agents that present no threat to people with healthy immune systems can cause serious damage in immunocompromised persons. Opportunistic infections (OIs) seen in children differ significantly from those seen in adults. For example, coccidioidomycosis and histoplasmosis almost never occur in children. Many OIs initially present as acute illness and then become chronic because of the weakened immune system and the body's inability to control the infection. Others develop more insidiously and cause more illness as the immune system becomes more damaged. Most infections will require lifelong suppressive therapy after the primary infection has been controlled (CDC, 1997a). There is no effective treatment for some infections and neoplasms, and supportive care is all that can be offered.

AIDS-INDICATOR DISEASES

Bacterial Infections

EPIDEMIOLOGY. Bacterial infections have been noted at many sites in HIV-infected children and are often recurrent. In 1996 bacterial infections in children with HIV infection accounted for 20% of initial AIDS diagnoses (CDC, 1996).

PATHOGENESIS. Because of their impaired humoral response, HIV-infected children are susceptible to both gram-positive and gram-negative bacterial infections, which can become acute if treatment is absent or incomplete (Dankner, 1995). Bacterial infections affect a variety of organ systems, including the skin, respiratory system, gastrointestinal tract, and blood. For unknown reasons, bone and joint infections are not increased in HIV-infected children.

CLINICAL MANIFESTATIONS. Common infections include cellulitis and abscesses caused by *Staphylococcus* and *Streptococcus;* the latter is the bacterial pathogen most frequently identified in children with HIV disease and is often implicated in pneumonia and bacteremia (Hauger & Powell, 1990). Skin infections may follow bites, eczema, or the insertion of intravenous catheters. Sinus and pulmonary complications include chronic otitis media, sinusitis, and pneumonia; chronic recurrent pneumonia predisposes some children to chronic lung diseases such as bronchiectasis. In the gastrointestinal tract, diarrhea is the most common symptom, and infectious agents are usually opportunistic, including cytomegalovirus (CMV), *Salmonella, Cryptosporidium, Mycobacterium avium-intracellulare* complex (MAC) and *Giardia.* In addition, any of these bacteria can cause sepsis, which often occurs secondarily in children who are hospitalized for acute infections, especially when a central venous catheter is in place.

DIAGNOSIS. The AIDS-defining diagnosis of bacterial infection in an HIV-infected child includes at least two multiple or recurrent bacterial infections within 2 years, excluding the skin and otitis media (Centers for Disease Control [CDC]), 1994). Bacterial infections are diagnosed by culture whenever possible. Roentgenography, other visualizing techniques and biopsies are also used to diagnose bacterial infection. Cultures are necessary to determine the causative organism and to choose the appropriate therapy. Evaluation of culture results is made difficult by the fact that normal flora have the potential to cause a bacterial infection in the immunocompromised HIV-infected child. Recurrent *Salmonella* (nontyphoid) septicemia (salmonellosis) is considered an AIDS-defining diagnosis.

TREATMENT. Bacterial infections are treated with appropriate antibiotics guided by culture and sensitivity results and administered for the maximum "normal" time with follow-up to ensure that the infection has been resolved. Treatment with intravenous immune globulin (IVIG) has been shown to reduce bacterial infections and hospitalizations in some HIV-infected children (National Institute of Child Health and Human Development, 1991). IVIG is used in the treatment of HIV-infected infants and children with hypogammaglobulinemia, poor functional antibody, or recurrent bacterial infections, including chronic sinusitis and bronchiectasis. Parenteral infusion of IVIG can be given in ambulatory care or home settings. IVIG does not appear to be of significant benefit in children receiving trimethoprim-sulfamethoxazole (TMP-SMX) for *Pneumocystis carinii* pneumonia (PCP) prophylaxis or in the presence of severe immunodeficiency (CD4+ T-cell count less than 200/mm³). For prophylaxis for recurrence, see Table 4–1.

CONSIDERATIONS FOR CARE. When care is given at home, clinicians must teach parents or other caregivers to administer required antibiotics. Caregivers must be instructed to complete a full course of medication, even if the child appears better. They should also be taught the signs and symptoms of acute infection and instructed to seek medical help early to assure an immediate and successful response to treatment. Caregivers should also be taught to discard old antibiotics and not to use them for a subsequent infection. When the family or caregivers prefer, and the health insurance will cover the services, home infusions of antibiotics or IVIG can save the child and family or caregivers many hours in the clinic. When a child is to receive parenteral therapy at home, a willing and able caregiver must be available during the infusion, there must be good intravenous access for the home care nurse to insert the catheter, and the child should have received initial therapy in the hospital or clinic setting to ensure that he or she can tolerate the treatment without any significant adverse reactions.

Candidiasis

EPIDEMIOLOGY. Candidiasis is the most common oral OI occurring in children with HIV, with a reported prevalence of 20% to 72% (Kline, 1996). It is most prevalent in children with a definitive diagnosis of AIDS. *Candida* esophagitis is also a common OI in children, but the incidence is not as well defined. In 1996, *Candida* infection in children with HIV infection accounted for 16% of initial AIDS diagnoses (CDC, 1996).

PATHOGENESIS. *Candida* is a commensal organism that is normally found in the oropharynx, vagina, large intestine, and skin. Most infections are endogenous, but exogenous infection can occur (e.g., nosocomial infection related to an intravenous catheter). Human-to-human infection can also occur (e.g., oral candidiasis in a newborn infant after vaginal delivery). Oral candidiasis is a fungal (yeast) infection seen in patients with low CD4+ T-cell counts and symptomatic disease. It has been associated with a poorer prognosis and more rapid progression of disease in children, especially between the ages of 3 and 5 years; oral candidiasis is rarely seen in children identified as long-term survivors (Katz et al., 1993).

CLINICAL PRESENTATION. Although most infection caused by *Candida albicans* is localized, in some instances it may be disseminated. The symptoms vary with the site. Along with herpes simplex virus (HSV) and CMV, it is among the causes of dysphagia (difficulty in swallowing) and odynophagia (pain in swallowing), both of which adversely affect feeding behaviors. Erythematous candidiasis is seen most commonly on the tongue and palate with inconspicuous erythematous changes. Pseudomembranous candidiasis is marked by white or yellow plaques that can involve any oral mucosal surface. The plaque can be easily removed, revealing erythema or bleeding of the underlying mucosa. *Candida* esophagitis may be seen with or without oral candidiasis and is usually manifested by dysphagia, odynophagia, substernal pain, and fever and is often associated with decreased oral intake and weight loss.

DIAGNOSIS. Diagnosis of *Candida* infection is made by gross inspection of the lesions or by microscopic examination of a specimen of tissue. Esophagitis is best diagnosed by clinical symptoms, endoscopy, or biopsy.

TREATMENT. Treatment of *Candida* infection is site specific. When it occurs on the skin, mucous membranes, or diaper area, it calls for an antifungal cream. Oral thrush is generally treated with an antifungal agent such as nystatin or clotrimazole troches or vaginal cream. If no improvement occurs in 5 to 7 days, short courses of ketoconazole or fluconazole can be prescribed. *Candida* infection in the esophagus or trachea can be treated with intravenous doses of fluconazole or amphotericin B. Primary prophylaxis is not indicated. Secondary prophylaxis can be considered when there have been two or more episodes of oral candidiasis or one episode of esophagitis. For prophylaxis for recurrence, see Table 4–1.

CONSIDERATIONS FOR CARE. Clinicians need to teach caregivers good oral care, including daily inspection with a flashlight, wiping the oral mucosa regularly with a wet cloth, rinsing after food and liquids, and avoidance of sleeping with a bottle. When there is pain and discomfort, it can be helpful to encourage cold beverages and food and avoidance of hot, spicy, or acidic foods and beverages.

Coccidioidomycosis

EPIDEMIOLOGY. Coccidioidomycosis is caused by *Coccidioides immitis,* a fungus found primarily in desert soil of the San Joaquin Valley in California, Southern Arizona, Southern New Mexico, West Texas, and Northern Mexico (Kirkland & Fierer, 1996). Coccidioidomycosis is rarely diagnosed in children and in 1996 was identified in only one HIV-infected child as the initial AIDS-defining illness (CDC, 1996).

PATHOGENESIS. *C. immitis* becomes airborne, especially during dust storms and dry periods, and enters the respiratory tract. Most persons with HIV who develop coccidioidomycosis manifest pulmonary disease. Dissemination often occurs, and extrapulmonary disease involving the meninges, lymph nodes, liver, spleen, bone marrow, and skin is common.

CLINICAL MANIFESTATIONS. The signs and symptoms of coccidioidomycosis vary and may be nonspecific, e.g., fever, malaise, weight loss, cough, and fatigue, or may present as pneumonia (Kirkland & Fierer, 1996). Extrapulmonary signs and symptoms appear according to the site of infection, e.g., meningitis, peritonitis.

DIAGNOSIS. Definitive diagnosis is established by microscopic study, culture, or direct examination of the infected tissues or fluid from the affected sites.

TREATMENT. Both fluconazole and itraconazole have been used successfully to treat nonmeningeal coccidioidomycosis. Amphotericin B is recommended for extremely ill patients. For prophylaxis for recurrence, see Table 4–1.

Table 4–1 ▪ Secondary Prophylaxis of AIDS-Defining Opportunistic Disease (After Chemotherapy for Acute Disease) in HIV-Infected Infants and Children

Pathogen	Indication	First Choice	Alternatives
RECOMMENDED FOR LIFE AS A STANDARD OF CARE			
Cytomegalovirus	Prior end-organ disease	Ganciclovir or foscarnet or, for retinitis, ganciclovir sustained-release implant	None
Coccidioides immitis	Documented disease	Fluconazole	Amphotericin B
Cryptococcus neoformans	Documented disease	Fluconazole	Itraconazole, amphotericin B
Histoplasma capsulatum	Documented disease	Itraconazole	Fluconazole, amphotericin B
Mycobacterium avium complex	Prior disease	Clarithromycin plus either ethambutol or rifabutin	None
Pneumocystis carinii	Prior episode of *P. carinii* pneumonia	TMP-SMZ	Pentamidine (aerosol or intravenous), dapsone
Salmonella species (nontyphi)	Bacteremia	TMP-SMZ	Antibiotic chemoprophylaxis with another active agent (determined by drug susceptibility of organism isolated)
Toxoplasma gondii	Prior toxoplasmic encephalitis	Sulfadiazine, plus pyrimethamine, plus leucovorin	Clindamycin, plus pyrimethamine, plus leucovorin
RECOMMENDED ONLY IF SUBSEQUENT EPISODES ARE FREQUENT OR SEVERE			
Bacterial infections, invasive	>2 infections in 1-year period	TMP-SMZ	Antibiotic chemoprophylaxis with another active agent (determined by drug susceptibility of organism isolated)
Candida species	Frequent or severe recurrences	Fluconazole or ketoconazole	None
Herpes simplex virus	Frequent or severe recurrences	Acyclovir	None

From Centers for Disease Control and Prevention. (1997). 1997 USPH/IDSA Guidelines for the Prevention of Opportunistic Infections in Persons Infected with Human Immunodeficiency Virus. *Mortality and Morbidity Weekly Report, 46*(RR-12), 1–46.

CONSIDERATIONS FOR CARE. Travel and migration history is extremely important when a diagnosis of coccidioidomycosis is suspected. HIV-infected persons who relocate to areas in which the disease is endemic are extremely vulnerable to this infection. Although HIV-infected persons living in or visiting endemic areas cannot completely avoid exposure to *C. immitis,* they should avoid activities that entail increased risk, e.g., extensive exposure to native soil, dust storms (CDC, 1997a).

Cryptococcosis

EPIDEMIOLOGY. *Cryptococcus neoformans* is a fungus that is frequently found in bird droppings and soil. It is most commonly seen in immunosuppressed patients. Although cryptococcosis is diagnosed less frequently in children, as survival increases, the number of cases of crytococcal meningoencephalitis will probably escalate. In 1996, cryptococcosis in children with HIV infection accounted for 1% of initial AIDS diagnoses (CDC, 1996).

PATHOGENESIS. The organism is aerosolized and enters the respiratory tract, with subsequent extrapulmonary spread due to the depletion of CD4+ T-cells. The most frequent site of infection is the central nervous system (CNS). *Cryptococcus neoformans* is the cause of meningoencephalitis in both adults and children with HIV infection. Extrapulmonary disease in children has also been reported (Leggiadro et al., 1991).

CLINICAL PRESENTATION. The symptoms of cryptococcal meningitis can occur slowly over a few weeks or months and include fever, headache, and altered mental status. Few focal neurologic signs are seen, and early in the course of infection, patients may not demonstrate any overt symptoms.

DIAGNOSIS. Diagnosis of *Cryptococcus neoformans* is made by examination of cerebral spinal fluid with the use of cryptococcal antigen, India ink preparation, and culture. When lumbar puncture is not possible, a negative serum cryptococcal antigen may help rule out cryptococcosis.

TREATMENT. Initial therapy is with amphotericin B, with or without flucytosine, until clinical response is achieved, followed by an 8- to 10-week course with fluconazole to complete initial treatment. For prophylaxis for recurrence, see Table 4–1.

CONSIDERATIONS FOR CARE. The insidious onset of cryptococcus means that clinicians must be alert for the early signs of meningitis in children with HIV. Reports of headache by children with HIV infection should be taken seriously and with appropriate work-up. Children and families should be taught to avoid pigeons, pigeon roosts, and other places where many birds gather together. Since maintenance therapy is lifelong, clinicians must help children and their caregivers with the issue of adherence to the treatment plan. Frequently adolescents like to experiment and try abstaining from their medications to see what will happen. Maintaining a supportive, nonjudgmental approach to the child and family or caregivers will encourage open communication about medication adherence and facilitate problem solving.

Cryptosporidiosis

EPIDEMIOLOGY. *Cryptosporidium* is an enteric protozoan that causes acute, self-limited disease in immunocompetent children but severe and persistent enteritis in the HIV-infected child (Van Dyke, 1995). It is transmitted by ingestion of oocysts excreted in the feces of infected animals and humans. The organism can be transmitted by contact with infected adults and diaper-age children, contact with infected animals, drinking contaminated water, and contact with contaminated water, e.g., swimming pools, during recreational activities. Outbreaks are often seen in day care centers (Cordell & Addiss, 1994). Since chlorine does not kill *Cryptosporidium,* municipal water supplies can be contaminated. In 1996, cryptosporidiosis in children with HIV infection accounted for 3% of initial AIDS diagnoses (CDC, 1996).

PATHOGENESIS. The most common site of infection is the small intestine. In patients who are severely immunosuppressed it is possible to find cryptosporidia throughout the gastrointestinal tract. *Cryptosporidium* causes a noninflammatory malabsorption in the small intestine, resulting in watery diarrhea and decreased absorption of carbohydrates.

CLINICAL MANIFESTATIONS. Symptoms of cryptosporidiosis include fever, frequent and voluminous watery diarrhea, bloody or mucoid stools, cramps and abdominal pain, weight loss and dehydration, and lactose intolerance.

DIAGNOSIS. The diagnosis of cryptosporidiosis is made by finding the organism in stool or tissue samples. At least three stool samples should be submitted for oocyst evaluation.

TREATMENT. There is no proven therapy for cryptosporidiosis in patients with AIDS. Certain medications such as azithromycin and paromomycin are being used but are somewhat ineffective. Supportive care with hydration and nutritional supplementation is recommended. Antidiarrheal agents such as loperamide can be used cautiously. Total parenteral hyperalimentation may be beneficial and can be decreased or discontinued once the child is able to eat and absorb nutrients.

CONSIDERATIONS FOR CARE. Families or caregivers should be educated and counseled about the many ways *Cryptosporidium* can be transmitted. Teaching children and caregivers to wash their hands before eating and after toileting is important as is the safe preparation of food. Drinking water and recreational water facilities may pose a risk for infection, and the use of bottled or boiled water is a preventive measure in selected areas (Ritchie & Becker, 1994). The purity of bottled water is not guaranteed because filtration processes vary. Water that is bottled by distillation is the only type that is presumably free of contaminants.

Since there are no effective treatments, clinicians must focus on symptom management and the prevention of the complications of unremitting diarrhea and abdominal pain. Interventions such as good skin care and hygiene, fluid replacement, nutritional support, and pain management can help a patient maintain a better quality of life. Infection control measures to prevent spread should include the wearing of protective clothing and gloves by caregivers, proper waste disposal, good hand-washing technique, and the implementation of enteric precautions. Because cryptosporidiosis is communicable, only toilet-trained children with symptoms should be permitted in group settings. Boiling drinking water for at least 1 minute will kill the oocysts.

Cytomegalovirus (CMV) Disease

EPIDEMIOLOGY. Human CMV is ubiquitous and can be transmitted by contact with virus-containing secretions (horizontal) or in utero (vertical). Horizontal transmission is most often caused by contact with infected saliva and is easily spread by young children in group situations. Nearly 60% of children with AIDS have either systemic CMV or viral shedding without symptoms (Whitley & Whitley, 1994). Infants born to women who are infected with both HIV and CMV stand a higher risk of being infected with CMV perinatally. While CMV infection in adults is usually a secondary reactivation of an earlier infection that occurred before HIV infection, children are more likely than adults to contract CMV as a primary infection after becoming infected with HIV. In 1996, CMV infections in children with HIV infection accounted for 1% of initial AIDS diagnoses (CDC, 1996).

PATHOGENESIS. In the immunosuppressed person, CMV can replicate in many body sites, including salivary glands, prostate, cervix, testes, and in some instances the peripheral blood lymphocytes. Common CMV infections in children include chorioretinitis, enteritis, interstitial pneumonitis, hepatitis, neutropenia, thrombocytopenia, and encephalitis.

CLINICAL MANIFESTATIONS. CMV chorioretinitis is found on ophthamologic examination when white perivascular exudates and hemorrhages with a cottage cheese or catsup appearance are seen in the retina. Colitis results in bloody diarrhea malabsorption and failure to thrive. CMV pneumonia presents with a diffuse interstitial appearance radiographically, hypoxemia, shortness of breath, and dry, nonproductive cough. The symptoms of encephalitis include fever, altered mental status, headaches, somnolence, behavior changes, and confusion.

DIAGNOSIS. Since so many normal children are infected with CMV, it is important to distinguish infection from disease. Therefore CMV is diagnosed by laboratory tests looking for isolation of the virus, detection of antigen, or an increase in CMV serum antibodies and by pathologic examination of infected tissue.

Some experts recommend that a CMV urine culture be obtained at birth for all HIV-infected or exposed infants to diagnose congenital CMV infection (CDC, 1997a). HIV-infected infants and children who are severely immunosuppressed and CMV-negative may benefit from annual CMV antibody testing. Those identified as having acquired CMV could then be screened for retinitis. Children with severe immunosuppression may benefit from a dilated retinal eye examination every 4 to 6 months.

TREATMENT. Antiviral treatment for CMV infection includes intravenous ganciclovir; foscarnet may be used as alternative therapy. For prophylaxis for recurrence, see Table 4–1.

CONSIDERATIONS FOR CARE. Clinicians should teach patients and caregivers the importance of good hand-washing in preventing the spread of CMV. Parents need to be counseled about the possibility of infants and children being exposed to CMV in day care centers, although this is not considered a reason to advise against day care for HIV-infected children. Older children can be taught to report floaters in the eye.

Patients who are receiving ganciclovir and zidovudine must be monitored for neutropenia. Children who have suffered vision loss from chorioretinitis should be referred to organizations for the blind for assistance with activities of daily living. Special educational placement may be necessary.

Encephalopathy

EPIDEMIOLOGY. Many children with HIV/AIDS have neurologic involvement. In the early years of the epidemic, the percentage of children being reported with progressive encephalopathy was high because the children being observed had advanced HIV disease. Neurodevelopmental delays in infants, as well as neuropsychological deficits in older children, have been noted in 75% to 90% of children with HIV (Butler et al., 1991). In 1996 HIV encephalopathy in children with HIV infection accounted for 17% of initial AIDS diagnoses (CDC, 1996).

PATHOGENESIS. The neurologic problems seen in pediatric patients are believed to be a result of direct damage caused by the HIV in brain tissue (Brouwers et al., 1994). The most common computed tomography (CT) finding is cerebral atrophy. HIV-1 has been cultured from the cerebrospinal fluid in children with encephalopathy. The brains of children with encephalopathy have shown atrophy and ventricular enlargement.

CLINICAL MANIFESTATIONS. Children can manifest either static or progressive encephalopathy. Common signs and symptoms include inability to achieve developmental milestones or loss of milestones, impaired brain growth, weakness with bilateral pyramidal tract signs, ataxia, and (less commonly) seizures and coma. Many children also manifest hypertonicity, spasticity, rigidity, and hyperreflexia. Static encephalopathy is characterized by nonprogressive cognitive or motor deficits, hyperactivity, or attention deficits.

DIAGNOSIS. Diagnosis is made by neurodevelopmental evaluation, computerized tomography, and examination of cerebrospinal fluid. Since other organisms such as *Toxoplasma gondii,* CMV, HSV, varicella-zoster virus (VZV), and Epstein-Barr virus (EBV) can cause encephalitis, differential diagnosis is necessary. Toxoplasmosis is relatively uncommon in young HIV-infected children, although it does occur in older, school-age children and adolescents.

TREATMENT. The best treatment for HIV encephalopathy appears to be antiretroviral therapy. Zidovudine has been shown to cause an improvement in neurodevelopmental functioning, and newer antiretroviral drugs used in combination therapy may further alter the course of HIV encephalopathy. Other identified underlying CNS infections are treated with the appropriate medications. Children with delays in motor, language, or cognitive development need rehabilitative services, such as physical therapy, speech therapy, and special education. Infants should be referred to early intervention programs as soon as any delays are noted.

CONSIDERATIONS FOR CARE. Because of the prevalence of HIV-related neurologic deficits in children with HIV, each child with HIV infection must be monitored frequently for changes in cognitive and motor functions. Every physical examination should include a basic neurologic evaluation; in addition, it is advisable for children to undergo neuropsychological testing at 6-month intervals. CNS involvement can occur at any time in the course of the disease and may start out quite discretely, with families reporting subtle to obvious changes. It is sometimes difficult for families to come to terms with their child's developmental delay, and they may deny that their child is any different from his or her normal peers. Understanding and acceptance of the consequences of the encephalopathic syndrome is a gradual process that can best be facilitated by the clinician who provides careful and simple explanations of the child's level of development and the benefits of rehabilitation therapies.

Herpes Simplex Virus (HSV) Disease

EPIDEMIOLOGY. Herpes simplex virus type 1 (HSV-1) is transmitted primarily by oral secretions. Most infections affect the skin and mucous membranes. Children living in lower socioeconomic situations are at higher risk of getting HSV-1. Recurrent episodes of severe ulcerative herpetic lesions develop in 5% to 10% of children who have HIV infections and primary gingivostomatitis (Whitley & Whitley, 1994). In 1996, HSV infections in children with HIV infection accounted for 5% of initial AIDS diagnoses (CDC, 1996).

PATHOGENESIS. HSV-1 can be asymptomatic, or it can present as gingivostomatitis. The virus then becomes latent and recurs in response to fever, menstruation, sun exposure, or trauma. Herpes labialis (also known as cold sores or fever blisters) is the most common form of recurrent HSV-1 infection. Immunosuppressed patients can develop viremia and disseminated disease.

CLINICAL MANIFESTATIONS. Primary HSV-1 gingivostomatitis causes fever, mucosal ulceration, drooling, pain, and anorexia. The lesion first appears as a painful vesicle with an erythematous base and then becomes an ulcer, which crusts over. Frequently there is tingling or burning for hours or days at the site where the lesion will develop. HSV-1 can also cause esophagitis with pain on swallowing, encephalitis, and widely disseminated disease in the liver, spleen, adrenal glands, lungs, kidney, and brain.

DIAGNOSIS. Diagnosis is based on clinical findings and laboratory examination of material obtained from gentle scraping of the vesicles.

TREATMENT. Acyclovir is the drug of choice for treatment of HSV-1 disease. It can be given orally for primary gingivostomatitis or intravenously for severe or unresponsive episodes or for disseminated disease. For prophylaxis for recurrence, see Table 4–1.

CONSIDERATIONS FOR CARE. Comfort measures such as analgesics, cold liquids, or ice packs for pain can be offered. Caregivers should wear gloves when in contact with oral secretions or lesions. Patients and caregivers should use good handwashing techniques. Children should be engaged in distracting activities to keep them from picking at the lesions and self-inoculating and spreading the virus to other parts of the body.

Histoplasmosis

EPIDEMIOLOGY. Histoplasmosis is caused by a fungus, *Histoplasma capsulatum,* and is endemic to certain geographic regions of the United States, including the Ohio and Mississippi river valleys. In addition, the organism is endemic to countries in the Caribbean and Central and South America. The spores are found in soil that contains bird or bat droppings. Although histoplasmosis is listed as an AIDS-defining illness in children with HIV infection, it is rarely diagnosed. In fact, in 1996 only one case of histoplasmosis was reported as the initial AIDS diagnosis in an HIV-infected child (CDC, 1996).

PATHOGENESIS. *H. capsulatum* is aerosolized, and the spores are inhaled and enter the bloodstream via the alveoli. In most HIV-infected adults, the development of histoplasmosis is a reactivation of a previous infection or is due to reinfection in persons living in endemic areas. Thus it is possible to see latent infection due to *H. capsulatum* develop in an HIV-infected person in New York who migrated from the Caribbean, e.g., Puerto Rico. Disease can also occur in immunocompromised persons who travel to endemic regions and are exposed to the organism.

CLINICAL MANIFESTATIONS. Data on the manifestations of histoplasmosis in HIV-infected children are limited. In adults the signs and symptoms of histoplasmosis include fever, weight loss, abdominal pain, diarrhea, cough, fatigue, lymphadenopathy, hepatomegaly, splenomegaly, oral ulcers, and skin lesions.

DIAGNOSIS. Diagnosis is suspected from travel history and confirmed by isolation of the fungus from respiratory secretions, blood, or bone marrow or by detecting *H. capsulatum* antigen in serum or urine (Ampel, 1996).

TREATMENT. For severe disseminated infection the drug of choice is amphotericin B. For less severe infections, itraconazole may be useful. For clients who cannot tolerate either of these agents, fluconazole may be of benefit (Ampel, 1996). For prophylaxis for recurrence, see Table 4–1.

CONSIDERATIONS FOR CARE. Travel history is an integral part of the suspicion of a diagnosis of histoplasmosis in nonendemic areas. Although persons living in or visiting endemic areas cannot be completely protected from exposure, the CDC (1997) recommends that HIV-infected persons avoid activities known to be associated with increased risk, e.g., cleaning chicken coops, disturbing the soil beneath bird-roosting sites, and exploring caves.

Lymphoid Interstitial Pneumonitis (LIP)

EPIDEMIOLOGY. Lymphoid interstitial pneumonitis (LIP) is a pulmonary disease that frequently occurs in HIV-infected children (Hauger, 1991). Despite the fact that the 1994 revised classification system for pediatric HIV infection lists LIP in category B (moderately symptomatic conditions), it remains an AIDS-defining condition (CDC, 1994). LIP is sometimes associated with hyperplasia of bronchus-associated lymphoid tissue (pulmonary lymphoid hyperplasia [PLH]). In the years since primary antiretroviral therapy for children became available, the incidence of LIP has decreased from 27.7% to 20.6% (Connor & Andiman, 1994). In 1996, LIP in children with HIV infection accounted for 20% of initial AIDS diagnoses (CDC, 1996).

PATHOGENESIS. LIP is an insidious, slowly progressive disease that is seen in the second or third year of life. Usually there is no fever, and the short-term effects are far less serious than those of PCP. LIP is often accompanied by wheezing, marked lymphadenopathy and hepatosplenomegaly, sharply elevated serum gamma globulin levels, and occasional parotitis.

CLINICAL MANIFESTATIONS. LIP-PLH causes chronic nonproductive cough and exertional dyspnea, leading to dyspnea and finally to hypoxemia at rest (Pitt, 1991). Chronic hypoxemia causes digital clubbing, mild lactate dehydrogenase elevation, and a widened alveolar-arterial oxygen gradient.

DIAGNOSIS. Pulmonary examinations of HIV-infected children should include roentgenographs of the chest, quantification of blood oxygenation (arterial blood gases or transcutaneous pulse oximetry), and in selected cases a CT scan of the chest. A roentgenograph of the chest may help in the diagnosis, although the definitive diagnosis is based on lung biopsy.

TREATMENT. LIP-PLH responds to corticosteroid therapy, but this therapy should be withheld until there is evidence of significant hypoxemia. Then treatment should begin with prednisone. If there is accompanying reactive airway disease, bronchodilator therapy becomes part of the treatment plan. The long-term management of LIP, when there is bronchiectasis or multiple episodes of bacterial pneumonia, includes admission of the patient to the hospital every 3

months for intravenous infusion of antibiotics, frequent bronchodilator treatments, and frequent chest physiotherapy for 10 to 14 days. This regimen is similar to that offered to patients with cystic fibrosis. As chronic hypoxemia develops, oxygen therapy is given.

CONSIDERATIONS FOR CARE. Initially, LIP is a quiet disease with few symptoms. It is hard for the child and the family or caregivers to understand that the child is sick, when he or she may feel well and the only evidence of LIP is found on roentgenographs. One of the most difficult things for families to understand is that LIP remains an AIDS-defining disease, even though it is put in the moderate classification of clinical symptoms. Parents should be taught that, even though the diagnosis of LIP now gives their child an AIDS diagnosis, children in whom LIP develops actually do better with their HIV infection than others. Given the strong and frightening meaning the word *AIDS* has for so many families, this distinction will have to be repeated more than once.

When reactive airway disease (RAD) is part of the child's clinical picture, families must be taught the management of acute and chronic asthma: the use of inhalers and nebulizers and the early signs of wheezing. As the disease progresses, the child will need more and more respiratory support (see also Respiratory Distress).

Mycobacterium tuberculosis

EPIDEMIOLOGY. In 1987 rates of tuberculosis (TB) began to increase, and by 1991 more than 26,000 cases had been reported in the United States (Gutman, 1993). These cases, primarily in young adults, represent an increasing risk of exposure for children. At present there are few reported studies regarding TB in HIV-infected children, although clinicians around the country are reporting increasing cases of TB in HIV-infected children. Active TB is diagnosed in more than 1000 children annually in the United States.

PATHOGENESIS. TB infection without disease is the preclinical stage of infection with *Mycobacterium tuberculosis*. The tuberculin skin test reaction is positive, but the chest radiograph is normal and the child is free of signs or symptoms. Disease occurs when clinical manifestations of pulmonary or extrapulmonary TB become apparent, either on a chest radiograph or by clinical signs and symptoms. In adults there is a clear time distinction of weeks or years between asymptomatic infection and clinical disease. In young children, however, the two stages are less distinct (Starke et al., 1992). Younger children (less than 4 years of age), children whose exposure occurs within a household, and those who are immunocompromised are considered at greatest risk of progression to the disease. Some experience suggests that HIV-infected children who acquire TB may also have worse pulmonary disease, more rapid progression, and possibly increased rates of extrapulmonary disease (Gutman, 1993).

CLINICAL MANIFESTATIONS. The clinical presentation of TB in HIV-infected children is nonspecific. The commonly known symptoms of fever, night sweats, weight loss, and fatigue are seen in other complications of HIV. In pulmonary TB, cough, dyspnea, chills, and hemoptysis may be present. Extrapulmonary presentation is related to site of infection.

DIAGNOSIS. Although pulmonary TB is not an AIDS-defining illness in children, extrapulmonary TB is an AIDS-indicator disease (CDC, 1994). The diagnosis of TB may be hampered by cutaneous anergy and difficulty in obtaining adequate sputum samples for culture. It is recommended that HIV-infected children who are household contacts of adults with diagnosed TB receive preventive therapy regardless of the results of intradermal skin testing or radiographic examination of the chest. Children whose intradermal tuberculin skin test result is positive are presumed to be infected. In the child with documented immunocompromise, a negative skin test result does not rule out infection. At present, clinicians consider Mantoux skin test results showing 2 to 10 mm of induration to be positive in certain children.

Because some HIV-infected persons may have a suppressed cell-mediated immunity, referred to as anergy, they may not react to a tuberculin skin test, even in the presence of mycobacterial infection or disease. For several years, anergy testing to delayed-type hypersensitivity (DTH) skin test antigens, along with the tuberculin skin test, had been recommended. However, recent studies have demonstrated a lack of standardization of

reagents and inconsistent results in repeat tests in HIV-seropositive persons (CDC, 1997b). Consequently, the routine use of anergy testing in conjunction with PPD testing is no longer recommended (CDC, 1997b). If anergy testing is performed by the primary care provider, at least two skin test reagents should be used, including *Candida* and mumps (CDC, 1997b).

TREATMENT. Standardized regimens for treatment of TB have been complicated by the emergence of strains resistant to therapy. The role of such strains in the infection of children is not yet known. Choice of a drug for treatment can be guided by the sensitivity patterns of the infecting strain. When the treatment is "preventive" or the strain is not known, treatment should include at least three drugs initially and should be continued for at least 9 months (Committee on Infectious Diseases, Academy of Pediatrics, 1992).

CONSIDERATIONS FOR CARE. Adherence to treatment is critical to prevention of complications in the HIV-infected child receiving treatment for TB. Noncompliance can be anticipated because of the long-term nature of treatment. It is critical to assess the ability of family members or caregivers to obtain medication, their understanding of what is expected of them, and their recognition that therapy must be completed. From the start of therapy the clinician should discuss all aspects of the administration of medications, develop a dosing schedule and routine, and show the caregiver how to manage relapse in adherence to the prescribed regimen. Missed appointments should be followed up by the health care team. Directly observed therapy, if available within the community, should be considered if the child's parent is ill or if the family or caregiver demonstrates problems with adhering to the plan of care.

Mycobacterium avium-intracellulare Complex (MAC)

EPIDEMIOLOGY. Nontuberculous or atypical mycobacterial disease has been reported in 10% and 18% of children with AIDS (Hoyt et al., 1992). It is usually extrapulmonary, most often affecting the gastrointestinal tract. Infection with *M. avium-intracellulare* complex (MAC) is responsible for more than 85% of atypical, nontubercular, mycobacterial infections in HIV-infected children (Horsburgh et al., 1993). MAC has been seen most frequently in patients with low CD4+ T-cell counts (see Chapter 3, Table 3–5).

PATHOGENESIS. *M. avium-intracellulare* is a ubiquitous organism found in soil and water, and in persons in whom MAC infection develops, colonization usually occurs before dissemination. The course of disease progresses from infection to bacteremia to multiple organ involvement. The predominant sites of infection include the lymph nodes, spleen, liver, and intestinal tract.

CLINICAL MANIFESTATIONS. The clinical presentation is often nonspecific, involving recurrent fever, chills, night sweats, abdominal pain, diarrhea, failure to gain or maintain weight, hepatosplenomegaly, transfusion-dependent anemia, neutropenia, anorexia, malaise, and diarrhea (Hoyt et al., 1992).

DIAGNOSIS. Definitive diagnosis can be made by cultures of blood, sputum, bone marrow, or stool or by tissue biopsy. Presence of the organism in organ tissue is indicative of dissemination. Identification of MAC in stool or respiratory tract secretions indicates colonization, with or without disease. All organisms should be specifically identified in the laboratory.

TREATMENT. Combination therapy with two drugs is recommended to prevent resistance. Clarithromycin and azithromycin, together with ethambutol, rifabutin, or ciprofloxacin, are the medications considered to be most efficacious (VanDyke, 1995). Treatment success is marked by resolution of fever and night sweats and an increase in weight. Children who are severely immunosuppressed should be offered prophylaxis to prevent primary MAC disease (see Chapter 3, Table 3–5). For prophylaxis for recurrence, see Table 4–1.

CONSIDERATIONS FOR CARE. In addition to treating with antimicrobials, clinicians must also treat the distressing symptoms of MAC. Antipyretics and analgesics should be given for fevers and pain, and caregivers should be taught the correct administration of these medications. Frequently children with MAC experience pain while eating, and if left untreated, they refuse to eat or take medications. This increases their malnutrition and leaves them susceptible to many other problems. Caregivers need to be taught to provide frequent small meals to anorexic children.

Neoplastic Disorders

EPIDEMIOLOGY. Malignant neoplasms occur less frequently in HIV-infected children than in infected adults, although this difference in incidence may not necessarily continue as survival times for children with HIV increase. The most common malignant lesions described are non-Hodgkin's lymphomas (NHL), Burkitt's lymphoma, and smooth muscle tumors (Mueller et al., 1994). Although Kaposi's sarcoma (KS) is listed in the pediatric HIV/AIDS classification system as an AIDS-defining illness in children, it is in fact rarely seen. In 1996 no cases of KS were reported as the initial AIDS-defining illness in an HIV-infected child (CDC, 1996). Both B-cell and T-cell lymphomas have been identified in children infected with HIV (McClain & Rosenblatt, 1990; Wiznia & Nichols, 1990). In 1996 lymphoma in children with HIV infection accounted for 1% of initial AIDS diagnoses (CDC, 1996).

PATHOGENESIS. The mechanisms thought to contribute to the development of malignant neoplasms in HIV are immune suppression along with chronic stimulation by oncogenic viruses such as EBV, human T-cell lymphotropic virus types 1 and 2, CMV, human papilloma virus (HPV), and hepatitis B virus. The uncontrolled growth of malignant cells may also be connected to the HIV-induced production of growth factors such as interleukin-1, interleukin-6, and tumor necrosis factor. Most NHL tumors are usually B-cell types and progress very aggressively. They can appear as systemic processes or as primary CNS lymphomas.

CLINICAL MANIFESTATIONS. In the few cases reported in the literature, there do appear to be differences in the clinical presentation seen in children as compared to adults. The appearance of KS skin lesions is extremely rare in children (McKinney & Prose, 1996). However, one report describes a 6-day-old infant with cutaneous KS lesions (Gutierrez-Ortega et al., 1989). Additionally, although KS in pediatric patients infected with HIV is usually limited to lymphadenopathic form, diffuse nodular skin lesions have been observed (O'Connor et al., 1990). See Chapter 6 for a detailed discussion of clinical manifestations.

Symptoms of lymphoma in children include fever, weight loss, diffuse adenopathy, jaundice, hepatomegaly, abdominal distention, and pain. CNS lymphoma is manifested by developmental delay, confusion, lethargy, memory loss, seizures, hemiparesis, and other focal neurologic signs.

DIAGNOSIS. Diagnosis of neoplastic disorders in children is established by clinical evaluation, imaging techniques, routine laboratory tests, and pathologic examination of tissue.

TREATMENT. Early institution of intravenous chemotherapy with combinations of Cytoxan, methotrexate, vincristine, and prednisone has been somewhat successful in treatment of lymphoma in HIV-infected children. However, the course of lymphomas in some children is so rapid and severe that chemotherapy and radiation therapy may be precluded.

Attempts to treat KS in pediatric patients are limited by the paucity of clinical experience and data available on this topic. Various treatment modalities, including localized radiation therapy, cryotherapy, electrocauterization, surgical excision, chemotherapy, and administration of interferon-alfa may help to control the lesions. No treatment has been shown to increase survival. At best, clinicians are forced to prudently use the treatment experiences that have been gained with adult patients.

CONSIDERATIONS FOR CARE. Although the decision as to whether to treat the child with a neoplastic disorder is based on the clinical and immunologic status of the patient, as well as the type and stage of malignancy, it may be difficult for some families or caregivers to forgo any attempts to treat this disease. Careful explanations of the choices must be provided so that the risks and benefits are clearly understood.

Pneumocystis carinii Pneumonia (PCP)

EPIDEMIOLOGY. *Pneumocystis carinii* is ubiquitous in nature; it is found in air, water, and soil, with worldwide distribution, and is carried by many domestic animals and people. Most children are exposed to *P. carinii* by the age of 4 years and form specific antibodies to it. PCP is the most common OI in children with HIV, accounting for 24% of AIDS-defining diseases in children during 1996 (CDC, 1996). Before the use of prophylaxis, both adults and children had a high mortality rate from PCP, with about half of the deaths among children occurring during the first episode of disease. Most cases of PCP in infants and children occur in the first 3 to 6 months of life (Simonds et al., 1993). With prophylaxis, the prognosis has improved substantially, although PCP remains the most serious OI in children and is often observed in conjunction with a failure to thrive, encephalopathy, and renal disease.

PATHOGENESIS. In children the onset of PCP is quicker and its progression is more fulminant than in adults (Hauger & Powell, 1990). Correlates of death from PCP in children include young age, depleted CD4+ T-cell counts, and the associated clinical manifestations, including failure to thrive, oral or esophageal candidiasis, and encephalopathy. Survival times of children with PCP are shorter than those of adults. The primary site of PCP infection is the lungs, although disseminated infection is also found in the spleen, lymphatic system, and blood (referred to as pneumocystosis).

CLINICAL MANIFESTATIONS. Clinical symptoms of disease include acute tachypnea, dyspnea, fever, dry cough, hypoxemia, and bilateral pulmonary infiltrates. PCP in children frequently progresses to respiratory failure with the need for ventilatory support in the pediatric intensive care unit.

DIAGNOSIS. Definitive diagnosis can be made by lung biopsy or bronchofibroscopy performed with bronchoalveolar lavage. The most prominent laboratory finding is a large alveolar-arterial oxygen gradient, denoting hypoxemia. The roentgenographic pattern is similar to that seen in diffuse interstitial lung disease. PCP should be suspected when hypoxemia is out of proportion to the abnormalities noted on chest radiographs. Isomorphic elevation of lactate dehydrogenase levels is sensitive to PCP but not specific. However, given the high mortality rates associated with untreated PCP, a presumptive diagnosis based on clinical symptoms is preferable to waiting for a definitive diagnosis.

TREATMENT. PCP is generally treated with TMP-SMX and appears to be better tolerated in children than in adults. For children whose condition fails to improve within a few days or who cannot tolerate TMP-SMX because of rash, fever, leukopenia, acute hypoglycemia, or a drop in blood pressure, an alternative treatment is intravenous infusion of pentamidine. However, this regimen has been associated with a high incidence of side effects, including renal insufficiency. Coadministration of corticosteroids has helped to improve outcomes (McLaughlin et al., 1995; Sleasman et al., 1993). For prophylaxis for recurrence, see Table 4–1. Given the high mortality rate associated with PCP in young infants, all clinicians caring for HIV-exposed infants should be knowledgeable about the CDC recommendations for PCP prophylaxis (see Chapter 3, Table 3–5).

CONSIDERATIONS FOR CARE. Oxygen saturations should be obtained on all infants in respiratory distress, and clinicians should have a high index of suspicion whenever an infant presents with respiratory distress and hypoxemia. Caregivers need to have the importance of PCP prophylaxis reinforced periodically; they should be taught to recognize the early signs of respiratory distress and to seek medical care promptly.

Progressive Multifocal Leukoencephalopathy

EPIDEMIOLOGY. The etiologic agent implicated in the development of progressive multifocal leukoencephalopathy (PML) is a neurotropic polyomavirus known as the JC virus (JCV). *J* and *C* are the initials of the first patient in whom the virus was isolated and should not be confused with Jakob Creutzfeldt disease. JCV has a worldwide distribution, and by middle adulthood most persons have been infected with this virus (Chaisson & Griffin, 1990).

PML occurs predominately in persons with severe immunocompromise and impaired cell-mediated immunity. It rarely is diagnosed before death in HIV-infected children, and in 1996 only one case of pediatric PML was reported to the CDC as the initial AIDS-defining illness (CDC,

1996). Kloss and associates (1993) suggest that, although the incidence of PML in HIV-infected children is extremely low, this may change as survival increases.

PATHOGENESIS. PML is a subacute demyelinating disease of the CNS, forming lesions in the white matter of the cerebrum, especially the parieto-occipital region, and may involve the brain stem and cerebellum.

CLINICAL MANIFESTATIONS. In adults the clinical course has resulted in dementia, blindness, paralysis, and death. In children the clinical presentations have included dysarthria, paresthesias of the tongue and chin, dementia, aphasia, muteness, hemiparesis, and severe spastic quadriparesis (Berger et al., 1992).

DIAGNOSIS. CT scan and magnetic resonance imaging (MRI) demonstrate white matter lesions without a mass lesion effect or ring enhancement; definitive diagnosis is established by brain biopsy or postmortem examination (Price, 1997).

TREATMENT. There is no proven effective treatment for PML. There are reports of remission in adult cases after zidovudine monotherapy or combination antiretroviral therapy with zidovudine, didanosine, and indinavir (Elliot et al., 1997; Singer et al., 1994). Cytarabine may also be helpful in some patients (Price, 1997).

CONSIDERATIONS FOR CARE. Most of the accumulated experience in the treatment of adults has demonstrated that the response to attempted therapies has been very poor. Clinicians should be aware that significant psychological support is needed for the family or caregivers as they watch someone they love change from a mobile, socially interactive person into a noncommunicative, paralyzed person with bladder and bowel incontinence. Most of the care is focused on prevention of HIV-related complications and the sequelae of immobility and dementia.

Toxoplasmosis

EPIDEMIOLOGY. Toxoplasmosis is caused by ingestion of a protozoan parasite *Toxoplasmosis gondii*. Most horizontal infection comes from ingestion of undercooked meat, contamination of other foods, and contact with cats. Cats are the known definitive hosts for *T. gondii.* Compared with its occurrence in adults, toxoplasmosis is generally seen sporadically and infrequently in HIV-infected children. In 1996, toxoplasmosis in children with HIV infection accounted for fewer than 1% of initial AIDS diagnoses (CDC, 1996).

Congenital toxoplasmosis that occurs in infants born to immunocompetent women is a result of primary infection during pregnancy. It is possible that when a woman has HIV and is severely immunocompromised, latent toxoplasmosis could be reactivated, resulting in congenital infection. The risk of an HIV-infected infant acquiring congenital toxoplasmosis from an HIV-positive mother has been reported to be low (Minkoff et al., 1997).

PATHOGENESIS. Once the organism has been ingested, sporozoites and bradyzoites are released in the intestine and infection of the epithelium of the gut takes place. Hematogenous dissemination follows, and the organism is spread to other organs, including the brain, heart, and skeletal muscle. In immunocompetent hosts the organism remains latent within the tissue cysts during the chronic phase. As the immune system deteriorates, reactivation of clinical disease is possible. Reactivation of tissue cysts in the central nervous system may explain the high incidence of toxoplasmosis encephalitis in immunosuppressed persons.

CLINICAL MANIFESTATIONS. Toxoplasmosis in older children and adults is believed to be reactivation of chronic infection. The most common presentation is encephalitis. The signs of CNS toxoplasmosis in older children and adults are focal neurologic abnormalities such as hemiparesis, ataxia, cranial nerve palsies, sensory deficits, fever, abnormal level of consciousness, and psychomotor retardation. Symptoms include headache, seizures, confusion, lethargy, impaired coordination, focal weakness, and vomiting. It is also possible to have *Toxoplasma* pneumonitis, which presents with hypoxemia, dyspnea, bilateral infiltrates, and fever.

Congenital toxoplasmosis in infants born to HIV-positive mothers usually is asymptomatic at birth. In the few cases that have been reported, those in whom symptoms later developed had chorioretinitis, cerebritis, pneumonitis, myocarditis, lymphadenopathy, and hepatosplenomegaly. Infants in whom toxoplasmosis was not diagnosed at birth and who were not treated went on to have severe symptoms. Those infants in whom toxoplasmosis was diagnosed before the eighth week of life because of known maternal infection and who were treated early survived the longest.

DIAGNOSIS. There are several different assays for *Toxoplasma* antibodies. The Sabin-Feldman dye test is considered the best one for detecting *Toxoplasma*-specific IgG, but because it is difficult to use in a clinical laboratory, the enzyme-linked immunosorbent assay (EIA) is often used. It is believed to have a 95% overall agreement with the Sabin-Feldman test. *Toxoplasma* IgM is detected by the indirect immunofluorescent IgM antibody test, a conventional IgM-EIA, a double-sandwich IgM-EIA, or an immunosorbent agglutination assay. Only the double-sandwich EIA and the immunosorbent agglutination assay are sensitive enough to diagnose congenital toxoplasmosis.

Serologic testing often is not helpful in distinguishing active toxoplasmosis from chronic toxoplasmosis in patients with AIDS because of immunosuppression or the fact that many cases are caused by reactivation of infection. Congenital toxoplasmosis in infants of HIV-positive mothers can be diagnosed on the basis of a positive IgM at birth and an elevated IgG.

Toxoplasma encephalitis is diagnosed by computed tomography (CT) with contrast, which shows intraparenchymal ring-enhancing lesions in various regions of the brain.

TREATMENT. The standard treatment for toxoplasmosis is pyrimethamine, sulfadiazine, and supplements of folinic acid (leucovorin). After a 6-week course of primary treatment is completed, suppressive therapy should be continued indefinitely to prevent relapse. For prophylaxis for recurrence, see Table 4–1. Steroids can be used if there is evidence of cerebral edema. HIV-exposed infants with congenital toxoplasmosis are also treated with pyrimethamine, sulfadiazine, and folinic acid. The length of treatment is not certain, although a minimum of 6 months is advisable.

Children more than 12 years old who receive PCP prophylaxis with TMP-SMX are usually protected against toxoplasmosis. If they are taking another prophylactic agent, then they may need annual serologic testing for *Toxoplasma* antibody.

CONSIDERATIONS FOR CARE. Education of patients and family or caregivers is very important in preventing toxoplasmosis. Pregnant women should be taught to wash their hands before eating or touching their faces, to cook meat thoroughly, and to avoid contact with cat feces. The same is true for all HIV-infected patients (see Appendix I for food safety and pets).

Since lifelong suppressive therapy may be necessary for patients with AIDS, the clinician must explore with the child and family or caregivers ways to assist with adherence to the treatment plan. Since most of the pediatric patients who get toxoplasmosis are adolescents, the clinician must pay special attention to the patient's beliefs and attitudes about illness and medications. Frequently adolescents will stop taking medications as a way of testing whether they are sick or in an effort to gain some control over their lives.

Wasting Syndrome

EPIDEMIOLOGY. In 1989 Kotler and associates studied the relationship between wasting and death in HIV-infected adults. These investigators found that body cell mass (a measure of the amount of functional protoplasm in muscles and viscera of the body) had a linear relationship to survival. The implication is that death from wasting may be due to the degree of wasting rather than the specific cause of wasting. In theory, therefore, maintenance of nutritional status should lead to prolonged survival. In 1996 the CDC reported that wasting syndrome was diagnosed in 15% of HIV-infected children.

PATHOGENESIS. The mechanisms that underlie wasting and growth failure are discussed in Chapter 3. Potential mechanisms for wasting in HIV-infected children include impaired or inadequate oral intake, impaired nutrient absorption or gastrointestinal malabsorption, and metabolic derangements or abnormal energy utilization (Kotler & Grunfeld, 1996; Miller, 1996).

The possible causes of inadequate oral intake (Miller, 1996) include

1. Oral/esophageal infection, e.g., candidiasis
2. Oral/esophageal ulcers, e.g., HSV, CMV, or idiopathic ulcers

3. Peptic disease, e.g., gastroesophageal reflux/ esophagitis, gastritis/ulcers
4. Abnormalities of taste
5. Encephalopathy
6. Primary anorexia

Other factors that may contribute to inadequate food intake include limited financial resources, unavailability of food, pain, fatigue, dyspnea, depression, or other psychosocial barriers (Ungvarski, 1996).

Gastrointestinal absorption is affected by infections of the gastrointestinal tract, malnutrition alone, or direct or indirect effects of HIV on the intestinal epithelial cell. Infections that are known to promote malabsorption include *Cryptosporidium*, microsporidia, MAC, *Giardia lamblia,* and rotavirus. Kotler and colleagues (1995) have also described a chronic bacterial enteropathy in adults with AIDS, which results in diarrhea and wasting. Malabsorption and wasting have also been identified in adults with AIDS, who have pathogen-negative diarrhea. Similarly, although not as yet seen in children, studies have reported bile acid malabsorption with chronic diarrhea and weight loss in adults with AIDS (Cramp et al., 1996; Steuerwald et al., 1995).

In 1987, McLoughlin and colleagues described gastrointestinal disease in children with HIV infection and theorized that idiopathic villus atrophy and bacterial or opportunistic infections may be causing the abdominal pain, diarrhea, and progressive weight loss. Miller and associates (1993) found that 60% of HIV-infected children had some degree of carbohydrate malabsorption and 40% had lactose malabsorption. The carbohydrate malabsorption was not associated with nutritional status or gastrointestinal symptoms, but abnormal d-xylose absorption was associated with active enteric infection.

The Italian Paediatric Intestinal/HIV Study Group (1993) also reported a high prevalence of intestinal dysfunction in HIV-infected children. Fat malabsorption was identified in 30%, carbohydrate malabsorption in 32%, and protein loss in 17% of the children observed in the study. Disaccharide intolerance in children infected with HIV has also been noted (Yolken et al., 1991).

Several aspects of intermediary metabolism have been studied in HIV-infected persons, and it is generally believed that metabolic alterations may play an important role in malnutrition and the wasting process. Caloric demands are increased during infection and fever, and resting energy expenditure has been shown to be higher in patients with advanced disease (Slusarczyk, 1994). This increased metabolic rate can contribute to caloric deprivation or weight loss. Children also have added metabolic needs related to growth.

It has also been theorized that altered metabolic rates are due in part to chemical messengers such as cytokines. Cytokines such as interleukin-1 (IL-1), interleukin-6 (IL-6), and tumor necrosis factor (TNF) are produced as a metabolic response to acute injury or infection. These cytokines communicate with somatic tissues in the presence of inflammation. This accelerated protein catabolism and gluconeogenesis of injury is, up to a point, an advantageous response to meet the increased metabolic demands. With HIV infection, a chronic viremic condition, the net effect of cytokines is the nonproductive use of substrates. This cachectic response, first described by Cerami and associates (1985), is also associated with hypertriglyceridemia and reduced clearance of triglycerides by lipoproteins. These investigators theorized that a decrease in triglyceride clearance would lead to an inability to use fats as a reserve source of energy, with consequent wasting of lean body mass. Increased levels of TNF have also been shown to produce severe weight loss, diarrhea, and anorexia (Buetler et al., 1985; Kawakami & Cerami, 1981).

DIAGNOSIS AND CLINICAL PRESENTATION. Wasting syndrome, an AIDS-defining illness, is defined in children as the absence of concurrent illness other than HIV infection that could explain any the following findings (CDC, 1994):

1. Persistent weight loss >10% of baseline
2. Downward crossing of at least two of the following percentile lines on the weight-for-age chart (95th, 75th, 50th, 25th, 5th) in a child ≥1 year of age
3. <5th Percentile on weight-for-height chart on two consecutive measurements ≥30 days apart
4. Chronic diarrhea, i.e., at least two stools per day for ≥30 days
5. Documented fever, intermittent or constant, for ≥30 days

TREATMENT. Ideally, nutrition intervention should be provided as soon as the diagnosis of HIV infection is established in order to prevent weight loss and wasting syndrome (see Chapter 3). Reversal of the wasting syndrome may involve the use of drugs, such as growth hormone or appetite stimulants. Growth hormone has shown efficacy in increasing both weight and lean body mass in adults, and its use is being investigated in children (Mulligan et al., 1993; Schanbelan et al., 1996). Appetite stimulants have been shown to produce weight gain in HIV-infected children (Clarick et al., 1997). Current management involves increasing the frequency of nutrition assessment and counseling and becoming more aggressive with nutrition interventions as disease progresses and weight loss occurs.

Nutrition screening and assessment should take place every 3 months. With altered nutrition and gastrointestinal symptoms, nutrition assessment and counseling should take place monthly. Nutrition interventions generally progress as follows:

1. Preventive nutrition counseling that focuses on
   a. Increasing nutrient density of diet
   b. Increasing food availability and minimizing food wastage
   c. Food safety
   d. Taking a multivitamin with minerals
   e. Promoting feeding development
   f. Meal psychology
2. With altered nutrition status (defined as weight growth velocity <5% in one major growth percentile for weight, or weight-for-height standard <90%, or loss of >5% lean body mass) the goal is to increase calorie and protein intake to 150% of the recommended daily allowance (RDA).
3. Evaluate for malabsorption by assessing d-xylose, fecal fat, amylase/lipase.
4. Provide oral enteral supplementation if dietary modification does not produce weight gain. May have to prescribe a specialized supplement, e.g., an elemental product, one with medium-chain triglyceride (MCT) oil, or lactose free, depending on the outcome of the malabsorption evaluation.
5. Consider prescribing an appetite stimulant for the loss of appetite when there is adequate absorption, food availability, and adequate oral/motor skills for eating.
6. Consider nasogastric or gastrostomy tube enteral feedings if oral enteral feedings fail to promote weight gain.

7. Consider parenteral nutrition if enteral nutrition fails to promote weight gain.

CONSIDERATIONS FOR CARE. The following case studies illustrate the multifactorial nature of nutritional problems seen in children with HIV/AIDS. Outcome measures for evaluating nutritional interventions include (1) increased appetite, (2) weight gain, and (3) increased lean muscle mass.

CASE STUDIES

■ GASTROINTESTINAL MANIFESTATIONS AND WASTING SYNDROME

Medical History HIV wasting syndrome, cryptosporidiosis, CD4 <2%, chronic sinusitis, urinary tract infection due to *E. coli,* shigella enteritis, hepatitis, anemia, thrombocytopenia.

Summary J. was an 11-year-old boy who had an acute weight loss of 23% of his highest body weight when *Cryptosporidium* was diagnosed. He had chronic diarrhea, consisting of 8 to 12 watery stools per day. J. had a good appetite and good oral intake despite the infection-related malabsorption. Requirements were met orally.

Nutrition Interventions Provided
by the Health Care Team
1. Estimate calorie and protein intake and requirements
2. Make recommendations for increasing soluble fiber for chronic diarrhea management
3. Assess diet for foods or beverages that would exacerbate diarrhea
4. Maintain adequate hydration
5. Assess for malabsorption
6. Recommend nutrition support (TPN) with a varied and nutrient-dense diet
7. Assess the family or caregivers' comfort level with nutrition support in the home
8. Arrange for at-home care services
9. Monitor liver enzymes and electrolytes regularly
10. Determine whether the nutrition plan fits into the lifestyle of the family or caregivers and the child, e.g., school
11. Assure that the caregiver and child, when appropriate, have been involved in the decision-making process

Outcome J. was started on nasogastric tube feedings with an elemental supplement but did not have adequate weight gain. Therefore TPN was initiated. The calories provided by TPN met about 60% of J.'s caloric requirement for catch-up growth. The re-mainder of his caloric needs were met orally. On a regularly scheduled basis, J.'s nutritional status and blood chemistries were monitored. In addition, the caregiver was taught to increase nutrient density in the diet, how to manage diarrhea, and how to follow food safety guidelines. J. continued to have three to four watery stools per day and gradually showed progressive weight loss.

■ NEPHROPATHY AND CARDIAC DISEASE

Medical History Cryptosporidiosis, pneumococcal sepsis (three episodes), CD4 <15%, meningitis, recurrent oral candidiasis, hypertension, cardiomegaly, hypothyroidism, hematuria, immune complex–mediated glomerulonephritis, compression fractures.

Summary K. was an 11½-year-old girl with an oral intake that fluctuated, depending on how much pain (due to compression fractures) she was experiencing. She had a recent deterioration in cognitive function. K. had both hematuria and proteinuria, and her serum albumin level before aggressive nutritional intervention was 3.7 g/dl (average range is 3.9 to 5.2 g/dl). Her blood urea nitrogen and creatinine levels are within normal range.

Both K.'s weight and height were below the fifth percentile on the National Center for Health Statistics (NCHS) growth curve. Her height z score was −4.3, weight z score was −2.5, and weight-for-age median was 58%; thus she was severely malnourished according to the Gomez classification system. Weight-for-height indices did not reflect wasting because her growth was so severely stunted.

Nutrition Interventions Provided
by the Health Care Team
1. Provide effective pain management
2. Estimate calorie and protein intake and requirements
3. Teach K. about meeting her nutritional needs by involving her in meal planning and food preparation
4. Monitor growth closely; in this case z scores and growth-velocity calculations may provide more useful information than the NCHS growth curve because the child is so far below the fifth percentile
5. Assess the efficacy of the appetite stimulant and evaluate whether it is increasing lean body mass or fat
6. Determine whether the nutrition plan fits into the lifestyle of the family or caregivers and the child, e.g., school
7. Assure that the caretaker and child, when appropriate, have been involved in the decision-making process

Outcome Since K. was more likely to drink fluids when she did not feel well, nutrition management was based on optimizing intake when K. was in pain. Both an appetite stimulant and an oral supplement were prescribed. She has no dietary restrictions, e.g., protein, sodium, potassium, or fluids. Weight stabilized for a period of time.

▪ NEUROLOGIC MANIFESTATIONS AND WASTING SYNDROME

Medical History Progressive encephalopathy, wasting syndrome, CD4 <15%, acute deterioration of neurologic status associated with carnitine deficiency (which improved after the discontinuation of zidovudine), pneumonia, anemia, neutropenia, tachycardia, recurrent otitis media.

Summary R. was a 3½-year-old girl with a rapidly deteriorating neurologic status. She could no longer walk or talk, and her oral and motor feeding skills were impaired. Nutrition interventions were adapted to her neurologic status by modifying food textures, working on positioning, and using adaptive feeding equipment. This was done in conjunction with a speech therapist to teach feeding therapy. Home visits were made to teach the child's mother how to increase nutrient density of foods by modifying preparation methods. An intact supplement (1.5 kcal/ml) was also prescribed.

R. has continued to cross downward on the growth curve, and over the course of 1 year she dropped from the 75th percentile on the NCHS growth curve weight-for-age to the 5th percentile weight-for-age. Her weight-for-height was greater than the 75th percentile the previous year, and decreased to the 25th percentile. When nutrition support (a feeding tube) was suggested R.'s mother was resistant. However, with continued counseling and information, she consented to try tube feedings.

Nutrition Interventions Provided by the Health Care Team
1. Provide ongoing nutrition surveillance/monitoring
2. Provide nutrition counseling for increasing nutrient density of diet, food safety, textures, etc.
3. Monitor the child's oral and motor skills for neurologic deterioration
4. Estimate calorie and protein intake and requirements
5. Plan nutrition support to prevent severe wasting syndrome
6. Assess the economic and social needs of the family or caregivers, e.g., food, housing, cooking facilities, support system
7. Assess the caretaker's and child's willingness and ability to manage high-tech nutrition support
8. Assess the need and payment source for home-based nursing

Outcome Nasogastric enteral tube feedings were initiated, and weight gain was appropriate. For long-term enteral nutrition support, a gastrostomy tube was placed and R. continued to gain weight at a rate appropriate for her age.

▪ HEMATOLOGIC MANIFESTATIONS AND WASTING SYNDROME

Medical History Wasting syndrome, CD4 <15%, severe transfusion-dependent anemia, pneumonia, clinical esophagitis, persistent oral thrush, generalized atrophy of the brain on CT scan.

Summary H. is a 13-year-old girl whose HIV infection was diagnosed when she was 11 years of age. She presented as severely malnourished; her 1-hour D-xylose value was 4%. Nasogastric (NG) tube feedings were started, and she received 100 ml/h of Peptamen for 12 hours each day. Antiretroviral therapy and PCP prophylaxis were also initiated. After 1 month, H.'s NG feedings were reduced to 4 days per week. She remained on this regimen 3 more months, and then the NG tube was removed. Her appetite improved, and she began to consume about 60% of her estimated caloric need orally; estimated caloric need was based on a formula for catch-up growth. A few months later, megesterol acetate was prescribed.

Nutrition Intervention Provided by the Health Care Team
1. On the basis of biochemical reports, recommend an appropriate oral supplement
2. Estimate calorie and protein intake and requirements
3. Recommend soft, warm (not hot), bland foods when oral thrush is present
4. Assess how the adolescent feels about having an NG tube
5. Strategize with an adolescent about compliance issues
6. Provide support for adolescent in her self-care management
7. Determine whether the nutrition plan fits into the lifestyle of the family or caregivers and the child, i.e., school, etc.
8. Assure that the caretaker and the child (when appropriate) are involved in the decision-making process

Outcome H. continued to have appropriate weight gain, and her weight-for-age on the NCHS growth curve was at the 25th percentile, up from below the fifth percentile when nutritional interventions were started. Her height-for-age has improved as well. Follow-up nutrition counseling was provided on a monthly basis with focus on increasing nutrient density of the diet, food safety, and involving H. in her own nutrition management.

ORGAN SYSTEM PROBLEMS

In addition to the complications associated directly with immune system dysfunction such as OI's and neoplasms, HIV can also have a direct cytopathic effect on various organ systems in children with AIDS. Most, but not all, complications are associated with advanced disease and poor immune function. Frequently children with AIDS will have more than one organ problem at a time. The following section presents a brief description of these organ complications.

Cardiac Problems

EPIDEMIOLOGY. Left ventricular dysfunction is becoming the most significant manifestation of cardiac disease in children with HIV disease. It has been observed in 29% of children with HIV disease and is seen more commonly in children with symptomatic disease (Lipshultz et al., 1989). In addition, cardiomyopathy has been noted in 14% of children with HIV disease (Scott et al., 1989).

PATHOGENESIS. Various factors that may contribute to the cardiomyopathy seen in pediatric HIV disease include HIV infection of cardiac tissues, myocardial inflammation, cardiotoxicity due to some medications used to treat HIV infection, cardiac infection, anemia, and malnutrition, or the cardiomyopathy may be a consequence of longer survival. It has been noted that hemodynamic abnormalities, dysrhythmias, and unexplained or sudden death are not uncommon in children with HIV disease and may be related to an autonomic dysfunction related to underlying disease of the CNS.

CLINICAL MANIFESTATIONS. Decreased left ventricular contractility and dilatation can result in congestive heart failure. Signs and symptoms of heart failure include tachycardia, gallop rhythm, tachypnea, hepatosplenomegaly, diaphoresis, hypoxia, poor peripheral circulation, edema, growth

failure, and fatigue. Other symptoms of cardiac failure include poor feeding in infants, mottled extremities, decreased urine output, decreased blood pressure, and activity intolerance. Patients with HIV disease can also experience arrhythmias, abnormalities of blood pressure (high or low), pericardial disease, and pulmonary hypertension.

DIAGNOSIS. Baseline evaluation should include careful measurement of vital signs and weight, a thorough physical examination, electrocardiographs, radiographs of the chest, and echocardiographs (Lane-McAuliffe & Lipshultz, 1995). A complete blood count will identify anemia, measurement of arterial blood gases or transcutaneous pulse oximetry will show an oxygen saturation indicative of hypoxia, and a blood culture may be needed if cardiac infection is suspected. A formal cardiac assessment should be sought when patients exhibit unexpected or unexplained respiratory symptoms, signs of congestive heart failure (CHF), arrhythmias, cyanotic episodes, or seizures.

TREATMENT. Treatment is aimed at providing cardiac support, since a cure is not possible. CHF is managed with inotropic agents (e.g., digoxin), after-load-reducing therapy such as angiotensin-converting enzyme inhibitors (e.g., captopril), diuretics, oxygen, and transfusion for anemia. Antiarrhythmic therapy and correction of electrolyte abnormalities can treat arrhythmias, and antihypertensives are used for symptomatic hypertension. For patients with severe malnutrition and worsening cardiac disease, it is recommended that the levels of micronutrients, selenium, and carnitine, which may play a role in ventricular dysfunction, be checked. If they are found to be low, replacement therapy may prove helpful (Lipshultz, 1994).

CONSIDERATIONS FOR CARE. Clinicians should be alert for the early signs of cardiac disease. It is recommended that a baseline cardiac evaluation be conducted at the time of diagnosis, with follow-up cardiac examinations at 12-month intervals. Children and families will require teaching about the need for tests, the medications prescribed, and the monitoring of the child in the home for signs of acute heart failure. The measurement and administration of cardiac medications must be thoroughly reviewed with the family or caregivers so that no mistakes in dosing are made. Some cardiologists prefer to have the caregiver check the apical pulse before giving each dose of digoxin and report any heart rate outside the parameters established by the doctor before administering any medication. Again, as with other chronic problems, when the need is identified, a visiting nurse can be requested to monitor the child's response to therapy by assessing vital signs, weight, and overall condition and by teaching the family or caregivers how to assess and manage the child's condition and reinforce the safe administration of medications.

Hematologic Problems

EPIDEMIOLOGY. Moderate anemia is present in nearly all perinatally infected infants and has been found in 94% of patients with symptoms (Ellaurie et al., 1990). Thrombocytopenia occurs in 19% of HIV-infected children and is often the initial sign of HIV infection (Mueller, 1994). Neutropenia has been seen in 43% of untreated children with HIV infection (Pizzo et al., 1988).

PATHOGENESIS. Hematologic disease may result directly from cytopathic effects of HIV or appear as a secondary consequence of immune system dysfunction. Certain drugs, including zidovudine and TMP-SMZ, cause anemia and neutropenia. Anemia can be caused by iron deficiency and acute parvovirus infection, and neutropenia is seen frequently with MAC. Thrombocytopenia is not well understood but may be a result of increased platelet destruction by immune-mediated mechanisms.

DIAGNOSIS. The diagnosis of hematologic problems is established by monitoring the complete blood count regularly. In complex situations, consultation with a hematologist is needed to definitively diagnose and treat the problem. Occasionally a bone marrow aspirate can be helpful in identifying the cause of a specific problem.

TREATMENT. Iron deficiency anemia is treated with ferrous sulfate. Chronic anemia sometimes requires transfusions of packed red blood cells to maintain hemoglobin levels above 8 g/dl. Erythropoietin has been helpful in adults and can be used in children. Granulocyte-macrophage colony–stimulating factor (GM-CSF) and granulocyte colony–stimulating factor (G-CSF) have been successful in raising the neutrophil count. G-CSF has been noted to be helpful for zidovudine-induced neutropenia, allowing patients to continue taking zidovudine. Thrombocytopenia is treated with corticosteroids and intravenous immune globulin, and in a few difficult cases vincristine has been used.

CONSIDERATIONS FOR CARE. The complete blood counts (CBC) of patients should be monitored routinely. Families should be taught the importance of this monitoring, especially when the patient is receiving bone marrow–suppressing medications. Parents of children receiving erythropoietin or G-CSF must be taught how to administer the medication and to rotate the injection sites. It may be necessary to have a visiting nurse administer the injections if adherence to the plan is a problem or if the caregiver is unwilling or unable to learn to perform the procedure safely. For children with neutropenia and fever, blood cultures should be performed and broad-spectrum antibiotics should be started. Caregivers should also be taught to watch for and report any unusual bruising or bleeding. In the presence of thrombocytopenia, caregivers should be cautioned not to administer aspirin or nonsteroidal anti-inflammatory agents.

Renal Problems

EPIDEMIOLOGY. HIV-associated nephropathy has been described in 15% of children with perinatally transmitted HIV infection (Strauss et al., 1989).

PATHOGENESIS. The most common renal lesions seen in patients with HIV infection are acute tubular necrosis, interstitial nephritis, and mesangial hyperplasia with glomerulosclerosis. HIV nephropathy is diagnosed when the patient has evidence of heavy proteinuria or nephrotic syndrome. The mechanism leading to kidney disease is unknown; it is speculated that the renal dysfunction seen may result from the presence of HIV.

Patients with HIV infection have also been observed with B- and T-cell lymphomas infiltrating the kidney. A number of drugs used to treat HIV infection, when used in combination, increase the risk of renal damage. Likewise, agents known to be nephrotoxic can cause renal problems. Other problems, such as vomiting, diarrhea, decreased fluid intake, and infections, can also contribute to renal dysfunction.

CLINICAL MANIFESTATIONS. The clinical manifestations of HIV nephropathy include electrolyte abnormalities, hyponatremia, hypokalemia, hyperkalemia, and metabolic acidosis. Proteinuria, edema, hypoalbuminemia, azotemia, and hypertension are also seen. Children rarely have renal failure, except when renal damage is due to nephrotoxic medications.

DIAGNOSIS. Children should be monitored routinely for early signs of renal disease. Baseline tests include urinalysis, CBC, and creatinine and blood urea nitrogen (BUN) determinations. If there is blood or protein in the urine or if urinary tract abnormalities are suspected, a urine culture should be obtained and a renal ultrasound examination performed. A renal biopsy may be necessary to diagnose the severity of renal disease and to rule out the possibility of lymphoma.

TREATMENT. Treatment of HIV nephropathy includes replacement of alkali and other electrolytes. Urinary tract infections should be treated with appropriate antibiotics. When the patient has nephrotic syndrome, sodium intake must be restricted and diuretics must be used carefully. Hypertension is treated with antihypertensive agents. The decision to implement dialysis needs to be considered in the light of the generally poor prognosis of patients with HIV renal failure.

CONSIDERATIONS FOR CARE. Pediatric HIV renal disease often is seen only in abnormal laboratory findings. Patients do not always exhibit overt symptoms, but they may have to take medications to prevent the development of symptoms. Once again, considerable teaching must be provided to help the child and the caregivers understand the need for ongoing treatment. When hypertension develops in a child, the family or caregivers may have to be taught how to take blood pressure readings at home. A visiting nurse referral is required to help reinforce the teaching that is done and to periodically monitor the pa-

tient's condition. A nutritionist should be included in the plan of care to provide nutritional counseling and to assist the caregiver in planning a low-sodium diet.

SYMPTOM MANAGEMENT IN CHILDREN

Many adverse symptoms are experienced by children with AIDS. Although frequently the cause of a particular symptom can be identified, sometimes no cause is uncovered. The uncomfortable and untreated symptoms of AIDS can negatively effect the quality of life of the child and the family or caregivers.

It is imperative to treat the symptom while attempting to determine the cause. Many of the complications of AIDS that cause untoward symptoms cannot be fully cured or take a long time to resolve when treated, prolonging the time of suffering for the child. Although there are few studies aimed at understanding the role of adverse symptoms in disease progression, one might speculate that untreated symptoms such as pain or nausea might interfere with a patient's other health-promoting behaviors, such as eating or exercising. Likewise, untreated symptoms that the family or caregivers suspect are related to certain medications can lead to noncompliance with prescribed regimens or alterations in the prescribed dosages. It is not uncommon to see symptom management offered only at the end of life. It is critical for clinicians to consider palliative care, including symptom management, throughout the course of HIV/AIDS. The following section contains a review of some of the more common symptoms experienced by children with AIDS.

Pain

In studies of adults with HIV/AIDS, it has been reported that pain is a frequently reported symptom during all stages of the disease (Hewitt et al., 1997; O'Neill & Sherrard, 1993). Types of pain include headaches, mouth and throat pain, chest pain, myalgia, peripheral neuritis, arthralgia, and the pain associated with medical procedures (Lebovitz et al., 1989; O'Neill & Sherrard, 1993; Singer et al., 1993). Pain in patients with HIV has been severely undertreated (Breitbart et al., 1996).

Unfortunately, the pain experiences of children with HIV/AIDS have received less attention. A few studies document that, compared with adults, children appear to have similar types of pain related to their HIV illness trajectory. A recent study reported a pain incidence of 59% in children with HIV infection, compared to an incidence of 47% in children with cancer (Hirschfeld et al., 1996). Types of pain experienced by children with HIV include headache, abdominal pain, oral cavity pain, neuromuscular pain, peripheral neuropathy, chest pain, earache, odynophagia, myalgia, and arthralgia (Czarniecki et al., 1993, 1994).

Pain in children with HIV infection poses several unique problems. As the survival of children with perinatally acquired HIV infection lengthens, the potential that multiple complications will create pain increases. Children who are nonverbal because of age or neurologic complications cannot report their own pain. Parents and health care providers may deny a child's pain because it represents progression of disease. Families who have a history of substance abuse may be very resistant to the use of opioid analgesics for fear of addiction.

For effective management of pain in children with HIV infection, the symptom must be acknowledged by all involved in the child's care. This can occur only if pain is consistently assessed. Reports of pain should be taken at face value, and the pain should be treated while a cause is being determined; certainly, it should be treated even if a cause is never identified.

It is frequently found that patients with HIV infection have pain of unknown cause. If there is a reason to suspect pain but the patient cannot tell anyone about it, it is within reasonable treatment guidelines to begin a trial of pain management to see how the patient responds. Frequently, children's chronic pain will be manifest by depressed affect, lack of activity, or anorexia, rather than by crying or grimacing.

The backbone of good pain management should be appropriate use of analgesics with a pain ladder (Pediatric Supportive Care/Quality of Life Committee, 1995):

1. Mild pain: nonsteroidal anti-inflammatory drugs (NSAIDs) or acetaminophen
2. Moderate pain: continue NSAIDs or acetaminophen and add a mild opioid such as codeine
3. Severe pain: continue NSAIDs or acetaminophen and add a strong opioid, morphine being the first choice

There is no ceiling on the dose of opioids used to achieve pain relief, and doses can go very high. Longer-acting opioids, such as liquid methadone or time-released morphine, can be used once the correct dose is determined with the use of short-acting morphine. The fentanyl patch, a transdermal system that provides timed-released fentanyl over 3 days, has been extremely helpful for non-opioid-naive patients who cannot tolerate oral medications. Whenever a long-acting agent is given, the patient must also be given prescriptions for a short-acting opioid for breakthrough pain, often referred to as a "rescue dose."

As tolerance develops, the clinician can calculate the 24-hour requirement for short-acting medication and adjust the long-acting opioid upward. Certain adjuvant medications such as anticonvulsants and antidepressants have been found useful for neuropathic pain. Hydroxyzine, which can help with nausea, also has an analgesic affect and can reduce the amount of opioid required. Side effects of opioids should be anticipated and treated aggressively.

Families must be educated about the difference between physical dependence and addiction. The clinician should explore with the patient and the family or caregivers the meaning of pain to them and their previous experience with pain and pain medications. The issue should be discussed directly with families in which substance abuse exists, and there must be mutual understanding and agreement about the administration of opioid prescriptions.

All children with chronic illnesses undergo multiple painful procedures for both diagnostic and treatment purposes. In many children this becomes the worst part of having a chronic disease. Children dread encounters with their health care providers because they realize, from a very early age, that pain will be involved. As children with HIV infection progress in the illness and AIDS develops, this situation may become worse. There are both pharmacologic and nonpharmacologic interventions that can eliminate the pain and anxiety from these painful procedures. A topical analgesic, eutectic mixture of local anesthesia (EMLA), applied to venipuncture and injection sites 45 to 60 minutes in advance, can eliminate the pain associated with these procedures. Conscious sedation should be employed whenever an extremely painful procedure such as a lumbar puncture, bone marrow aspiration, or placement of a central line, is planned or whenever a child has become severely sensitized to more routine procedures.

In addition to analgesics, other nonpharmacologic measures such as distraction, visualization, hypnosis, relaxation, and music therapy can be helpful. Children respond well to techniques that encourage the use of their imaginations.

Ideally, if children never have to experience their first painful procedure, they will be able to participate and cooperate and will avoid unnecessary trauma. When children are unafraid and able to cooperate, the staff can perform the procedure more quickly and safely. Clinicians should familiarize themselves with these techniques or call on those professionals who have such experience in order to have a range of interventions to offer each child.

Nausea and Vomiting

Nausea and vomiting are frequently seen in children with HIV/AIDS. There are multiple possible causes, including opportunistic infections of the gastrointestinal tract, side effects of medications, pain, and anxiety (Winter & Miller, 1994). Gastroesophageal reflux has been seen as a cause of vomiting, especially in children with encephalopathy. Although nausea can cause some children to become anorexic, in other instances some children will eat and drink the very things that cause nausea.

Interventions are multifaceted. Treatment of any underlying cause, such as infection, is the first goal. Other strategies can include a range of dietary changes such as smaller and more frequent feedings, feeding of thickened foods, upright positioning after meals, avoidance of certain foods that are greasy or whose odor causes nausea, and withholding of nausea-inducing medications for ½ hour before or ½ hour after feedings. Antiemetic medications given around the clock rather than only as needed (prn) may be helpful. Other medications to control reflux, pain, spasticity, and anxiety may also be helpful. Older receptive children can be taught such techniques as relaxation, distraction, and visualization.

Diarrhea

Diarrhea, like nausea and vomiting, is most commonly caused by opportunistic or bacterial organisms and side effects of medication. Protease inhibitors frequently cause diarrhea, especially during the initial induction period. Other causes are lactose intolerance, food or dietary supplement intolerance, and HIV enteropathy. Treatment of the underlying cause, if known, is the first goal. Severe diarrhea requires treatment in the hospital with replacement fluid and electrolytes to prevent dehydration.

Chronic diarrhea is best managed with dietary manipulations. It is advisable to offer a lactose-free diet for lactose intolerance, a low-fat diet with MCT oil additive for fat malabsorption, an elemental formula to maximize absorption, an osmotic formula for osmotic diarrhea, and soluble fiber for chronic diarrhea. Antimotility medications can be offered and given around the clock (Ferris et al., 1995). Since diarrhea can cause skin irritation, caregivers must be taught good skin care and hygiene. If the diarrhea is accompanied by cramps, children may also become anorexic, adding to their weight loss.

School-age children and adolescents often suffer from severe embarrassment and altered body image when they have diarrhea, especially if it is sudden, unpredictable, explosive, or malodorous. Sometimes children have stool leakage, which is also a cause of embarrassment. They may refuse to attend school or to go out of the house for fear of having an episode of fecal incontinence. Having children and families keep a diary of their stool patterns can sometimes help them identify the time of day they are likely to pass a stool or a particular food or beverage that may induce diarrhea. Then they can arrange their schedule and intake accordingly. Parents of older children who are incontinent may need assistance in acquiring disposable diapers for their children.

Fever

Fever is a very common problem in children with AIDS. Causes include infections, malignant neoplasms, dehydration, reactions to medications, and HIV viremia. Because fever is so commonly associated with infection, some of which might be life-threatening in an immunocompromised host, each fever should be worked up appropriately with a physical examination, CBC, blood cultures, and other tests for opportunistic infections. Chest radiographs, lumbar punctures, and other diagnostic tests are performed as indicated by the clinical condition of the patient. Frequently children with OIs will have recurrent predictable fevers at a particular time of the day. When other causes have been ruled out and the pattern is established, treatment can be offered without an extensive work-up.

Antipyretics, such as ibuprofen or acetaminophen, are given for fever as needed. In addition, the patient should be covered with a sheet or loose woven blanket to prevent chilling and shivering, which increase temperature. One should provide increased fluids and calories to meet the increased metabolic needs associated with fever and promote comfort by keeping the patient dry.

Caregivers must be able to demonstrate taking a correct temperature and should have a thermometer available in the home. Parents should be taught that the rectal route is preferred, especially when fever is present. Oral and axillary routes are acceptable for afebrile patients. Caregivers need to know that the axillary temperature is about 1° less than temperatures measured by other routes. Parents should be taught to use the type of thermometer that will be used in the home. For caregivers who have trouble learning to read a glass thermometer, assistance should be provided in obtaining an electronic one that gives a digital reading.

Most important, parents need to know the importance of reporting fever to their health care provider as soon as possible. If the patient has recurrent fevers, parents need to be taught to report changes in the degree or frequency of the fever.

Respiratory Distress

Patients with LIP/PLH, PCP, or pneumonia often have dyspnea, tachypnea, wheezing, cough, chest pain, and fatigue. Hypoxia is often present. As the lung disease progresses, these symptoms can increase in severity and have a negative impact on the child's comfort and quality of life.

Infectious causes of respiratory distress can be controlled or treated with antibiotics. When the underlying problem is progressive (as in LIP/PLH), supportive care must be provided. Supportive care measures can include bronchodilators, steroids, oxygen, antitussive agents, chest physiotherapy, and artificial ventilation. Frequent paroxysmal cough may require opioids (Woodruff, 1996).

Children and families need to be taught how to administer all supportive therapies to be given in the home. Respiratory therapy consults may be indicated to make home visits to set up and teach the safe use of therapeutic equipment. Families should be taught to help the child pace his or her activities, building in rest periods throughout the day. The child may need to sleep in a semisitting position for maximum oxygenation. A wheelchair may be necessary for excursions outside the home that would entail a lot of walking. If, at the end of life, the child develops respiratory failure and is not going to be artificially ventilated, attention must be paid to the anxiety that can develop from air hunger. Medications such as opioids and anxiolytics can relieve some of this distress.

Altered Mental State

HIV infection can have serious effects on the CNS. In children, this is most frequently seen as developmental delay or loss of developmental milestones (see also Encephalopathy). Less often, usually in older school-age children and adolescents, changes in mental functioning are seen. These changes can include memory loss, confusion, paranoia, hallucinations, seizures, and coma. In many instances the cause of these changes may be related to the direct effects of HIV or OI on the central nervous system.

If a diagnosis of a known OI such as toxoplasmosis or central nervous system CMV infection is made, treatment of those infections is begun and maintained throughout the patient's life. In many cases in which the cause is unknown or there are no effective treatment options (e.g., PML), therapeutic goals are directed toward preventing injury, maintaining function for as long as possible, and providing the caregivers with as much support as possible. Rehabilitation services, such as physical, occupational, and speech therapy, provide the patient with interventions to prevent further complications and assistive devices to facilitate activities of daily living. Mental health professionals can help when there is depression, altered personality, or psychosis. Occasionally the patient is treated with antipsychotic medication.

Skin Lesions

Several types of skin problem can occur in children with HIV infection. These include fungal infections of the skin, scalp, and nailbeds, herpes simplex and zoster, molluscum contagiosum, diaper candidiasis, bacterial infections, rashes due to medications, and rashes of unknown origin. These skin problems can cause itching, pain, secondary infection, and embarrassment for the child.

In healthy persons, molluscum contagiosum is commonly seen as yellow or skin-colored, clustered, umbilicated papules that usually occur on the torso or in the anogenital region. In children with HIV infection, the lesions often involve atypical areas such as the face and may disseminate or form a giant molluscum. If lesions are not extensive, treatment by local destruction may be attempted; however, recurrence is common. Lesions have been noted to clear after the initiation of antiretroviral therapy. In immunosuppressed persons, skin lesions associated with histoplasmosis or cryptococcosis may mimic molluscum. Therefore biopsy is recommended for definitive diagnosis (Whitworth et al., 1995).

The first goal is to treat the underlying problem, if possible. Treatments can be both topical and systemic. The related symptoms should be treated concomitantly. Pain medication, antipruritics, steroids, hydrating creams or ointments, cool oatmeal baths, and massage may be beneficial. It is important to prevent skin breakdown related to scratching, infection, or immobility. Children will frequently scratch or pick at skin lesions. Helpful interventions to discourage this include distracting activities, covering the affected area with clothing or loose dressings, and covering the hands with gloves or mittens at night. Immobilized children should be repositioned every 2 hours or less to prevent the development of pressure sores. Good hygiene to the skin is essential in preventing secondary infections. Bathing should be gentle, with a mild soap, thorough rinsing, and application of an emollient cream after the bath to retain skin moisture.

PSYCHOSOCIAL CARE OF THE CHILD WITH AIDS

Throughout the course of HIV disease, many psychosocial issues involving the child and family or caregivers have to be addressed. As the disease progresses and more and more complications develop, the stress for everyone increases. Each new diagnosis brings fear, grief, anger, and the need to make more decisions. The physical care of the child becomes more of a burden for the family or caregivers. Likewise, the child's emotional reactions to being sicker also present challenges. The following discussion highlights some of the common psychosocial problems the child and the family or caregivers may be forced to confront.

Decision Making

The family or caregivers must learn about each new problem that is identified, its effects on the child, and its possible treatments. The family or caregivers will have to make decisions about whether to use one treatment or another. Even when professionals believe that a certain treatment must be started, the person responsible for the child's care must deal with the fear that adding another medication to the child's treatment plan might cause other problems or complications. Frequently the proposed treatment, while deemed necessary to control a problem and to prolong life, interferes in a major way with the child's and the family's or caregivers' quality of life. The treatment may involve increased pain or suffering for the child or may even involve some added risk, e.g., surgery and general anesthesia. The fear of making a decision that will result in an adverse outcome for the child is always present.

Clinicians must be sensitive to these feelings and give the family or caregivers time to absorb the new information and understand all of its ramifications. Explore with the child and the family or caregivers what the presence of this new problem means to them. Do they believe it heralds the beginning of the end, or are they in some degree of denial about it? Children who are capable of understanding what is happening to them can also have feelings similar to those of the family or caregivers. The child is the one who must ultimately undergo the new treatment, and it is absolutely necessary to take the time to explain the problem, as often as necessary, clearly identifying the effects on the body and the benefits and risks of the treatment being offered. Age-appropriate teaching tools, such as body books and dolls, should be used. If the treatment involves some kind of permanent device, such as a tube or catheter, the child and the family or caregivers should be shown the device and given a chance to touch and hold it. Printed materials such as booklets and drawings should also be used.

Caring for the Child in the Community

As children become sicker, they frequently cannot engage in their previous daily routine. This means that the family or caregivers must either care for them at home or find help to do it. Children who were able to attend day care or school for long periods may no longer be able to endure full schedules but still may be able to participate for shorter periods of time. This is a major problem for the family or caregivers who need to maintain full-time employment. One family member or caregiver may have to stay home to care for the child, at the risk of losing his or her job, income, and heath insurance coverage. When the family or caregivers have not disclosed the diagnosis to other family members, friends, or their religious organization, they have limited their available support network and it is difficult for them to ask for help. The worsening condition of the child may require them finally to let others know about the diagnosis. Sometimes when families are offered home care, such as home health aide or private duty nursing services, they are fearful of using them for fear that the person who comes to the home will be someone from their community who might know them or be acquainted with someone they know. In some instances, despite the fact that they need home care services, the family or caregivers view the presence of the home care staff as intrusive and an invasion of their privacy.

Clinicians can be of enormous help to individual families or caregivers by listening, helping them explore all their options, suggesting the words to use when disclosing the diagnosis, and even offering to participate in the disclosure encounter. Social workers and nurses can help families obtain whatever community-based assistance is available and for which they are eligible. If the family has disclosed the child's diagnosis to school officials, the health care providers can work with the school to make an adjusted schedule or, if necessary, arrange for home-based education. It is important for the child to continue with normal childhood activities, such as school, play, and religious participation, for as long as possible. Often families or caregivers will be afraid to let their children participate in activities for fear of causing more medical problems; this can evoke feelings of isolation and resentment in the child.

Facilitating openly candid discussions regarding these issues can lead to mutually satisfactory agreements and ease the stress for everyone.

When the family or caregivers do receive home care services, the HIV primary care providers must maintain close communication with the home care staff. This is important because now even more participants are involved with the plan of care, offering information and advice to the family or caregivers. Home care providers and HIV clinicians must be sure that all know what is happening with the child and the family or caregivers and that each is communicating accurate information to the family or caregivers. This prevents confusion and misunderstandings that can undermine the support the family or caregivers need. Case conferences at the start of a service and at intervals thereafter offer one way to achieve this (see Chapter 11, Case Management).

Adherence to the Treatment Plan

With advancing disease, more medications and treatments are added to the child's life. This can be physically difficult and emotionally draining for all involved in the child's care. The more medication the child has to take, the more difficult his or her daily schedule becomes and the harder it is to maintain a sense of normalcy. Older school-age children and adolescents, who so desperately need to "fit in" and appear to be just like their peers, find that taking multiple medications and losing time from school make them appear different. This is embarrassing and can lead to social isolation. Teenagers will go to extraordinary lengths to maintain the appearance of conformity, skipping medication doses at school or hiding symptoms in order to remain one of the crowd. Learning about all the medications, their names, actions, administration, and side effects can be a daunting task. Keeping track of medication schedules and the need for prescription renewals is also challenging. If clinicians are honest with themselves and think of how hard it is to take or give just one medication, it is not hard to imagine what children and their families or caregivers are going through. Health care providers should employ as many tools as necessary to facilitate adherence to the treatment plan.

The first thing the clinician must do is explore with the child and the family or caregivers how they feel about these medications, one medication at a time. Ask the family or caregivers which medications they think are most or least important, which ones the child has the most difficulty taking or tolerating, and which ones the child misses most often. Ask about the daily routine of the child and the family or caregivers and how the medication regimen affects it. When this is done in a nonjudgmental way, it is possible for clinicians to work flexibly with the child and the family or caregivers to solve problems and work out a reasonable plan. Such tools as calendars and schedules can be helpful. A few older children have liked recording each time they take their medication on a form similar to ones used by nurses in hospitals. Helping parents and children to remember to take medications by using something in their daily schedule as reminders (e.g., meals, schooltime, television programs) can also be useful (Czarniecki, 1996).

Sometimes as children become sicker, the family or caregivers begin to believe that the medications are the cause of the new problems and they want to stop treatment. In some instances this is, in fact, the case, when an adverse effect of a medication is experienced. Sometimes they want to seek alternative treatments outside the conventional health care system. Clinicians must respect the child and the family or caregivers as they make treatment decisions. Even when they are making decisions with which the health care provider disagrees, it is important for the clinician to avoid communicating his or her judgment of that decision and jeopardizing the provider's relationship. Encourage the child and the family or caregivers to be open and honest about what they are or are not taking or about alternative treatments they are seeking. Use of these approaches allows for an open dialogue and continuing interest in learning.

Multiple Hospitalizations

Children with HIV/AIDS are hospitalized frequently because of acute and chronic problems. When this happens, the child and the family or caregivers must interact with another group of health care providers, including different physicians and nurses. If they are fortunate, they will still be able to have contact with their own primary care providers or HIV specialists. Unfortunately, however, this is an infrequent occurrence.

Issues of communication, knowledge, and trust can arise. Chronic treatment plans can be changed, overlooked, or disrupted. Different or even erroneous information may be given by an inexperienced professional. The child and the family or caregivers may become confused or frightened by what is happening or may not agree to a new plan because they do not fully trust those who are offering it to them.

To avoid some of these problems, clinicians can remember some basic rules about caring for a child with AIDS in the hospital (Oleske & Boland, 1997):

1. Make sure that all of the child's chronic medications and treatments are ordered.
2. Help the family or caregivers receive a consistent message by conferring with the child's hospital care team throughout the acute care stay.
3. Obtain agreement from the team about any new treatments to be offered.
4. Begin discharge planning as soon as the child's condition is stable and his or her home care needs have been identified.
5. Work with the hospital team or the child's case manager to develop a realistic and achievable home care plan.

END-OF-LIFE ISSUES AND CARE

As the child with HIV/AIDS is nearing the end of life, attention must be paid to helping the child and the family or caregivers move through this time period with the least amount of suffering and with the most support and dignity possible. To accomplish this, there are tasks which the child, the family or caregivers, and the health care providers must achieve together.

Recognizing the End of Life

The unpredictability of the course of the HIV illness, along with the development of new antiretroviral agents, makes it difficult to know with any degree of certainty that the HIV-infected child is nearing the end of life. Unlike other diseases, in which certain signs herald the terminal phase of the disease, HIV infection presents a challenge for everyone. Since children do still die of AIDS, it is important for clinicians to be able to recognize when a child may be entering the terminal stage of the disease. Usually, when a child begins to experience multiple progressive organ complications that cannot be controlled, has multiple OIs for which there are few or no effective treatments, and has experienced HIV treatment failure, even with salvage therapy, he or she is approaching or is in the end stage of HIV disease. This is the time when the child's quality of life is greatly compromised by the need for multiple medications, frequent clinic visits, frequent painful procedures, and multiple hospitalizations and when pain and symptoms are increasing.

At the same time, the child, the family or caregivers, and the health care providers are grappling with understanding what is happening and struggling to keep the child alive with the best quality of life possible. It is not uncommon for any one of these persons to come to an understanding about the nearness of death before the others. Sometimes it is the child who begins to realize that he or she can no longer fight, or it is the parent who recognizes that the child's suffering is too great. Different members of the health care team may come to this realization at different times.

When the family or caregivers remain in deep denial and want everything provided, including high-technology aggressive treatments, and clinicians believe that offering such care would be ultimately futile and increase the child's suffering, the potential for conflict exists. Similarly, the potential for conflict again arises when a child or the family or caregivers decide that they would rather stop some treatments or forgo others so that the child can be at home and as comfortable as possible, and the health care providers are unable to admit that this time has come.

All the people involved in the child's care must communicate as openly as possible about what is happening. The primary care providers must speak clearly and explain the child's condition to family or caregivers so that they can make informed decisions about the child's care and the remaining time. Euphemisms can be confusing and can send double messages. Most parents do not want professionals to "give up" on their child, but if it is explained that, rather than giving up, there is simply no further treatment available that will significantly postpone death, parents will understand the difference and begin to make decisions. Parents need to be constantly reassured that all efforts possible will be made to keep the child com-

fortable and that those treatments that enhance comfort will be continued.

Decision Making

As the terminal stage of AIDS approaches, the child who is able to comprehend the situation and the family or caregivers need to make some very difficult decisions. These decisions involve choices about how the child will die, where the child will die, and what plans will be made for the funeral and autopsy.

The decision about how the child will die will involve deciding whether extraordinary means, such as resuscitation, artificial ventilation, and intravenous inotropic therapy, will be used. Discussions about "do not resuscitate" (DNR) orders need to take place before a crisis arises. This discussion is a process in which families are helped to understand their child's medical condition, the treatment options that still remain, and the most likely consequences of those treatments. For example, a child with end-stage cardiomyopathy might live awhile longer with intravenous infusions of cardiac inotropic medications and mechanical ventilation. However, it is improbable that the child would ever be weaned from those therapies and would die slowly while connected to a machine in the intensive care unit. In this instance, the family or caregiver could also be given the option of foregoing the inotropic agents and ventilator and have the child die peacefully at home.

Even when a DNR decision is made, families have to decide which other therapies they will continue, initiate, or forgo. This can include decisions about the continued use of long-term therapies and the administration of other therapies such as blood transfusions or intravenous antibiotics. The benefits to the child in terms of efficacy and comfort need to be weighed against any potential risk or discomfort involved. These discussions are never easy, and families and health care providers can have ambiguous feelings and vacillate in the decision-making process. It is important to keep communication open at all times and to assure families that there are no "wrong" decisions but only those that are right for the child and the family or caregivers. Respecting the wishes of the family or caregivers to be aggressive or to forgo some treatments may be difficult for health care providers when they disagree with the decisions made. It is vitally important to remember that the family or caregivers must cope with the consequences of their decision for the rest of their lives and need as much support as possible.

If a decision has been made to stop any further treatment of the disease and to focus only on comfort and quality of life, then certain interventions can be very helpful to patients and families. First, the family or caregivers can decide whether to have the child die at home or in the hospital. If the home is chosen, referrals to hospice programs or home health agencies can be made. Hospice programs offer a wide array of services, including nursing care, volunteers, spiritual support, support groups, and expertise in symptom management. If the family or caregivers opt for in-hospital care, then every effort should be made to provide hospicelike services.

If they are able to do this in advance of the death, families can be assisted in deciding on the location and type of funeral they will want. Older children who have expressed a desire to be involved in this process should be allowed to do so. Families may need to explore resources for assistance with the financial part of the funeral, and it is easier for this to be worked out in advance than during the time of acute grief.

Similarly, the decision about having an autopsy is best made ahead of time if at all possible. It is a difficult thing to discuss at the time of death when families are in such intense crisis, so clinicians should try to bring it up before the child's death. Autopsies continue to be one of the best ways for us to learn about the disease. Even when the cause of death is known, more can usually be learned from an autopsy. Despite these valid reasons for having an autopsy performed, it is still the right of the family or caregivers to decline this procedure, and pressure should not be placed on them to consent. Rather, the benefits of autopsy for the future care of children with HIV/AIDS should be explained and the actual procedure described in simple terms so that parents understand that the child's body will not be mutilated.

Some families or caregivers consent to autopsy because they see it as a way of giving additional meaning to their child's life or as a gift to others. Some want to know all that they can about what happened to their child. Meetings should be held with such parents to go over the results of the autopsy when they are able to deal with it. Other parents feel strongly that their child has been through enough suffering and they do not want anything more done to him or her, or there may be religious proscriptions against autopsy. The wishes of the family or caregivers should always be respected.

Developing a Plan for the End of Life

If the decisions previously discussed have been made, then the plan flows from those decisions. The child and the family or caregivers may have "business" they need to conclude before the child dies. This may include sharing certain feelings, resolving certain issues, making provisions for the giving away of certain belongings, and exploring certain psychological and spiritual concerns to achieve acceptance of death and peace. HIV clinicians can help the child and the loved ones to complete their business by offering their presence and listening to each individual as he or she makes this journey. There is no right or wrong way to die, only that way that is best for the individual child and the family or caregivers.

Helping families prepare in advance for the death, including teaching them how their child might look and act, can decrease their fear of the unknown. Talking openly with the child about what is happening to him or her, reading stories about death, and talking about his or her feelings and beliefs about death can reduce the child's fears and sense of isolation. Families who had previously not participated in religious practices may now want certain spiritual rituals performed.

When the decision is made to have the child die at home, a plan should be made in advance for having the child pronounced dead in the home and transported to either a funeral parlor or a hospital (if an autopsy is to be performed). Parents who have provided excellent home care may wish to place a child in the hospital as death approaches; some may refuse home-based hospice care because they do not want new people introduced into their lives. Rehospitalization should remain an option for terminally ill children.

Clinicians caring for the child in the home or hospital can make sure that the child is kept clean and smelling as good as possible, that no needless tests are performed, that parents are involved in their child's care as much as they desire, and that the child is as free of pain as possible, with other symptoms adequately controlled. When death occurs, parents and other family members need adequate time to say good-bye, which may involve bathing the child's body or fixing his or her hair. Although such time is seldom provided in busy hospital settings, these hours are invaluable to parents. The family or caregivers cannot be rushed; nurses who provide such support can help them begin the mourning process.

SUMMARY

Caring for sick, suffering, and dying children is never easy. Clinicians need to seek their own support systems. They need to examine their own belief systems and feelings about sickness, suffering, and death and be in touch with these feelings enough to communicate empathy while not imposing their own beliefs on the family or caregivers. They need to walk the fine line between being totally objective and uninvolved emotionally to overidentifying with what the family or caregivers are going through. A clinician who can remain separate from the family while communicating empathy and compassion will be effective and will avoid burning out. The clinician who can reframe his or her sense of "success" from one of total cure to one of optimal care and support will derive much satisfaction and reward from caring for children with AIDS.

REFERENCES

Ampel, N.M. (1996). Emerging disease issues and fungal pathogens associated with HIV infection. *Emerging Infectious Diseases, 2*(2), 109–116.

Berger, J.R., Scott, G., Albrecht, J., et al. (1992). Progressive multifocal leukoencephalopathy in HIV-1-infected children. *AIDS, 6*(8), 837–841.

Beutler, B., Milsark, I.W., Cerami, A.L. (1985). Passive immunization against cachectin/tumor necrosis factor protects mice from lethal effect of endotoxin. *Science, 229*, 869–871.

Breitbart, W., Rosenfeld, B.D., Passik, S.D., et al. (1996). The undertreatment of pain in ambulatory AIDS patients. *Pain, 65*, 243–249.

Brouwers, P., Belman, A., Epstein, L. (1994). Central nervous system involvement: Manifestations, evaluation and pathogenesis. In P. Pizzo, C. Wilfert (Eds.), *Pediatric AIDS: The challenge of HIV infection in infants, children and adolescents* (pp. 433–455). Baltimore: Williams & Wilkins.

Butler, C., Hittelman, J., Hauger, S. (1991). Approach to neurodevelopmental and neurologic complications in pediatric HIV infection. *Journal of Pediatrics, 119*, S41–S46.

Centers for Disease Control and Prevention. (1994). Revised classification system for HIV infection in children less than thirteen years of age. *Mortality and Morbity Weekly Report, 43*(RR-12), 1–19.

Centers for Disease Control and Prevention. (1996). *HIV/AIDS Surveillance Report, 8*(2), 1–39.

Centers for Disease Control and Prevention. (1997a). 1997 USPH/IDSA guidelines for the prevention of opportunistic infections in persons infected with human immunodeficiency virus. *Mortality and Morbidity Weekly Report, 46*(RR-12), 1–46.

Centers for Disease Control and Prevention. (1997b). Anergy skin testing and preventive therapy for HIV-infected persons: Revised recommendations. *Mortality and Morbidity Weekly Report, 46*(RR-15), 1–12.

Cerami, A., Ikeda, Y., Latrang, N., et al. (1985). Weight loss associated with endotoxin induced mediator form peritoneal macrophages: The role of cachectin (tumor necrosis factor). *Immunology Letters, 11*, 173–177.

Chaisson, R.E., Griffin, D.E. (1990). Progressive multifocal leukoencephalopathy in AIDS. *Journal of the American Medical Association, 264*(1), 79–82.

Clarick, R.H., Hanekom, W.A., Yogev, R., Chadwick, E.G. (1997). Megestrol acetate treatment of growth failure in children infected with human immunodeficiency virus. *Pediatrics, 99*(3), 354–357.

Committee on Infectious Diseases, Academy of Pediatrics. (1992). Chemotherapy of tuberculosis in infants and children. *Pediatrics, 89*, 161–165.

Connor, E.M., Andiman, W.A. (1994). Lymphoid interstitial pneumonitis. In P. Pizzo, C. Wilfert (Eds.), *Pediatric AIDS: The challenge of HIV infection in infants, children and adolescents* (pp. 467–481). Baltimore: Williams & Wilkins.

Cordell, R.L., Addiss, D.G. (1994). Cryptosporidiosis in child care settings: A review of the literature and recommendations for prevention and control. *Pediatric Infectious Disease Journal, 13*, 310–317.

Cramp M.E., Hing M.C., Marriott D.J., et al. (1996). Bile acid malabsorption in HIV infected patients with chronic diarrhea. *Australian New Zealand Journal of Medicine, 26*(3), 368–371.

Czarniecki, L. (1996). Advanced HIV disease in children. *Nursing Clinics of North America, 31*, 207–219.

Czarniecki, L., Boland, M.G., Oleske, J. (1993). Pain in children with HIV disease. *PAAC Notes, 5*, 492–495.

Czarniecki, L., Dollfus, C., Strafford, M. (1994). Children with pain and HIV/AIDS. In D. Carr (Ed.), *Pain in HIV/AIDS* (pp. 48–52). Washington, D.C.: France-USA Pain Association.

Dankner, W.M. (1995). Bacterial infections in HIV infected children. *Seminars in Pediatric Infectious Diseases, 6*, 10–16.

Delfraissy, J.F., Blanche, S., Rouzioux, C., Mayaux, M.J. (1992). Perinatal HIV transmission facts and controversies. *Immunodeficiency Reviews, 3,* 305–327.

Ellaurie, M., Burns, E.R., Rubinstein, A. (1990). Hematologic manifestations in pediatric HIV infection: Severe anemia as a prognostic marker. *American Journal of Pediatric Hematology Oncology, 12*(4), 449–453.

Elliot, B., Aromin, I., Gold, R., et al. (1997). 2.5 year remission of AIDS-associated progressive multifocal leukoencephalopathy with combined antiretroviral therapy. *Lancet, 349,* 1554–1555.

Falloon, J., Eddy, J., Wiener, L., Pizzo, P. (1989). Human immunodeficiency virus infection in children. *Journal of Pediatrics, 115,* 1–30.

Ferris, F.D., Clannery, J.S., McNeal, H.B., et al. (1995). A comprehensive guide for the care of persons with HIV disease, Module 4: Palliative care. Toronto: Mt. Sinai Hospital/Casey House Hospice.

Grubman, S., Gross, E., Lerner-Weiss, N., et al. (1995). Older children and adolescents living with perinatally acquired human immunodeficiency acquired infection. *Pediatrics, 95*(5), 657–663.

Gutierrez-Ortega, P., Hierro-Orozco, S., Sanchez-Cisneros, R., Montano, L.F. (1989). Kaposi's sarcoma in a 6-day-old infant with human immunodeficiency virus [Letter]. *Archives of Dermatology, 125*(3), 432–433.

Gutman, L.T. (1993). Recent developments in the intersection of the epidemics of tuberculosis and HIV in children. *Pediatric HIV Forum, 1*(1), 1–5.

Hauger, S.B. (1991) Approach to the pediatric patient with HIV infection and pulmonary symptoms. *Journal of Pediatrics, 119,* S25–S33.

Hauger, S.B., Powell, K.R. (1990). Infectious complications in children with HIV infection. *Pediatric Annals, 19,* 421–436.

Hewitt, D.J., McDonald, M., Portenoy, R., et al. (1997). Pain syndromes and etiologies in ambulatory AIDS patients. *Pain, 70,* 117–123.

Hirschfeld, S., Moss, H., Dragisic, K., et al. (1996). Pain in pediatric human immunodeficiency virus infection: Incidence and characteristics in a single-institution pilot study. *Pediatrics, 98,* 449–456.

Horsburgh, C.R., Caldwell, M.D., Simonds, R.J. (1993). Epidemiology of disseminated nontuberculous mycobacterial disease in children with acquired immunodeficiency syndrome. *Pediatric Infectious Disease Journal, 12,* 219–221.

Hoyt, L., Oleske, J., Holland, B., Connor, E. (1992). Nontuberculous mycobacteria in children with acquired immunodeficiency syndrome. *Pediatric Infectious Disease Journal, 11,* 354–360.

Italian Paediatric Intestinal/HIV Study Group. (1993). Intestinal malabsorption of HIV-infected children: Relationship to diarrhea, failure to thrive, enteric microorganisms and immune impairment. *AIDS, 7,* 1435–1440.

Katz, M.H., Mastrucci, H.T., Leggott, P.J., et al. (1993). Prognostic significance of oral lesions in children with perinatally acquired human immunodeficiency virus. *American Journal of Diseases of Children, 147,* 45–48.

Kawakami, M., Cerami, A. (1981) Studies of endotoxin-induced decrease in lipoprotein lipase activity. *Journal of Experimental Medicine, 154,* 631–639.

Kirkland, T.N., Fierer, J. (1996). Coccidioidomycosis: A reemerging infectious disease. *Emerging Infectious Diseases, 2*(3), 192–199.

Kline, M.W. (1996). Oral manifestations of pediatric human immunodeficiency virus infection: A review of the literature. *Pediatrics, 97,* 380–388.

Kloss, S., Kropp, S., Fuchs, A., et al. (1993). Unusual manifestations of pediatric AIDS [abstract PO-B05-1018]. *International Conference on AIDS, 9*(1), 305.

Kotler, D.P., Giang, T.T., Thiim, M., et al. (1995). Chronic bacterial enteropathy in patients with AIDS. *Journal of Infectious Disease, 171,* 552–558.

Kotler, D.P., Grunfeld, C. (1996). Pathophysiology and treatment of the AIDS wasting syndrome. *AIDS Clinical Review 1995–96, 229*–275.

Kotler, D.P., Tierney, A.R., Francisco, A., et al. (1989). The magnitude of body cell mass depletion determines the timing of death from wasting in AIDS. *American Journal of Clinical Nutrition, 50,* 444–447.

Lambl, B.B., Federman, M., Pleskow, D., Wanke, C.A. (1996). Malabsorption and wasting in AIDS patients with microsporidia and pathogen-negative diarrhea. *AIDS, 10*(7), 739–744.

Lane-McAuliffe, E., Lipshultz, S.E. (1995). Cardiovascular manifestations of pediatric HIV infection. *Nursing Clinics of North America, 30*(2), 291–316.

Lebovitz, A., Lefkowitz, M., McCarthy, D., et al. (1989). The prevalence and management of pain in patients with AIDS: A review of 134 cases. *Clinical Journal of Pain, 5,* 245–248.

Leggiadro, R., Kline, M.W., Hughes, W. (1991). Extrapulmonary cryptococcosis with acquired immunodeficiency syndrome. *Pediatric Infectious Disease Journal, 10*(9), 658–662.

Lipshultz, S.E. (1994). Cardiovascular problems. In P. Pizzo, C. Wilfert (Eds), *Pediatric AIDS: The challenge of HIV infection in infants, children and adolescents* (pp. 483–511). Baltimore: Williams & Wilkins.

Lipshultz, S.E., Chanock, S., Sanders, S.P., et al. (1989). Cardiovascular manifestations of human immunodeficiency infection in infants and children. *American Journal of Cardiology, 63,* 1489–1497.

McClain, K.L., Rosenblatt, H. (1990). Pediatric HIV infection and AIDS: Clinical expression of malignancy. *Seminars in Pediatric Infectious Diseases, 1*(1), 124–129.

McKinney, R.E., Prose, N.S. (1996). Mucocutaneous manifestations of pediatric HIV infection. In A.E. Friedman-Kien, C.J. Cockerell (Eds.), *Color atlas of AIDS* (2nd ed., pp. 169–180). Philadelphia: Saunders.

McLaughlin, G.E., Virdee, S.S., Schleien, C.L., et al. (1995). Effect of corticosteroids on survival of children with AIDS and *Pneumocystis carinii* related respiratory failure. *Journal of Pediatrics, 12,* 821–824.

McLoughlin, L.C., Nord, K.S., Joshi, V.J., et al. (1987). Severe gastrointestinal involvement in children with acquired immunodeficiency syndrome. *Journal of Pediatric Gastroenterology and Nutrition, 6,* 517–524.

Miller, T. (1996). Malnutrition: Metabolic changes in children, comparisons with adults. *Journal of Nutrition, 126,* 2623s–2631s.

Miller, T.L., Evans, S.J., Orav, E.J., et al. (1993). Growth and body composition in children infected with the human immunodeficiency virus. *American Journal of Clinical Nutrition, 57,* 588–592.

Minkoff, H., Remington, J.S., Holman, S., et al. (1997). Vertical transmission of toxoplasma by human immunodeficiency virus-infected women. *American Journal of Obstetrics and Gynecology, 176*(3), 555–559.

Mitchell, C. (1994). Toxoplasmosis. In P. Pizzo, C. Wilfert (Eds.), *Pediatric AIDS: The challenge of HIV infection in infants, children, and adolescents* (pp. 419–431). Baltimore: Williams & Wilkins.

Mueller, B. (1994). Hematological problems and their management in children with HIV infection. In P. Pizzo, C. Wilfert (Eds.), *Pediatric AIDS: The challenge of HIV infection in infants, children, and adolescents* (pp. 591–601). Baltimore: Williams & Wilkins.

Mueller, B., Shad, A.T., Magrath, I.T., Horowitz, M.E. (1994). Malignancies in children with HIV infection. In P. Pizzo, C. Wilfert (Eds.), *Pediatric AIDS: The challenge of HIV infection in infants, children, and adolescents* (pp. 603–622). Baltimore: Williams & Wilkins.

Mulligan, K., Grunfeld, C., Hellerstein, M.K., et al. (1993). Anabolic effects of recombinant human growth hormone in patients with wasting associated with human immunodeficiency virus infection. *Journal of Clinical Endocrinology Metabolism, 77*(4), 956–962.

National Institute of Child Health and Human Development. (1991). Intravenous immune globulin for the prevention of bacterial infections in children with symptomatic human immunodeficiency virus infection. *New England Journal of Medicine, 325,* 73–80.

O'Connor, E., Boccon-Gibod, L., Joshi, V., et al. (1990). Cutaneous acquired immunodeficiency syndrome-associated Kaposi's sarcoma in pediatric patients. *Archives of Dermatology, 126*(6), 791–793.

Oleske, J., Boland, M. (1997). When a child with a chronic condition needs hospitalization. *Hospital Practice, 32,* 167–181.

O'Neill, W., Sherrard, J. (1993). Pain in human immunodeficiency disease: A review. *Pain, 54,* 3–14.

Pediatric Supportive Care/Quality of Life Committee for the NIAID's Pediatric ACTG. (1995). Enhancing supportive care and promoting quality of life: Clinical practice guidelines. *Pediatric AIDS and HIV infection: Fetus to Adolescent, 6,* 187–203.

Pitt, J. (1991). Lymphocytic interstitial pneumonia. *Pediatric Clinics of North America, 38*(1), 89–96.

Pizzo, P.A., Eddy, J., Falloon, J. (1988). Effect of continuous intravenous infusion of zidovudine (AZT) in children with symptomatic HIV infection. *New England Journal of Medicine, 319,* 889–896.

Price, R.W. (1997). Management of the neurological complications of HIV-1 infection and AIDS. In M.A. Sande, P.A. Volberding (Eds.), *The medical management of AIDS* (pp. 197–216). Philadelphia: Saunders.

Ritchie, D.J., Becker, E.S. (1994). Update on the management of intestinal cryptosporidiosis in AIDS. *Annals of Pharmachemotherapy, 28*(6), 767–778.

Schanbelan, M., Mulligan, K., Grunfeld, C., et al. (1996). Recombinant growth hormone in patients with HIV-associated wasting. *Annals of Internal Medicine, 125*(11), 873–882.

Scott, G.B. (1991). HIV infection in children: Clinical features and management. *Journal of Acquired Immune Deficiency Syndromes, 4,* 109–115.

Scott, G.B., Hutto, C., Makuch, R.W., et al. (1989). Survival in children with perinatally acquired human immunodeficiency virus type I infection. *New England Journal of Medicine, 321,* 1791–1796.

Simonds, R.J., Oxtoby, M.J., Caldwell, M.B.K., et al. (1993). *Pneumocystis carinii* pneumonia among United States children with perinatally acquired HIV infection. *Journal of the American Medical Association, 270,* 470–473.

Singer, E.J., Stoner, G.L., Singer, G.L., et al. (1994). AIDS presenting as progressive multifocal leukoencephalopathy with clinical response to zidovudine. *Acta Neurologica Scandinavia, 90*(6), 443–447.

Singer, B.J., Zorilla, C., Fahy-Chandon, B., et al. (1993). Painful symptoms reported by ambulatory HIV infected men in a longitudinal study. *Pain, 54,* 15–19.

Sleasman, J.W., Hemenway, C., Klein, A.S., Barrett, D.J. (1993). Corticosteroids improve survival of children with AIDS and *Pneumocystis carinii* pneumonia. *American Journal of Diseases in Children, 147,* 30–34.

Slusarczyk, R. (1994). The influence of human immunodeficiency virus on resting energy expenditure. *Journal of Acquired Immune Deficiency Syndrome, 7,* 1025–1027.

Starke, J.R., Jacobs, R.F., Jereb, J. (1992). Resurgence of tuberculosis in children. *The Journal of Pediatrics, 120,* 839–855.

Steuerwald, M., Bucher, H.C., Muller-Brand, J., et al. (1995). HIV enteropathy and bile acid malabsorption: Response to cholestyramine. *American Journal of Gastroenterology, 90*(11), 2051–2053.

Strauss, J., Abitol, C., Zilleruelo, G., et al. (1989). Renal disease in children with the acquired immunodeficiency syndrome. *New England Journal of Medicine, 321*(10), 625–630.

Ungvarski, P.J. (1996). Waging war on HIV wasting. *RN, 15*(20), 26–33.

VanDyke, R.B. (1995). Opportunistic infections in HIV-infected children. *Seminars in Pediatric Infectious Diseases, 6*(1), 10–16.

Whitley, R.J., Whitley, S.J. (1994). Herpes virus infections in children with human immunodeficiency virus. In P. Pizzo, C. Wilfert (Eds.), *Pediatric AIDS: The challenge of HIV infection in infants, children, and adolescents* (pp. 346–352). Baltimore: Williams & Wilkins.

Whitworth, J.M., Jannifer, C.K., Oleske, J.M., Schwartz, R.A. (1995). Cutaneous manifestations of childhood acquired immunodeficiency syndrome and human immunodeficiecy virus infection. *Cutis, 55,* 62–72.

Winter, H.S., Miller, T.L. (1994). Gastrointestinal and nutritional problems in pediatric HIV disease. In P. Pizzo, C. Wilfert (Eds.), *Pediatric AIDS: The challenge of HIV infection in infants, children, and adolescents* (pp. 513–533). Baltimore: Williams & Wilkins.

Wiznia, A., Nichols, S. (1990). Organ system involvement in HIV-infected children. *Pediatric Annals, 19,* 475–476, 479–481.

Woodruff, R. (1996). *Palliative medicine: Symptomatic and supportive care for patients with advanced cancer and AIDS* (2nd ed.). Melbourne: Asperula.

Yolken, R.H., Hart, W., Oung, I., et al. (1991). Gastrointestinal dysfunction and disaccaride intolerance in children infected with human immunodeficiency virus. *Journal of Pediatrics, 118,* 359–363.

5

Adolescents and Adults

HIV DISEASE CARE MANAGEMENT

PETER J. UNGVARSKI ■ JAMES ANGELL ■ DANNY J. LANCASTER ■ JULIANA P. MANLAPAZ

Scientific progress in quantifying HIV activity and the ability to provide effective combination antiretroviral therapy early in the course of the disease have provided a challenge to primary care providers. Although in many persons HIV disease is easily diagnosed at later stages of the illness, it is more difficult to make a diagnosis at the time of primary HIV infection with an acute retroviral syndrome.

Some persons may be free of symptoms after their initial exposure to HIV, but in the majority symptoms develop within 5 to 30 days, with a median duration of symptoms of 14 days (Rosenberg & Cotton, 1997). The majority of newly infected persons appear to seek medical attention (Rosenberg & Cotton, 1997). In a review of the literature on signs and symptoms manifested during primary HIV infection (N = 365 cases), Katsufrakis & Daar (1997) noted fever (94%), adenopathy (69%), sore throat (66%), rash (54%), myalgia/arthralgia (48%), headache (39%), diarrhea (32%), and nausea/vomiting (29%). Other manifestations of primary HIV infection include aphthous ulcers, leukoplakia, thrombocytopenia, elevated liver enzyme levels, and neurologic symptoms ranging from aseptic meningitis to encephalitis (Katsufrakis & Daar, 1997). Differential diagnoses include influenza, Epstein-Barr or cytomegalovirus virus infection, toxoplasmosis, rubella, and syphilis (Rosenberg & Cotton, 1997).

The initial burst of HIV-1 activity can produce an intense viremia that can result in drastically reduced CD4+ cell counts. A healthy, uninfected person usually has between 500 and 1500 CD4+ cells per cubic millimeter of blood. This initial attack can, in some instances, reduce the CD4+ cell count to less than 100/mm^3 (or less than 7.5% of total lymphocytes), leaving the patient vulnerable to the development of an opportunistic infection. In fact, primary infection may cause illness that requires hospitalization, and both esophageal candidiasis and *Pneumocystis carinii* pneumonia (PCP) have been reported in patients with primary HIV-1 infection (Tindall & Cooper, 1991; Vento et al., 1993). The most important aspect of the initial work-up is the health history, which, when taken in detail, may reveal clues to HIV exposure.

BASELINE EVALUATION

The initial assessment focuses on an organized, systematic approach to health appraisal in order to (1) identify risk behaviors associated with HIV exposure, (2) detect signs and symptoms that may indicate the presence of HIV disease or a related illness that is indicative of AIDS, and (3) determine the person's needs for health teaching and follow-up care. The Box contains a detailed outline for taking a health history.

Social History

Sexual activity as a principal mode of HIV transmission accounts for the majority of AIDS cases worldwide. To identify persons who may be at risk of HIV infection through sexual activity, clinicians must obtain careful sexual histories from their clients. However, numerous studies of

▪ BASELINE HEALTH HISTORY AND REVIEW OF SYSTEMS ▪

A. Social history
   1. Sexual activities
     a. Sex with men, women, or both
     b. Preferred sexual activities
     c. Absolutely safe behavior: abstinence or mutual monogamy with a noninfected partner
     d. Very safe behavior: noninsertive sexual practices
     e. Probably safe behavior: insertive sexual practices with the use of condoms and spermicide
     f. Risky behavior: everything else
     g. Use of condoms (both male and female) including application, removal, use of lubricants, and difference in condom efficacy
     h. Engaging in sex with multiple partners
     i. Use of mood-affecting drugs before or during sexual activities
     j. Whether HIV disease has been diagnosed in anyone with whom the client has had sex
   2. Needle exposure
     a. Use of drugs by intravenous route, sharing of needles, syringes and other drug paraphernalia
     b. Other needle-exposure activities such as tattoos, acupuncture, treatment by unskilled persons or "folk doctors," or sharing of prescribed drugs between friends
     c. Whether HIV disease has been diagnosed in anyone with whom client has shared needles
   3. Tobacco use, including cigars, cigarettes, pipes, and chewing tobacco
   4. Occupational history
     a. Current employment status
     b. Client's occupation and responsibilities in relation to risk potential for HIV exposure
     c. Whether client experienced any exposures
     d. What type of health care follow-up the client has pursued since exposure
     e. Client's knowledge level regarding the signs and symptoms or seroconversion and need for follow-up
   5. Health insurance
     a. Is present coverage linked to employment status
     b. Does the client need social work referral to determine Medicaid or Medicare eligibility
   6. Travel
     a. Within the past 10 years
     b. Sexual activities when traveling in areas where the number of AIDS cases is high, such as New York, California, New Jersey, Texas, Florida, or such countries as Haiti or Zaire
     c. Treatment of illnesses or accidental injuries while traveling
     d. Immigration history and potential exposures in country of origin
B. Family history of medical and mental health problems, including but not limited to substance use in the home or by other family members, tuberculosis, and HIV infection
C. Medication history: Current or previous use of medication such as steroids that may suppress the immune system; current treatment for chemical dependence if applicable
D. History of nutrition and use of mood-affecting agents
   1. Nutrition history: See Tables 5–4 and 5–5
   2. Use of mood-affecting drugs
     a. Drugs such as alcohol, marijuana, cocaine, crack, LSD, Quaalude, amphetamines, barbiturates, tranquilizers, amyl or butyl nitrate (called "poppers"), heroin, crystal meth, ecstasy
     b. Route of administration: oral, inhalation (including sniffing, snorting, and smoking), intravenous, or subcutaneous ("skin-popping")
     c. Any current or previous treatment for substance abuse

■ BASELINE HEALTH HISTORY AND REVIEW OF SYSTEMS *Continued* ■

E. Medical history
   1. Usual source and patterns of seeking health care
   2. HIV testing in the past: has it ever been recommended; where was it done and what were the results; does the client have documentation
   3. Major diseases including (but not limited to) tuberculosis, hepatitis (specific type), mononucleosis, and hemophilia and treatment with clotting replacements such as factor VIII; cancer; tuberculosis
   4. Treatment for psychiatric/emotional disorders
   5. Transfusion donor or recipient
   6. Date of last chest x-ray
   7. Date of last tuberculin test and results
F. Surgical history
G. Childhood illnesses, including but not limited to varicella and immunization history including measles, mumps, rubella (MMR), last tetanus booster, hepatitis A or B vaccination, Pneumovax, influenza, Bacillus Calmette-Guérin (BCG), as well as anergy panel testing
H. Sexually transmitted diseases (STDs), including (but not limited to) syphilis; gonorrhea; amebiasis; herpes simplex (oralis or genitalis); *Giardia lamblia* enteritis and *Chlamydia* infection, condyloma, trichomoniasis, pelvic inflammatory disease (PID)
I. Gynecologic history
   1. Menstrual history
   2. Pregnancy history
   3. Methods of birth control
   4. Date of last Papanicolaou (Pap) smear and results
J. Review of systems
   1. General: a comment from the client concerning a self-appraisal of current state of health should be elicited
   2. Skin: eruptions, lesions, itching, dryness, redness, rashes, lumps, color changes, changes in hair or nails
   3. Head: headaches, light-headedness, or other sensations
   4. Eyes: blurred vision, diplopia, loss of visual fields, or "floaters"
   5. Ears: impaired hearing or tinnitus
   6. Nose and sinuses: obstruction, pain, discharges, or nosebleed
   7. Mouth and throat: creamy white patches, lesions, bleeding gums, dysphagia, odynophagia, changes in taste or sore throat
   8. Respiratory: dyspnea with or without certain activities, coughing, wheezing, chest pain, "cold" or "flu-like" symptoms
   9. Cardiovascular: chest pain, palpitations, edema, or known hypertension or hypotension
   10. Gastrointestinal: changes in appetite, involuntary weight loss, abdominal pain or cramping, changes in bowel habits, loose stools, diarrhea, blood in stool, rectal or perianal pain or itching
   11. Genitourinary: dysuria, nocturia, pain, itching, discharges, or lesions
   12. Gynecologic: changes in menstruation, dyspareunia, vaginal discharge, breast abnormalities, obstetrical history, abortions, and chronic infections
   13. Musculoskeletal: arthralgia or myalgia
   14. Neurologic and emotional: problems with memory, nervousness, personality changes, confusional states, stiff neck, photophobia, tremors, paresthesias, seizures, or syncope
   15. Endocrine: polyuria, polyphagia, polydipsia, fevers, or night sweats
   16. Hematopoietic: lymphadenopathy, bruising or bleeding, history of anemia

both physicians and nurses reveal that the sexual history–taking practices of health care providers appear to be lacking (Ferguson et al., 1991; Gemson et al., 1991; van Servellen et al., 1988; Weinrich et al., 1997). According to Asch and associates (1997), screening of HIV risk in the primary care setting remains inadequate.

Human sexuality is inextricably woven into the fabric of all human beings, and the promotion of sexual health is a legitimate, essential function of both physicians and nurses (Fogel, 1990). Sexual history taking may be uncomfortable for both the client and the clinician, and questions may delve into areas that both perceive as socially unacceptable. The client may be reluctant to discuss sexual activities in the presence of judgmental attitudes for fear of discrimination if confidentiality is breached (Hecht & Soloway, 1993a).

A prerequisite to effective sexual history taking is self-evaluation and clarification of individual attitudes toward various sexual behaviors (Andrist, 1988; Fogel, 1990). In a survey of senior medical students, Benevedes and Abrams (1997) found that 50% thought they were poorly trained in obtaining sexual histories, and 25% of the sample were embarrassed by the task. It was noted that students who stated that a sexual history was of limited importance were more likely to be homophobic and authoritarian and had the greatest fear of acquiring HIV infection. The first necessary step to overcoming fear is to practice sexual history taking with friends or colleagues. It is imperative that the health care professional maintain a nonjudgmental demeanor during the actual interview process and avoid a shocked expression in response to answers given. Clinicians should examine their feelings and responses regarding oral sex, anal sex, masturbation, homosexuality, heterosexuality, bisexuality, transvestism, transsexualism, casual sex, commercial sex, use of birth control methods and devices, and sexual encounters outside alleged monogamous relationships. It should be emphasized that the health care provider taking the sexual history does not in anyway relinquish his or her own values in the process of acknowledging the values of others (Hogan, 1980).

Andrist (1988) and Kelly and Holman (1993) offer some helpful suggestions for health care providers taking sexual histories. The clinician should begin by ensuring privacy; should appear warm, open, and empathetic; and should main-

tain eye contact. It is advisable to introduce the topic by making a general statement that concerns about sexual issues are universal. The clinician should assist the client in identifying risk-related sexual activities and should try to determine how much knowledge the client has regarding the HIV-related risk behaviors of his or her sexual partner(s). Finally, the clinician should offer information that specifically addresses the client's concerns. Printed material that is sexually explicit and directed toward specific lifestyles is available from most nonprofit, community-based AIDS organizations. Sexual history taking should be inclusive and detailed and should be performed universally with all clients. A major error to avoid with sexual history taking is to make assumptions regarding sexual behaviors of clients on the basis of preconceived ideas of certain lifestyles. All gay men are not at risk of HIV infection. Even gay men with multiple sexual partners who exclusively practice mutual masturbation are unlikely to acquire HIV infection. Conversely, although rare, the clinician should not assume that lesbians are not at risk of HIV since woman-to-woman sexual transmission has been reported (Perry et al., 1989; Rich et al., 1993).

The concept of monogamy is likewise elusive. Both men and women have little control over the sexual activities of their partners. The biased perception that casual sex versus monogamy intrinsically increases the risk of HIV can be misleading. Rodrigues and Moreno (1991) note that HIV transmission can and does occur in women in a stable relationship or marriage. Smeltzer and Whipple (1991) point out that women are often unaware of the risks of HIV because they may not associate themselves with so-called high-risk groups but may, in fact, participate in high-risk behaviors.

Sexual history taking should not be omitted because of age. By 1997, 8% of the women and 11% of the men with AIDS were over the age of 50 years (CDC, 1996a). The incidence of AIDS and STDs is increasing in older Americans (Tichy & Talashek, 1992; Wallace et al., 1993). Nokes (1996) noted that older persons may participate in episodic encounters with commercial sex workers. The failure to identify HIV infection in older clients has led to the misdiagnosis of Alzheimer's disease in the presence of HIV dementia and delayed diagnosis of *Pneumocystis carinii* pneumonia in elderly persons (Fillit et al., 1990; Hargreaves et al., 1988; Weiler et al., 1988). Persons over the age of 50 are less likely than younger people (1) to perceive any risk for acquiring HIV, (2) to use condoms when engaging in high-risk sexual behaviors, and (3) to be tested for HIV (CDC, 1998). Hinkle (1991) concludes that health care professionals have been guilty of complacency when it comes to screening and educating the elderly population regarding HIV infection.

Exploration of the use of mood-affecting agents should be conducted objectively, and assumptions on the direct causal effects of alcohol or drugs on risky sexual behavior should be avoided. Temple and colleagues (1993) found that although sexual encounters with new partners were more likely to involve alcohol, the presence of alcohol was not significantly associated with risky sexual behaviors. Those authors concluded that the relationship between drinking and risky sex is the result of a complex reaction among personality, situational, and behavioral factors. Weiner and associates (1992) reported that crack-cocaine users who primarily engage in oral sex are more likely to become infected with HIV than those who primarily engage in vaginal intercourse. The authors speculate that crack smoking itself, possibly because of damage from the heat of the crack pipe causing oral trauma, may be a factor in making fellatio a risky behavior. Other problems noted to be associated with crack use were hypersexuality, trading of sex for drugs, and impaired judgment leading to inconsistent condom use.

It is important to use open-ended questions to obtain accurate information on substance use. Given the psychological defense mechanisms that substance users employ, direct questions such as "Do you use drugs?" are too threatening and are unlikely to elicit truthful responses (Blum, 1987). Although many standard assessment forms place alcohol and drug use in the section with tobacco, it may be better to ask about substance use during the nutrition assessment (see Table 5–5). Questions such as the following minimize potentially judgmental queries: "What do you usually eat in a day? What do you drink? Could you tell me about your use of alcohol and drugs?" Primary care providers need to know which substances are being used and the route of adminis-

tration, but it is not necessary to know the amounts used unless the client is being treated for detoxification.

Questions concerning drug use will lead to questions about needle exposure. Although some exposures, such as those of an intravenous-heroin addict, are obvious, other types of needle exposure, such as tattooing and body piercing, may put people at risk (Aylward et al., 1995; Long & Rickman, 1994). Anecdotal reports have also revealed needle sharing among persons who self-administer and share estrogens intramuscularly because they plan eventually to have transsexual surgery. In the early years of the AIDS epidemic, epidemiologic studies in Haiti traced HIV transmission to dirty needles used by untrained persons to give intramuscular injections (Pape & Johnson, 1989). Other reports from the World Health Organization indicated that contaminated injection equipment in health care settings in Romania and the former U.S.S.R. (Mann et al., 1992) was a primary source of large-scale epidemics of HIV disease.

The health history used to identify persons at risk of HIV disease should also include occupational history and accidental exposure to blood, needles, or instruments (Hecht & Soloway 1993a). It might be difficult to sort out the occupational groups at risk. Although the more obvious ones include physicians, nurses, laboratory workers, and phlebotomists, selective questioning of only a few occupational groups may overlook others such as police officers, paramedics, and sanitation workers. Therefore questioning should include all persons who might be at risk.

Travel history and potential risk exposure should be explored. Emphasizing the need to explore travel, Rowbottom (1993) noted that STDs and HIV infections were being diagnosed in an increasing number of Australians after international travel. Along with travel history, immigration history is equally important.

Health History and Review of Systems

When reviewing the client's health history, the clinician should note the presence of recurrent infections, such as bacterial infections, sexually transmitted diseases (STDs), pneumonia, tuberculosis, or such refractory fungal infections as vulvovaginal candidiasis. These infections, often referred to as sentinel diseases in HIV infection, may reflect an underlying immunodeficiency, especially if they did not respond well to treatment, are chronic in nature, or occur repeatedly.

The last part of the health history, the review of systems, is a detailed examination for signs and symptoms indicating HIV disease or the possibility of an associated AIDS-indicator disease. After completion, a careful review of the history with the client should conclude with questions regarding whether the client is satisfied with the history or wishes to change any responses. This will provide the basis for developing a plan of care and health teaching.

Physical Examination

The physical examination findings are as diverse as is the spectrum of HIV disease. Findings range from normal in an asymptomatic HIV-infected person to evidence of the presence of an opportunistic disease or infection that is associated with a diagnosis of AIDS. HIV-related conditions have demonstrated the ability of HIV to affect virtually every anatomic structure and organ site (Hernandez, 1990). Therefore, a complete physical examination should be performed, and any deviations from normal findings should be considered significant in relation to HIV infection. The early detection of complications related to HIV disease are often treatable, and treatment can sometimes prevent or slow progression to more serious disease (Hecht & Soloway, 1993a). The elements of a baseline physical examination of the person with HIV infection are outlined in the Box.

▪ **BASELINE PHYSICAL EXAMINATION OF THE HIV-POSITIVE CLIENT** ▪

A. General: weight and height, temperature, respiratory rate, pulse, blood pressure
B. Neurologic examination
   1. Cerebral functions: impaired cognitive functions, decreased level of consciousness, anger, inattentiveness, depression, denial
   2. Cranial nerve (CN) examination
      a. CN II (optic nerve): papilledema, white retinal spots, yellow-white retinal infiltrates, retinal hemorrhage; visual field deficiencies, blurred vision
      b. CNs III, IV, VI (oculomotor, trochlear, abducens nerves): impaired extraocular movements, unequal pupils, diplopia, ptosis, nystagmus
      c. CN V (trigeminal nerve): photophobia
      d. CN VII (facial nerve): hemiparesis
      e. CN VIII (acoustic nerve): tinnitus, vertigo, impaired hearing
      f. CNs IX, X (glossopharyngeal and vagus nerves): dysphagia, dysarthria
   3. Motor examination: motor weakness, hemiparesis, paraparesis
   4. Sensory examination: dysesthesias, paresthesia, areas of anesthesia
   5. Cerebellar examination: ataxia, dysmetria, tremors
   6. Reflexes: abnormal reflexes, a positive Babinski's sign
   7. Meningeal signs: nuchal rigidity, Brudzinski's sign, Kernig's sign
C. Mouth and throat examination: lesions, discoloration exudates
D. Cardiovascular examination
   1. Heart: disturbances in cardiac rate and rhythm and presence of pericardial friction rub
   2. Peripheral vascular: edema, decrease in peripheral pulse(s)
E. Respiratory examination: tachypnea, lag of excursion on palpation, dullness to percussion, presence of rales (crackles) or rhonchi (wheezes)
F. Lymphatic examination: lymphadenopathy
G. Abdominal examination: masses, tenderness, hepatomegaly, splenomegaly, hyperactive bowel sounds
H. Breast examination: lesions, masses, discoloration, tenderness, discharges
I. Examination of genitalia (both men and women) and perianal region: lesions, discharges
J. Musculoskeletal examination: pain on range of motion, evidence of muscle wasting
K. Skin examination: lesions or discolorations, dryness, thinning of hair, alopecia, body piercing, tattoos

Confirming the Diagnosis of HIV Infection

Serologic testing for HIV should be performed on all persons to provide concrete evidence of disease as well as to rule out factitious or psychogenic HIV infection. The term *factitious HIV infection* has been applied to situations in which the clinical presentation of the client mimics HIV disease but the underlying cause is another disease process (Craven et al., 1994). Psychogenic or malingering HIV infection has been reported in the literature, identifying persons who present themselves for health care and give a verbal history of having a previous diagnosis of HIV infection without providing any printed evidence (Craven et al., 1994; Sno et al., 1991). This may occur in situations where services and entitlements for persons living with HIV exceed those of other populations.

The standard test used to establish the diagnosis of HIV infection is the enzyme-linked immunosorbent assay (EIA). All HIV-positive tests should be followed by a confirmatory Western blot test. The average "window period" for seroconversion, after which HIV antibodies are detectable, is approximately 4 to 12 weeks (Bartlett, 1997; Brodie & Sax, 1997). The accuracy of the these testing methods ranges from 99.3% to 99.9% (Burke et al., 1988; Lackritz et al., 1995; MacDonald et al., 1989). There are limitations to the use of the EIA and Western blot tests in the United States: (1) not all commercial laboratories use screening assays to detect both HIV-1 and HIV-2, (2) many assays do not detect HIV-1 subtype "O", and (3) the HIV-1 Western blot may fail to detect subtype "O" and HIV-2 in approximately 10% to 20% of the specimens (Bartlett, 1997). Likewise, false-negative results will occur when the test is performed before the period of seroconversion. False-positive results are extremely rare but may occur in patients with autoimmune disorders, such as lupus erythematosus, or in persons who have participated in HIV vaccine studies (Barthel & Wallace, 1993; Bartlett, 1997). Indeterminate results may be attributed to (1) testing during the process of seroconversion, (2) low titers of antibodies, which can occur in advanced infection, (3) cross-reacting alloantibodies from pregnancy, blood transfusions, and organ transplantation, (4) autoantibodies encountered with autoimmune diseases, collagen-vascular diseases, cancer, (5) HIV-2 infection, and

(6) participants in HIV vaccine studies (Bartlett, 1997). Repeat testing should be performed at 3- to 6-month intervals. Most persons with indeterminate test results and absent risk factors for HIV infection usually have negative findings on follow-up testing. Patients with indeterminate test results who have HIV risk factors and who are in the process of seroconversion will usually test positive within 1 month after the indeterminate test (Barlett, 1997).

According to Bartlett (1997), other tests to establish a diagnosis of HIV infection, such as detection of p24 antigen, viral isolation, or polymerase chain reaction (PCR) techniques, are not considered superior to routine serologic tests but may have a limited role in establishing a diagnosis in a complicated case. Three rapid tests have been licensed by the Food and Drug Administration: the Single-Use-Diagnostic-System (SUDS), the Recombigen HIV-1 Latex Agglutination Test, and the Genie HIV-1 test. These tests have the advantage of providing results within 30 minutes and may be useful in situations in which the clinician cannot wait several days or weeks for standard serologic test results. These situations may involve (1) emergent blood or organ donations, (2) occupational exposure of health care workers for whom immediate treatment decisions are needed, or (3) unknown HIV status in pregnant women in labor (Brodie & Sax, 1997). The accuracy is estimated to parallel the EIA test results. Positive results should still be confirmed by EIA and Western blot.

Additional methods for detecting HIV infection include home test kits, salivary tests, and urine tests. Home test kits, available to the consumer without health care professional supervision, include Confide HIV Testing Service and the Home Access Express Test. Instructions for these kits include using a lancet to obtain a blood specimen and blotting the blood on a filter strip, which is then mailed back to the company with an anonymous identification number. The accuracy of these tests is nearly 100% (Bartlett, 1997). However, their marketability and popularity appear to be less than anticipated, and in the summer of 1997 the Confide test kit was withdrawn from the market because of lack of demand and low sales.

Primary care providers may also now use Ora-Sure by collecting saliva on a specially impregnated cotton pad on a stick and then sending it for testing. Results are available within 3 days, and the accuracy is comparable to that of standard serologic testing. The sentinel HIV-1 urine EIA can also be used by the primary care provider to detect antibodies in the urine. Urine testing is less accurate than serologic testing (Brodie & Sax, 1997). Whatever the testing method, all primary care providers have the ethical responsibility to provide adequate pretest and posttest counseling (see Chapter 2 for an in-depth discussion of the issues and process of HIV testing).

All clinicians should avoid speculating with the client on the probability of positive or negative test results on the basis of the health history findings. This is especially important when, for example, the sexual history reveals obscure or rare experiences with possible exposure to HIV and when the review of symptoms alludes to an underlying immunodeficiency. In rare instances, idiopathic CD4+ T-lymphocytopenia (ICL) or profound depletion of CD4+ T-lymphocytes in the absence of HIV infection has been reported. This may be a consideration in the absence of HIV positivity (Fauci, 1993).

Laboratory Testing

Initial laboratory testing of the HIV-infected person is important not only to establish baseline data on the patient with newly diagnosed HIV infection but also to serve as an indicator of disease progression, as a means of identifying complications of HIV disease, and to provide possible evidence of drug toxicity (Bartlett, 1993). Table 5–1 outlines initial laboratory screening. Appendix III describes common laboratory studies performed on HIV-infected persons and the interpretations of test results.

CD4+ T-lymphocytes have been the most widely used laboratory method of evaluating persons with HIV infection. The CD4+ T-lymphocyte count is considered a surrogate marker to determine HIV-related immune dysfunction and, along with HIV RNA serum levels, is used to monitor disease progression and guide treatment decisions, such as institution of antiretroviral therapy and of chemoprophylaxis for certain opportunistic infections. Problems that exist with the interpretation of the absolute CD4+ T-cell count include interlaboratory variability, diurnal variations, and intercurrent variations (Bartlett,

1993; CDC, 1992; Malone et al., 1990; Choi et al., 1993). According to Murphy and Chmiel (1992), a more consistent measurement is the percentage of lymphocytes that are CD4+ T-cells. Hecht and Soloway (1993b) recommend that evaluation of surrogate markers of immune function include the absolute CD4+ T-cell count, the CD4+ T-cell percentage, and the CD4+ to CD8+ ratio. Clinical decisions should never be based on one laboratory report, but on baseline data, trends, and changes, and, when used for treatment decisions, serial CD4+ T-cell counts.

Careful explanations of CD4+ T-cell measurements must be provided for the client. Hypervigilant behaviors regarding their CD4+ T-cell counts may develop with some persons. Variations in absolute numbers as a result of laboratory reporting differences, as well as intrapersonal variations, must be explained. Many HIV-infected persons have friends who are HIV-positive or attend HIV-positive support groups and exchange information. Lack of understanding CD4+ T-cell count variables can lead to unnecessary anxiety and worry. Other markers of immune status, such as serum neopterin, beta-2 microglobulin, HIV p24 antigen, soluble interleukin-2 receptors, immunoglobulin A, and delayed-type hypersensitivity (DTH) skin-test reactions, may be useful in the evaluation of HIV-infected patients but are not as strongly predictive of HIV disease progression as are measurements of CD4+ T-cell and HIV RNA viral load (CDC, 1992; U.S. Department of Health and Human Services, 1997).

A more direct method of measuring HIV activity has been developed to quantify viral load, also referred to as viral burden. By measuring the amount of HIV RNA in plasma, clinicians can more accurately assess the amount of HIV activity that is taking place in the body and can treat the patient appropriately. RNA is the substance that programs HIV reproduction. HIV RNA viral load tests

- Measure the amount of HIV RNA in plasma
- Quantify HIV activity
- Determine prognosis
- Indicate the need for antiretroviral treatment
- Evaluate the efficacy of prescribed antiretroviral therapy
- Identify treatment failure

Table 5–1 ▪ Initial Laboratory Studies for the HIV-Infected Person*

Tests	Comments
CD4+ T-cell count/percentage and CD4+/CD8+ ratio	Absolute numbers may vary significantly from test to test; percentage is considered a more stable numeric value
HIV RNA viral load test	Should not be performed if acute illness, e.g., bacterial pneumonia, tuberculosis, herpes simplex infection is present or the client has recently received an immunization, since these events can cause increases in serum plasma HIV RNA lasting for 2–4 weeks
Complete blood cell count with differential	Complications frequently seen in HIV disease
Multichannel chemistry panel	
Urinalysis	
Tuberculin skin test (Mantoux test) with or without anergy panel testing	See text
Chest x-ray examination	Repeat for signs and symptoms of pulmonary disease for clients newly identified as having positive PPD results and for newly identified anergic clients
Pregnancy test	
Papanicolaou (Pap) test	For abnormal or uninterpretable results, a colposcopy should be performed
Venereal Disease Research Laboratory (VDRL) test or rapid plasma reagin (RPR) screening test	High rates of coinfection in HIV populations; false-negative and false-positive results, although rare, do occur; clients with negative results who are sexually active should be tested yearly; clients with positive test results should have fluorescent treponema antibody absorption (FTA-ABS) test performed for confirmation; sexual partners should be evaluated
Gonorrhea culture	Screen all women (even if free of symptoms); test all men with symptoms; evaluations should include possibility of pharyngeal and/or rectal infection; sexual partners should be evaluated
Chlamydia culture	Screen all women (even if free of symptoms); test all men with symptoms; sexual partners should be evaluated
Hepatitis A panel	Prevalence is high in sexually active men who have sex with men, injecting and noninjecting illegal drug users, and persons who have clotting-factor disorders; for these individuals who test negative HAV vaccination is recommended
Hepatitis B panel	Prevalence of past exposure is high in most HIV-infected populations in the United States; if result is negative and the client is at continued risk of having HBV infection, vaccination is recommended
Hepatitis C panel	Especially indicated for intravenous drug users and patients with abnormal liver function tests
Toxoplasmosis serologic test	Repeat testing may be considered for seronegative patients when the CD4+ T-cell count is less than $100/mm^3$ and patients are unable to tolerate trimethoprim-sulfamethoxazole
Cytomegalovirus tests	May be performed initially for baseline data on previous exposure, current disease, or both
Varicella serologic test	May be considered for baseline data in patients who cannot provide a history of chickenpox or shingles
Glucose-6-phosphate dehydrogenase level (G-6-PD)	May be considered for certain populations; African-Americans and Mediterraneans (see text)

*See Appendix III for interpretation of results.
Data from AIDS Institute (1997), Bartlett (1997), CDC (1996b, 1997a), Cornelson (1997).

Three tests that are being used include

1. RT-PCR (quantitative polymerase chain reaction)
2. bDNA (branched-chain DNA)
3. NASBA (nucleic acid sequence-based amplification)

The test results are reported in number of copies per milliliter. Copy counts fewer than 10,000/ml indicate a low risk of advancing disease. Test results showing copy counts between 10,000 and 100,000/ml indicate a medium risk of advancing disease, and copy counts more than 100,000/ml indicate a high risk of advancing disease (Sax, 1996). Testing is usually performed as part of the initial work-up, when CD4+ cell counts indicate a clinical problem, and 3 to 4 weeks after starting or changing antiretroviral

therapy. Illnesses such as influenza, herpes, or pneumonia can temporarily increase the viral load. Immunizations such as those for influenza or tetanus can also cause a temporary increase; thus testing should not be performed in the presence of any of these conditions.

Although high viral loads are generally correlated with a low CD4+ cell count and low loads with a high count, the correlation is weak and inconsistent. Some patients with low CD4+ cell counts have low viral loads, and vice versa (Mellors et al., 1996). Therefore CD4+ cell counts are not reliable substitutes for viral load tests when one is trying to determine the degree of HIV disease activity or evaluating the efficacy of treatment. Table 5–2 contains the recommended schedule for HIV RNA testing.

The complete blood count is necessary to

Table 5–2 ▪ Indications for Plasma HIV RNA Testing

Clinical Indication	Information Provided	Clinical Importance
Syndrome consistent with acute, primary HIV infection	Establishes a diagnosis when HIV antibody test is negative or indeterminate	Diagnosis of HIV disease
Initial evaluation of newly diagnosed HIV infection	Baseline viral load, also referred to as "set point"	Use to make a decision as to whether to start antiretroviral therapy
Every 3-4 months in patients not on therapy	Detects changes in viral activity	Use to make a decision as to whether to start antiretroviral therapy
Four to 8 weeks after starting antiretroviral therapy	Initial assessment of efficacy of prescribed therapy	Provides information as to whether the prescribed therapy should be continued or changed
Three to 4 months after starting antiretroviral therapy	To determine maximum effects of antiretroviral therapy	Provides information as to whether the prescribed therapy should be continued or changed
Every 3-4 months while on antiretroviral therapy	To monitor durability of antiretroviral therapy effect	Provides information as to whether the prescribed therapy should be continued or changed
A clinical event occurs, e.g., an infection, or a decline in CD4+ T-cells	To determine whether there is a correlation with the clinical event or a decline in CD4+ T-cells with the viral load	Provides information as to whether the prescribed therapy should be continued or changed

1. Viral load testing should not be performed during an acute illness (e.g., bacterial pneumonia, tuberculosis, HSV infection, PCP, etc.) or near the time immunizations are administered, since these types of situations can cause increases in the plasma HIV RNA for 2-4 weeks.
2. When changes are noted in either HIV RNA or CD4+ T-cell test results, they should be verified with a repeat test before starting or making any changes in therapy.
3. The HIV RNA should be measured by using the same assay method and the same laboratory to prevent intralaboratory or intramethod variations in test results.
4. When plasma HIV RNA testing identifies HIV infection, the definitive diagnosis should be confirmed by EIA and Western blot testing (performed 1-2 weeks after the initial indeterminate of negative test).

From U.S. Department of Health and Human Services, Public Health Service. (1997). *Guidelines for the use of antiretroviral agents in HIV-infected adults and adolescents.* Rockville, MD: Author.

identify three common problems in HIV disease: anemia, thrombocytopenia, and leukopenia. From a clinical perspective, client complaints about being tired or having profound fatigue may often be related to varying degrees of anemia. The increasing severity of anemia may also lead to shortness of breath as well as impaired cognition. Decreasing platelet counts may increase the propensity for bleeding. Clinicians should always monitor the use of commonly used over-the-counter medications such as aspirin, which could further complicate the clinical picture. Severe leukopenia (fewer than 1000 granulocytes) may place the client at increased risk of infection. These three frequently coexisting problems are often aggravated by the toxic effects of medications, and careful monitoring is required.

Baseline information on liver and kidney function from serum chemistry determinations will often dictate which medications will be chosen to treat HIV disease and the related complications. Once again, clinicians should be aware not only of the over-the-counter medications the clients are taking but also of the alternative/complementary therapies they may be using (see Chapter 11). Clients may be taking self-prescribed therapies, in combination with certain clinician-prescribed medications, thus increasing the potential for hepatotoxicity.

Persons with HIV disease are particularly vulnerable to reactivation of latent tuberculosis (TB) infections, as well as to disease caused by new TB infections. The potential for TB transmission is increased when HIV-infected persons are placed in congregate living arrangements, such as hospitals, prisons, residences, and shelters. Since 1986, the CDC has recommended that HIV-infected persons who have not had a prior reaction to purified protein derivative (PPD) undergo tuberculin testing annually. This applies to all HIV-infected persons. Clinicians should not attempt to distinguish which persons are at risk of TB as a basis for determining who should be tested. This point is emphasized by studies in which TB caused by tubercle bacilli resistant to multiple drugs was diagnosed in persons not typically recognized to have a high prevalence of TB and in patients without traditional risk factors for drug-resistant TB (Fischl et al., 1992; Pearson et al., 1992).

Because some HIV-infected persons may have a suppression of cell-mediated immunity, referred to as anergy, they may not react to a tuberculin skin test, even in the presence of mycobacterial infection or disease. For several years, anergy testing to delayed-type hypersensitivity (DTH) skin test antigens, along with the tuberculin skin test, had been recommended. However, recent studies have demonstrated a lack of standardization of reagents and inconsistent results in repeat tests in HIV seropositive persons (CDC, 1997d). Consequently, the routine use of anergy testing in conjunction with PPD testing is no longer recommended (CDC, 1997d). If anergy testing is performed by the primary care provider, at least two skin test reagents should be used, including *Candida* and mumps (CDC, 1997d).

Initial screening for STDs such as syphilis, gonorrhea, or *Chlamydia* infections is appropriate to detect occult disease in HIV-infected persons. Many HIV-infected women come from populations with a high incidence of *Chlamydia* infection and gonorrhea (U.S. Preventive Services Task Force, 1989a, 1989b). The need for repeated testing for these diseases is determined by the clinician and by the client's current history of sexual activities. However, because the client may not always provide complete or accurate information, some clinicians may choose to screen routinely for these STDs in all sexually active persons.

Gynecologic abnormalities, such as infection with human papillomavirus and cervical intraepithelial neoplasia, tend to occur at higher rates in HIV-infected women (Jewitt & Hecht, 1993). Therefore routine evaluation of women for these problems is warranted. Papanicolaou (Pap) tests should be performed twice during the first year after HIV diagnosis and, if both tests are negative, then annually (CDC, 1997a). Some specialists in the care of HIV-infected women recommend that Pap tests be performed every 6 months.

Initial laboratory evaluation of all HIV-infected persons should include screening for hepatitis B virus (HBV) (AIDS Institute, 1997; Bartlett, 1997). Many experts also recommend routine screening for hepatitis C virus (HCV), especially for persons who engage in high-risk behaviors or who have abnormal liver function test results (AIDS Institute, 1997; Bartlett, 1997). Although not yet specifically recommended for all HIV-infected persons, serologic testing for hepatitis A virus is recommended for populations at risk of HIV infection, including (1) sexually ac-

---

▪ SPECIAL CONSIDERATIONS FOR THE BASELINE EXAMINATION
OF THE HIV-POSITIVE ADOLESCENT ▪

1. Sexual history should include exploration of situations in which sexual activity may have taken place when the client did not consent (sexual abuse by peers or within the family)
2. Needle-exposure risk should explore the practice of peer tattooing or the sharing of needles and hormones with transgender youth
3. Mental health and social history should assess for
   a. Perceived sexual orientation and adjustment difficulties
   b. Peer relationships both in the community and at school
   c. Episodes of depression or suicidal attempts or ideation
   d. Legal status, e.g., under 18 years of age but emancipated, immigration status
   e. Sources of financial support
   f. Access to and payment source for health care
   g. Home environment including substance use and HIV disease in parents, siblings, or both
   h. HIV confidentiality: who will the client allow the primary care provider to share information
4. Physical examination considerations
   a. General growth parameters (plotted on growth charts)
   b. Genitalia: Tanner stage
   c. Pelvic examination: limited to girls with a history of sexual intercourse

---

Data from AIDS Institute (1997).

tive men who have sex with men, (2) injection and noninjection illegal drug users, and (3) persons who have clotting-factor disorders (CDC, 1996b).

Serologic testing for cytomegalovirus (CMV) is now also recommended for HIV-infected persons who may be considered at low risk of CMV infection (Bartlett, 1997; CDC, 1997a). Testing for previous exposure to varicella in patients who can not provide a history may prove useful in latter determining the need for treatment of postexposure prophylaxis (Bartlett, 1997; CDC, 1997a). Serologic testing for previous infection due to *Cryptococcus neoformans, Histoplasma capsulatum,* or *Coccidioides immitis* has not proved useful in identifying patients at risk but may be useful in the assessment of clinical disease (Bartlett, 1993; Dismukes, 1988; Galgiani & Ampel, 1990; Wheat et al., 1992). Most physicians continue to advocate testing for serologic evidence of toxoplasmosis in HIV disease, although a negative serologic status does not exclude the potential diagnosis of toxoplasmosis in persons with AIDS (Bartlett, 1997; Porter & Sande, 1992).

Bartlett (1997) recommends testing of African-Americans and Mediterranean people, especially men, for glucose-6-phosphate dehydro-

genase (G-6-PD) deficiency. Both these populations are at high risk of this genetic deficiency, which may predispose them to hemolytic anemia when exposed to oxidant drugs, such as dapsone or primaquine and sulfonamides.

Initial Evaluation of the HIV-Seropositive Adolescent

The challenges of providing care for the adolescent with HIV infection differ in many ways from those of providing care to an adult. Internal conflicts may be numerous, and primary care providers should anticipate the need for more emotional support than may be encountered with adult clients. The Box above contains an overview of some of the special considerations for caring for the HIV-infected adolescent. Chapter 8 includes an in-depth discussion of the needs of this special population.

CLASSIFICATION OF HIV DISEASE IN ADULTS AND ADOLESCENTS

The current classification system for HIV-1 infection/AIDS in adults and adolescents was implemented in January, 1993 (CDC, 1992). Three major changes occurred with the 1993 revision: (1) instead of simply identifying clinical cate-

Table 5–3 ■ 1993 Revised Classification System for HIV Infection and Expanded AIDS Surveillance Case Definition for Adolescents and Adults

	Clinical Categories*		
CD4+ T-cell Categories	**(A) Asymptomatic, Acute (Primary) HIV or PGL**	**(B) Symptomatic, Not (A) or (C) Conditions**	**(C) AIDS-Indicator Conditions**
(1) ≥500/mm³	A1	B1	**C1**
(2) 200–499/mm³	A2	B2	**C2**
(3) <200/mm³ (AIDS-indicator T-cell count)	**A3**	**B3**	**C3**

*Boldface type indicates AIDS-defining categories.
From Centers for Disease Control and Prevention. (1992). 1993 Revised classification system for HIV infection and expanded surveillance case definition for AIDS among adolescents and adults. *Morbidity and Mortality Weekly Report, 41*(RR-17), 1–19.

gories, CD4+ T-lymphocyte counts were also emphasized; (2) a CD4+ T-cell count of less than 200/mm³ (14% of total lymphocytes) was added to the AIDS case surveillance definition; and (3) three new AIDS-indicator diseases were added, including pulmonary tuberculosis, recurrent pneumonia, and invasive cervical cancer. Table 5–3 presents the 1993 revised classification system.

CD4+ T-lymphocyte Categories

The three CD4+ T-lymphocyte categories are defined by cell counts: category 1, >500/mm³; category 2, 200 to 499/mm³; and category 3, 200/mm³. These categories correspond to CD4+ T-lymphocyte counts per microliter of blood and guide clinical and therapeutic actions in the management of adolescents and adults infected with HIV-1.

HIV-1–infected persons should be classified on the basis of existing guidelines for the medical management of HIV-1–infected persons. Thus the lowest accurate but not necessarily the most recent CD4+ T-lymphocyte count should be used for classification purposes.

Clinical Categories

CLINICAL CATEGORY A. Category A includes adults or adolescents who exhibit asymptomatic infection, persistent generalized lymphadenopathy (PGL) , or acute (primary) HIV-1 infection with accompanying illness or a history of acute HIV-1 infection. Many clinicians recommend antiretroviral therapy for persons in category A.

CLINICAL CATEGORY B. Category B consists of symptomatic conditions in HIV-1–infected ado-

lescents or adults that are not included among conditions listed in clinical category C and that meet at least one of the following criteria: (a) the conditions are attributed to HIV-1 infection or are indicative of a defect in cell-mediated immunity or (b) the conditions are considered by physicians to have a clinical course or to require management that is complicated by HIV-1 infection. Examples of conditions in clinical category B include but are not limited to those listed in the Box below.

■ **SYMPTOMATIC CONDITIONS IN HIV-1-INFECTED ADULTS AND ADOLESCENTS** ■

- Bacillary angiomatosis
- Candidiasis, oropharyngeal (thrush)
- Candidiasis, vulvovaginal; persistent, frequent, or poorly responsive to therapy
- Cervical dysplasia (moderate or severe/ cervical carcinoma in situ)
- Constitutional symptoms, such as fever (38.5° C) or diarrhea >1 month
- Hairy leukoplakia, oral
- Herpes zoster (shingles) involving at least two distinct episodes or more than one dermatome
- Idiopathic thrombocytopenia purpura
- Listeriosis
- Pelvic inflammatory disease, particularly if complicated by tubo-ovarian abscess
- Peripheral neuropathy

From Centers for Disease Control and Prevention. (1992). 1993 Revised classification system for HIV infection and expanded surveillance case definition for AIDS among adolescents and adults. *Morbidity and Mortality Weekly Report, 41*(RR-17), 1–19.

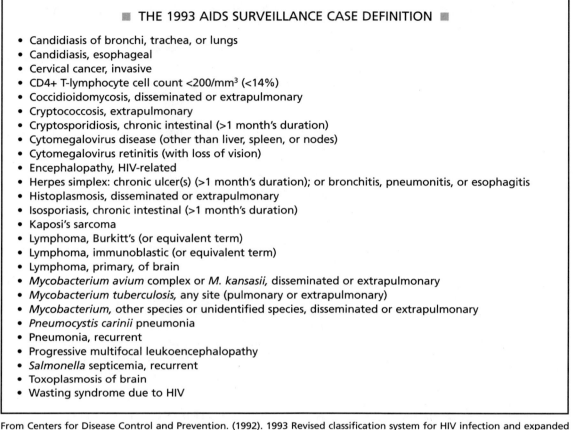

▪ THE 1993 AIDS SURVEILLANCE CASE DEFINITION ▪

- Candidiasis of bronchi, trachea, or lungs
- Candidiasis, esophageal
- Cervical cancer, invasive
- CD4+ T-lymphocyte cell count <200/mm³ (<14%)
- Coccidioidomycosis, disseminated or extrapulmonary
- Cryptococcosis, extrapulmonary
- Cryptosporidiosis, chronic intestinal (>1 month's duration)
- Cytomegalovirus disease (other than liver, spleen, or nodes)
- Cytomegalovirus retinitis (with loss of vision)
- Encephalopathy, HIV-related
- Herpes simplex: chronic ulcer(s) (>1 month's duration); or bronchitis, pneumonitis, or esophagitis
- Histoplasmosis, disseminated or extrapulmonary
- Isosporiasis, chronic intestinal (>1 month's duration)
- Kaposi's sarcoma
- Lymphoma, Burkitt's (or equivalent term)
- Lymphoma, immunoblastic (or equivalent term)
- Lymphoma, primary, of brain
- *Mycobacterium avium* complex or *M. kansasii,* disseminated or extrapulmonary
- *Mycobacterium tuberculosis,* any site (pulmonary or extrapulmonary)
- *Mycobacterium,* other species or unidentified species, disseminated or extrapulmonary
- *Pneumocystis carinii* pneumonia
- Pneumonia, recurrent
- Progressive multifocal leukoencephalopathy
- *Salmonella* septicemia, recurrent
- Toxoplasmosis of brain
- Wasting syndrome due to HIV

From Centers for Disease Control and Prevention. (1992). 1993 Revised classification system for HIV infection and expanded surveillance case definition for AIDS among adolescents and adults. *Morbidity and Mortality Weekly Report, 41*(RR-17), 1–19.

For classification purposes, category B conditions take precedence over those in category A. For example, someone previously treated for oral or persistent vaginal candidiasis (and who has not developed a category C disease) but is now free of symptoms should be classified in clinical category B.

CLINICAL CATEGORY C. Category C includes the clinical conditions listed in the AIDS surveillance case definition (see the Box above). For classification purposes, once a category C condition has occurred, the person will remain in category C. Chapter 6 discusses the AIDS-indicator diseases listed in category C.

PLANNING FOR CARE AND FOLLOW-UP

Nutritional Assessment

Maintenance of optimal nutritional status not only is critical to the health and well being of the person with HIV disease but also can have a direct effect on survival. Kotler and colleagues (1989) provided important evidence that maintaining body mass can prolong survival in AIDS. Changes in nutritional status often take place early in the course of HIV disease. Nutritional deficiency has the potential to (1) directly affect body organs such as the heart, lungs, and liver, (2) influence the host's susceptibility to opportunistic infections, and (3) contribute to the severity of illness (Timbo & Tollefson, 1994). In addition, inadequate or improper dietary intake can affect absorption and excretion of many of the medications prescribed for HIV disease and related illnesses. Conditions such as anorexia, infection, diarrhea, and drug side effects often result in poor nutritional status, which can diminish the effective functioning of an already failing immune system (Hyman & Kaufman, 1989). Weight loss and cachexia, accompanied by the loss of lean muscle mass, as well as specific nutrient deficiencies are commonly seen throughout the course of HIV infection (Bandy et al., 1993; Cimoch, 1997). The severity of nutritional deficiency seen in HIV infection appears to be related to the degree of immunodeficiency, with severe malnutrition occurring when the person is diagnosed with AIDS in the latter stages of disease (Babameto & Kotler, 1997). See chapter 6 for an in-depth discussion of the AIDS diagnosis of HIV wasting.

Weight loss and malnutrition seen in HIV disease are thought to be multifactorial and are often attributable to decreased food intake, malabsorption, and hormonal or metabolic abnormalities (Cimoch, 1997; Kotler, 1992; von Roenn, 1994). In many instances, the causes overlap. For example, during HIV infection, a metabolic problem occurs when the level of tumor necrosis factor (TNF), a cytokine that helps regulate the immune system, rises. The increase in TNF results in anorexia and decreased food intake and also in malabsorption, which allows for the sparing of fat and acceleration of muscle breakdown (Coodley et al., 1994). Hormonal abnormalities, such as low testosterone levels, which are associated with malnutrition and loss of muscle mass in HIV disease, have been noted in approximately 30% to 50% of HIV-infected men and women (Engelson et al., 1996; Grinspoon et al., 1996, 1997).

Hypermetabolic states, such as acute episodes of an opportunistic infection, have been thought to be a major causative factor in weight loss since it has been assumed that metabolism increases and, in turn, requires an increased intake of protein and calories for energy. However, Macallan and associates (1995), in a study of HIV-infected men, found

1. The total energy expended by the HIV-infected men was no more than that expended by HIV-negative men
2. During rapid weight loss, total energy expenditure was reduced primarily as a result of reduced physical activity (due to the protective mechanism of fatigue)
3. During rapid weight loss the negative energy balance was primarily the result of the reduction in energy intake
4. The rate of weight change was strongly correlated with energy (food) intake.

The authors concluded that reduced energy intake, not an elevated energy expenditure, was the prime determinant in HIV-associated wasting.

Comorbid symptoms that have been associated with decreased food intake include (1) hyperosmia (increased sensitivity to odors), (2) hyposmia (decreased sensitivity to odors), (3) anosmia (absence of the sense of smell), (4) nausea, (5) diarrhea, (6) oral lesions or disease, (7) dysphagia (difficulty swallowing), and (8) odynophagia (painful swallowing). Associated symptoms often seen in HIV illness, such as cognitive impairment, dyspnea, and fatigue, may impede a person's ability to obtain or prepare food (Ungvarski, 1996). Other factors that may contribute to malnutrition include lack of money to buy food, the absence of cooking facilities, and selection of complementary nutritional therapies such as a macrobiotic diet, which is known to promote protein-energy malnutrition and vitamin and mineral deficiencies (U.S. Department of Health and Human Services, 1996; Ungvarski, 1996).

Weight loss, wasting, and malnutrition should not be viewed as inevitable consequences of HIV infection, since they can be diminished with early aggressive nutritional intervention and education (Cimoch, 1997; McKinley et al., 1994). HIV-positive persons may have episodes of periodic weight loss followed by partial or complete recovery. The American Dietetic Association (ADA) recommends early proactive nutrition intervention and education at all stages of HIV disease in order to minimize complications (ADA, 1994). Nutrition counseling, intervention, and follow-up care should begin as soon as HIV infection is diagnosed, since malnutrition and wasting often begin insidiously early in the course of disease (Ly, 1991). In addition, with nutrition counseling that requires a client to change dietary patterns it will take some time before the desired outcomes are achieved. Simply telling the HIV-infected person what is nutritionally best may increase the person's knowledge but result in minimal behavior change. Primary care providers can realistically expect to achieve an improved dietary pattern with their clients only when they provide ongoing counseling and follow-up that include emotional support and encouragement. Appendix I contains the essential elements to be covered in nutritional counseling as well as important concerns about nutrition for HIV-infected women.

The nutritional needs across the spectrum of illness are

1. In the early stages, information on food and water safety and the need for balanced intake of macronutrients (calories, protein, carbohydrates, fat) and micronutrients (vitamins and minerals)
2. In later stages, managing symptoms that have an impact on nutritional status such as fatigue, fever, and diarrhea, so as to prevent weight loss
3. In advanced stages, strategies that diminish the effects of malnutrition (Skurnick et al.,1996; U.S. Department of Health and Human Services, 1996)

Nutrient deficiencies commonly seen in HIV disease include decreases in total kilocalories, vitamin A, vitamin B_6, vitamin B_{12}, vitamin C, vitamin E, folic acid, magnesium, selenium, and zinc (Cimoch, 1997). It is important to note that protein-calorie malnutrition has a negative effect on cellular immunity.

Table 5–4 describes the essential components for nutritional assessment. Table 5–5 presents a quick nutrition screen (QNS) containing 20 questions that are designed to capture the most common nutritional concerns associated with HIV disease. For the initial nutritional assessment, the clinician should (1) have the client complete the QNS, (2) at a minimum, measure height and weight, (3) review the results of the QNS with the client, focusing on "yes" responses, and (4) focus on one issue at a time (U.S. Department of Health and Human Services, 1996). Above all, the clinician should be realistic, since the client may have many problems that have higher priority at the time of the assessment. Management strategies for the identified problems are contained in the following section, Symptom Management.

Immunizations

In general, persons with HIV infection should not receive live virus or live bacteria vaccines (CDC, 1993). However, since limited studies of both patients with and those without symptoms of HIV infection who have received measles-mumps-rubella (MMR) vaccine have not documented serious or unusual adverse events, MMR vaccination is recommended when indicated (Onorato et al., 1988; Sprauer et al., 1993). Regardless of prior vaccination status, all HIV-infected persons who are exposed to measles should receive immune globulin. Other live attenuated

vaccines, such as oral polio vaccine (OPV), bacille Calmette-Guérin (BCG), typhoid vaccine, and vaccinia, should not be administered to HIV-infected persons. Yellow fever vaccine should be given HIV-infected persons only when potential exposure cannot be avoided (CDC, 1993).

In most cases the use of killed or inactivated vaccines in HIV-infected persons is relatively safe. CDC (1993) recommends that the decision to administer *Haemophilus influenzae* B (Hib) conjugate vaccine should be based on the patient's risk of Hib disease and the effectiveness of the vaccine. Steinhart and associates (1992), although they do not recommend routine use, suggest that since Hib vaccine is safe and inexpensive, administration of the vaccine to HIV-infected persons may be worthwhile.

Routine administration of influenza vaccine is recommended (CDC, 1993; CDC, 1997b). This vaccine is given annually, usually in November (AIDS Institute, 1997; Hecht & Soloway, 1993c). Studies examining the effect of influenza vaccination on HIV RNA viral loads have yielded conflicting results as to whether the vaccine increases viral replication (Fowke et al., 1996; Fuller et al., 1996; O'Brien et al., 1993; Yerly et al., 1993). Although influenza vaccine has produced protective antibody titers in HIV-infected persons with minimal AIDS-related symptoms and a high CD4+ cell count, the vaccine may not always have the same effect in HIV-infected persons with advanced HIV disease and low CD4+ cell counts (CDC, 1997b). Because influenza can result in serious illness and complications, and because influenza vaccination may result in protective antibody titers, current recommendations are that influenza immunization be offered to HIV-infected persons. Alternatives for influenza prophylaxis include oral therapy with either rimantadine or amantadine (CDC, 1997b)

Since Schuchat and colleagues (1991) identified increased risk of pneumococcal disease, pneumococcal vaccine has been recommended for HIV-infected persons. Persons with either asymptomatic or symptomatic HIV disease should be vaccinated as soon as their HIV diagnosis is confirmed (CDC, 1997c). Revaccination 5 years after the initial dose is recommended for high-risk persons such as those infected with HIV (CDC, 1997c). Although the vaccine is not as effective for immunocompromised patients as it is for immunocompetent patients, and it may cause

Table 5–4 ▪ Nutrition Assessment

Assess	Important Findings
ANTHROPOMETRICS Height: take measurement rather than rely on self-report Weight: actual weight, usual adult weight, weight during previous 6–12 months, ideal body weight (IBW) Assessment of protein stores: Triceps Skinfold (TSF), Body Mass Index (BMI), Bioelectrical Impedance Analysis (BIA)	Significant weight loss is a common first diagnosis before an AIDS diagnosis A significant weight loss is one that is involuntary and recent (within the last 6–12 months) Weight measurements are only gross indicators of nutritional status since weight can be affected by abnormalities in body composition Standards such as Metropolitan weight tables and TSF are based on healthy adults and designed for detecting obesity BIA, when available, is a more reliable indicator of lean body mass
BIOCHEMICAL (BASELINE FASTING) Albumin, total iron-binding capacity (TIBC), prealbumin Cholesterol, triglycerides Liver enzymes, renal panel Hemoglobin, serum iron, magnesium, folate Vitamin B_{12}, serum retinol (vitamin A)	Useful indicators of current status and can warn of changes when at risk of wasting Key indicators of visceral protein or specific nutrient status Measurements of cholesterol, albumin, and serum retinol may be predictive of mortality and morbidity in HIV-infected persons Albumin, TIBC, and prealbumin are excellent markers of nutritional status and good indicators of protein status and wasting Triglyceride levels are elevated in HIV disease as result of alterations in fat metabolism. Sudden elevations may indicate secondary infections, wasting, or drug side effects
CLINICAL Physical examination Current medications Current medical diagnoses Alternative or complementary therapies Neuropsychiatric status	Current health status, including acute infection, may impact the ability to eat and food choices Multiple medications and dosage schedules may make adequate intake of food difficult Side effects of medications and dosage schedules may make adequate food intake difficult Side effects of medications may alter intake patterns Symptoms such as depression are often associated with poor nutrition Limited mobility may impede the person's ability to prepare food; assess the client's ability to physically obtain and prepare food
DIETARY Use screening tool such as Quick Nutrition Screen (QNS), food-intake record Explore additional factors that will impact eating such as dysphagia, odynophagia, hyposmia, diarrhea, nausea	Appetite: Knowing what to eat and when to eat is not enough. Client must want to eat enough food daily Early signs of developing illness may be a sudden loss of interest in food Symptoms such as hyposmia, diarrhea, bloating, dysphagia, will result in reduced food intake
ECONOMIC/SOCIAL Living conditions and support systems Financial resources Access to food Primary spoken language Literacy and the ability to read English Cultural and religious practices Use of community-based AIDS nutrition programs	Client's ability to obtain food, distance for shopping, resources, and income as well as eligibility for subsidized food programs Living environment—stove, refrigerator, running water, etc. Support systems—family, life partner, primary care partner Illiteracy and inability to read English Cultural practices that can be incorporated into the nutritional plan Religious dietary restrictions Need for social work referral to determine eligibility for Medicaid or Medicare

Data from U.S. Department of Health and Human Services, Public Health Service, Health Resources Administration (1996).

Table 5–5 ▪ Quick Nutrition Screen

Question	Yes	No
1. Without wanting to, I have lost 10 pounds or more in the last 6 months		
2. I have problems eating because of my current health status		
3. I eat less than 3 times a day		
4. I eat meat or other proteins like beef, poultry, peanut butter, and dried beans less than 3 times a day		
5. I eat bread, cereals, rice, pasta, less than 4 times a day		
6. I eat fruits or vegetables or drink juice less than 4 times a day		
7. I drink/eat milk products like milk, cheese, and yogurt less than 3 times a day		
8. I have 3 or more drinks of beer, liquor, or wine almost every day		
9. I do not always have enough money to buy the food I need		
10. I do not have any place to cook or to keep my foods cold		
11. I do not take any vitamin and mineral supplements		
12. I often have one or more of the following: *circle all that apply:* diarrhea, nausea, heartburn, bloating, vomiting, no/poor appetite, feel too tired, pain		
13. When I take my medicines I get: *circle all that apply:* diarrhea, nausea, heartburn, bloating, vomiting, no/poor appetite, feel too tired		
14. I smoke cigarettes or cigars or chew tobacco every day		
15. I often do not feel like eating, food shopping, or cooking		
16. I have problems when I eat or drink milk products (like cramps or bloating)		
17. I have a problem when I eat high-fat or greasy foods (like a stomachache, pain in my belly, or diarrhea)		
18. I have tooth, swallowing, or mouth problems		
19. I have to watch what I eat because of certain health problems like: *circle all that apply:* diabetes, high blood pressure, kidney or liver problems		
20. I am pregnant or breast-feeding		

Data from U.S. Department of Health and Human Services, Public Health Service, Health Resources Administration (1996).

a transient rise in viral load, the potential benefits and the safety of the vaccine justify its use.

If there is no evidence of prior infection or current immunity, administration of HBV vaccine is recommended, especially in the case of intravenous drug users (AIDS Institute, 1997; Bartlett, 1997; CDC, 1997a; Hecht & Soloway, 1993b). Because of the high cost of the vaccine, laboratory screening should be performed first. After HBV vaccine has been administered, antibody response should be tested, and those who have not responded should be revaccinated with one to three additional doses (CDC, 1993). Although not as yet specifically recommended for HIV-infected persons, hepatitis A vaccine is recommended for populations at risk of HIV infection including (1) sexually active men who have sex with men, (2) injection and noninjection illegal drug users, and (3) persons who have clotting-factor disorders (CDC, 1996b).

Other vaccines containing killed or inactivated antigens, such as diphtheria-tetanus-pertussis vaccine, enhanced inactivated polio vaccine, meningococcal vaccine, rabies vaccine, cholera vaccine, plague vaccine, and anthrax vaccine may be used for the same indications as for persons with healthy immune systems (CDC, 1993). In general, it should be noted that response rates to vaccinations are lower in the HIV-infected person, and declines in response appear to be related to progressive immunodeficiency (Hecht & Soloway, 1993c).

HIV-infected persons may benefit from protection by passive immunization through the use of immune globulin preparations (CDC, 1993). Immune globulin (IG) is recommended to prevent measles after exposure. Symptomatic HIV-infected persons should receive IG regardless of their previous vaccination status because measles vaccine may not be effective in such patients and the disease may be severe. IG should also be used when the person with HIV disease has been exposed to hepatitis A (CDC, 1996b).

Varicella-zoster immune globulin (VZIG) is indicated for severely immunocompromised persons after significant exposure to chickenpox or zoster. Significant exposure is defined as household contacts, close contact indoors of more than 1 hour, sharing the same hospital room, or prolonged direct face-to-face contact such as occurs with nurses or doctors who care for these infected patients (CDC, 1993). An alternative drug for HIV-infected persons with significant exposure to varicella zoster is a 3-week course of therapy with oral acyclovir (CDC, 1997a).

Other immune globulins should be administered for the same indications and in the same doses as in immunocompetent persons. These include hepatitis B immune globulin (HBIG), vaccinia immune globulin (VIG), tetanus immune globulin (TIG), and human rabies immune globulin (HRIG).

Health Teaching

The primary purpose of health teaching is to assist the client with decision making regarding health protection in the presence of HIV disease. Although some clients may choose to improve their own health by adopting all suggestions provided by the health care professional, many will not and others will select only a few areas in which to initiate change. It is important to remember that the choice belongs to the individual client, not to the clinician. Appendix I contains an outline of topics and content to be covered with HIV-infected clients for maintaining and improving their health.

If the client permits, the health teaching encounters should include the client's lover, spouse, friends, or family (whomever the client designates as significant others) and should include the provision of printed materials for later use as a reference source. This is especially true when teaching is implemented soon after the initial diagnosis of HIV infection. Weisman (1979) best describes this period as one of existential plight. The overwhelming impact of the initial diagnosis precipitates psychologic turmoil that can last for weeks. Although clients are unlikely to retain much information given at this time, this may be the only contact the health care professional will have with them for a long time. Providing printed material and sharing information with the client and significant others will at least ensure that the infor-

mation has been made available. At this time it is also important that the clinician provide a printed schedule and information for health care follow-up, as well as a list of community-based organizations for professional and peer support.

Antiretroviral Therapy

Until 1995, the mainstay of antiretroviral therapy was the use of nucleoside analog reverse transcriptase inhibitors (NRTIs), commonly referred to as nucleoside analogs. When incorporated into the DNA of HIV during viral replication, the NRTI terminates the DNA chain preventing viral replication and results in viral stasis (Lipsky, 1996). These agents will prevent the spread of HIV to new cells, but they do not interfere with viral replication in cells that are already infected (Hirsch & D'Aquila, 1993). Examples of NRTIs include zidovudine (Retrovir, AZT), didanosine (Videx, ddI), zalcitabine (Hivid, ddC), stavudine (Zerit, d4T), and lamivudine (Epivir, 3TC).

In 1995 a second group of drugs known as proteinase or, more commonly, protease inhibitors (PIs) were approved for treatment of HIV infections. Proteins that are necessary for viral replication include protease, reverse transcriptase, integrase, and structural proteins. PIs inhibit protease, acting on chronically infected cells and resulting in noninfectious viral particles (Lipsky, 1996). Examples of PIs include saquinavir (Fortovase, Invirase), indinavir (Crixivan), ritonavir (Norvir), and nelfinavir (Viracept).

A third class of antiretroviral drugs consists of nonnucleoside reverse transcriptase inhibitors (NNRTIs). Reverse transcriptase is a part of HIV required to infect cells in the body and make more virus. Although NNRTIs do not actually terminate the DNA chain, they are similar to NRTIs and act by stopping the process of reverse transcription. Examples of NNRTIs include delavirdine (Rescriptor) and nevirapine (Viramune). Other agents under study include hydroxyurea, integrase inhibitors, and nucleotides.

Over the past few years, scientists have learned that a major factor in decreasing the durability and efficacy of antiretroviral therapy is the use of one drug at a time (monotherapy). Combination therapy, also referred to as highly active antiretroviral therapy (HAART), results in a more sustained antiviral effect in a person with HIV infection, decreases the emergence of drug resistance, and has more effect on a wider range of cellular and tissue reservoirs of HIV (Caliendo & Hirsch, 1994). Combination therapy using NRTIs with either a PI or an NNRTI has caused the viral load to drop below detectable levels and dramatically improved the overall health and well-being of HIV-infected persons (Carpenter et al., 1997).

The most significant threat to the longevity of effective therapy is the development of drug resistance (the ability of the virus to grow in the presence of the drug). Two types of drug resistance can occur: genotype and phenotype. With genotype resistance the virus mutates, and with phenotype resistance there is a decrease in the sensitivity of the virus to the drug. In addition, cross-resistance can occur when the virus develops resistance to one drug and is then resistant to other drugs in the same family. Cross-resistance has been identified as an emerging problem with HIV antiretroviral therapy (Carpenter et al., 1997).

Drug susceptibility assays to detect the presence of HIV viral phenotype and genotype resistance have been developed to assist the primary care provider in determining which antiretroviral agents will be most effective for an individual client. However, the tests are expensive and limited in their susceptibility spectrum. Phenotypic assays, measuring the ability of HIV to grow in the presence of various drug combinations, work well in determining zidovudine susceptibility, but they are less effective in determining the susceptibility of other NRTIs, have a low correlation for predicting clinical response, and may fail to detect small but significant resistant populations that can cause drug failure, and the results are difficult to replicate between different laboratories (Jackson, 1997). In addition, they are expensive, costing between $750 and $1000 per test, and take up to 6 weeks to perform. Genotypic resistance assays can detect multiple mutations and approximate the percentage of mutant virus but are limited in detecting subtle mutations, are unreliable in instances in which the viral load is low, and do not always yield definitive answers (Jackson, 1997). According to Jackson (1997), although these assays show some promise, data from well-controlled trials regarding their validity and reliability are lacking, and clinicians should continue to make assumptions about resistance and efficacy of the antiretroviral agents they are prescrib-

ing on the basis of the patient's history of prior drug therapy and CD4+ T-cell and viral load responses to the drugs prescribed.

Clinicians and patients can minimize the potential for the development of drug resistance. Primary care providers prescribing antiretroviral therapy should

1. Avoid monotherapy
2. Order only optimal doses of the drugs
3. Not reduce dosages because of minor side effects or compliance problems
4. Avoid "drug holidays" in which all the drugs or any one of the drugs is stopped for brief periods of time and then restarted
5. Evaluate and screen all prescribed medications for interactions with the antiretroviral drugs ordered
6. Avoid prescribing drugs that will lower the serum plasma levels of the antriretroviral agents
7. Switch all the antiretroviral agents when changing combinations
8. Monitor and evaluate patient compliance

Clinicians should exercise caution when writing prescriptions for antiretroviral therapy. Ungvarski and Rottner (1997), in a review of medical orders for protease inhibitors, found incorrect dosing schedules written on 40% of client records ($N = 202$). Additional findings included orders for suboptimal dosages and orders for protease inhibitor monotherapy.

Clinicians should explain to patients the necessary behaviors to optimize the effectiveness and durability of these drugs, including

1. Taking the prescribed dose of the drug at the specified intervals
2. Not skipping doses
3. Not increasing or decreasing the number of pills taken each day
4. Following meal and daily fluid intake instructions
5. Storing medications as instructed
6. Reporting side effects of medications to their primary care provider and asking for information on managing side effects
7. If they decide to stop taking the drugs, informing their primary care provider rather than having the clinician think the drugs are no longer effective

---

▨ PRINCIPLES OF HIV ANTIRETROVIRAL THERAPY ▨

1. Ongoing HIV replication leads to immune system damage and progression to AIDS. HIV infection is always harmful, and true long-term survival, free of clinically significant immune system dysfunction, is unusual.

2. Plasma HIV RNA levels indicate the magnitude of HIV replication and its associated rate of CD4+ T-cell destruction, while CD4+ T-cell counts indicate the extent of HIV-induced immune system damage already suffered. Regular, periodic measurements of plasma HIV RNA levels and CD4+ T-cell counts are necessary to determine the risk of disease progression in an HIV-infected individual and to determine when to initiate or modify antiretroviral treatment regimens.

3. As rates of disease progression differ among individuals, treatment decisions should be individualized by level of risk indicated by plasma HIV RNA and CD4+ T-cell counts.

4. The use of potent combination antiretroviral therapy to suppress HIV replication to below the levels of detection of sensitive plasma HIV RNA assays limits the potential for selection of antiretroviral-resistant variants, the major factor limiting the ability of antiretroviral drugs to inhibit virus replication and delay disease progression. Therefore maximum achievable suppression of HIV replication should be the goal of therapy.

5. The most effective means to accomplish durable suppression of HIV replication is the simultaneous initiation of combinations of effective anti-HIV drugs with which the patient has not been previously treated and that are not cross-resistant with antiretroviral agents with which the patient has been treated previously.

6. Each of the antiretroviral drugs used in combination therapy regimens should always be used according to optimum schedules and dosages.

7. The available effective antiretroviral drugs are limited in number and mechanism of action, and cross-resistance between specific drugs has been documented. Therefore any change in antiretroviral therapy increases future therapeutic constraints.

8. Women should receive optimal antiretroviral therapy regardless of pregnancy status.

9. The same principles of antiretroviral therapy apply to both HIV-infected children and adults, although the treatment of HIV-infected children involves unique pharmacologic, virologic, and immunologic considerations.

10. Persons with acute primary HIV infection should be treated with combination antiretroviral therapy to suppress virus replication to levels below the limit of detection of sensitive HIV RNA plasma assays.

11. HIV-infected persons, even those with viral loads below detectable limits, should be considered infectious and should be counseled to avoid sexual and drug-use behaviors that are associated with transmission or acquisition of HIV and other infectious pathogens.

From U.S. Deparment of Health and Human Services, Public Health Service. (1997). *Guidelines for the use of antiretroviral agents in HIV-infected adults and adolescents.* Rockville, MD: Author.

See also Medication Management in Chapter 10.

The Box contains the principles of antiretroviral therapy for HIV infection. Although the consensus is that all patients who meet the 1993 classification of HIV disease for adults and adolescents, both category B (symptomatic disease) and category C (AIDS-indicator conditions), should be treated with combination antiretroviral therapy, considerable discussion continues on whether or not to treat persons in category A (acute infection and asymptomatic) (U.S. Department of Health and Human Services, 1997). Table 5–6 contains considerations and recommendations for initiation of antiretroviral therapy.

Many experts recommend treating newly infected persons when there is clinical evidence of acute HIV infection such as detectable HIV RNA in plasma, even with a negative or indeterminate HIV antibody test, since the person may be in the process of seroconversion (1997d). Therefore when suspicion of acute infection is high, as when there is a history of recent HIV-risk behavior in association with signs and symptoms of acute infection, a test for HIV RNA should be performed in addition to HIV antibody testing. Many ex-

Table 5–6 ▪ Indications for Antiretroviral Therapy

Clinical Category	CD4+ T-cell Count and HIV RNA Copy Count	Recommendation
Acute primary infection	Any value	Although based upon theoretical considerations, many experts recommend treatment
Asymptomatic	CD4+ T-cells >500/mm^3 *and* HIV RNA copies <10,000/ml (bDNA); HIV RNA copies <20,000/ml (RT-PCR)	Many experts would delay therapy and observe; however, some experts would treat
Asymptomatic	CD4+ T-cells <500/mm^3 *or* HIV RNA copies >10,000/ml (bDNA); HIV RNA copies >20,000/ml (RT-PCR)	Treatment should be offered*
Symptomatic	Any value	Treat

*Some experts would observe patients with CD4+ T-cell counts between 350 and 500/mm^3 and HIV RNA copy counts <10,000 (bDNA) or <20,000 (RT-PCR).
From U.S. Department of Health and Human Services, Public Health Service. (1997). *Guidelines for the use of antiretroviral agents in HIV-infected adults and adolescents.* Rockville, MD: Author.

perts would also treat any person in whom HIV antibody seroconversion has been documented to have occurred within the previous 6 months (U.S. Department of Health and Human Services, 1997). The rationale for treating a person with acute infection includes

1. Suppression of the initial burst of viral replication and decrease of the magnitude of virus dissemination throughout the body
2. Potential decrease in the severity of acute disease
3. Potential decrease in the initial viral "set point," which may ultimately affect the rate of disease progression
4. Possible reduction in the rate of viral mutation due to the suppression of viral replication (U.S. Department of Health and Human Services, 1997)

Once therapy is initiated, many clinicians recommend that antiretroviral therapy be continued indefinitely since the optimal duration and composition of therapy are unknown and viremia has been documented to reappear or increase after discontinuation of therapy.

The decision to initiate therapy in an asymptomatic person involves a discussion between the primary care provider and the client regarding the risks and benefits. Factors that should be considered before initiation of therapy in an asymptomatic antiretroviral-naive person (one who has never taken HIV antiretroviral agents) include

1. The willingness of the client to begin therapy
2. The degree of existing immunodeficiency as determined by the CD4+ cell count
3. The risk of disease progression as determined by the level of plasma HIV RNA
4. The potential benefits and risks of initiating therapy
5. The likelihood, after counseling and education, of adherence to the prescribed medication regimen (U.S. Department of Health and Human Services, 1997)

Potential benefits of early antiretroviral therapy include

1. Control of viral replication and mutation and reduction in viral load
2. Prevention of progressive immunodeficiency and possibly maintenance of a normal immune system
3. Delayed progression to an AIDS-defining illness
4. Decreased risk of the development of viral resistance
5. Decreased risk of drug toxicity
6. Most important, increased survival with HIV disease

Potential risks include

1. Reduction in the quality of life because of adverse drug effects and inconvenience of current maximally suppressive regimens
2. Earlier development of drug resistance

3. Limitation in the future choices of antiretroviral agents due to the development of resistance
4. Unknown long-term toxicity of antiretroviral drugs
5. Unknown duration of the effectiveness of current antiretroviral therapies (U.S. Department of Health and Human Services, 1997)

Perhaps the most compelling evidence in favor of treating persons with asymptomatic HIV infection is the fact that in the absence of any treatment, HIV continues to destroy not only CD4+ cells but also the lymphatic structures in which these cells are formed. Consequently, over time, not only the quantity but also the quality of CD4+ cells changes dramatically (Connors et al., 1997). Essentially, certain types of CD4+ cell that are programmed to fight different pathogens are destroyed and appear to be lost permanently, and when antiretroviral therapy is started only the existing repertoires of CD4+ T-cells are increased. Even immunomodulator therapy with interleukin-2, which increases CD4+ T-cell counts, leads to only minor changes in previously disrupted repertoires (Connors et al., 1997). Therefore, if antiretroviral combination therapy is initiated after the CD4+ T-cell count has dropped to levels that require therapy to prevent opportunistic infections, the therapy should be continued even when the CD4+ T-cell count rises to higher levels. Despite the fact that HAART reduces plasma HIV RNA levels, a low degree of HIV replication continues and contributes to the maintenance of a reservoir of infected CD4+ T-cells (National Institute of Allergy and Infectious Diseases, 1997).

The guidelines for antiretroviral therapy and for the initiation of therapy in pregnant HIV-infected women should generally be the same as those outlined for nonpregnant adults (U.S. Department of Health and Human Services, 1997). For HIV-infected antiretroviral-naive pregnant women, the primary care provider and the patient may consider delaying therapy during the first 14 weeks of pregnancy, since this is the period of organogenesis when the embryo is most susceptible to potential teratogenic effects of drugs and the risks to the fetus are unknown. However, the decision should include assessment of the woman's health status and the risks and benefits of delaying therapy for several weeks. Some women who become pregnant after therapy has

been initiated may choose to stop their therapy until after the first 14 weeks to decrease the potential for teratogenicity. However, a rebound in viral load can be anticipated with such an interruption and could be associated with an increased risk of early in utero HIV transmission or could potentiate disease progression in the women. Therefore many experts suggest continuation of combination antiretroviral therapy during the first trimester (U.S. Department of Health and Human Services, 1997).

Clinical experience with PIs and NNRTIs in adolescents has been limited. Dosages of medications used to treat both HIV and opportunistic infections in adolescents should be based on the Tanner staging of puberty and not on specific age (U.S. Department of Health and Human Services, 1997). Adolescents in early puberty (Tanner I-II) should be dosed under pediatric guidelines, whereas those in late puberty (Tanner V) should be dosed by adult guidelines. Youth who are in the midst of their growth spurt (Tanner III females and Tanner IV males) should be closely monitored for medication efficacy and toxicity when adult or pediatric dosing guidelines are chosen.

Although prophylaxis after sexual exposure is considered by many to be controversial, the fact is that many physicians are treating patients for accidental sexual exposure to HIV. Although there is no scientific evidence that such treatment will, in fact, prevent HIV infection, many primary care providers are following the same guidelines for postexposure prophylaxis after an occupational exposure and prescribing combination antiretroviral therapy for cases of sexual assault or accidental condom breakage (Daily, 1997). Primary care providers should be prepared for such an encounter, especially when they are caring for discordant couples (person HIV-positive and the other negative). See Appendix IV for details of postexposure prophylaxis.

Follow-up Care

Health care follow-up for a person whose HIV disease has just been diagnosed should be scheduled immediately, rather than waiting until problems develop. Continuous monitoring of clinical status is also important if antiretroviral therapy and chemoprophylaxis for opportunistic infections are to be instituted at the appropriate time. Symptom-free clients should be seen at 3- to 6-month intervals, and clients with symptoms

---

▪ CONSIDERATIONS FOR PLANNING CLINICAL FOLLOW-UP FOR THE HIV-INFECTED PERSON ▪

1. **History and physical examination:** Should be performed at least annually unless client is on antiretroviral therapy, then checked with every visit.
2. **CD4+ T-cell count/percentage and CD4+/CD8+ ratio:** Check every 3 to 4 months or 4 weeks after starting therapy. For significant changes, a repeat test should be performed before making treatment decisions.
3. **HIV RNA plasma levels:** Check every 3 to 4 months or 4 weeks after starting therapy. For significant changes, a repeat test should be performed before making treatment decisions.
4. **Complete blood cell count with differential:** At least annually unless client is on antireroviral therapy, which requires more frequent checks for toxicity.
5. **Multichannel chemistry panel:** At least annually unless client is on antireroviral therapy, which requires more frequent checks for toxicity.
6. **Urinalysis:** At least annually unless client is on antireroviral therapy, which requires more frequent checks for toxicity.
7. **Tuberculin skin test:** At least annually.
8. **Papanicolaou (Pap) smear:** At least annually. Some experts recommend every 3 to 6 months in HIV-infected women who have symptoms.
9. **VDRL test:** At least annually if client is sexually active.
10. **Gonorrhea/*Chlamydia* test:** Every 6 to 12 months if client is sexually active.
11. **Toxoplasmosis serologic test:** Annually for IgG antibody negative persons.
12. **Other serologic tests:** As clinically indicated.

Data from Bartlett (1997), CDC (1997a), Cornelson (1997).

should be evaluated at 1- to 3-month intervals, depending on the severity of illness. Follow-up testing should be performed at this time (see the Box above).

Physical assessment at follow-up visits should be inclusive, with particular attention given to

1. General appearance, including weight changes, evidence of muscle wasting, and adenopathy
2. Eye examination, including visual impairment and exudates
3. Oral examination for lesions, thrush, or both
4. Skin examination for general condition and for lesions
5. Neurologic examination for mental status and sensorimotor changes
6. Pelvic/genitourinary examination

An updated history should include a review of systems (signs and symptoms) and notation of any illness that has occurred since the last visit, where the patient was treated, and how the problem was managed. Health teaching performed in the past or currently needed should be evaluated at follow-up visits. The client's knowledge of current prescribed medications and his or her ability to comply with the medication regimen should also be assessed.

Follow-up visits should routinely include nutritional assessment. The clinician should

1. Ask the client to complete the quick nutrition screen
2. Follow up on previously identified problems, noting whether they are better or worse, have resolved, or are under control
3. Identify new problems and their management
4. For recurrent problems, suggest that the client keep a nutrition diary and bring it to the next visit to help identify the source of the problem (U.S. Department of Health and Human Services, 1996)

Evaluation of the effectiveness of antiretroviral therapy is based on clinical presentation, HIV RNA viral load, and CD4+ cell counts. The primary reasons that a primary care provider would consider changing antiretroviral therapy are treatment failure, toxic effects, intolerance, noncompliance, or current use of a suboptimal regimen (Carpenter et al., 1997). Treatment failure should be considered when there is

1. Less than a 0.5 to 0.75 log reduction in plasma HIV RNA 4 weeks after starting therapy or less than 1 log reduction by 8 weeks
2. Failure to suppress HIV RNA plasma to undetectable levels within 4 to 6 months of initiating therapy
3. Repeated detection of HIV RNA in plasma after initial suppression to undetectable levels
4. Any reproducible significant increase (threefold or greater from the nadir) of plasma HIV RNA that is not attributable to intercurrent infection, vaccination, or testing methods
5. Persistently declining CD4+ cell counts, measured on two separate occasions
6. Clinical deterioration (Carpenter et al., 1997; U.S. Department of Health and Human Services, 1997)

Considerations for changing a failing regimen include

1. Recent history and physical examination findings that indicate disease progression
2. Plasma HIV RNA levels measured on two separate occasions
3. Absolute CD4+ T-cell count and changes in counts
4. Remaining treatment options in terms of potency, potential resistance patterns from prior antiretroviral therapies, and potential for compliance or tolerance
5. Assessment of adherence to medications
6. Preparation of the patient for the implications of the new regimen, including side effects, drug interactions, dietary requirements, and possible need to alter other concomitant medications (U.S. Department of Health and Human Services, 1997)

Ideally, in the presence of treatment failure all current antiretroviral agents in the combination should be changed. When this is not feasible because of the patient's past experience with antiretroviral therapy, at least two drugs should be removed and replaced with new agents. Addition of a single drug to a failing regimen should be avoided, since this practice is considered to be similar to sequential monotherapy and will lead to more rapid emergence of drug resistance (Carpenter et al., 1997).

Additional treatment decisions include the initiation of chemoprophylactic therapy to prevent opportunistic infections. Current recommendations include prophylactic therapy to prevent *Pneumocystis carinii* pneumonia in HIV-infected persons with CD4+ T-cell counts less than $200/mm^3$ and prophylaxis for disseminated *Mycobacterium avium* complex infection in HIV-infected persons with CD4+ T-cell counts less than $50/mm^3$ (CDC, 1997a). Guidelines for primary prophylaxis to prevent development of opportunistic infections are contained in Table 5–7. If antiretroviral therapy is started after the CD4+ T-cell count has dropped and drug therapy to prevent opportunistic infections has been started, continuation of the chemoprophylaxis should be considered, given the fact that repertoires of CD4+ T-cells change over the course of HIV disease (Connors et al., 1997).

MANAGING ADVANCING DISEASE

As HIV infection progresses, the focus of follow-up care shifts to treatment of symptomatic conditions associated with HIV disease and to symptom management. Table 5–8 describes symptomatic conditions seen in HIV-infected adults and adolescents. The major challenge for clinicians in managing advanced disease is symptom control, and the goal is to maintain or improve the quality of life for clients in the later stages of the illness trajectory. Chapter 6 discusses the diagnosis and treatment of AIDS-indicator diseases.

Giardino and Wolf (1993) noted that symptoms serve as intervention foci for clinicians in planning the care of patients and emphasized that the patients' subjective experiences with symptoms and their desire for specific treatment may contrast sharply with the clinician's objective assessment of both the presence and the severity of symptoms. Symptoms are the subjective phenomena regarded as indicators of a condition that is departing from normal function. Signs are defined as objective indicators of disease that are verifiable by physical findings or the results of technology (Giardino & Wolf, 1993).

For the measurement of symptoms, numerous instruments have been developed and tested for reliability and validity. The problem with many tools is that they are of limited usefulness in the clinical setting in which most health care providers work, given the time constraints associ-

Table 5–7 ▪ Primary Prophylaxis of AIDS-Indicator Opportunistic Infections in HIV-Infected Adults and Adolescents

Pathogen	Indication	First Choice	Alternatives
STRONGLY RECOMMENDED AS STANDARD OF CARE			
Mycobacterium avium complex	CD4+ count <50/mm^3	Clarithromycin, **or** azithromycin	Rifabutin, **or** azithromycin
Mycobacterium tuberculosis			
Isoniazid (INH)-sensitive	Tuberculin skin test (TST) reaction ≥5 mm **or** prior TST result without treatment **or** contact with an active case	INH **plus** pyridoxine	Rifampin
INH-resistant	Same; high probability of exposure to INH-resistant TB	Rifampin	Rifabutin
Mutlidrug resistant (INH and rifampin resistant)	Same; high probability of exposure to multidrug-resistant TB	Choice of drugs requires consultation with public health authorities	None
Pneumocystis carinii	CD4+ count <200/mm^3; **or** oropharyngeal candidiasis **or** unexplained fever ≥2 wk	Trimethoprim-sulfamethoxazole (TMP-SMZ)	Dapsone, **or** dapsone **plus** pyrimethamine, **plus** leucovorin, **or** aerosolized pentamidine every month via Respirgard II nebulizer
Toxoplasma gondii	IgG antibody to *toxoplasma* and CD4+ count <100/mm^3	TMP-SMZ	Dapsone **plus** pyrimethamine **plus** leucovorin
NOT RECOMMENDED FOR MOST PATIENTS: INDICATED FOR USE ONLY IN UNUSUAL CIRCUMSTANCES			
Bacteria	Neutropenia	Granulocyte-colony stimulating factor (G-CSF), **or** granulocyte-macrophage colony-stimulating factor (GM-CSF)	None
Candida species	CD4+ count <50/mm^3	Fluconazole	None
Cryptococcus neoformans	CD4+ count <50/mm^3	Fluconazole	Itraconazole
Cytomegalovirus (CMV)	CD4+ count <50/mm^3 and CMV antibody positive	Ganciclovir	None
Histoplasma capsulatum	CD4+ count <100/mm^3, endemic geographic area	Itraconazole	None

1. Dosages are listed in Appendix II.
2. For information on preventing other non-AIDS-defining infections such as hepatitis A and B, influenza, pneumococcal disease, refer to the section on Immunizations in this chapter.
From Centers for Disease Control and Prevention. (1997). 1997 USPHS/IDSA guidelines for the prevention of opportunistic infections in persons infected with human immunodeficiency virus. *Morbidity and Mortality Weekly Report, 46*(RR-12), 1–46.

Table 5–8 ▪ Management of Symptomatic Conditions in HIV Disease

Condition (Etiology)	Manifestations	Management
Bacillary angiomatosis (*Bartonella henselae, Bartonella quintana:* spread by ticks, lice, cat bites or scratches)	Erythematous papules and nodules on the skin, which may resemble Kaposi's sarcoma; may also involve bone, liver, lymph nodes, lungs, gastrointestinal tract, and cause bacteremia	**Treatment:** erythromycin, doxycycline, tetracycline **Health teaching:** see Appendix I, Pets
Candidiasis, oropharyngeal (*Candida albicans:* endogenous in origin)	1. Pseudomembranous: creamy white plaques on an erythematous base on the tongue, palate, or buccal mucosa 2. Erythematous: spotty or confluent erythematous patches 3. Hyperplastic: white patches that do not wipe off 4. Angular cheilitis: fissures and erythematous areas in the corners of the mouth All may be associated with *Candida* esophagitis	**Treatment:** clotrimazole, nystatin (pastilles or suspension), ketoconazole, fluconazole, itraconazole, amphotericin B oral suspension or intravenous **Health teaching:** see Appendix I, Mouth Care
Cervical dysplasia (multifactorial risk factors for cervical intraepithelial neoplasia (CIN) include 1. Early age at first intercourse 2. Multiple sex partners 3. Sex with men with multiple sex partners 4. Cigarette smoking 5. Dietary deficiencies 6. Use of oral contraceptives 7. Immunosuppression 8. Low socioeconomic status 9. Lack of access to health care 10. History of sexually transmitted diseases, especially infection with human papillomavirus (HPV)	In HIV-infected women, the frequency and severity of CIN as well as cervical carcinoma have been correlated with the degree of immunosuppression as well as coinfection with HPV; early stages of CIN are asymptomatic	**Treatment:** depending on the results of the Pap smear, cervical biopsy, and colposcopy, treatment may include laser therapy, conization, cryosurgery, electrocautery, or simple hysterectomy **Health teaching:** the need to have a Pap smear annually
Constitutional symptoms (either HIV or developing infection or neoplasm)	Fever (temperature ≥38.5° C) or diarrhea >1 month in duration	See Symptom Management, Fever and Diarrhea
Hairy leukoplakia, oral (Epstein-Barr virus: secondary infection, reappearance of previously acquired pathogen)	White plaques on lateral borders of tongue; may involve dorsum of tongue and pharynx; may be asymptomatic or cause pain, difficulty chewing, or altered taste	**Treatment:** acyclovir **Health teaching:** see Appendix I, Mouth Care

Table continued on following page

Table 5–8 ▪ Management of Symptomatic Conditions in HIV Disease *Continued*

Condition (Etiology)	Manifestations	Management
Herpes zoster, shingles (varicella zoster virus: secondary infection, reappearance of previously acquired pathogen)	Painful vesicular lesions on an erythematous base that follow unilateral dermatomal distribution; often involves the trigeminal nerve, and delay in treatment can result in blindness; may also cause pneumonia or disseminated disease	**Treatment:** famciclovir, acyclovir, foscarnet, analgesics **Health teaching:** in immunocompromised persons, contagiousness may persist as long as new lesions are appearing; VZV can also be shed from encrusted lesions; inform contacts who might have been exposed so they may seek appropriate treatment
Idiopathic thrombocytopenic purpura (platelet-associated immunoglobulin; infectious or neoplastic conditions involving bone marrow, alcohol use, medications that cause myelosuppression)	May be symptomatic; prolonged bleeding from minor cuts or venipuncture sites; ecchymosis or petechiae; blood in urine or feces; frank bleeding from other sites, e.g., gums	**Treatment:** antiretrovirals, e.g., high-dose zidovudine, prednisone, or intravenous immune globulin; splenectomy; for severe forms, transfusion of packed red blood cells or platelets; discontinue drug-related cause; attempt to offer treatment for alcoholism; alternatives may include splenectomy, irradiation, danazol, vincristine, interferon **Health teaching:** avoid aspirin and non-steroidal anti-inflammatory drugs; use electric razors for shaving, exercise caution when using sharp objects
Listeriosis (*Listeria monocytogenes*—contaminated food, e.g., vegetables, meats, dairy products, and congenital transmission)	Fever, myalgia, nausea, diarrhea, headache, nuchal rigidity, ataxia, confusion, seizures, bacteremia	**Treatment:** ampicillin, erythromycin, penicillin G **Health teaching:** see Appendix I, Food Safety
Pelvic inflammatory disease (*Neisseria gonorrhoeae*, *Chlamydia trachomatis*)	Fever, chills, malaise, lower abdominal tenderness, adnexal tenderness, cervical motion tenderness; vaginal secretions may be mucopurulent	**Treatment:** ofloxacin, clindamycin, metronidazole, cefoxitin ceftriaxone, doxycycline, amoxicillin/clavulanic acid, gentamycin **Health teaching:** the development of PID in an HIV-infected woman usually indicates the lack of use of barriers, e.g., condoms, during sexual activities. The patient, as well as her sexual partners, should be tested for STDs. Sexual practices and prevention should be discussed; see Appendix I, Sexual Practices
Peripheral neuropathy (HIV-induced sensory neuropathy, or toxic neuropathy due to medications, e.g., ddI, ddC, d4T)	Tingling, numbness, pain in feet, hands, and extremities; contact hypersensitivity, reduced pinprick/vibratory sensation, and reduced or absent ankle jerks	Discontinue neurotoxic medication; see Symptom Management; Pain, Neuropathic

Data from Bartlett (1997), Cassell et al. (1997), CDC (1990), Hambelton (1997), Koehler (1997).

ated with the delivery of health care services. In addition, many tools are not user-friendly and require training in proper use.

Giardino and Wolf (1993), in a review of symptom experiences, identified several useful tools that may be used for symptom assessment. The Duke-UNC Health Profile (DUHP) measures adults' ongoing health status in the primary care setting and assesses symptom experience, physical function, and emotional and social function (Parkerson et al., 1981). The DUHP, considered too lengthy, was revised by Parkerson and colleagues (1990) into the Duke Health Profile (DUKE) and is considered useful for monitoring health as an outcome of health promotion interventions. The briefest, yet effective measure of wellness and dysfunction is a modified version of the DUHP, the mini-DUHP (Blake & Vandiver, 1986). McCorkle and Young (1978) developed the Symptom Distress Scale (SDS) to measure the degree of physical distress the patient experiences with nausea, insomnia, pain, fatigue, cough, changes in appetite, bowel habits, concentration, appearance, breathing, and outlook. Rhodes and Watson (1987) adopted the SDS for use in evaluation of nausea and vomiting associated with chemotherapy. The Cornell Medical Index (CMI) is also considered a reliable measure of the patient's perception of illness and the reported presence of symptoms (Abramson et al., 1965, 1966).

The most convenient tool for symptom assessment is the Visual Analog Scale (VAS) (Freud, 1923). It is a self-reporting measure of subjective experiences of symptoms. The VAS provides a rapid way for the patient to identify the severity of the symptom and to monitor trends in symptom presentation and symptom control evaluation (Freud, 1923; Gift, 1989). The vertical scale has been found to be more sensitive for measuring symptoms and easier for patients to use (Gift et al., 1986).

The next section focuses on symptom management. Although interventions specific to the identified symptoms seen in PLWA have not been studied, it is reasonable to expect that symptom management strategies developed empirically for other patient populations may be effective. For example, the topic of dyspnea and the related nursing care is based on research conducted on patients with lung disease, cardiac disease, and cancer. Much of the knowledge gained regarding fever has been obtained from afebrile persons or persons with febrile conditions associated with neurologic disorders. An exception is the topic of weight loss, which has been studied extensively in PLWA.

Symptom Management

FEVER

Etiology
A. Chronic HIV infection
B. Secondary opportunistic infection(s) or malignant conditions
C. Autoimmune disorders
D. Diarrhea
E. Dehydration
F. Allergic response to medications (drug fever)
G. Infections of intravenous lines, catheters, drains, and incisions

Assessment
A. Subjective data
   1. History of symptom
   2. Associated symptoms
   3. 24-hour dietary history, including fluid intake
   4. Medical and surgical history
   5. Current drug therapy
B. Objective data
   1. Vital signs
   2. Mental status, including alertness, cognition, and orientation
   3. Skin assessment, including integrity, temperature, turgor, appearance, and signs of injury or infection
   4. Assessment for dehydration, including the preceding plus fluid intake and output estimates and urine color, quantity, and consistency
   5. Laboratory evaluation (CBC, culture)
   Note well: Mackowiak and associates (1993), in a study of normal body temperatures, suggests that 37.2° C (98.9° F) in the early morning and 37.7° C (99.9° F) overall should be regarded as the upper limit of the normal body temperature range in healthy adults 40 years of age or younger. This study used an electronic digital thermometer for measuring oral temperatures. It is important for clini-

cians to remember that, because of the underlying immunodeficiency resulting in an impaired inflammatory response, clinical manifestations of infection, including fever, may be greatly muted (Hibberd & Rubin, 1991).

C. Assessment tools (Holtzclaw, 1992)
1. In euthermia and low-grade fever, oral or axillary modes can be used
2. Rectal temperature, although often undesirable, is more reliable than oral temperature in afebrile persons (no studies of linear relationships between rectal and other measures in febrile patients are available)
3. Statistically significant differences have been found in electronic thermometer readings when the probe is placed in the posterior sublingual versus the front sublingual regions. Negligible differences were seen when mercury thermometers were used (Erickson, 1980)
4. Continuous pulmonary artery and tympanic membrane temperatures are ideal
5. Hot and cold liquids can influence oral temperatures for as long as 9 minutes
6. Although oxygen administration has no effect on oral temperature, tachypnea and mouth breathing can cause lower readings (Dressler et al., 1983)
7. Liquid crystal "stick-on" patches to measure temperature are inaccurate in febrile patients (Ilsley et al., 1983)
8. The same instrument, technique, and placement should be used for each measurement to assure that trends in temperature change are accurately detected

Goals. After discussing the assessment findings, the client or care partner and the clinician will select interventions to control fever and maintain or replace fluid loss.

Planning Care and Health Teaching
A. Nonpharmacologic interventions (Holtzclaw, 1992)
1. Promote heat loss by
   a. Allowing heat to escape from trunk by applying a sheet and a loosely woven blanket
   b. If no skin lesions are present and the patient is ambulatory, immersion in a tub bath with water temperature at 39° C (102.2° F), avoiding chilling when emerging from bath
2. Avoid counterproductive treatments such as
   a. Tepid water sponge bathing, which causes defensive vasoconstriction. This has not been shown to be an effective coolant in persons with fever, can cause shivering, and is also distressful (Morgan, 1990; Newman, 1985)
   b. Alcohol sponging causes vasoconstriction, shivering, and toxic fumes and may be absorbed cutaneously, causing hypoglycemia (McCarthy, 1991; Morgan, 1990; Newman, 1985)
3. Holtzclaw (1992) recommends that the use of cooling blankets and ice packs be reserved for conditions in which core temperature is rising uncontrollably to potentially damaging levels. Goodman and Knochel (1991) suggest that hypothermia blankets and similar devices not be used in interleukin-1–mediated temperature elevations (pyrogenic fever), since the associated shivering is counterproductive to reduction of core temperature.
4. Prevent febrile shivering by
   a. Keeping patient in a warm room to avert shivering (Palmes & Park, 1965)
   b. Avoiding fanning bedcovers, skin exposure, or rapid removal of clothing, all of which might cause chilling
5. Control febrile shivering by wrapping the arms from fingertips to axillae and the legs from toes to groin with three layers of terry cloth toweling (Abbey et al., 1973; Caruso et al., 1992; Holtzclaw, 1990a, 1990b).
6. Increase caloric and fluid intake by
   a. Providing a plan for six feedings distributed over a 24-hour period
   b. Providing high-protein, high-calorie nutritional supplements, especially in the presence of anorexia
   c. Provide at least 2 to 2.5 liters of fluid to drink daily
7. Record intake and output
8. Maintain comfort and safety by:
   a. Providing dry clothes and bed linens; use cotton materials rather than synthetics

b. Using emollient creams for dry skin
c. Monitoring mental status frequently, especially when client is febrile
d. Evaluating the client's need for assistance with all activities of daily living
9. For chronic recurrent night fever and night sweats
   a. Suggest that client take the antipyretic agent of choice before going to sleep
   b. Have a change of bedclothes nearby in case a change is necessary
   c. Keep a plastic cover on pillow
   d. Place a towel over pillow in case of profuse diaphoresis
   e. Keep liquids at bedside to drink
B. Pharmacologic interventions
1. Aspirin, nonsteroidal anti-inflammatory agents, and acetaminophen may be prescribed, with consideration given to recent laboratory tests that evaluate hepatic and hematologic abnormalities, as well as taking into account potential drug interactions with currently prescribed medications
2. Although concern has been expressed about concomitant administration of zidovudine and acetaminophen, Steffe and associates (1990) and Sattler and colleagues (1991) found no significant interaction between the two drugs. However, Shriner and Goetz (1992) reported severe hepatotoxicity in a patient taking both drugs and cautioned clinicians to be aware of this potential problem, especially in patients who are malnourished and have hepatic disease
C. Complementary therapy may include the use of homeopathic remedies such as belladonna (Ferris et al., 1995)

Referrals
A. Clinical nurse specialist (CNS) in HIV disease
B. Dietitian
C. Visiting nurse

Evaluation. The client or care partner will
A. Identify appropriate measures to be taken in the presence of fever
B. Demonstrate the ability to initiate and maintain adequate hydration and nutrition
C. Demonstrate the ability to take and record the temperature accurately

FATIGUE

Etiology
A. Chronic HIV infection
B. Secondary opportunistic infection(s) or cancers and associated symptoms, e.g., fever and dyspnea
C. Anemia
D. Malnutrition
E. Diarrhea
F. Prolonged immobility
G. Psychological factors
H. Metabolic disorders, e.g., low testosterone levels
I. Situational factors

Assessment
A. Subjective data
1. History of symptoms
2. Associated symptoms
3. Current ability to perform activities of daily living safely and to exercise
4. Factors that increase fatigue, e.g., weather, alcohol
5. Medical and surgical history
6. Current drug therapy
7. Nutrition history
B. Objective data
1. Assess activity tolerance by taking vital signs before and immediately after the performance of an activity such as dressing or ambulating
2. Assess for associated signs and symptoms such as pallor, diaphoresis, or complaints of dyspnea or dizziness
C. Assessment tools
1. Symptom Distress Scale (SDS) (McCorkle & Young, 1978)
2. Visual Analog Scale to Measure Fatigue Severity (VAS-F) (Lee et al., 1991)
3. Piper Fatigue Scale (PFS) (Piper et al., 1989)
4. Pearson and Byars' Fatigue Feeling Tone Scale (Pearson & Byars, 1956)

Goals. After discussing and validating the assessment findings, the client or care partner and the clinician will select interventions to
A. Increase self-awareness of fatigue, associated symptoms, environmental factors affecting fatigue, and activity tolerance

B. Identify the importance of resting when needed
C. Develop a plan for activity and rest
D. Accept assistance when needed
E. Develop a life-style that keeps client involved in ADL, independent, and socially active

Planning Care and Health Teaching
A. Nonpharmacologic interventions (Gift & Pugh, 1993; Hart et al., 1990; Piper, 1993)
   1. Promote self-care and self-awareness
      a. Have client keep a daily fatigue diary for at least 1 week to identify sources of fatigue and appropriate interventions, as well as patterns of peak fitness
      b. Use an assessment tool to evaluate fatigue
   2. Promote adequate sleep
      a. Increase the amount of sleep
      b. Reduce the amount of sleep cycle interruptions by preparing for sleep and keeping needed items, e.g., iced water, urinal, towel to absorb perspiration, at bedside
      c. See Insomnia
   3. Encourage adequate nutrition
      a. Substances such as coffee, tobacco, or alcohol may increase fatigue
      b. Abstain from or curtail foods to which the client may be sensitive
      c. See Weight Loss
   4. Assist the patient in learning to pace activities
      a. Plan a written 24-hour schedule for activities of daily living that alternates short activities with rest periods
      b. Assist in identifying activity priorities such as eating breakfast and then resting before bathing in the morning as opposed to the reverse
      c. Evaluate the person's needs and point out ways to conserve energy, such as sitting down while dressing, shaving, or preparing food, sitting in a shower chair while bathing, and using disposable items for eating so that no cleanup is needed
   5. Write up a plan, progressing from daily to weekly, for rest and activities
   6. Always plan activities ahead of time

   7. Several short periods of rest may be more effective than long rest periods
   8. Plan an exercise schedule (immobility may lead to increased fatigue as a result of decreased endurance)
      a. Plan exercise at peak energy times (after a rest period)
      b. Follow exercise with rest
      c. Have physical therapist assess and plan an exercise program
      d. Aerobic exercise, which increases endurance, has been shown to reduce fatigue (MacVicar & Winningham, 1986; Pardue, 1984; Thayer, 1987)
B. Pharmacologic interventions are used for treatable underlying causes, e.g., epoetin alfa for severe anemia, vitamin B_{12} replacement for an identified deficiency, or testosterone for low testosterone levels
C. Complementary therapies may include progressive muscle relaxation, accupressure, massage, reflexology, imagery and visualization, autogenic relaxation, reframing and positive affirmations, therapeutic touch, and social support and support groups (Ferris et al., 1995)

Referrals
A. Physical therapist
B. Occupational therapist
C. CNS in HIV disease or rehabilitation
D. Visiting nurse
E. Community-based AIDS program that provides visitors or "buddies"

Evaluation. The client and care partner will
A. Identify causative factors that increase fatigue
B. Demonstrate the ability to plan a schedule of paced activity for a 24-hour period
C. Demonstrate the ability to participate in a program of exercise
D. Verbalize a decrease in the fatigue experienced over a 24-hour period

WEIGHT LOSS

Etiology
A. Increased nutrient requirements resulting from primary systemic infection with HIV or secondary systemic (opportunistic) infection causing hypermetabolism, fever, or catabolism

B. Decreased food intake resulting from side effects of medication or systemic infection causing anorexia, nausea, vomiting, or alterations in taste
C. Oral or esophageal infection causing impaired chewing, dysphagia, or odynophagia
D. Decreased assimilation of food because of primary intestinal infection with HIV or secondary (opportunistic) gastrointestinal infection causing malabsorption diarrhea
E. Inability to obtain food because of fatigue or lack of money
F. Lack of facilities to store and prepare food
G. Lack of knowledge of the importance of nutrition in HIV infection and its impact on survival
H. Neuropsychiatric problems such as depression, impaired cognition, or paralysis

Assessment. See Tables 5–4 and 5–5

Goals. After discussing and validating the assessment findings, the client or care partner and the clinician will select interventions to stimulate appetite, increase weight, preserve lean muscle mass, and provide adequate levels of all nutrients.

Planning Care and Health Teaching
A. Nonpharmacologic interventions (Life Sciences Research Office, 1990; Newman, 1992; Task Force on Nutrition Support in AIDS, 1989):
  1. For alterations in the sense of smell
     a. Hyperosmia (increased sense of smell): Avoid cooking odors by keeping windows open and the home well aerated; encourage meals that include cold foods
     b. Hyposmia (decreased sense of smell): use spices such as basil, oregano, rosemary, thyme, cloves, mint, cinnamon, or lemon juice to enhance smell
  2. For alterations in sense of taste (especially related to distaste for red meat)
     a. Marinate meat before cooking in commercial marinade, wine, or vinegar
     b. As substitutes for red meat, use other protein sources such as eggs, peanut butter, tofu, cheeses, poultry, or fish
  3. For persons living alone or experiencing fatigue or depression

     a. Eat small meals frequently throughout the day; try to eat by the clock
     b. Include high-calorie snacks or commercially prepared supplements (liquids or bars)
     c. Indulge desires for favorite foods
     d. Consume more nutrient-dense foods and beverages, rather than filling up on low-calorie items
     e. Drink liquids ½ hour before eating instead of with meals
     f. Prepare meals (such as soups or casseroles) ahead of time so that they can be divided into individual servings and frozen until needed
     g. Keep easy-to-prepare foods, such as frozen dinners, canned foods, and eggs, on hand
     h. Make food presentation and service appealing
     i. Encourage dining with friends or family in pleasant surroundings
     j. Get family members and friends involved in meal preparation; the warm atmosphere they can provide may stimulate the patient's appetite
     k. Use home food delivery service, e.g., "meals on wheels" programs
     l. Direct the patient to support services in the community; sources of information on available food programs may include outpatient dietitians at local hospitals or public health department nutritionists
     m. When traveling, carry powdered forms of dietary supplements because they are easier to carry than ready-to-use forms in cans
  4. See Nausea
  5. For difficulty in chewing, dysphagia (difficulty in swallowing), or odynophagia (painful swallowing), avoid
     a. Rough foods such as raw fruits and vegetables
     b. Spicy, acidic, or salty foods
     c. Alcohol or tobacco
     d. Excessively hot or cold foods
     e. Sticky food such as peanut butter and slippery foods such as gelatin, bologna, and elbow macaroni

6. For difficulty in chewing, dysphagia (difficulty in swallowing), or odynophagia (painful swallowing) encourage
   a. Eating foods at room temperature
   b. Choosing mild foods and drinks, e.g., apple juice rather than orange juice
   c. Eating dry grain foods such as breads, crackers, and cookies softened in milk, tea, etc.
   d. Eating nonabrasive, easy-to-swallow foods such as ice cream, pudding, well-cooked eggs, noodle dishes, baked fish, and soft cheese
   e. Eating Popsicles to numb pain
   f. Using a straw when drinking
   g. Tilting head back or moving it forward to make swallowing easier
7. Evaluate financial resources and the need for referral for Medicaid, food stamps, etc.
8. Evaluate the home and the client's ability to prepare and obtain food, looking for such factors as absence of cooking facilities
9. Explore community resources that provide free meals
10. Discuss nutritional requirements for persons with HIV disease, including
    a. High-protein sources and ways to increase protein intake by
       (1) Adding skim milk powder to regular whole milk
       (2) Preparing canned creamed soups with heavy cream instead of water or milk
       (3) Increasing intake of peanut butter and eating it on whole wheat bread
       (4) Adding pasteurized processed cheeses to soups and vegetables
       (5) Eating hard-boiled eggs for snacks
    b. Increasing caloric intake by
       (1) Using extra peanut butter, cream cheese, sugar, honey, sour cream, and mayonnaise
       (2) Substituting heavy creams for milk in coffee, tea, soups, etc.
       (3) Eating sweets for snacks
       (4) Drinking commercially prepared liquid dietary supplements

       (5) Making a liquid nutritional supplement at home by mixing a 1-quart packet of powdered milk with 1 quart of whole milk and adding four packets of a flavored instant breakfast mix
       (6) Eating small frequent meals instead of a few large meals
11. Reviewing a balanced diet selection for a 24-hour menu plan
12. Review essential elements of a low-microbial diet and food safety and preparation (see Appendix I)
13. See Diarrhea
Note well: The nutritional teaching should as much as possible follow the client's usual pattern of food intake rather than expecting the client to follow a totally new, unfamiliar prescription for meal planning.
B. Pharmacologic interventions include cyproheptadine, dronabinol, human growth hormone, megestrol acetate, nandrolone decanoate, oxandrolone, serostim, testosterone, and thalidomide (Bartlett, 1997; Cimoch, 1997)
C. Complementary therapies that may be used include acupuncture (may boost energy), aroma therapy, massage, therapeutic touch, and traditional Chinese medicine (Ferris et al., 1995)

Referrals
A. Dietician
B. Social worker
C. CNS in HIV disease
D. Visiting nurse
E. Community-based AIDS program that provides meals

Evaluation. The client and care partner will
A. Demonstrate weight maintenance or gain
B. Identify factors related to anorexia, difficulty in chewing, dysphagia, or odynophagia
C. Identify sufficient resources to obtain and prepare food or report that social work intervention has been established to obtain food stamps or public assistance
D. Identify means of increasing protein and calorie intake

E. Identify key concepts in planning a low-microbial diet

F. Select a balanced 24-hour menu

NAUSEA

Etiology

A. Opportunistic infections either in the gastrointestinal tract or disseminated

B. Neoplasms in the gastrointestinal tract or hepatobiliary disease

C. Side effects of medications

D. Associated with pain, anorexia, vomiting, fear, and anxiety

E. Psychologically induced when the person is exposed to noxious odors, tastes, sights

F. Anticipatory nausea and vomiting (ANV), a learned phenomenon where nausea or vomiting precedes the administration of a chemotherapeutic agent

Assessment

A. Subjective data
   1. History of symptom
   2. Associated symptoms, e.g., cough-induced nausea
   3. Current drug therapy
   4. Nutrition history
   5. Impact of symptom on activities of daily living
   6. Factors that increase or decrease symptom

B. Objective data
   1. Height and weight
   2. Vital signs
   3. Anthropometric measurements
   4. Laboratory tests for serum albumin, total protein, transferrin, complete blood count with differential, and serum electrolytes (to detect malnutrition and dehydration)

C. Assessment tools
   1. Rhodes Index of Nausea and Vomiting (INV) Form 2 (Rhodes et al., 1986)
   2. The Morrow-Assessment of Nausea and Emesis (MANE) (Morrow, 1984)
   3. Adapted Symptom Distress Scale (ASDS) Form 2 (Rhodes, 1990)
   4. Self-care journal (SCJ) (Rhodes, 1990)

Goals. After discussing the assessment findings, the client or care partner and the clinician will select interventions to manage nausea and maintain adequate nutrition and hydration.

Planning Care and Health Teaching

A. Nonpharmacologic interventions (Briscoe, 1989; Grant, 1987; Jablonski, 1993; Life Sciences Research Office, 1990; Rhodes, 1990; U.S. Department of Health and Human Services, 1996)
   1. Eat larger meals at times when feeling better
   2. Reschedule meals if nausea consistently occurs at the same time of day
   3. Avoid favorite foods during nausea to prevent development of taste aversions for these foods
   4. Eat saltier foods
   5. Avoid very sweet foods
   6. Avoid greasy or fatty foods
   7. Try cold entrees rather than hot ones; they are less aromatic and often are better tolerated
   8. Eat smaller portions of food throughout the day
   9. Stay out of the kitchen while food is being prepared if food odors provoke nausea
   10. Eat dry foods, such as toast or crackers, especially if nausea occurs in the morning (unless oral or esophageal lesions are present or salivary flow is impaired)
   11. Eat soft, bland foods that are easier to tolerate, such as rice, soft-cooked or poached eggs, apple juice, nectars, and custards
   12. Time meals and medications to avoid anticipatory vomiting
   13. Take antiemetic drugs before meals
   14. Replace fluid and salt by consuming broths, ginger ale, and juices if vomiting occurs
   15. Drink fluids through a straw between meals, rather than with meals
   16. Chew foods thoroughly and eat slowly
   17. Rest after meals but avoid reclining or lying down immediately after eating

B. Pharmacologic interventions (Bartlett, 1997; Bernstein et al., 1996; Martin, 1994)
   1. Agents that may be prescribed include prochlorperazine haloperidol, meclizine, dimenhydrinate, ondansetron, methobenzamide, metoclopramide, or promethazine

2. The use of cannabinoids such as dronabinol for antiemetic purposes may be of benefit in some HIV-positive persons, since it may also act as an appetite stimulant and result in weight gain (Plasse et al., 1991)
3. For severe nausea, it may be more effective to take an antiemetic on a regularly scheduled basis rather than only as needed
4. Because of the continuous development of new antiretroviral therapies to treat HIV infection, information on drug interactions is often limited
5. Benzodiazepines that may be used as antiemetics may alter the pharmacokinetics of zidovudine, potentially increasing toxicity (Burger et al., 1993)

C. Complementary therapies (Burish & Carey, 1984; Ferris et al., 1995; Lyles et al., 1982; Redd, 1984)
1. Relaxation using videotape; soothing music, environmental sounds, and images of nature have been used effectively
2. Distraction or relaxation, including, rest, reading or audio relaxation tapes, television, music, exercise, games, imagery, laughter or humor, conversations or storytelling, massage, and therapeutic touch

Referrals
A. Dietician
B. CNS in HIV disease
C. Visiting nurse

Evaluation. The client or care partner will
A. Identify causative factors
B. Identify appropriate management strategies
C. Report decreasing episodes of nausea
D. Maintain weight

DIARRHEA

Etiology
A. Gastrointestinal infection caused by bacteria (e.g., *Salmonella, Shigella, Mycobacterium avium-intracellulare, Campylobacter, Clostridium difficile,* small-bowel overgrowth after antibiotic treatment), fungi (e.g., *Candida*), or protozoa (e.g., *Cryptosporidium, Isospora belli,* Microsporidia, *Entamoeba histolytica, Giardia*), or viruses (e.g., cytomegalovirus, herpes simplex, adenovirus, astrovirus, picornavirus)
B. Kaposi's sarcoma in the gastrointestinal tract
C. Reaction to medications (antiretrovirals that may lead to loose stools or diarrhea include didanosine, nelfinavir, and ritonavir)
D. Lactose intolerance
E. Intolerance to dietary supplements with high osmolarity
F. Malnutrition with secondary villous atrophy
G. Metabolic disorders such as zinc deficiency or inadequate digestive enzymes (Anastasi & Sun Lee, 1996)

Assessment
A. Subjective data
1. Usual pattern of elimination
2. Usual pattern of nutrition
3. Food intolerance, especially lactose intolerance as evidenced by cramping, flatulence, and diarrhea after consumption of milk or milk products
4. History of diarrhea
5. Associated symptoms, e.g., tenesmus
6. Current drug therapy
7. Sexual activities involving anal intercourse or oral-anal contact
8. Current and past medical and surgical history
B. Objective data
1. Observation of fecal material for steatorrhea, mucus, and blood
2. Assessment of mucocutaneous surfaces (hydration status)
3. Assessment of blood pressure for orthostatic hypotension
4. Auscultation and palpation of abdomen
5. Examination of perianal region
6. Baseline serum albumin, total iron-binding capacity, blood urea nitrogen, and creatinine levels (Roberts, 1993)
C. Assessment tools include nutritional diary and record of bowel patterns
1. Record of intake and output

Goals. After discussing and validating the assessment findings, the client or care partner will select interventions to reduce symptoms, facilitate the restoration of usual bowel patterns, and prevent associated complications such as dehydration and skin breakdown.

Planning Care and Health Teaching

A. Nonpharmacologic interventions (Culhane, 1984; Task Force on Nutrition Support in AIDS, 1989; U.S. Department of Health and Human Services, 1996)
  1. Low-residue, high-protein, high-calorie diet including
     a. Cottage cheese, cream cheese, and mild processed cheeses
     b. Cooked eggs
     c. Boiled low-fat milk, yogurt, and buttermilk
     d. Clear broth and bouillon
     e. Baked, broiled, or roasted fish, poultry, or lean ground beef
     f. Gelatin, pudding, custard
     g. Cooked Cream of Wheat or Cream of Rice cereal
     h. Bananas, applesauce, peeled apples, apple juice, grape juice, or avocados
     i. White bread, toast, or crackers made from refined flour
     j. Noodles, pasta, or white rice, cooked vegetables such as baked potatoes, carrots, squash, peas, and green or wax beans
     k. Cream soups
  2. Foods to avoid include
     a. Whole-grain bread, cereals, or brown rice
     b. Nuts, seeds, popcorn, pretzels, potato chips, and similar snacks
     c. Fried foods
     d. Fresh fruits (except those listed previously) and dried fruits
     e. Raw vegetables and fresh salads
     f. Rich pastries
     g. Strong spices such as chili powder or curry
     h. Foods that increase flatus, such as cabbage, broccoli, and onions
     i. Coffee, tea, colas, chocolate
     j. Carbonated beverages
     k. Alcoholic beverages
     l. Tobacco
  3. Hydrate with at least 2.5 to 3 liters of fluid per day, including
     a. Water
     b. Gatorade
     c. Noncarbonated drinks or soda that has been opened and is relatively "flat" (with minimum carbonation left)
     d. Caffeine-free drinks
     e. Diluted fruit juices
  4. Provide frequent small meals and dietary supplements
  5. Avoid foods that are very hot, very cold, or spicy
  6. In the presence of lactose intolerance, use lactose-free dairy products such as Lactaid
  7. Provide skin care (Lincoln & Roberts, 1989):
     a. Clean the skin thoroughly and gently (water alone usually is not an adequate means of cleansing; commercial spray cleaner, e.g., Peri Wash, UniWash, and Hollister Skin Cleanser contain substances that emulsify the stool and aid in its removal)
     b. If skin is intact, after cleansing, apply a petroleum-based protective ointment to limit further contact of stool on the skin
     c. If skin denuded, after cleansing, apply a coat of protective powder such as Stomahesive and then apply a petroleum-based protective ointment
  8. For ambulatory persons:
     a. Use plastic squeeze bottle filled with warm water and spray cleaner to wash perianal area while sitting on toilet after each bowel movement
     b. Carry Tucks to cleanse perianal area when not at home
     c. Wear absorbent "shields" to line underwear to prevent embarrassment and protect clothing from incontinence or staining of fecal liquid or from creams applied to perianal region; if incontinence is severe, an adult diaper may be used
  9. Assess for orthostatic hypotension and teach gradual assumption of upright position
  10. For bed-bound patients with large volume or continuous diarrhea, a fecal incontinence pouch connected to gravity

drainage can be used (Lincoln & Roberts, 1989)

11. Teach client to avoid anal intercourse or oral-anal sexual activities

B. Pharmacologic interventions include kaolin and pectate or psyllium hydrophilic mucilloid for mild diarrhea, diphenoxylate hydrochloride with atropine, loperamide, codeine, tincture of opium, or octreotide for severe diarrhea, Lactaid tablets for lactose intolerance, and treatment for specific pathogens (Bartlett, 1997; Friedman, 1994; Martin, 1994)

C. Complementary therapies that may be used include relaxation therapy, therapeutic touch, and homeopathic remedies (Ferris et al., 1995)

Referrals

A. Dietitian

B. CNS in HIV disease or ostomy care

C. Visiting nurse

Evaluation. The client and the care partner will

A. Identify factors that contribute to diarrhea

B. Plan a 24-hour menu of low-residue, high-protein, high-calorie foods and adequate hydration

C. Demonstrate the ability to provide proper skin care after each bowel movement

D. Verbalize the need to avoid anal sexual practices

E. Verbalize a decrease in the number of bowel movements over a 24-hour period

PAINFUL OR DRY MOUTH

Etiology

A. Primary infection of HIV (diffuse infiltrative lymphocytosis syndrome

B. Secondary infections caused by bacteria (e.g., *Mycobacterium avium-intracellulare*), fungi (e.g., *Candida albicans, Cryptococcus neoformans, Histoplasma capsulatum*), viruses (e.g., herpes simplex, herpes zoster, papillomavirus, Epstein-Barr virus [causing oral hairy leukoplakia])

C. Malnutrition

D. Dehydration

E. Reaction to drug therapy or local radiation therapy

F. Neutropenia

G. Dentures that fit poorly because of weight loss

H. Mouth breathing

I. Inadequate oral hygiene

J. Continued alcohol and tobacco use

K. Periodontal disease, e.g., linear gingival erythema, necrotizing ulcerative gingivitis, necrotizing ulcerative periodontitis

L. Vitamin B_{12} deficiency

M. Autoimmune response, e.g., recurrent aphthous ulcers, salivary gland disease, immune thrombocytopenia

Assessment

A. Subjective data

1. History of symptoms
2. Associated symptoms, e.g., dysphagia, odynophagia, oral pain
3. History of recent nutritional intake
4. History of oral hygiene habits
5. Use of alcohol and tobacco
6. Medical, surgical, and dental history
7. Current drug therapy

B. Objective data

1. Examination of the lips, tongue, buccal mucosal surfaces, teeth, and dental appliances
2. Laboratory test to evaluate serum vitamin B_{12} level (Grbic & Lamster, 1997)

C. Assessment tools include the Oral Assessment Guide (Eilers et al., 1988)

Goals. After discussing the assessment findings, the client or care partner and the nurse will select interventions to

A. Establish a routine oral hygiene regimen

B. Minimize the potential for or severity of stomatitis

C. Maintain adequate nutrition

Planning Care and Health Teaching

A. Nonpharmacologic interventions (Greifzu et al., 1990; Liebman, 1992):

1. Implement an oral hygiene regimen by having client

   a. Perform oral hygiene with a mirror over sink

   b. Remove dental appliances

   c. Examine oral cavity with adequate lighting

   d. Brush teeth with a small, soft toothbrush

e. Avoid brushing mucosal surfaces

f. Rinse thoroughly with cool water

g. Floss between teeth and avoid flossing near gum line

2. Use a foam swab or large cotton swab instead of toothbrush if the platelet count falls below 50,000/mm³

3. Advise against commercial mouthwashes that contain alcohol or glycerin; substitute mouthwash with a solution of 1 quart warm water with ½ teaspoon each of salt and baking soda (change solution daily)

4. For profound fatigue or the client who is not capable of complying with a regimen of oral hygiene, consider saline mouth rinses after meals and wiping teeth with a paper napkin

5. For oral pain
   a. Use straws
   b. Popsicles and ice cream can temporarily numb painful lesions
   c. Avoid very hot or spicy foods
   d. Apply topical agents to control pain before meals
   e. Evaluate the need for systemic analgesia

6. For xerostomia (dryness of mouth)
   a. Avoid tobacco, alcohol, spicy foods, very hot or very cold foods, citrus juices, commercial mouthwashes, coarse or hard foods
   b. Use salt and baking soda rinse solution
   c. Take frequent sips of fluid, keep water at the bedside
   d. Use commercially prepared artificial saliva
   e. Suck on sugarless hard candies or chew sugarless gum
   f. Use lip balms to keep lips moist

7. Provide adequate nutrition; see Weight Loss

B. Pharmacologic interventions (Grbic & Lamster, 1997; Holmstrup & Westergaard, 1994; Jacobson et al., 1997; Martin, 1994; National Institutes of Health, 1990; Skaare et al., 1996):

1. When adequate oral hygiene is a problem, chlorhexidine oral rinse may be ordered

2. For oral pain, agents that may be used include viscous lidocaine, dyclonine and diphenhydramine elixir mouth rinse, tetracaine gel, benzocaine gel, and cocaine gel; for severe pain, systemic analgesics may be indicated

3. For aphthous ulcers (often referred to as canker sores) fluocinonide 1:1 Orabase, or halobetasol 1:1 orabase may be ordered; mouth rinses containing triclosan have also been found to reduce the incidence of recurrent aphthous ulcers; short-term thalidomide therapy has also been successful, although HIV RNA has been noted to rise during therapy

4. For linear gingival erythema, povidone-iodine rinse, chlorhexidine rinse, metronidazole, or amoxicillin may be effective

5. For necrotizing ulcerative gingivitis and periodontitis chlorhexidine rinse, metronidazole and amoxicillin may be effective

C. Complementary therapies that may be used include relaxation therapy and therapeutic touch (Ferris et al., 1995)

Referrals

A. Dentist or dental hygienist

B. CNS in HIV disease

C. Visiting nurse

Evaluation. The client or care partner will

A. Demonstrate the ability to assess oral cavity before and after hygiene

B. Demonstrate the ability to perform an oral hygiene routine

C. Demonstrate moist, pink, intact mucosal surfaces

D. Verbalize a decrease in perceived symptoms

DRY SKIN AND SKIN LESIONS

Etiology

A. Commonly seen skin conditions in HIV diseases (Herpes simplex, herpes zoster [shingles], *Candida albicans* infection, *Mycobacterium avium-intracellulare* infection, staphylococcal folliculitis, bacillary angiomatosis, molluscum contagiosum, insect bite reactions, photosensitivity, eosinophilic folliculitis, seborrheic dermatitis, psoriasis, Reiter's syndrome

B. Dry skin secondary to diaphoresis and febrile states associated with HIV disease

C. Anemia

D. Cutaneous invasion by Kaposi's sarcoma
E. Immobility
F. Malnutrition
G. Cutaneous reactions to drug therapy
H. Vitamin and essential fatty acid deficiency

Assessment
A. Subjective data
   1. History of symptoms
   2. Associated symptoms
   3. Usual patterns of bathing and skin care
   4. Bathing facilities in home
   5. Current nutritional history
   6. Past medical and surgical history
   7. Exercise and rest patterns
   8. Current drug therapy
   9. Continence patterns
   10. Client and care partner's knowledge of risks and prevention strategies related to dry skin and skin lesions
B. Objective data
   1. Examination of skin, with particular attention to areas under skin folds, pressure points, sites of invasive procedures, e.g., incisions, biopsy sites, venipuncture sites, and genital, perineal, and perianal regions
   2. Palpate skin for temperature, texture, pain, turgor, moisture, circulation, and edema
   3. Observe for redness, scaling, cracking, flaking
   4. Perform motor and sensory examination and evaluate ability to transfer, change position, and ambulate
C. Assessment tools
   1. To monitor and evaluate the client for dry skin, the Modified Skin Condition Data Form (SCDF) can be used (Hardy, 1992)
   2. To monitor potential or actual development of pressure ulcers, the Braden Scale or Norton Scale can be used (Panel for the Prediction and Prevention of Ulcers in Adults, 1992)

Goals. After discussing and validating the assessment findings, the client or care partner and the clinician will select intervention to
A. Add moisture to the skin through bathing

B. Maintain and improve tissue tolerance to pressure in order to prevent injury
C. Protect against the adverse effects of external mechanical forces: pressure, friction, and shear

Planning Care and Health Teaching
A. Nonpharmacologic interventions (Hardy, 1992; Panel for the Prediction and Prevention of Ulcers in Adults, 1992)
   1. Keep skin clean and well moisturized:
      a. Shower with a continuous spray over all body parts for 10 minutes (facilitated by the use of handheld showerhead)
      b. Maintain water temperature of 90° F to 105° F
      c. Use a superfatted soap for cleansing
      d. Pat the skin dry with a cotton towel rather than by rubbing
      e. Apply an emollient over all body parts while skin is damp
      f. Maintain a humid environment
      g. Use clothing and linen that have been thoroughly rinsed of detergent without antistatic rinses or dryer products
      h. Wear cotton clothing
   2. Prevent dissemination of infection or development of secondary infection:
      a. Avoid tub baths or sitz baths if skin lesions are present
      b. Avoid bar soap
      c. Use separate washcloth to bathe areas with infectious lesions
      d. Explain dangers of scratching and extension of infection and lesions
   3. Establish a plan to prevent skin breakdown
      a. Inspect skin at least once a day
      b. Individualize bathing schedule
      c. Minimize environmental factors such as low humidity and cold air
      d. Avoid massage over a bony prominence
      e. Use proper positioning, transferring, and turning techniques
      f. Use lubricants (corn starch and creams) to reduce friction injuries
      g. Assess the need for physical therapy consult to institute a plan for rehabilitation

4. Reduce the potential for injury for bed-bound persons:
   a. Reposition at least every 2 hours
   b. Use pillows or foam wedges to keep bony prominence from direct contact
   c. Use devices that totally relieve pressure on the heels; do not use donut-shaped devices (more likely to cause pressure ulcers than to prevent them)
   d. Avoid positioning directly on the trochanter
   e. Elevate the head of the bed as little as possible and for as short a time as possible
   f. Use lifting devices to move rather than drag patients during transfers and position changes
   g. Place at-risk patients on pressure-reducing mattresses; do not use donut-type devices
5. Reduce the potential for injury for chair-bound persons:
   a. Reposition at least every hour
   b. Have patient shift weight every 15 minutes if capable
   c. Use pressure-reducing devices for seating surfaces; do not use donut-type devices
   d. Consider postural alignment, distribution of weight, balance and stability, and pressure relief when positioning persons in chairs or wheelchairs
6. Minimize skin exposure to moisture due to incontinence:
   a. Cleanse skin at time of soiling
   b. Assess for treatment of urinary incontinence
   c. When moisture cannot be controlled, use underpads or briefs (or shields) that are absorbent and present a quick-drying surface to the skin
7. Identify related factors such as nutritional deficits, especially protein and calories (see Weight Loss), and memory deficits (see Impaired Cognition)
B. Pharmacologic interventions to treat associated pruritus may include topical steroids such as hydrocortisone or systemic agents such as cyproheptadine
C. Complementary therapies may include aroma therapy, massage, or homeopathic remedies (Ferris et al., 1995)

Referrals
A. Physical therapist
B. CNS in HIV disease or dermatologic disorders
C. Visiting nurse

Evaluation. The client or care partner will
A. Verbalize causes and risk factors for skin breakdown and pressure ulcers
B. Demonstrate the ability to perform a skin and risk assessment, use support devices, and position properly
C. Show evidence that the plan of care is being followed
D. Demonstrate that skin surfaces remain intact without evidence of redness, dryness, or infection

PAIN

Etiology
A. Localized pain in bone, nerve, and viscera caused by tumor invasion, opportunistic infection(s), or organomegaly
B. Generalized arthralgia and myalgia associated with chronic HIV disease
C. Autoimmune response to HIV disease resulting in vasculitis, chronic demyelinating neuropathy, or inflammatory myopathy
D. Pain related to surgery, radiation therapy, chemotherapy, diagnostic procedures, or medications
E. Pain related to other conditions such as diabetic neuropathy or postherpetic pain (Breitbart & McDonald, 1996)

Assessment
A. Subjective data (Acute Pain Management Guideline Panel, 1992)
   1. Significant previous or ongoing instances of pain and its effect on the patient
   2. Previously used methods for pain control that the patient has found either helpful or unhelpful
   3. The patient's attitude toward the use of opioid, anxiolytic, or other medications, including any history of substance abuse
   4. The patient's typical coping response to stress or pain, including more broadly the presence or absence of psychiatric disorders such as depression, anxiety, or psychosis

5. Family expectations and beliefs concerning pain and stress
6. Ways the patient describes or shows pain
7. The patient's knowledge of, expectations about, and preferences for pain management methods and for receiving information about pain management
8. Self-report about pain, including description, location, intensity/severity, and aggravating and relieving factors

B. Objective data
1. Assess heart rate, blood pressure, and respiratory rate
2. Observe the ability and willingness to participate in activities of daily living

Note well: The Acute Pain Management Guideline Panel (1992), in a review of the literature, concluded that (1) the single most reliable indicator of the existence and intensity of acute pain and any related discomfort or distress is the patient's self-report; (2) neither behavior nor vital signs can substitute for self-report; and (3) patients may be experiencing excruciating pain even while smiling or using laughter as coping mechanisms.

C. Assessment tools (Acute Pain Management Guideline Panel, 1992)
1. A numerical rating scale (NRS)
2. A visual analog scale (VAS)
3. An adjective rating scale (ARS)
4. McGill (MPQ) Short Form (Melzack, 1987)

Goals. After discussing and validating the assessment findings, the client or care partner and the clinician will seek interventions to
A. Reduce the incidence and severity of pain
B. Communicate effectively about pain experiences
C. Enhance comfort and satisfaction

Planning Care and Health Teaching
A. Nonpharmacologic interventions (Acute Pain Management Guideline Panel, 1992)
1. Identify activities of daily living that appear to increase the intensity and severity of the pain experience
2. Provide additional comfort measures such as using a pressure-relieving mattress, positioning and supporting limbs comfortably when in bed or sitting up in chair,

and using a "pull-sheet" to move patient or to change position
3. When client is institutionalized, encourage family or significant other to bring in familiar objects such as pillows and blankets, favorite photographs, religious articles, personal clothing, colognes, makeups, face powders, and other cosmetics
4. Physical therapy to provide
a. Exercise to maintain or increase physical activity levels and endurance
b. Ultrasound, as well as physical agents such as application of heat or cold, especially for musculoskeletal pain
c. Therapeutic massage
d. Instruction and supervision for using a transcutaneous electrical nerve stimulation (TENS) device

B. Pharmacologic treatments should include the following considerations (Breitbart & McDonald, 1996; Carr et al., 1994; Reiter & Kudler, 1996):
1. For nociceptive pain (e.g., mucocutaneous, visceral, deep somatic, headache) using the World Health Organization's (1986) Guidelines for cancer pain, which is an analgesic stepladder:
a. Step 1 (nonopioid analgesics), for mild pain, agents that may be used include acetaminophen, aspirin, fenoprofen, ibuprofen, indomethacin, meclofenamate, mefenamic acid, naproxen, piroxicam, sulindac, tolmetin, diflunisal, or choline magnesium trisalicylate
b. Step 2 (weak opioids), for moderate pain, agents that may be used include codeine, codeine with acetaminophen, hydrocodone with acetaminophen or aspirin, or oxycodone with acetaminophen or aspirin. Step 1 agents may also be used concomitantly as adjuvant agents
c. Step 3 (strong opioids), for severe pain, agents that may be used include morphine sulfate (parenteral or elixir), morphine sulfate sustained release, hydromorphone, fentanyl transdermal, levorphanol, or methadone. Step 1 agents may also be used concomitantly as adjuvant agents

2. For neuropathic pain (e.g., HIV-associated polyneuropathy, acute and postherpetic neuralgia, nucleoside toxicity with didanosine, zalcitabine, stavudine), adjuvants such as ibuprofen may be used as well as amitriptyline, desipramine, nortriptyline, doxepin, carbamazepine, divalproex, phenytoin, gabapentin, or mexilitene

3. Primary care providers should anticipate several changes in prescriptions for analgesics when initiating a pain-control regimen. A major error in initial pain management occurs when a clinician prescribes a 2-week supply of an analgesic, assumes that the prescription will work, and has no further contact until the patient returns 2 weeks later for follow-up. On the contrary, during the initial phase of pain control, the clinician should have daily contact with the patient, even if by telephone, and should anticipate schedule changes. Dosage frequency should be adjusted to prevent pain from recurring once the duration of analgesic action is determined. Likewise, it is a waste of money to prescribe large amounts of an analgesic, e.g., a 30-day supply, knowing that the orders will require a change

4. Orders for opioid analgesics should include "rescue" doses for "breakthrough" pain instances when regularly scheduled doses are insufficient

5. Orders for p.r.n. analgesics, result in delays in administration and intervals of inadequate pain control

6. Both patients and their care partners should be informed that during the first few days of a pain-control regimen, the patient may sleep for extended periods and appear very drowsy. Although some of this may be due to the initial effects of the medication, in many instances it also reflects exhaustion and the need for rest as a result of sleep deprivation caused by pain. This situation usually reverses itself within a few days after starting a scheduled pain-management regimen

7. The possibility exists that the patient may wish to refuse an analgesic if not in pain or to forego it if asleep. However, the clinician should explain that this may lower blood analgesia levels and may result in resurgence of pain and interfere with the pain-control plan

8. Although the anti-inflammatory effects of aspirin are highly effective as an analgesic adjuvant, since aspirin inhibits platelet function, it may be contraindicated in the presence of a low platelet count

9. For managing pain in the injection drug user Dal Pan and McArthur (1994) suggest that
   a. Single practitioners prescribe the medications
   b. "Lost" prescriptions not be refilled
   c. Narcotic prescriptions be carefully rationed
   d. Rescue doses of narcotic analgesics be limited on a monthly basis

10. Patients who are in recovery from narcotic addiction and are being treated with methadone maintenance will still experience pain and in most instances will require higher and more frequent doses of analgesia than a narcotic-naive person would

11. Since diarrhea is common in HIV disease, especially when protease inhibitors are prescribed, the constipating effects of analgesics may actually be beneficial. It is preferable to evaluate each patient for response to therapy instead of automatically ordering stool softeners when initiating the pain-control plan

C. Complementary therapies that may be used include cognitive-behavioral interventions such as education and instruction in pain control, relaxation exercises, imagery, music distraction, biofeedback, and therapeutic touch (Ferris et al., 1995; NIH Technology Assessment Panel, 1996)

Referrals

A. Occupational/physical therapist
B. CNS in HIV disease, hospice, or mental health
C. Pharmacist
D. Psychologist
E. Visiting nurse

Evaluation. The client or care partner will

A. Identify aggravating or precipitating factors related to the pain experienced
B. Identify measures to control pain
C. Verbalize a decrease in the amount and type of pain experienced over a 24-hour period

DYSPNEA

Etiology

A. Infections of the respiratory system caused by bacteria (e.g., *Mycobacterium tuberculosis*), fungi (e.g., *Coccidioides immitis*), protozoa (e.g., *Pneumocystis carinii*), or viruses (e.g., cytomegalovirus)
B. Respiratory tract invasion by neoplasms, e.g., Kaposi's sarcoma
C. Autoimmune manifestation of HIV infection, e.g., lymphocytic interstitial pneumonitis
D. Anemia
E. Exercise intolerance

Assessment

A. Subjective data
   1. History of problem
   2. Associated symptoms, e.g., fatigue, pain
   3. Situational factors that may precipitate dyspnea, e.g., bad weather, wind, pollens in the air, crowds, smoke, air pollution, stress
   4. Medical and surgical history
   5. Current drug therapy
   6. Self-evaluation by client of ability to dress, bathe, toilet, ambulate, etc.
B. Objective data
   1. Detailed respiratory assessment, including observation, palpation, and auscultation
   2. Cardiovascular assessment, including blood pressure, pulse, and skin color
   3. Evaluation of cardiovascular and respiratory system in relation to client's response to activities of daily living
   4. Situational assessment, including living arrangements, presence of significant other(s), and community and social support
   5. Laboratory evaluation of arterial blood gases (especially with pneumonia), pulse oximetry, or stress oximetry
   6. Pulmonary function testing
   7. Chest x-ray

C. Assessment tools
   1. A visual analog scale (VAS) (Gift, 1989)
   2. The Symptom Distress Scale (SDS) (McCorkle & Young, 1978)
   3. American Thoracic Society's Breathlessness Scale (American Thoracic Society, 1978)
   4. Borg scale (Borg, 1982)

Goals. After discussing the assessment findings, the client or care partner and the clinician will select interventions to identify factors that may precipitate dyspnea, identify strategies to prevent and control dyspnea, and develop a lifestyle that keeps the client involved in activities of daily living, independent, and socially active.

Planning Care and Health Teaching

A. Nonpharmacologic interventions (Butler, 1963, 1974; Carrieri & Janson-Bjerklie, 1986; Carrieri-Kohlman & Jansen-Bjerklie, 1993; Gift, 1993; Gift & Austin, 1992; Gift et al., 1992; Renfroe, 1988; Sharp et al., 1980)
   1. Teach physiologic therapies to control breathing patterns when dyspnea occurs
      a. Teach pursed-lips breathing: inhaling deeply and exhaling slowly through lips that are pursed
      b. Teach body positioning:
         (1) Sit upright
         (2) Lean forward
         (3) Elevate and support arms
      c. Encourage regular exercise and arrange for physical therapy consult for upper body extremity exercise training
      d. Explore physically efficient ways to perform self-care activities of daily living
   2. Teach psychologic therapies to control responses
      a. Coping with anxiety by using relaxation techniques either on a daily basis or when an acute attack of dyspnea occurs
      b. Prevent or control depression by encouraging patient to remain as active and independent as possible
      c. Encourage participation in support groups
      d. Structured Life Review, although used primarily with older adults, may be of

benefit in increasing life satisfaction and psychologic well-being in the HIV-infected person
  e. Coping with hostility when dyspnea occurs by understanding that hostility may occur with a sudden bout of dyspnea, especially if it interferes with planned activities
3. Social therapies to minimize social restrictions and prevent dyspnea
  a. Teach pacing of activities including:
    (1) Developing a written daily/weekly plan of activities
    (2) Performing activities at a slower pace
    (3) Planning frequent rest periods
    (4) Limiting the number of daily activities
  b. See Fatigue
  c. See Sexual Dysfunction
4. Cognitive therapies to restructure the patient's perception of dyspnea (Gift, 1993)
  a. Changing the perception of symptom by treating the underlying cause of dyspnea (if known) or exploring the patient's perception of dyspnea and his or her ability to cope with the symptom
  b. Altering the interpretation of dyspnea through desensitization by having the patient exercise to the point of dyspnea and then teaching control of the symptom
  c. Recalling past experiences in which dyspnea was handled effectively
5. Minimize factors contributing to the client's perception of dyspnea
  a. For smoking
    (1) Discuss the possibility of a smoking-cessation program
    (2) If client has a need to continue, discourage smoking before eating and before, during, and immediately after performing activities of daily living
    (3) Discuss a daily reduction schedule of cigarettes smoked
    (4) Consider use of commercial filters to reduce the amount of tar, nicotine, and carbon monoxide inhaled (especially if client uses marijuana)
  b. For inadequate pulmonary hygiene or immobility
    (1) Change position frequently
    (2) For immobilized client, develop a regimen of frequent coughing and deep breathing exercises
    (3) If necessary and not contraindicated, consider use of incentive spirometer and chest physical therapy
    (4) Provide adequate hydration: 2 to 2.5 L of fluid per day; monitor fluid intake and output
    (5) If client has productive cough or copious secretions, see Cough
  c. There is evidence that blowing of air on the face (with a fan) may have some beneficial effect in the reduction of dyspnea (Schwartzstein et al., 1987)
B. Pharmacologic interventions (Ferris et al., 1995; Huggins & Drascic, 1997; Martin, 1994)
  1. Oxygen therapy when indicated. In the home an oxygen concentrator is more cost-effective and safer than a tank of oxygen, is usually sufficient, and is especially needed if the patient or others in the home are smoking
  2. To relieve anxiety associated with dyspnea, lorazepam, diazepam, or midazolam may be prescribed
  3. In the presence of comorbid disease such as chronic obstructive lung disease, bronchodilator therapy may be indicated
  4. Dexamethasone may be ordered for dyspnea secondary to neoplastic obstruction in the lungs such as Kaposi's sarcoma
  5. For severe dyspnea in terminal stages, morphine may be prescribed
C. Complementary therapies that may be used include acupuncture, aroma therapy using eucalyptus, pine, or benzoin oils, and therapeutic touch (Ferris et al., 1995)

Referrals
A. Respiratory therapist
B. Physical therapist
C. Occupational therapist
D. CNS in HIV disease or respiratory disorders
E. Visiting nurse

Evaluation. The client or care partner will
A. Identify the contributing factors related to dyspnea
B. Develop a plan of self-care by pacing activities of daily living
C. Verbalize a decrease in the number of times a day dyspnea is experienced

COUGH

Etiology
A. See Dyspnea
B. Respiratory therapy or procedures
C. Gastroesophageal reflux
D. Aspiration
E. Sinusitis
F. Chemical and mechanical irritants
G. Anxiety
H. Allergic responses

Assessment
A. Subjective data: See Dyspnea
B. Objective data
   1. Abnormal breath sounds
   2. Use of respiratory accessory muscles
   3. Stridor
   4. Tachypnea

Goals. After discussing and validating the assessment findings, the client or care partner and the clinician will select interventions to promote optimum respiratory function and minimize the discomfort associated with chronic cough.

Planning Care and Health Teaching
A. Nonpharmacologic interventions
   1. Minimize discomfort associated with chronic nonrelieved cough:
      a. Encourage client to take cough medications on a scheduled basis rather than p.r.n. and to schedule doses appropriately between, not with, meals
      b. Encourage use of cough drops and tea with lemon and honey
      c. Consider warm saline gargle frequently to soothe sore throat
      d. Avoid oxygen administration without adequate humidification
   2. Minimize factors that contribute to cough suppression:
      a. If chest pain from chronic, nonrelieved cough is present, medicate on a scheduled basis rather than p.r.n.
      b. Demonstrate splinting techniques to minimize pain associated with coughing
   3. Minimize cough related to viscous secretions:
      a. Hydrate with 2 to 2.5 L of fluid per day
      b. Assist client in controlled coughing exercise schedule to clear secretions
B. Pharmacologic interventions (Ferris et al., 1995; Huggins & Drascic, 1997)
   1. Medications that may be prescribed include dextromethorphan hydrobromide or guaifenesin syrup, codeine, hydrocodone, and, for severe coughing in terminal stages, morphine
   2. In the presence of comorbid disease such as chronic obstructive lung disease, bronchodilator therapy may be indicated
C. Complementary therapies that may be employed include acupuncture, aroma therapy, e.g., eucalyptus or pine oils, and massage or chest physical therapy (Ferris et al., 1995)

Referrals
A. CNS in HIV disease or respiratory disorders
B. Visiting nurse

Evaluation. The client or care partner will
A. Identify effective cough remedies
B. Demonstrate the ability to cough effectively
C. Verbalize a decrease in the amount of cough experienced daily

IMPAIRED COGNITION

Etiology
A. HIV-induced conditions such as aseptic meningitis seen in primary HIV infection or subacute encephalitis such as HIV encephalopathy, also referred to as AIDS dementia complex
B. AIDS-related opportunistic infections caused by bacteria (e.g., *Mycobacterium tuberculosis* or atypical mycobacteria), fungi (e.g., *Cryptococcus neoformans, Histoplasma capsulatum*), protozoa (e.g., *Toxoplasma gondii*), viruses (e.g., cytomegalovirus, or JC virus)

C. Other central nervous system infections caused by varicella-zoster virus or *Treponema pallidum*
D. Malignant conditions, e.g., lymphoma, Kaposi's sarcoma
E. Cerebrovascular accidents resulting from infarction, hemorrhage, or vasculitis
F. Complications of HIV therapy such as drug side effects or irradiation side effects
G. Psychiatric disorders such as psychosis, depression, or anxiety
H. Other causes such as anemia, hypoxia, adrenal insufficiency, renal or liver disease, nutritional deficiencies, drug or alcohol use

Assessment (McArthur, 1990; Rasin, 1990; Ungvarski, 1989)
A. Subjective data (obtained from client and significant other)
   1. History of symptoms
   2. Associated symptoms
   3. Problems with memory, concentration, and conversation
   4. Problems with missing appointments or forgetting to do things
   5. Changes in leisure activities, e.g., loss of interest in reading printed materials or watching television
   6. Withdrawal from social activity
   7. History of lifestyle, including occupation, recreation and leisure interests, sleep patterns
   8. Coping patterns, including substance abuse
   9. Availability of support systems
   10. Ability and interest in performing activities of daily living
   11. History of a typical week of client's activities
   12. Self-assessment
   13. Changes in upper motor function, such as signature change, or in lower motor function, such as walking
   14. Behavior changes noticed by significant other
   15. Medical and surgical history
   16. Psychiatric history
   17. Current drug therapy
   18. Nutritional history
B. Objective data

   1. General appearance, including grooming and dress
   2. Examination of cerebral functioning, including level of consciousness and orientation, and cognitive function testing, including calculations, memory, and attention or distraction during the interview
   3. Behavior, e.g., apathetic, withdrawn, irritable
   4. Affect, e.g., appropriate or flat
   5. Cranial nerve examination
   6. Motor and sensory examination
   7. Cerebellar examination
   8. Reflexes
   9. Meningeal signs
   10. Laboratory studies, including complete blood count, multichannel chemistry panel, and urinalysis
   11. Lumbar puncture
   12. Neuroimaging studies such as MRI or CT scan
C. Assessment tools
   1. The Johns Hopkins Rating Scale (Mascolini, 1996; Power et al., 1995)
   2. Neurobehavioral Rating Scale (Hilton et al., 1990; Sultzer et al., 1992)
   3. Mattis Dementia Rating Scale (Kovner et al., 1992)
   4. AIDS Dementia Complex Rating Scale (van Gorp et al., 1992)
   Note well: According to Rasin (1990), "the value of using bedside cognitive instruments is not in the computation of a score so that the patient can be categorized as cognitively impaired or nonimpaired, it is in the ability to identify specific deficits in cognitive functioning" (p. 13).

Goals. After discussing and validating the assessment findings, the client or care partner and the clinician will select interventions to
A. Promote independence
B. Identify factors that contribute to sensory-perceptual alteration
C. Provide meaningful and sufficient sensory input
D. Minimize disorientation
E. Provide for safety

F. Improve the individual's ability to cope with reality

Planning Care and Health Teaching

A. Nonpharmacologic interventions (McArthur, 1990; Muwaswes, 1993; Rasin, 1990; Ungvarski, 1989)
1. Assess for causative factors in institutional care settings:
   a. Sleep interruption because of the facility routines such as taking vital signs during the night
   b. Auditory overload because of staff talking at night, alarms going off, and other noises
   c. New, unfamiliar staff providing care
   d. Social isolation because of infection-control practices such as isolation for pulmonary tuberculosis
   e. Restricted environment
   f. Lack of personal routine
   g. Lack of familiar visitors
   h. Fear, especially of loss of control
   i. Medication side effects
   j. Physiologic alterations
2. Assess for causative factors in the community:
   a. Lack of supervision or motivation
   b. Change in housing, e.g., placement in a nursing home or AIDS residence
   c. Lack of social support, e.g., visitors
   d. Lack of psychologic support, e.g., non-participation in peer support groups
   e. Lack of established routines
   f. Changes in home care staff
   g. Medication side effects
   h. Continued substance use
   i. Physiologic alterations
3. Reduce or eliminate causative factors:
   a. Provide a written schedule of activities for client and encourage all involved in care to adhere to schedule as much as possible
   b. Provide a copy of the routines for client to follow
   c. Avoid changes in staff assignment as much as possible
   d. Decrease noise input, especially at night
   e. Encourage regular visiting by friends

f. When friends visit, encourage them to take client out; in acute-care settings, take client for a walk to another area or to the cafeteria
g. Encourage participation in weekly peer support groups
h. When barrier precautions are necessary, put them on in front of the client, explaining their purpose
i. Discuss dangers of substance use with impaired cognition, especially with friends who may bring substances to client and with significant others
j. When external auditory stimuli cannot be controlled, consider use of personal radio with earphones
k. Keep pictures of loved ones nearby
4. Promote cognitive stimulation and orientation:
   a. Address client by name
   b. Always maintain face-to-face contact during interactions
   c. Identify self frequently (especially important with telephone conversations)
   d. Explain all care activities
   e. Engage client in areas of pleasure or interest such as board games, cards
   f. Encourage friends to watch television and read newspapers with client
   g. Keep calendar visible and cross off each day
   h. Have client wear wristwatch and check time with client periodically
5. Promote independence and self-esteem:
   a. Engage client in decision making
   b. Keep important telephone numbers next to telephone for client's use
   c. Prepour medications and evaluate client's ability to self-medicate
   d. Encourage client to perform, as much as possible, activities of daily living, including cleaning, shopping, and cooking
   e. Have client dress and groom daily; do not allow client to sit around in bed-clothes at home
   f. Encourage client to verbalize fears and concerns
6. Promote exercise:
   a. Include exercise as a part of each day's routine

b. Plan purposeful exercise such as shopping or visiting a friend

c. If client was previously engaged in a routine exercise program, continue within physical limitations of client's capabilities

7. Provide for safety:

a. Assist with potentially dangerous activities such as cooking and using appliances

b. Assess with client, significant other, and primary care provider the client's ability to continue to drive a motor vehicle

c. If client smokes, monitor safety and attempt to prohibit smoking in bed

d. Assess for hazards in the home and make necessary changes such as removing scatter rugs and breakable objects

e. Continually assess the need for assist devices such as a cane, walker, or bath bar

B. Pharmacologic interventions (Huggins & Drascic, 1997; Martin, 1994; Price, 1997)

1. Combination antiretroviral therapy may be effective in treating impaired cognition due to HIV

2. For palliative management, lorazepam, loxepine, and haloperidol may be prescribed

3. HIV-positive persons may be more prone to severe extrapyramidal symptoms when high-potency neuroleptics are used (Breitbart et al., 1988; Hriso et al., 1991; Swensen et al., 1989)

4. Benzodiazepines that may be prescribed may alter the pharmacokinetics of zidovudine, potentially increasing toxicity (Burger et al., 1993)

C. Complementary therapies that may be employed include aroma therapy, art therapy, massage, music therapy, and therapeutic touch (Ferris et al., 1995).

Note well: Because of the nature of cognitive impairment, it is extremely important to include the client's designated care partner in all planning and health teaching. Documentation on the client's record should reflect all instructions and concerns provided to both persons.

Referrals

A. CNS in HIV disease, neurologic disorders, or mental health

B. Physical therapist

C. Occupational therapist

D. Community-based AIDS organization for participation in a volunteer visitor program, support groups

E. Day care program for cognitively impaired persons (if available)

Evaluation

A. The client or significant other will

1. Identify causative factors contributing to sensory-perceptual alterations

2. Demonstrate the reduction or elimination of identified factors

3. Provide and maintain a safe home environment

B. The client will

1. Participate in decision making

2. Maintain or improve appearance

3. Participate in the plan of care

4. Verbalize fears and concerns

5. Be free from injury

IMPAIRED VISION

Etiology (Heinemann, 1992)

A. HIV infection of the eye

B. Ocular infection caused by bacteria (e.g., *Mycobacterium avium-intracellulare*), fungi (e.g., *Cryptococcus neoformans*), protozoa (e.g., *Toxoplasma gondii*), or viruses (e.g., cytomegalovirus, herpes simplex virus)

C. AIDS-related microangiopathy (noninfectious retinopathy)

D. Malignant disease, e.g., Kaposi's sarcoma

E. Complications of central nervous system disease, e.g., primary lymphoma of the brain

F. Side effects of medications

Assessment (Heinemann, 1992; Plona & Schremp, 1992)

A. Subjective data

1. Previous health history related to vision

2. History of visual impairment, noting progression of vision loss

3. Self-reported changes in visual acuity, e.g., blurred vision, floaters, or gaps in vision, unilateral or bilateral
4. Description of visual impairment, limitations on activities of daily living, especially noting housing, egress from home, assistance needed, ability to summon assistance, ability to feed, bathe, dress, toilet, and medicate self
5. Current drug therapy
6. Emotional response and concerns about vision loss
B. Objective data
   1. Examination of cranial nerves II (optic), III (oculomotor), IV (trochlear), V (trigeminal), and VI (abducens)
   2. Evaluation of ability to negotiate immediate surroundings, feed, bathe, dress, groom self, and manage self-medication
   3. Mental status examination
C. Assessment tools
   1. Snellen chart
   2. Self-reporting diary (tape recorder if client is unable to write)
   3. Teich Target (Teich & Saltzman, 1996)
Note well: Allen (1990) identifies three phases of adjustment to visual impairment: (1) preimpact, associated with an insidious loss of vision in which the person does not realize that vision changes are occurring, (2) impact, the point at which the person recognizes and acknowledges visual impairment (often at the time of diagnosis; may be accompanied by emotional responses such as anger, sadness, depression, insecurity, feelings of wanting to give up, or self-pity), and (3) learning to live with the impairment, coming to terms with the vision loss and adapting activities.

Goals. After discussing and validating the assessment findings, the client or care partner and the clinician will select interventions to identify potential hazards in the environment and methods to avoid injury, adjust to vision loss, and maintain maximum independence in activities of daily living.

Planning Care and Health Teaching
A. Nonpharmacologic interventions (Daly, 1990)
   1. Provide for safety in institutional settings
     a. Orient to unfamiliar surroundings

     b. Explain call system and assess client's ability to use it
     c. Keep bed in lowest position
     d. Assess frequently at night and keep a night-light on at all times
     e. Encourage client to ask for assistance at night, especially when first adjusting to impaired vision
     f. Accommodate client with unilateral visual loss by assignment to a bed in which client's intact visual field is toward the door and by placing over-bed table, telephone, and call light on appropriate side of bed
   2. Discuss general safety measures for the home:
     a. Avoid changing furniture arrangements
     b. Remove hazards such as small, unsecured area rugs, and exposed sharp objects
     c. Dangers of using mind-altering substances such as alcohol or illegal drugs
     d. Avoid smoking when alone or unsupervised
   3. Minimize sensitivity to light by
     a. Encouraging the use of sunglasses
     b. Keeping the environment dimly lit
     c. Encouraging client to wear brimmed hat when out of doors
     d. Keeping television at low level of brightness
   4. Promote independence and assist in relearning activities of daily living:
     a. Feeding self:
       (1) Describe location of utensils when serving food
       (2) Describe locations of food on a plate referring to clock (e.g., the potatoes are at 12 o'clock, meat at 6 o'clock)
       (3) Use "finger foods" for snacks
       (4) Use cups or mugs for liquids such as soups
     b. Bathing and grooming self:
       (1) Arrange equipment according to client's preference and replace in same location when finished with toilet
       (2) Consider use of assist devices such as bath bar or shower chair

(3) Provide supervision until client is comfortable performing alone

(4) Encourage short hair styles that require a minimum of care and grooming

(5) Encourage use of electric shaver

c. Dressing self:

(1) Assist client in planning location of clothing

(2) Place matching clothing on same hanger

d. Toileting self:

(1) If bedpan or urinal is necessary, keep accessible at all times

(2) If diarrhea is present, evaluate usefulness of bedside commode

(3) If confusion is present, consider use of external catheter with drainage bag on leg or use of adult diapers

e. Medicating self:

(1) Develop a plan for medication management

(2) Frequently review side effects of drugs, such as narcotic analgesics, that may further increase the potential for injury and the need to restrict activities

5. Use sensory support techniques for visually impaired:

a. Visual support (for color impairments and limited vision) includes printing medication and activity schedules in letter size in accordance with visual acuity; a magnifying glass is extremely useful, as is a red marker (Hi Marker, manufactured by Kentucky Industries for the Blind) that leaves a raised red dot on medication bottles and vials indicating frequency of dosing

b. Auditory support includes speaking to patient in a soft tone (loud auditory stimuli with visual loss may result in sensory overload) and, for client with complete vision loss, teaching and instructions should be recorded on audiotape

c. Provide tactile support when orienting, point out descriptively the temperature and texture of environmental furniture and surroundings

B. Pharmacologic interventions

1. Treatment for specific opportunistic infection or malignant disease

2. For mental health problems that may be associated with vision loss, psychotropic medications may be necessary, especially during the impact phase

Referrals

A. Occupational therapist

B. CNS in HIV disease or neurologic or ophthalmic disorders

C. Visiting nurse

D. Local organizations for the blind

E. Community-based support groups for people with AIDS

Evaluation. The client or care partner will

A. Identify potential hazards in the environment

B. Demonstrate the ability to move about the environment safely

C. Demonstrate the ability to feed, bathe, dress, and toilet self

D. Describe a plan for assistance with medication administration

E. Identify coping strategies to assist in adjusting to vision loss

INSOMNIA

Etiology

A. Organic mental disorders such as HIV encephalopathy

B. Psychological factors such as stress, anxiety, and depression

C. Side effects of medications, e.g., zidovudine, didanosine

D. Environmental conditions that are not conducive to sleep, e.g., noise, lights, interruptions for care

E. Drug or alcohol dependency or preexisting psychiatric problems

Assessment (Cohen & Merritt, 1992; Ferris et al., 1995)

A. Subjective data

1. History of symptom

2. Associated symptoms such as anxiety, depression, restlessness, irritability, lethargy, disorientation, pain, fever, night sweats

3. Usual patterns of sleep

4. Diet history and daily food intake patterns
5. Use of drugs, alcohol, and tobacco
6. Current ability to perform activities of daily living
7. Medical and psychiatric history
8. Current drug therapy

B. Objective data
1. Mild fleeting nystagmus
2. Slight hand tremors
3. Ptosis of eyelids
4. Expressionless face
5. Dark circles under eyes
6. Frequent yawning
7. Changes in posture
8. Thick speech with mispronunciation and incorrect words

C. Assessment tools
1. Sleep Pattern Questionnaire (SPQ) (Baekeland & Hoy, 1971)
2. Bedtime Routine Questionnaire (BRQ) (Johnson, 1986)

Goals. After discussing the assessment findings, the client or care partner will select interventions to promote healthy sleep and to increase energy levels and participation in activities of daily living.

Planning Care and Health Teaching
A. Nonpharmacologic interventions may include (Cohen, 1988; Cohen & Merritt, 1992; Golden and James, 1988; Jensen & Herr, 1993; Pulling, 1991; Reimer, 1987)
1. Establishing regular times for sleep
2. Avoidance close to bedtime of
   a. Strenuous exercise
   b. Heavy meals, but avoid going to bed hungry
   c. Spicy foods
   d. Caffeine-containing beverages and alcohol
   e. Smoking or other use of tobacco
3. Engaging in restful activities near bedtime, such as reading; avoid stimulating, anxiety-producing activities, e.g., watching the news on television
4. Providing a quiet, dark, comfortable environment

5. Teaching progressive muscular relaxation techniques to be used (use when first getting into bed)
6. If unable to sleep (after about 30 minutes), engage in a restful activity and avoid lying in bed thinking about insomnia
7. Using bed exclusively for sleeping; avoid using it for activities such as working or eating); to maintain an association with a restful place, rest during the day should be taken in other places such as a couch or chair
8. Interventions for patients in institutional settings include
   a. Providing medication for sleep or pain
   b. Providing a back rub
   c. Turning lights down
   d. Reminding the patient to void before retiring
   e. Leaving the patient alone for at least 90 minutes, without interruption, after he or she has fallen asleep
   f. Decreasing staff conversations
   g. Assuring the patient that the nurse is available when needed

B. Pharmacologic interventions (Bartlett, 1997; Ferris et al., 1995)
1. Drugs that may be prescribed for insomnia include lorazepam, oxazepam, diazepam, alprazolam, amitriptyline, trazodone, diphenhydramine, chloral hydrate, dimenhydrinate, and zopiclone
2. When selecting a drug to treat insomnia consideration should be given to a client's history of drug abuse or dependence

C. Complementary therapies that may be employed include aroma therapy, guided meditation, herbal treatment such as teas, homeopathy, massage, relaxation therapies, and therapeutic touch (Ferris et al., 1995)

Referrals
A. CNS in HIV disease or mental health
B. Community-based support groups
C. Visiting nurse

Evaluation. The client and care partner will
A. Identify strategies to improve sleep and prevent insomnia

B. Demonstrate increased participation in activities of daily living
C. Verbalize an improvement in sleep patterns

SEXUAL DYSFUNCTION

Etiology
A. Chronic genital lesions, e.g., herpes simplex or Kaposi's sarcoma
B. Chronic *Candida* vaginitis
C. Physical limitations, e.g., fatigue, shortness of breath, paralysis
D. Medication side effects
E. Partner unwilling, uninformed, or unavailable
F. Religious conflict
G. Lack of knowledge, e.g., fear of HIV transmission
H. Pain
I. Substance abuse
J. Fear of failure
K. Hypogonadotropism, e.g., low testosterone levels
L. Depression

Assessment
A. Subjective data
   1. History of problem
   2. Desire for sexual experience
   3. Changing patterns of sexual activity, e.g., increase or decrease
   4. Concern about adequacy
   5. Concerns about body image and desire to have sex
   6. Current sexual interactions with partner
   7. Initiation of sexual activity, including communication, both verbal and nonverbal, use of substances (drugs and alcohol), and use of enhancements, e.g., clothing, sexual devices, videotapes
   8. Use of fantasy during sexual activities
   9. Sexual dislikes
   10. Sexual experiences with multiple or different partners
   11. Male-specific questions: erections, quality, failure, and satisfaction with size of penis, orgasms, frequency, how achieved, e.g. by penetration, oral sex, masturbation, concern over partner reaching climax, and sexual experiences, degree of experimentation
   12. Female-specific questions: facility for vaginal lubrication, sufficient time for lubrication, vaginal pain with penile penetration, orgasms, frequency and method, e.g., masturbation, manual and oral manipulation by partners
   13. Situations that inhibit orgasms
   14. Presence, absence, or fear of pain
   15. Knowledge of safer sexual practices
   16. Fear of infection
   17. Comfort level with sexual orientation
   18. Sex-related fears, e.g., conflict with religious belief, concern about disease transmission
   19. Medical and surgical history
   20. Current drug therapy
B. Objective data
   1. Unwillingness to acknowledge problem
   2. Avoidance behaviors when topic is mentioned
   3. Presence of physical limitations, e.g., dyspnea, paralysis
   4. Serum testosterone levels in men

Goals. After discussing and validating the assessment findings, the client or sex partner and the clinician will select the interventions to encourage free expressions of concerns about sexual activities and minimize fear of sexual experience in the presence of HIV disease.

Planning Care and Health Teaching
A. Nonpharmacologic interventions (Annon, 1976)
   1. Permission: provide a milieu in which the client and significant other can freely discuss their sexual feelings and concerns by
      a. Assuring the client that sexuality is an expression of a person's identity
      b. Assessing for areas of concern and contributing factors of sexual problems, both psychological and physical
      c. Noting the knowledge deficits about sexual practices that may place the client at risk of disease transmission, e.g., exchange of body fluids
      d. Assessing for presence of conflicts in sexual practices with the client's spiritual beliefs

2. Limited information: provide information relevant to the client's concerns; explain effects of HIV disease and client's symptoms, as well as medication effects, on sexual desires and performance
3. Specific suggestions: offer suggestions that can facilitate sexual functioning:
   a. Concern about having sex with a partner in the presence of HIV disease:
      (1) Explain prevention of potential harm to client and others during sexual activity through discussion of specific sexual behaviors
      (2) Provide resource information on local AIDS support groups and events sponsored for HIV-positive persons
      (3) If having sex with a partner is unacceptable to client, consider masturbation
   b. Concern over genital lesions or infection:
      (1) For men, using colored condoms
      (2) For women, using a female condom
   c. Concern over sexual appeal related to weight loss or to lesions on legs, torso, or arms:
      (1) Wear garments that may stimulate sexual arousal in both client and partner (encourage client and significant other to identify garments that stimulate sexual arousal)
      (2) Consider reducing lighting in room when engaging in sexual activities
4. Managing shortness of breath:
   a. Client should remain passive in relation to position changes during sexual activities
   b. Avoid lying flat
   c. Use oxygen during sex if needed
   d. Avoid sexual practices such as fellatio that may interfere with breathing
5. Managing fatigue:
   a. Planning rest before sexual activity
   b. Teaching the client to remain passive in relation to positional changes
6. Managing pain:
   a. Assist client in determining the best time for medication in relation to sexual activities, e.g., 30 to 60 minutes before
      b. Using a water-soluble lubricant for intercourse
      c. For localized painful lesions, use anesthetic creams or ointments before sexual activity
7. When indicated, assist client with referral for counseling and therapy
B. Pharmacologic interventions
   1. Treatment of associated symptoms
   2. Drugs used to treat men with impotence include alprostadil injection and alprostadil urethral suppository
   3. Testosterone replacement for decreased levels
C. Complementary therapies that may be used
   1. Teaching sex partners to use massage as a sexual stimulant with use of oils for body rubs and colognes
   2. Consider use of sexually explicit and appealing videotapes
   3. Consider use of a sexual adjuvant such as vibrator or dildo

Referrals
A. CNS in HIV disease, human sexuality, or mental health
B. Psychologist or psychiatrist
C. Support groups for persons with HIV disease

Evaluation. The client and sex partner will
A. Discuss sexual concerns and feelings
B. Identify sexual activities that prevent exchange of bodily fluids during sex
C. Express concerns over changes in body image and identify strategies to cope with the changes
D. Discuss physiological limitations to having sex
E. Identify strategies to enhance sexual activity
F. When appropriate, identify the need for further counseling and seek out assistance with referral

RESEARCH NEEDED

Zeller and colleagues (1993) have made recommendations for clinical research related to symptom management in PLWA, including:

1. Respiratory symptoms
   a. Management of dyspnea associated with PCP
   b. Determining whether interventions developed for other types of patients with dyspnea are effective for PLWA
   c. Studying the effects of these interventions on survival
2. Malnutrition and gastrointestinal symptoms:
   a. Developing and testing interventions to manage reduced nutrient intake, malabsorption, altered taste sensations, dysphagia, odynophagia, nausea and vomiting, and diarrhea
   b. Evaluating the efficacy of oral rehydration therapies used for pediatric diarrhea in adult PLWA
   c. Comparing the benefits of enteral versus parenteral therapies
3. Neurologic symptoms: evaluation of the efficacy of strategies developed to maximize cognitive functioning in patients with Alzheimer's disease for PLWA
4. Opportunistic and nosocomial infections:
   a. Strategies to prevent opportunistic infections, e.g., *Candida* or *Cryptosporidium* infection
   b. Treatment protocols for managing venous access devices and urinary catheters
   c. Studies of health care workers' handwashing techniques and skin-cleansing agents
   d. Evaluation of the efficacy of low microbial diets in preventing infection
5. Pain:
   a. The efficacy of complementary therapies, e.g., therapeutic touch, relaxation, and hypnosis
   b. Comparative studies of delivering prescribed analgesia, e.g. controlled-released analgesia versus traditional methods of pain control

O'Brien and Pheifer (1993) have recommended the study of physical and psychological aspects of care, including

1. Examination of cultural variables associated with coping with HIV
2. Longitudinal research on surviving HIV over time

3. Intervention studies to test specific interventions in various settings such as hospital, home, and clinic
4. Descriptive research on the impact of HIV and AIDS on the family, functioning, and adaptation

Additional considerations for future research include:

1. Assessment
   a. Descriptive studies identifying the most frequent physiologic and psychological signs and symptoms experienced by PLWA
   b. Congruency studies to determine the similarities and differences in problems identified by clients as compared to those identified by clinicians
   c. Identification of the comorbidity of symptoms in PLWA
   d. Identification of problem differences in the different populations with HIV disease, e.g., gay men and drug users, as well as culture issues
   e. Development, testing, and validation of assessment tools that are practical and user-friendly for clinicians to use for symptom assessment
2. Symptom management
   a. Developing and testing interventions for symptoms identified in people with HIV disease/AIDS
   b. Identifying and testing nursing treatments that can be used in the presence of comorbid symptoms
3. Evaluation
   a. Evaluation of nonpharmacologic interventions and complementary therapies based on patient preferences and outcomes
   b. Comparative analysis of the costs of nonpharmacologic interventions, pharmacologic interventions, and complementary therapies and patient outcomes

SUMMARY

To provide adequate care for an HIV-infected person, the primary care provider must be knowledgeable about the illness trajectory and the appropriate interventions. Assisting the client in selecting health-promoting behaviors can prevent some of the complications associated with HIV disease. Both antiretroviral therapy and chemo-prophylaxis to prevent opportunistic infections result in a significant reduction in both morbidity and mortality.

The clinician's approach to symptom management should involve more than writing a prescription. It should be comprehensive and should incorporate nonpharmacologic and complementary therapies, as well as pharmacologic interventions when indicated. Symptom-management interventions should also be based on research findings, and evaluation of their efficacy should be based on the client's individual response to treatment as well as quantifiable outcomes.

REFERENCES

Abbey, J.C., Andrews, C., Avigliano, K., et al. (1973). A pilot study: The control of shivering during hypothermia by a clinical nursing measure. *Journal of Neuroscience Nursing, 5*(2), 78–88.

Abramson, J.H. (1966). The Cornell Medical Index as an epidemiological tool. *American Journal of Public Health, 56*(2), 287–298.

Abramson, J.H., Terespolsky, L., Brook, J.G., et al. (1965). Cornell Medical Index as a health measure in epidemiological studies. *British Journal of Preventive Social Medicine, 19*(3), 103–110.

Acute Pain Management Guideline Panel. (1992, February). *Acute pain management: Operative or medical procedures and trauma.* Clinical practice guideline (AHCPR Pub. No. 92-0032). Rockville, MD: Agency for Health Care Policy and Research, Public Health Service, U.S. Department of Health and Human Services.

AIDS Institute. (1997, July). HIV medical evaluation and preventive care. In *Protocols for the medical care of HIV infection* (7th ed.). Albany, NY: New York State Department of Health.

Allen, M. (1990). Adjusting to visual impairment. *Journal of Ophthalmic Nursing & Technology, 9*(2), 47–51.

American Dietetic Association. (1994). Position of the American Dietetic Association and the Canadian Dietetic Association: Nutrition intervention in the care of persons with human immunodeficiency virus infection. *Journal of the American Dietetic Association, 94,* 1042–1045.

American Thoracic Society. (1978). Recommended respiratory disease questionnaire for use with adults and children in epidemiological research. *American Review of Respiratory Disease, 118,* 16.

Anastasi, J.K., Sun Lee, V. (1994). HIV wasting: How to stop the cycle. *American Journal of Nursing, 94,* 18–24.

Andrist, L.C. (1988). Taking a sexual history and educating clients about safe sex. *Nursing Clinics of North America, 23*(4), 959–973.

Annon, J.S. (1976). The PLISS & model: A proposed conceptual scheme for the behavioral treatment of sexual problems. *Journal of Sex Education and Therapy, 2*(1), 211–215.

Asch, S.M., London, A.S., Barnes, P.F., Gelberg, L. (1997). Testing for human immunodeficiency virus infection among tuberculosis patients in Los Angeles. *American Journal of Respiratory Critical Care Medicine, 155*(1), 378–381.

Aylward, B., Kane, M., McNair-Scott, R., Hu, D.J. (1995). Model-based estimates of the risk of human immunodeficiency virus and hepatitis B virus transmission through unsafe injections. *International Journal of Epidemiology, 24*(2), 446–452.

Babameto, G., Kotler, D.P. (1997). Malnutrition in HIV infection. *Gastroenterology Clinics of North America, 26*(2), 393–415.

Baekeland, F., Hoy, P. (1971). Reported versus recorded sleep characteristics. *Archives of General Psychiatry, 24*(6), 548–555.

Bandy, C.E., Guyer, L.K., Perkin, J.E., et al. (1993). Nutrition attitudes and practices of individuals who are infected with human immunodeficiency virus and who live in south Florida. *Journal of the American Dietetic Association, 93*(1), 70–72.

Barthel, H.R., Wallace, D.J. (1993). False-positive human immunodeficiency virus testing in patients with lupus erythematosus. *Seminars in Arthritis and Rheumatology, 23*(1), 1–7.

Bartlett, J.G. (1993). Routine laboratory testing in asymptomatic infection. *PAAC Notes: The News Journal of the Physicians in AIDS Care, 5*(5), 192–197.

Bartlett, J. (1997). *Medical management of HIV infection.* Available: http://www.hopkins-aids.edu.

Benevedes, J.M., Abrams, D.I. (1997). Approach to the individual potentially infected with the human immunodeficiency virus. In V.T. DeVita, Jr., S. Hellman, S.A. Rosenberg (Eds.), *AIDS: Etiology, diagnosis, treatment and prevention* (4th ed., pp. 197–200). Philadelphia: Lippincott-Raven.

Bernstein, B.M., Brennan, T.G., Horowitz, H.W., et al. (1996). Managing active HIV disease. *Patient Care, 30*(9), 103–128.

Blake, R.L., Vandiver, T.A. (1986). The reliability and validity of a ten-item measure of functional status. *Journal of Family Practice, 23*(5), 455–459.

Blum, J. (1987). *When you face the chemically dependent patient: A practical guide for nurses.* St Louis: Ishiyaku Euro-America, Inc.

Borg, G. (1982). Psychophysical bases of perceived exertion. *Medicine and Science in Sports and Exercise, 14,* 337–381.

Breitbart, W., Marotta, R.F., Call, P. (1988). AIDS and

neuroleptic malignant syndrome [Letter]. *Lancet, 2*(8626–8627), 1488–1489.

Breitbart, W., McDonald, M.V. (1996). Pharmacologic pain management in HIV/AIDS. *Journal of the International Association of Physicians in AIDS Care, 2*(7), 17–26.

Briscoe, K. (1989). Optimal management of nausea and vomiting in clinical oncology. *Oncology, 3*(Suppl. 8), 11–15.

Brodie, S., Sax, P. (1997). Novel approaches to HIV antibody testing. *AIDS Clinical Care, 9*(1), 1–5, 10.

Burish, T.G., Carey, M.P. (1984). Conditioned responses to cancer chemotherapy: Etiology and treatment. In B.H. Fox, B.H. Newberry (Eds.), *Impact of psychoendocrine systems in cancer and community* (p. 147). Lewiston, NY: C.J. Hogrefe.

Burger, D.M., Meenhorst, P.L., Koks, C.H., et al. (1993). Drug interactions with zidovudine. *AIDS, 7*(4), 445–460.

Burke, D.S., Brundage, J.F., Redfield, R.R., et al. (1988). Measurement of the false positive rate in a screening program for human immunodeficiency virus infections. *New England Journal of Medicine, 319*(15), 961–964.

Butler, R.N. (1963). The life review: An interpretation of reminiscence in the aged. *Psychiatry, 256,* 65–76.

Butler, R.N. (1974). Successful aging and the role of the life review. *Journal of the American Geriatric Society, 22*(12), 529–535.

Caliendo, A.M., Hirsch, M.S. (1994). Combination therapy for infection due to human immunodeficiency virus type 1. *Clinical Infectious Diseases, 18*(4), 516–524.

Carpenter, C.C., Fischl, M.A., Hammer, S.C., et al. (1997). Antiretroviral therapy for HIV infection in 1997: Updated recommendations of the international AIDS Society—USA Panel. *Journal of the American Medical Association, 277*(24), 1962–1969.

Carr, D.B., Dubois, M., Luu, M., Shepard, K.V. (1994). Pharmacotherapy of pain in HIV/AIDS. In D.B. Carr (Ed.), *Pain in HIV/AIDS* (pp. 18–28). Washington, DC: France-USA Pain Association.

Carrieri, V.K., Janson-Bjerklie, S. (1986). Strategies patients use to manage the sensation of dyspnea. *Western Journal of Nursing Research, 8*(3), 284–305.

Carrieri-Kohlman, V.K., Janson-Bjerklie, S. (1993). Dyspnea. In V. Carrieri-Kohlman, A.M. Lindsey, C.M. West (Eds.), *Pathophysiological phenomena in nursing human responses to illness* (2nd ed., pp. 247–278). Philadelphia: Saunders.

Caruso, C.C., Hadley, B.J., Shukla, R., et al. (1992). Cooling effects and comfort of four cooling blanket temperatures in humans with fever. *Nursing Research, 41*(2), 68–72.

Cassell, J., Kell, P., Adler, M. (1997). Pelvic inflammatory disease: A review. *Journal of the International Association of Physicians in AIDS Care, 3*(10), 20–23.

Centers for Disease Control. (1990). Risk for cervical disease in HIV infected women. *Morbidity and Mortality Weekly Report, 39*(47), 846–849.

Centers for Disease Control. (1991). Update on adult immunization practices advisory committee (ACIP). *Morbidity and Mortality Weekly Report, 40*(RR-12), 1–94.

Centers for Disease Control and Prevention. (1992). 1993 Revised classification system for HIV infection and expanded surveillance case definition for AIDS among adolescents and adults. *Morbidity and Mortality Weekly Report, 41*(RR-17), 1–19.

Centers for Disease Control and Prevention. (1993). Recommendations of the advisory committee on immunization practices (ACIP): Use of vaccines and immune globulins in persons with altered immunocompetence. *Morbidity and Mortality Weekly Report, 42*(RR-4), 1–18.

Centers for Disease Control and Prevention. (1996a). *HIV/AIDS Surveillance Report, 8*(2), 1–39.

Centers for Disease Control and Prevention. (1996b). Prevention of hepatitis A through active or passive immunization: Recommendations of the advisory committee on immunization practices. *Morbidity and Mortality Weekly Report, 45*(RR-15), 1–30.

Centers for Disease Control and Prevention. (1997a). 1997 USPHS/IDSA guidelines for the prevention of opportunistic infections in persons infected with human immunodeficiency virus. *Morbidity and Mortality Weekly Report, 46*(RR-12), 1–46.

Centers for Disease Control and Prevention. (1997b). Prevention and control of influenza: Recommendations of the Committee on Immunization Practices (ACIP). *Morbidity and Mortality Weekly Report, 46*(RR-9), 1–25.

Centers for Disease Control and Prevention. (1997c). Prevention of pneumococcal disease: recommendations of the Committee on Immunization Practices (ACIP). *Morbidity and Mortality Weekly Report, 46*(RR-8), 1–24.

Centers for Disease Control and Prevention. (1997d). Anergy skin testing and preventive therapy for HIV-infected persons: Revised recommendations. *Morbidity and Mortality Weekly Report, 46*(RR-15), 1–13.

Centers for Disease Control and Prevention. (1998). AIDS among persons aged ≥50 years—United States, 1991–1996. *Morbidity and Mortality Weekly Report, 47*(2), 21–27.

Choi, S., Lagakos, S.W., Schooley, R.T. (1993). CD4+ lymphocytes are an incomplete surrogate marker for clinical progression in persons with asymptomatic HIV infection. *Annals of Internal Medicine, 118*(9), 674–680.

Cimoch, P.J. (1997). Nutritional health: Preventive and treatment of HIV-associated malnutrition, a case manager's guide. *Journal of the International Association of Physicians in AIDS Care, 3*(5), 28–40.

Cohen, F.L. (1988). Narcolepsy: A review of a common, life-long sleep disorder. *Journal of Advanced Nursing, 13*(5), 546–556.

Cohen, F.L., Merritt, S.L. (1992). Sleep promotion. In G.M. Bulechek, J.C. McCloskey (Eds.), *Nursing interventions* (2nd ed., pp. 109–119). Philadelphia: Saunders.

Connors, M., Kovacs, J.A., Krevat, S., et al. (1997). HIV infection induces changes in CD4+ T-cell phenotype and depletions within the CD4+ T-cell repertoire that are not immediately restored by antiretroviral or immune-based therapies. *Nature Medicine, 3*(5), 533–540.

Coodley, G.O., Loveless, M.O., Merrill, T.M. (1994). The wasting syndrome: A review. *Journal of Acquired Immunodeficiency Syndromes, 7*(7), 681–694.

Cornelson, B. (1997). HIV primary care evaluation and management. In M.M. Fanning (Ed.), *HIV infection: A clinical approach* (2nd ed., pp. 10–43). Philadelphia: Saunders.

Craven, D.E., Steger, K.A., LaChapelle, R., Allen, D.M. (1994). Factitious HIV infection: The importance of documenting infection. *Annals of Internal Medicine, 121*(10), 763–766.

Culhane, B. (1984). Diarrhea. In J.M. Yasko (Ed.), *Nursing management of symptoms associated with chemotherapy* (pp. 41–47). Reston, VA: Reston Publishing.

Daily, J.P. (1997). Postexposure prophylaxis for HIV. *AIDS Clinical Care, 9*(8), 59–61, 66.

Dal Pan, G., McArthur, J.C. (1994). Diagnosis and management of sensory neuropathies in HIV infection. *AIDS Clinical Care, 6*(2), 9–12, 16.

Daly, M.R. (1990). Sensory supports for the visually impaired. *Journal of Ophthalmic Nursing & Technology, 9*(6), 243–244.

Dismukes, W.E. (1988). Cryptococcal meningitis in patients with AIDS. *Journal of Infectious Diseases, 157*(4), 624–628.

Dressler, D.K., Smejkal, C., Ruffolo, M.L. (1983). A comparison of oral and rectal temperature measurement on patients receiving oxygen by mask. *Nursing Research, 32*(6), 373–375.

Eilers, J., Berger, A.M., Petersen, M.C. (1988). Development, testing, and application of the oral assessment guide. *Oncology Nursing Forum, 15*(3), 325–330.

Engelson, E.S., Goggin, K.J., Rabkin, J.G., Kotler, D.P. (1996). Nutrition and testosterone status in HIV+ women. *International Conference on AIDS* (abstract Tu.B.2382), *11*(1), 332.

Erickson, R. (1980). Oral temperature differences in relation to thermometer and technique. *Nursing Research, 29*(3), 157–164.

Fauci, A. (1993). CD4+ T-lymphocytopenia with HIV infection—No lights, no camera, just facts [editorial]. *New England Journal of Medicine, 328*(6), 429–431.

Ferguson, K.J., Stapleton, J.T., Helms, C.M. (1991). Physicians' effectiveness in assessing risk for human immunodeficiency virus infection. *Archives of Internal Medicine, 151*(3), 561–564.

Ferris, F.D., Flannery, J.S., McNeal, H.B., et al. (1995). *A comprehensive guide for the care of persons with HIV disease. Module 4: Palliative care.* Toronto, Canada: Mount Sinai Hospital and Casey House Hospice.

Fillit, H., Fruchtman, M.D., Sell, L., et al. (1990). AIDS in the elderly: A case and its implications. *AIDS Patients Care, 4*(1), 8–12.

Fischl, M.A., Uttamchandani, R.B., Daikos, G.L., et al. (1992). An outbreak of tuberculosis caused by multiple-drug-resistant tubercle bacilli among patients with HIV infection. *Annals of Internal Medicine, 117*(3), 177–183.

Fogel, C.I. (1990). Sexual health promotion. In C.I. Fogel, D. Lauver (Eds.), *Sexual health promotion* (pp. 1–18). Philadelphia: Saunders.

Fowke, K.R., D'Aimicon, R., Chernoff, D.N., et al. (1996). Immunologic and virologic evaluation of influenza vaccination of HIV-1-infected patients. *International Conference on AIDS* (abstract Tu.A.385), *11*(1), 226.

Freud, M. (1923). The graphic rating scale. *Journal of Educational Psychology, 14,* 83.

Friedman, S.L. (1994). Diarrhea. In M.A. Sande, P.A. Volberding (Eds.), *The AIDS knowledge base* (2nd ed., pp. 5.19.1–5.19.19). Boston: Little Brown.

Fuller, J.D., Chernoff, D., Steger, K., et al. (1996). The impact of influenza immunization of HIV-1 plasma RNA levels. *International Conference on AIDS* (abstract We.B.111), *11*(2), 17.

Galgiani, J.N., Ampel N.M. (1990). Coccidioidomycosis in human immunodeficiency virus-infected patients. *Journal of Infectious Diseases, 162*(5), 1165–1169.

Gemson, D.H., Colombotos, J., Elinson, J., et al. (1991). Acquired immunodeficiency syndrome prevention. Knowledge, attitudes, and practices of primary care physicians. *Archives of Internal Medicine, 151*(6), 1102–1108.

Giardino, E.R., Wolf, Z.R. (1993). Symptoms: Evidence and experience. *Holistic Nurse Practice, 7*(2), 1–12.

Gift, A.G. (1989) Visual analogue scales: Measurement of subjective phenomena. *Nursing Research, 38*(5), 286–288.

Gift, A. (1993). Therapies for dyspnea relief. *Holistic Nurse Practice, 7*(2), 57–63.

Gift, A.G., Austin, D.J. (1992). The effects of a program of systematic movement of COPD patients. *Rehabilitation Nursing, 17*(1), 6–10, 25.

Gift, A.G., Moore, T., Soeken, K. (1992). Relaxation to reduce dyspnea and anxiety in COPD patients. *Nursing Research, 41*(4), 242–246.

Gift, A.G., Plaut, S.M., Jacox, A.K. (1986). Psychologic and physiologic factors related to dyspnea in subjects with chronic obstructive pulmonary disease. *Heart & Lung, 15*(6), 595–601.

Gift, A.G., Pugh, L.C. (1993). Dyspnea and fatigue. *Nursing Clinics of North America, 28*(2), 373–384.

Golden, R.N., James, S.P. (1988). Insomnia. *Postgraduate Medicine, 83*(4), 251–258.

Goodman, E.L., Knochel, J.P. (1991). Heat stroke and other forms of hyperthermia. In P.A. Mackowiak (Ed.), *Fever: Basic mechanisms and management* (pp. 267–287). New York: Raven Press.

Grant, M. (1987). Nausea, vomiting, and anorexia. *Seminars in Oncology Nursing, 3*(4), 277–286.

Grbic, J.T., Lamster, I.B. (1997). Oral manifestations of HIV infection. *Patient Care and STDs, 11*(1), 18–24.

Greifzu, S., Radjeski, D., Winnick, B. (1990). Oral care is part of cancer care. *RN, 53*(6), 9–10.

Grinspoon, S., Corcoran, C., Lee, K., et al. (1996). Loss of lean body and muscle mass correlates with androgen levels in hypogonadal men with acquired immunodeficiency syndrome and wasting. *Journal of Clinical Endocrinology and Metabolics, 81*(11), 4051–4058.

Grinspoon, S., Cocoran, C., Miller, K., et al. (1997). Body composition and endocrine function in women with acquired immunodeficiency syndrome wasting. *Journal of Clinical Endocrinology and Metabolics, 82*(5), 1332–1337.

Hambelton, J. (1997). Hematologic complications of HIV infection. In M.A. Sande, P.A. Volberding (Eds.), *The medical management of AIDS* (5th ed., pp. 239–246). Philadelphia: Saunders.

Hardy, M.A. (1992). Dry skin care. In G.M. Bulechek, J.A. McCloskey (Eds.), *Nursing interventions: Essential nursing treatments* (2nd ed., pp. 34–47). Philadelphia: Saunders.

Hargreaves, M.R., Fuller, G.N., Gazzard, B.G. (1988). Occult AIDS: *Pneumocystis carinii* pneumonia in elderly people. *British Medical Journal, 297*(6650), 721–722.

Hart, L.K., Freel, M.I., Milde, F.K. (1990). Fatigue. *Nursing Clinics of North America, 25*(4), 967–976.

Hecht, F.M., Soloway, B. (1993a). Identifying patients at risk for HIV infection. In D.J. Cotton, G.H. Friedland (Eds.), *HIV infection: A primary care approach* (Rev. ed., pp. 3–7). Waltham, MA: Massachusetts Medical Society.

Hecht, F.M., Soloway, B. (1993b). Laboratory tests for monitoring HIV infection. In D.J. Cotton, G.H. Friedland (Eds.), *HIV infection: A primary care approach* (Rev. ed., pp. 16–18). Waltham, MA: Massachusetts Medical Society.

Hecht, F.M., Soloway, B. (1993c). Immunizations in HIV-infected patients. In D.J. Cotton, G.H. Friedland (Eds.), *HIV infection: A primary care approach* (Rev. ed., pp. 39–41). Waltham, MA: Massachusetts Medical Society.

Heinemann, M. (1992). Ophthalmic problems. *The Medical Clinics of North America, 76*(1), 83–97.

Hernandez, S.R. (1990). History and physical exam of HIV infected patients. In P.T. Cohen, M.A. Sande, P.A. Volberding (Eds.), *The AIDS knowledge base* (pp. 421.1–421.7). Waltham, MA: Medical Publishing Group.

Hibberd, P.L., Rubin, R.H. (1991). Fever in the immunocompromised host. In P.A. Mackowick (Ed.), *Fever: Basic mechanisms and management* (pp. 197–218). New York: Raven Press.

Hilton, G., Sisson, R., Freeman, E. (1990). The Neurobehavioral Rating Scale: An interrator reliability study in the HIV seropositive population. *Journal of Neuroscience Nursing, 22*(1), 36–42.

Hinkle, K. (1991). A literature review: HIV seropositivity in the elderly. *Journal of Gerontological Nursing, 7*(10), 12–17.

Hirsch, M.S., D'Aquila, R.T. (1993). Therapy for human immunodeficiency virus infection. *New England Journal of Medicine, 328*(23), 1686–1695.

Hogan, R. (1980). *Human sexuality: A nursing perspective.* New York: Appleton-Century-Crofts.

Hollander, H. (1997). Initiating routine care for the HIV-infected adult. In M.A. Sande, P.A. Volberding (Eds.), *The medical management of AIDS* (5th ed., pp. 107–112). Philadelphia: Saunders.

Holmstrup, P., Westergaard, J. (1994). Periodontal diseases in HIV-infected patients. *Journal of Clinical Periodontology, 21*(4), 270–280.

Holtzclaw, B.J. (1990a). Effects of extremity wraps to control drug induced shivering: A pilot study. *Nursing Research, 39*(5), 280–283.

Holtzclaw, B.J. (1990b). Control of febrile shivering during amphotericin B therapy. *Oncology Nursing Forum, 17*(4), 521–524.

Holtzclaw, B.J. (1992). The febrile response in critical care: State of the science. *Heart & Lung, 21*(5), 482–501.

Hriso, E., Kuhn, T., Masdey, J.C., et al. (1991). Extrapyramidal symptoms due to dopamine-blocking agents in patients with AIDS encephalopathy. *American Journal of Psychiatry, 148*(11), 1558–1561.

Huggins, M., Drascic, D. (1997). Palliative care and pain management. In M.M. Fanning (Ed.), *HIV infection: A clinical approach* (2nd ed., pp. 238–263). Philadelphia: Saunders.

Hyman, C., Kaufman, S. (1989). Nutritional impact of acquired immune deficiency syndrome: A unique counseling opportunity. *Journal of the American Dietetic Association, 89,* 520–527.

Ilsley, A.H., Rutten, A.J., Runciman, W.B. (1983). An evaluation of body temperature measurement. *Anesthesia Intensive Care, 11*(1), 31–39.

Jablonski, R.S. (1993). Nausea: The forgotten symptom. *Holistic Nursing Practice, 7*(2), 64–72.

Jackson, B. (1997). Assays for the detection of HIV resistance. *The Johns Hopkins AIDS Service Report, 9*(3). Available: http://www.hopkins-aids.edu.

Jacobson, J.M., Greenspan, J.S., Spritzler, J., et al. (1997). Thalidomide for the treatment of oral aphthous ulcers in patients with human immunodeficiency virus infection. National Institute of Allergy and Infectious Diseases AIDS Clinical Trials Group. *New England Journal of Medicine, 336*(21), 1468–1493.

Jensen, D.P., Herr, K.A. (1993). Sleeplessness. *Nursing Clinics of North America, 28*(2), 385–405.

Jewitt, J.F., Hecht, F.M. (1993). Preventive health care for adults with HIV infection. *Journal of the American Medical Association, 269*(9), 1144–1153.

Johnson, J. (1986). Sleep and bedtime routines in non-institutionalized aged women. *Journal of Community Health Nursing, 3*(3), 117–125.

Katsufrakis, P.J., Daar, E.S. (1997). HIV/AIDS assessment, testing, and natural history. *Primary Care Clinics in Office Practice, 24*(3), 479–496.

Kelly, P.J., Holman, S. (1993). The new face of AIDS. *American Journal of Nursing, 93*(3), 26–34.

Koehler, J.E. (1997). Bacillary angiomatosis and other unusual infections in HIV-infected individuals. In M.A. Sande, P.A. Volberding (Eds.), *The medical management of AIDS* (5th ed., pp. 239–246). Philadelphia: Saunders.

Kotler, D.P. (1992). Causes and consequences of malnutrition in HIV/AIDS. In G. Nary (Ed.), *Nutrition and HIV/AIDS* (Vol. 1, pp. 5–8). Chicago: PAAC Publishing.

Kotler, D.P., Tierney, A.R., Wang, J., et al. (1989). Magnitude of body-cell-mass depletion and timing of death from wasting in AIDS. *American Journal of Clinical Nutrition, 50*(3), 444–437.

Kovner, R., Lazar, J.W., Lesser, M., et al. (1992). Use of the Dementia Rating Scale as a test for neuropsychological dysfunction in HIV-positive i.v. drug users. *Journal of Substance Abuse Treatment, 9*(2), 133–137.

Lackritz, E.M., Satten, G.A., Aberle-Grasse, J., et al. (1995). Estimated risk of transmission of the human immunodeficiency virus by screened blood in the United States. *New England Journal of Medicine, 333*(26), 1721–1725.

Lee, K.A., Hicks, G., Nino-Murcia, C. (1991). Validity and reliability of a scale to assess fatigue. *Psychiatry Research, 36*(3), 291–298.

Liebman, M.C. (1992). Practice corner: Oral care. *Oncology Nursing Forum, 19*(6), 939–941.

Life Sciences Research Office, Federation of American Societies for Experimental Biology. (1990, November). *Nutrition and HIV Infection.* Washington, D.C.: Center for Food Safety and Applied Nutrition, Food and Drug Administration, Department of Health and Human Services.

Lincoln, R., Roberts, R. (1989). Continence issues in acute care. *Nursing Clinics of North America, 24*(3), 741–754.

Lipsky, J.J. (1996). Antiretroviral drugs for AIDS. *Lancet, 348,* 800–803.

Long, G.E., Rickman, L.S. (1994). Infectious complications of tattoos. *Clinical Infectious Diseases, 18*(4), 610–619.

Ly, L. (1991). Nutritional complications and incidence of malnutrition among AIDS patients. *Journal of the American Dietetic Association, 91,* 217–218.

Lyles, J.N., Burish, T.G., Krozely, M.G., et al. (1982). Efficacy of relaxation training and guided imagery in reducing the aversiveness of cancer chemotherapy. *Journal of Consulting and Clinical Psychology, 50*(4), 509–524.

Macallan, D.C., Noble, C., Baldwin, C., et al. (1995). Energy expenditure and wasting in human immunodeficiency virus infection. *New England Journal of Medicine, 333*(2), 123–124.

MacDonald, K.L., Jackson, J.B., Bowman, R.J., et al. (1989). Performance characteristics of serologic tests for human immunodeficiency virus type 1 (HIV-1) antibody testing among Minnesota blood donors: Public health and clinical implications. *Annals of Internal Medicine, 110*(8), 617–621.

Mackowiak, P.A., Wasserman, S.S., Levine, M.M. (1993). A critical appraisal of 98.6 degrees F, the upper limit of the normal body temperature, and other legacies of Carl Reinhold August Wunderlich. *Journal of the American Medical Association, 268*(12), 1578–1580.

MacVicar, A.G., Winningham, M.L. (1986). Promoting functional capacity of cancer patients. *Cancer Bulletin, 38,* 235–239.

Malone, J.L., Simms, T.E., Gray, G.C., et al. (1990). Sources of variability in repeated T-helper lymphocyte counts from human immunodeficiency virus type 1-infected patients: Total lymphocyte count of fluctuations and diurnal cycle are important. *Journal of Acquired Immune Deficiency Syndromes, 3*(2), 144–151.

Mann, J., Tarantola, D.J., Netter, T.W. (1992). *A global report: AIDS in the world.* Cambridge, MA: Harvard University Press.

Martin, J.P. (1994). Symptom management guidelines. In M.A. Sande, P.A. Volberding (Eds.), *The AIDS knowledge base* (2nd ed., pp. 4.8.1–4.8.9). Boston: Little Brown.

Mascolini, M. (1996). HIV dementia, neuropathy, & HIV: An interview with Justin C. McArthur, MB, B.S., MPH. *Journal of the International Association of Physicians in AIDS Care, 2*(6), 27–28, 31–34.

McArthur, J. (1990). AIDS dementia: Your assessment can make all the difference. *RN, 53*(3), 36–42.

McCarthy, P.L. (1991). Fever in infants and children. In P.A. Mackowiak (Ed.), *Fever: Basic mechanisms and management* (pp. 219–231). New York: Raven Press.

McCorkle, R., Young, K. (1978). Development of a symptom distress scale. *Cancer Nursing, 1*(5), 373–378.

McKinley, M.J., Goodman-Block, J., Lesser, M.L., Salbe, A.D. (1994). Improved body weight status as a result of nutrition intervention in adult HIV-positive outpatients. *Journal of the American Dietetic Association, 94,* 1014–1017.

Mellors, J.W., Rinaldo, C.R., Gupta, P., et al. (1996). Prognosis in HIV-1 infection predicted by the quantity of virus in plasma. *Science, 272*(5265), 1167–1170.

Melzack, R. (1987). The short form McGill Pain Questionnaire. *Pain, 30*(2), 191–197.

Morgan, S.P. (1990). A comparison of three methods of managing fever in the neurologic patient. *Journal of Neuroscience Nursing, 22*(1), 19–24.

Morrow, G.R. (1984). Methodology in behavioral and psychosocial cancer research. The assessment of nausea and vomiting. Past problems, current issues and suggestions for future research. *Cancer, 53*(Suppl. 10), 2267–2280.

Murphy, R., Chmiel, J. (1992). Prognostic value of the CD4 count and other surrogate markers. *HIV: Advances in Research and Therapy, 2*(2), 25–29.

Muwaswes, M. (1993). Alterations in consciousness. In V. Carrieri-Kohlman, A.M. Lindsey, C.M. West (Eds.), *Pathophysiological phenomena in nursing human responses to illness* (2nd ed., pp. 195–220). Philadelphia: Saunders.

National Institute of Allergy and Infectious Diseases. (1997, November 13). HIV persists and can replicate despite prolonged combination therapy. *NIAID News.*

National Institutes of Health. (1990). Oral complications of cancer therapies: Diagnosis, prevention and treatment. *Clinical Courier, 8*(3), 1–8.

Newman, C.F. (1992). The role of nutritional assessments and nutritional plans in the management of HIV/AIDS. In G. Nary (Ed.), *Nutrition & HIV/AIDS* (Vol. 1, pp. 57–106). Chicago: PAAC Publishing.

Newman, J. (1985). Evaluation of sponging to reduce body temperature in febrile children. *Canadian Medical Association Journal, 132*(6), 641–642.

NIH Technology Assessment Panel on Integration of Behavioral and Relaxation Approaches into the Treatment of Chronic Pain. (1996). Integration of behavioral and relaxation approaches into the treatment of chronic pain. *Journal of the American Medical Association, 276*(4), 313–318.

Nokes, K.M. (1996). Health care needs. In K.M. Nokes (Ed.), *HIV/AIDS and the older adult* (pp. 9–23). Bristol, PA: Taylor & Francis.

O'Brien, M.E., Pheifer, W.G. (1993). Physical and psychological nursing care for patients with HIV infection. *Nursing Clinics of North America, 28*(2), 303–316.

O'Brien, W.A., Ovcak, S., Kalhor, H., et al. (1993). HIV-1 replication can be increased in blood from seropositive patients following influenza immunization. *International Conference on AIDS* (abstract PO-A12-0209), *9*(1), 169.

Onorato, I.M., Markowitz, L.E., Oxtoby, M.J. (1988). Childhood immunization, vaccine-preventable diseases and infection with human immunodeficiency virus. *Pediatric Infectious Disease, 7*(8), 588–595.

Palmes, E.D., Park, C.R. (1965). The regulation of body temperature during fever. *Archives of Environmental Health, 11*(6), 749–759.

Panel for the Prediction and Prevention of Ulcers in Adults. (1992). *Pressure ulcers in adults: Prediction and prevention. Clinical practice guideline, Number 3* (AHCPR Pub. No. 92-0047). Rockville, MD: Agency for Health Care Policy and Research, Public Health Service, U.S. Department of Health and Human Services.

Pape, J.W., Johnson, W.D. (1989). HIV-1 infection and AIDS in Haiti. In R.A. Kaslow, D.P. Francis (Eds.), *The epidemiology of AIDS* (pp. 194–221). New York: Oxford University Press.

Pardue, N.H. (1984). Energy expenditure and subjective fatigue of chronic obstructive pulmonary disease patients before and after a pulmonary rehabilitation. Doctoral dissertation, Catholic University, Washington, DC.

Parkerson, G.R., Broadhead, W.E., Tse C-K.J. (1990). The Duke health profile: A 17 item measure of health and dysfunction. *Medical Care, 28*(11), 1056–1069.

Parkerson, G.R., Gehlbach, S.H., Wagner, E.H., et al. (1981). The Duke-UNC health profile: An adult health status instrument for primary care. *Medical Care, 19*(8), 806–823.

Pearson, M.L., Jereb, J.A., Frieden, T.R., et al. (1992). Nosocomial transmission of multidrug-resistant *Mycobacterium tuberculosis:* A risk to patients and health care workers. *Annals of Internal Medicine, 117*(30), 191–196.

Pearson, R.G., Byars, G.E., Jr. (1956). *The development and validation of a checklist for measuring subjective fatigue* (Report No. 56-115). Randolph AFB, TX: USAF School of Aviation Medicine.

Perry, S., Jacobsberg, L., Fogel, K. (1989). Orogenital transmission of human immunodeficiency virus (HIV) [Letter]. *Annals of Internal Medicine, 111*(11), 951–952.

Piper, B. (1993). Fatigue. In V. Carrieri-Kohlman, A.M. Lindsey, C.M. West (Eds.), *Pathophysiological phenomena in nursing human responses to illness* (2nd ed., pp. 279–302). Philadelphia: Saunders.

Piper, B.F., Rieger, P.T., Brophy, L., et al. (1989). Recent advances in the management of biotherapy-related side effects: Fatigue. *Oncology Nursing Forum, 16*(Suppl. 6), 27–34.

Plasse, T.F., Gorter, R.W., Krasnow, S.H., et al. (1991). Recent clinical experience with dronabinol. *Pharmacology, Biochemistry and Behavior, 40*(3), 695–700.

Plona, R.P., Schremp, P.S. (1992). Nursing care of patients with ocular manifestations of human immunodeficiency virus infection. *Nursing Clinics of North America, 27*(3), 793–805.

Porter, S., Sande, M.A. (1992). Toxoplasmosis of the central nervous system in the acquired immunodeficiency syndrome. *New England Journal of Medicine, 327*(23), 1643–1648.

Power, C., Selnes, O.A., Grim, J.A., McArthur, J.C. (1995). HIV dementia scale: A rapid screening test. *Journal of Acquired Immune Deficiency Syndromes and Human Retrovirology, 8*(3), 273–278.

Price, W.P. (1997). Management of the neurologic complications of HIV-1 infection and AIDS. In M.A. Sande, P.A. Volberding (Eds.), *The medical management of AIDS* (5th ed., pp. 197–216). Philadelphia: Saunders.

Pulling, C.A. (1991). The relationship between critical care nurses' knowledge about sleep, and the initiation of sleep promoting nursing interventions. *Axone, 13*(2), 57–62.

Rasin, J.H. (1990). Confusion. *Nursing Clinics of North America, 25*(4), 909–918.

Redd, W.H. (1984). Control of nausea and vomiting and vomiting in chemotherapy patients: Four effective behavior methods. *Postgraduate Medicine, 75*(5), 105–107.

Reimer, M. (1987). Sleep pattern disturbance: Nursing interventions perceived by patients and their nurses as facilitating nocturnal sleep in hospital. *Classification of Nursing Diagnoses: Proceedings of the seventh conference, North American Nursing Diagnosis Association* (pp. 372–376). St. Louis: North American Nursing Diagnosis Association.

Reiter, G.S., Kudler, N.R. (1996). Palliative care and HIV. Part II: Systemic manifestations and late-stage issues. *AIDS Clinical Care, 8*(4), 27–36.

Renfroe, K.L. (1988). Effect of progressive relaxation on dyspnea and state anxiety in patients with chronic obstructive pulmonary disease. *Heart & Lung, 17*(4), 408–413.

Rhodes, V.A. (1990). Nausea, vomiting and retching. *Nursing Clinics of North America, 25*(4), 885–900.

Rhodes, V.A., Watson, P.M., Johnson, M.H. (1986). Association of chemotherapy related nausea and vomiting with pretreatment and posttreatment anxiety. *Oncology Nursing Forum, 13*(4), 41–47.

Rhodes, V.A., Watson, P.M. (1987). Symptom distress—the concept: Past and present. *Seminars in Oncology Nursing, 3*(4), 242–247.

Rich, J.D., Buck, A., Tuomala, R.E., Kazanjian, P.H. (1993). Transmission of human immunodeficiency virus infection presumed to have occurred via female homosexual contact. *Clinical Infectious Diseases, 17*(6), 1003–1005.

Roberts, M.F. (1993). Diarrhea: A symptom. *Holistic Nurse Practice, 7*(2), 73–80.

Rodriques, L., Moreno, C.G. (1991). HIV transmission to women in stable relationships [Letter]. *New England Journal of Medicine, 325*(13), 966.

Rosenberg, E., Cotton, D. (1997). Primary HIV infection and the acute retroviral syndrome: The urgent need for recognition. *AIDS Clinical Care, 9*(3), 19, 23–25.

Rowbottom, J. (1993). STDs and the overseas traveler. *Australian Family Physician, 22*(2), 125–131.

Sattler, F.R., Ko, R., Antoniskis, D., et al. (1991). Acetaminophen does not impair clearance of zidovudine. *Annals of Internal Medicine, 114*(11), 937–940.

Sax, P. (1996). Viral load testing. *AIDS Clinical Care, 8*(4), 31–32.

Schuchat, A., Broome, C.V., Hightower, A., et al. (1991). Use of surveillance for invasive pneumococcal disease to estimate the size of the immunosuppressed HIV-infected population. *Journal of the American Medical Association, 265*(24), 3275–3279.

Schwartzstein, R.M., Lahive, K., Pope, A., et al. (1987). Cold facial stimulation reduces breathlessness induced in normal subjects. *American Review of Respiratory Disease, 136*(1), 58–61.

Sharp, J.T., Drutz, W.S., Moisan, T., et al. (1980). Postural relief of dyspnea in severe chronic obstructive pulmonary disease. *American Review of Respiratory Disease, 122*(2), 201–211.

Shriner, K., Goetz, M.B. (1992). Severe hepatotoxicity in a patient receiving both acetaminophen and zidovudine. *American Journal of Medicine, 93*(1), 94–96.

Skaare, A.B., Herlofson, B.B., Barkvoll, P. (1996). Mouth rinses containing triclosan reduce the incidence of recurrent aphthous ulcers (RAU). *Journal of Clinical Periodontology, 23*(8), 778–781.

Skurnick, J.H., Bogden, J.D., Baker, H., et al. (1996). Micronutrient profiles in HIV-1-infected heterosexual adults. *Journal of Acquired Immunodeficiency Syndromes and Human Retrovirology, 12*, 75–83.

Smeltzer, S.C., Whipple, B. (1991). Women and HIV infection. *Image, 23*(4), 249–256.

Sno, H.N., Storosum, J.G., Wortel, C.H. (1991). Psychogenic "HIV infection." *International Journal of Psychiatry in Medicine, 21*(1), 93–98.

Sprauer, M.A., Markowitz, L.E., Nicholson, J.K., et al. (1993). Response of human immunodeficiency virus-infected adults to measles-rubella vaccination. *Journal of Acquired Immune Deficiency Syndromes, 6*(9), 1013–1016.

Steffe, E.M., King, J.H., Inciardi, J.F., et al., (1990). The effect of acetaminophen on zidovudine metabolism in HIV-infected patients. *Journal of Acquired Immune Deficiency Syndromes, 3*(7), 691–694.

Steinhart, R., Reingold, A.L., Taylor, F., et al. (1992). Invasive *Haemophilus influenzae* infections in men with HIV infection. *Journal of the American Medical Association, 268*(23), 3350–3352.

Sultzer, D.L., Levin, H.S., Mahler, M.E., et al. (1992). Assessment of cognitive, psychiatric, and behavioral disturbances in patients with dementia: The Neurobehavioral Rating Scale. *Journal of the American Geriatric Society, 40*(6), 549–555.

Swensen, J.R., Erman, M., Labelle, J., et al. (1989). Extrapyramidal reactions: Neuropsychiatric mimics in patients with AIDS. *General Hospital Psychiatry, 11*(4), 248–253.

Task Force on Nutrition Support in AIDS. (1989). Guidelines for nutrition support in AIDS. *Nutrition, 5*(1), 39–45.

Teich, S.A., Saltzman, B.R. (1996). Evaluation of a new self-screening chart for cytomegalovirus retinitis in patients with AIDS. *Journal of Acquired Immune Deficiency Syndromes and Human Retrovirology, 13*(4), 336–342.

Temple, M.T., Leigh, B.C., Schafer, J. (1993). Unsafe sexual behavior and alcohol use at the event level: Results of a national survey. *Journal of Acquired Immunodeficiency Syndromes, 6*(4), 393–401.

Thayer, R.E. (1987). Energy, tiredness and tension effects of a sugar snack versus moderate exercise. *Journal of Personality and Social Psychology, 52*(1), 119–125.

Tichy, A.M., Talashek, M.L. (1992). Older women: Sexually transmitted diseases and acquired immunodeficiency syndrome. *Nursing Clinics of North America, 27*(4), 937–949.

Timbo, B.B., Tollefson, L. (1994). Nutrition: A cofactor in HIV disease. *Journal of the American Dietetic Association, 94*, 1019–1022.

Tindall, B., Cooper, D.A. (1991). Primary infection: Host responses and intervention strategies. *AIDS, 5*(1), 1–14.

Ungvarski, P.J. (1989). AIDS dementia complex: Considerations for nursing. *Journal of the Association of Nurses in AIDS Care, 1*(1), 10–12.

Ungvarski, P.J. (1996). Waging war on HIV wasting. *RN, 59*(2), 26–32.

Ungvarski, P.J., Rottner, J.E. (1997). Errors in prescribing HIV-1 protease inhibitors. *Journal of the Association of Nurses in AIDS Care, 8*(4), 55–61.

U.S. Department of Health and Human Services, Public Health Service, Health Resources Administration. (1996). *Health care and HIV. Nutrition Guide for Providers and Clients.* Rockville, MD: Author.

U.S. Department of Health and Human Services, Public Health Service. (1997). *Guidelines for the use of antiretroviral agents in HIV-infected adults and adolescents.* Rockville, MD: Author.

U.S. Preventive Services Task Force. (1989a). Screening for chlamydia infectious. In M. Fisher (Ed.), *Guide to clinical prevention services: An assessment of the effectiveness of 169 interventions* (pp. 147–150). Baltimore: Williams & Wilkins.

U.S. Preventive Services Task Force. (1989b). Screening for gonorrhea. In M. Fisher (Ed.), *Guide to clinical prevention services: An assessment of the effectiveness of 169 interventions* (pp. 135–138). Baltimore: Williams & Wilkins.

van Gorp, W.G., Mandelkern, M.A., Gee, M., et al. (1992). Cerebral metabolic dysfunction in AIDS: Findings in a sample with and without dementia. *Journal of Neuropsychiatry and Clinical Neuroscience, 4*(3), 280–287.

van Servellen, G.M., Lewis, C.E., Leake, B. (1988). Nurses' responses to the AIDS crisis: Implications for continuing education programs. *The Journal of Continuing Education in Nursing, 19*(1), 4–8.

Vento, S., DiPerri, G., Garofano, T., et al. (1993). *Pneumocystis carinii* pneumonia during primary HIV-1 infection. *Lancet, 342*(8862), 24–25.

von Roenn, J.H. (1994). Management of HIV-related bodyweight loss. *Drugs, 47*(5), 774–783.

Wallace, J.I., Paauw, D.S., Spack, D.H. (1993). HIV infection in older patients: When to suspect the unexpected. *Geriatrics, 48*(6), 69–70.

Weiler, P.G., Mungas, D., Pomerantz, S. (1988). AIDS: A cause of dementia in the elderly. *Journal of the American Geriatric Society, 36*(2), 139–141.

Weiner, A., Wallace, J.I., Steinberg, A., et al. (1992). Intravenous drug use, inconsistent condom use, and fellatio in relationship to crack smoking are risk behaviors for acquiring AIDS in streetwalkers. *International Conference on AIDS* (abstract PoC 4560), *8*(2), C338.

Weinrich, M.D., Curtis, J.R., Carline, J.D., et al. (1997). HIV risk screening in the primary care setting: Assessment of physician's skills. *Journal of General Internal Medicine, 12*(2), 107–113.

Weisman, A.D. (1979). A model for psychological phasing in cancer. *General Hospital Psychiatry, 1*(1), 187–195.

Wheat, L.J., Connolly-Stringfield, P., Williams, B., et al. (1992). Diagnosis of histoplasmosis in patients with the acquired immunodeficiency syndrome by detection of *Histoplasma capsulatum* polysaccharide antigen in bronchoalveolar lavage fluid. *American Review of Respiratory Disease, 145*(6), 1421–1424.

World Health Organization. (1986). *Cancer pain relief.* Geneva: World Health Organization.

Yerly, S., Wyler, C.A., Kaiser, L., et al. (1993). Antigenic stimulation by immunization does not increase HIV viral load. *International Conference on AIDS* (abstract PO-B22-1929), *9*(1), 457.

Zeller, J.M., Swanson, B., Cohen, F.L. (1993). Suggestions for clinical nursing research: Symptom management in AIDS patients. *Journal of the Association of Nurses in AIDS Care, 4*(3), 13–17.

6

Adolescents and Adults

CARE MANAGEMENT OF AIDS-INDICATOR DISEASES

Jo Anne Staats ■ Michael Sheran ■ Roger Herr

In the early years of the AIDS epidemic, the disease was considered essentially fatal and emphasis was placed on compassionate, low-technology care aimed at improving the quality rather than the length of life (Cotton, 1989). What many hoped would be a limited endemic among homosexual men in large urban centers in the United States has rapidly evolved into a major pandemic resulting in widespread human suffering with devastating socioeconomic consequences (Lange & Tapper, 1993).

Over the past few years the incidence of AIDS-related opportunistic infections (OIs) has been stabilized, delaying the diagnosis of AIDS in many HIV-infected persons (CDC, 1997a). This decline in disease progression has been attributed to improved medical care, the use of antiretroviral combination therapy, and an increasing use of prophylactic drugs to prevent AIDS-related OIs (Hogg et al., 1998; Palella et al., 1998).

To understand the clinical aspects of the development of OIs associated with AIDS, the reader should be aware of some generalizations that can be made about their presence in an HIV-infected person (Glatt et al., 1988; National Institute of Allergy and Infectious Diseases, 1990). OIs are caused by a wide spectrum of diverse pathogens, many of which are ubiquitous in nature and rarely cause disease in healthy hosts (persons with an intact immune system). In many cases, these infections represent a secondary occurrence of a previous primary infection or, in other words, a reactivation of a previously acquired pathogen. The OIs associated with AIDS are rarely curable

and, at best, can be controlled during an acute episode; long-term suppressive therapy is required to prevent recurrence. Complicating the issue of long-term therapy is the resistance to standard therapies that some opportunistic pathogens develop.

A single OI is rare in persons with AIDS; concurrent or consecutive infections with different organisms are common. Infections associated with HIV, because of the coexisting immunodeficiency, are often severe and difficult to treat and require extended initial treatment regimens. Furthermore, many infections become disseminated, with a high density of organisms in the affected tissues. By understanding the epidemiologic characteristics of certain pathogens, the clinician can provide clients with information on preventing some of these infections. Progress in research on AIDS-related OIs has led to the development of prophylactic measures to prevent some infections.

The information that follows focuses on the most frequently diagnosed AIDS-indicator diseases and their clinical manifestations. Appendix II contains a list of drugs frequently prescribed for AIDS-related conditions and their common side effects.

CANDIDIASIS

EPIDEMIOLOGY. *Candida* organisms are yeasts (that is, fungi) that exist predominantly in unicellular forms. Although there are more than 150 species of *Candida*, *Candida albicans* is the most common. *Candida tropicalis, Candida krusei,*

Candida glabrata (formerly *Torulopsis glabrata*), and a newly discovered strain, *Candida dubliniensis,* are other non–*Candida albicans* strains that cause disease in persons infected with HIV (Coleman et al., 1997; Greenspan & Greenspan, 1996; McCreary et al., 1996; Reef & Mayer, 1995; Sullivan et al., 1995, 1996). *C. albicans* is ubiquitous. It has been found in soil, food, inanimate objects, and hospital environments. *Candida* is a commensal organism that can be found on teeth, gingiva, and skin and in the oropharynx, vagina, and large intestine.

The majority of infections caused by *Candida* are endogenous and are related to interruption of normal defense mechanisms. Immunosuppression secondary to HIV infection and in persons receiving chemotherapy is a major cause of candidal infections. In addition, broad-spectrum antibiotics, invasive surgical procedures, and indwelling central venous catheters leave patients susceptible to infection by *Candida* (Coleman et al., 1997).

Human-to-human transmission is possible. Examples include congenital transmission in infants, in whom thrush develops after vaginal delivery; development of balanitis in uncircumcised men who do not wear condoms during intercourse with women who have candidal vaginitis; and nosocomial spread in hospital settings (Edwards, 1995). Infections caused by *Candida* species are estimated to occur at some time in the course of HIV disease in 90% to 95% of patients with HIV infection (Coleman et al., 1997; HIV Hotline, 1997). Oropharyngeal candidiasis is frequently the initial indicator of HIV infection and has been noted to occur in some patients at the time of seroconversion to HIV (Rolston, 1993).

PATHOGENESIS. The likelihood of mucosal *Candida* infection increases with progressive cellular immunodeficiency associated with HIV disease and is often associated with a decreased number of circulating CD4+ lymphocytes (Greenspan & Greenspan, 1996; Maiello et al., 1996; Reef & Mayer, 1995). Most clinicians now believe that oral candidiasis is an accurate predictor of disease progression and of the development of other AIDS-related infections (CDC, 1992a). The frequent use of broad-spectrum antibiotics to treat infections associated with HIV disease suppresses normal bacterial flora and allows *Candida* to pro-

liferate, especially in the gastrointestinal tract (Edwards, 1995). Skin alterations caused by poor nutrition, dehydration, poor hygiene, or indwelling catheters can also provide a portal of entry for Candida.

Most *Candida* infections in persons with HIV are mucocutaneous, whereas other fungal infections are disseminated. Candidemia, or disseminated infection, is seen in persons with HIV infection who have neutropenia because of antineoplastic or antiviral therapy, as well as in those with central venous access lines (Rolston, 1993).

CLINICAL PRESENTATION. Oral candidiasis has several clinical presentations. Pseudomembranous candidiasis is characterized by creamy or white plaques that can appear anywhere on the oral or pharyngeal mucosa. The patches can be wiped off, leaving an erythematous or even bleeding mucosal surface that may be painful. Erythematous candidiasis, the most frequent, is less obvious, with smooth depapillated areas on the palate and on the dorsal surface of the tongue (Coleman et al., 1997; Greenspan & Greenspan, 1996). Angular cheilitis presents with erythema, cracks, fissures, and maceration that may be bilateral at the corners of the mouth (Coleman et al., 1997).

Another oral form of candidiasis is hyperplastic candidiasis, which appears as white lesions on the buccal mucosa, tongue, or hard palate and cannot be wiped off (Greenspan & Greenspan, 1996). This can be confused with hairy leukoplakia. Oral candidiasis can be superimposed on other oral lesions, such as herpes simplex, and can cause secondary infections. Pindborg (1994) considers the term *thrush* to be unscientific and suggests that clinicians use the term *pseudomembranous candidiasis* to describe oral candidiasis seen in HIV-infected persons. Pindborg (1994) also divides the condition into the erythematous stage (often seen in symptom-free patients), pseudomembranous (seen in patients with AIDS), chronic (which is rare and seen on the margins of the tongue), and angular cheilitis.

Complaints of dysphagia in persons with HIV disease are most commonly associated with candidal esophagitis, the most common cause of esophageal disease in persons with AIDS (Coleman et al., 1997; Wilcox & Schwartz, 1996). Oropharyngeal and esophageal candidiasis are not necessarily present concurrently; therefore the absence of oral candidiasis does not preclude the possibility that an HIV-infected person may have candidal esophagitis (Greenspan & Greenspan, 1996). Cello (1992) defined the dysphagia associated with candidal esophagitis as difficulty in swallowing with a sensation of food sticking in the throat. Although pain on swallowing (odynophagia) and episodic retrosternal pain without swallowing may be present with the complaint of dysphagia, they are more commonly associated with ulcerations of the esophagus caused by herpesvirus or cytomegalovirus (Cello, 1992; Wilcox & Schwartz, 1996).

Intertrigo can occur at any site where the proximity of skin surfaces provides a warm, moist environment. This cutaneous form of candidiasis can involve the groin, axillary vault, or areas surrounding the breasts and appears as a vivid red, slightly eroded eruption with a wrinkled surface coated with a white membrane (Edwards, 1995). Clients with cutaneous candidiasis usually complain of burning and itching.

Candidal infection of the nails is usually manifested as paronychia (inflammation of the tissues surrounding the nails) but can also involve the nail itself (Edwards, 1995). In addition to the inflamed appearance, the patient complains of tenderness in the area. Frequent exposure to water is a significant predisposing factor in candidal nail infection.

Vulvovaginal candidiasis is characterized by intense pruritus of the vulva and a white, curdlike vaginal discharge. This infection usually results in erythema of the vagina and labia, which may extend into the perineum. In the early years of the HIV epidemic, small studies reported that vaginal candidiasis was more frequently seen in women with HIV infection. More recent studies have demonstrated that the incidence of vaginal candidiasis in women with HIV infection has not increased (Coleman et al., 1997; Giraldo et al., 1996; Sobel et al., 1996). White (1996) defines recurrent vaginal candidiasis as at least four microbiologically proven symptomatic episodes of acute vaginal candidiasis within a 12-month period.

Although rare, disseminated candidiasis almost always occurs late in the course of AIDS. Other sites of *Candida* infection in HIV disease that have been reported include the trachea, bronchi, lungs, heart, central nervous system (CNS), eyes, joints, and testes (Daar & Meyer, 1992).

DIAGNOSIS. Diagnosis of oropharyngeal candidiasis is usually based on clinical presentation and a positive response to treatment. Definitive diagnosis of esophageal candidiasis is made by endoscopic gross inspection or at autopsy or by microscopic examination of a specimen of affected tissues. Diagnosis based on culture is unreliable because cultures may remain positive despite clinical improvement (HIV Hotline, 1997). With culture, however, it is possible to identify the strain of *Candida* and its susceptibility to various antifungal agents, which may be of benefit in patients who are not responding to treatment. Isolation of *Candida* from blood may also be questionable in a patient with an indwelling intravenous catheter, since transient candidiasis is possible and often clears without treatment once the device is removed (Chernoff & Sande, 1990).

TREATMENT. Mucocutaneous candidiasis is treated locally or systemically with clotrimazole troches, nystatin suspension, nystatin pastilles, ketoconazole, fluconazole, miconazole, and in some cases itraconazole or amphotericin B. Both fluconazole and itraconazole have been found to be effective in the treatment of *Candida* infection, and some studies have shown fluconazole to be more effective than ketoconazole (Barbaro et al., 1996; Cartledge et al., 1997; Darouiche et al., 1996; De Wit et al., 1989; Laine et al., 1992; Moskovitz et al., 1996). Generally, for oropharyngeal candidiasis, clotrimazole, fluconazole, or nystatin is used initially; if there is no response, alternative therapy may include itraconazole or amphotericin B (oral suspension or parenteral therapy). Itraconazole is the preferred therapy for fluconazole-resistant candidiasis (Cartledge et al., 1997). For candidal vaginitis, topical treatment with miconazole or clotrimazole or systemic therapy with fluconazole or ketoconazole is usually effective.

Fluconazole is usually effective in treating esophageal candidiasis. Alternatives for refractory cases include ketoconazole, itraconazole, or amphotericin B. Candidal esophagitis is usually associated with dysphagia and, in some cases, odynophagia, both of which lead to decreased food and fluid intake. For severe weight loss associated with these symptoms, it is advisable to request a speech-language-pathology consult to teach the patient how to swallow with these symptoms and how to make the necessary dietary modifications to maintain adequate nutrition (Rogers, 1992).

The development of azole-resistant candidiasis has become a significant problem in HIV disease. Some risk factors that may lead to resistance include a low CD4+ cell count, prolonged exposure to the azoles, nontherapeutic doses of medication, poor patient compliance, and drug interactions (Fichtenbaum et al., 1997; HIV Hotline, 1997; Maenza et al., 1996). Heald and associates (1996) found that continuous fluconazole therapy, which created sterile cultures, led to less resistance than intermittent fluconazole therapy. It has also been shown that use of fluconazole is associated with a higher incidence of *Candida* non-albicans colonization (Heald et al., 1996; Palmieri et al., 1996). When the azoles fail to control candidiasis, amphotericin B (either oral or intravenous) may be the drug of last resort. However, there have been cases of candidiasis that did not respond to amphotericin therapy, leaving the patient and the provider with symptom management only (Kelly et al., 1996). There are reports of resolution of resistant candidiasis with the initiation of antiretroviral therapy (didanosine plus saquinavir) and subsequent improvement of immune status (Zingman, 1996).

Cutaneous candidiasis may respond to topically applied clotrimazole, miconazole, or ketoconazole or to systemically administered ketoconazole or fluconazole. Topically applied imidazole may be used to treat candidiasis of the nails, and

Table 6–1 ■ Secondary Prophylaxis of AIDS-defining Opportunistic Disease (after Chemotherapy for Acute Disease) in HIV-infected Adults and Adolescents

Pathogen	Indication	First choice	Alternatives
RECOMMENDED FOR LIFE AS A STANDARD OF CARE			
Cytomegalovirus	Prior end-organ disease	Ganciclovir, *or* Foscarnet, *or* cidofovir, *or* for retinitis, ganciclovir sustained-release implant every 6–9 months	None
Coccidioides immitis	Documented disease	Fluconazole	Amphotericin B, *or* itraconazole
Cryptococcus neoformans	Documented disease	Fluconazole	Amphotericin B, *or* itraconazole
Histoplasma capsulatum	Documented disease	Itraconazole	Amphotericin B, *or* fluconazole
Mycobacterium avium complex	Documented disseminated disease	Clarithromycin *plus* one or more of the following: ethambutol, rifabutin	Azithromycin, *plus* one or more of the following: ethambutol, rifabutin
Pneumocystis carinii	Prior episode of *P. carinii* pneumonia	TMP-SMZ	TMP-SMZ, *or* dapsone *plus* pyrimethamine *plus* leucovorin, *or* dapsone, *or* aerosolized pentamidine
Salmonella species (nontyphi)	Bacteremia	Ciprofloxacin	None
Toxoplasma gondii	Prior episode of *Toxoplasma* encephalitis	Sulfadiazine *plus* pyrimethamine *plus* leucovorin	Clindamycin *plus* pyrimethamine *plus* leucovorin
RECOMMENDED ONLY IF SUBSEQUENT EPISODES ARE FREQUENT OR SEVERE			
Herpes simplex virus	Frequent or severe recurrences	Acyclovir	None
Candida (vaginal or esophageal)	Frequent or severe recurrences	Fluconazole	Ketoconazole, *or* itraconazole

Note: For information on primary prophylaxis see Chapter 5.
From Centers for Disease Control and Prevention. (1997). 1997 USPHS/IDSA guidelines for the prevention of opportunistic infections in persons infected with human immunodeficiency virus. *Morbidity and Mortality Weekly Report, 46*(RR-12), 1–46.

itraconazole may also be effective for this condition (Torres, 1993).

The first-line treatment for vaginal candidiasis should be a topical cream or suppository. The older imidazoles (e.g., clotrimazole) may be less effective against non-albicans species of *Candida* than the newer triazole agent (terconazole) (Tobin, 1995). Systemic therapy should be reserved for vaginal candidiasis that does not respond to topical agents.

PREVENTION. Since acute treatment for *Candida* infection is effective, since mucosal candidiasis has a low mortality rate, and since there is the potential for the development of resistant *Candida,* primary prophylaxis is not recommended (CDC, 1997c). However, Schuman and associates (1996) demonstrated the effectiveness of weekly fluconazole in the prevention of vaginal candidiasis in women with a CD4+ cell count of less than 300/mm^3 without the development of resistance. Health care workers should routinely take precautions to prevent nosocomial infection by using gloves for care, meticulous hand-washing techniques, and extreme care when handling and manipulating intravenous therapy equipment. In addition, since *Candida* flourishes under moist dressings, the risks and benefits of using occlusive dressings should always be evaluated when such dressings may be indicated. Measures to minimize the potential for and the severity of candidiasis are contained in Appendix I (see Mouth Care and Skin Care). Secondary prophylaxis is indicated for vaginal or esophageal candidiasis if subsequent episodes are frequent or severe (see Table 6–1).

Hilton and associates (1992), in a study of women with recurrent candidal vaginitis (who were not infected with HIV), found that daily ingestion of 8 ounces of yogurt containing *Lactobacillus acidophilus* decreased both the colonization and the infection. Anecdotal reports from clinicians caring for patients with HIV/AIDS have noted an overall decrease in *Candida* infections when *L. acidophilus* in yogurt or capsule form is consumed daily.

CERVICAL CANCER (INVASIVE)

EPIDEMIOLOGY. Although 1.3% of women with AIDS reported to the Centers for Disease Control

and Prevention (CDC) in 1993 had an initial AIDS diagnosis of invasive cervical cancer, other studies offer conflicting data regarding the true incidence of invasive cervical cancer (Chaisson et al., 1996; Gates et al., 1997; Klevens et al., 1996; Weber & Sidhu, 1997).

Cervical intraepithelial neoplasia (CIN), also referred to as cervical dysplasia, consists of precursor lesions to carcinoma of the cervix. The progression of CIN to invasive cancer in immunocompetent women usually is a slow process, taking several years. On average, CIN occurs in women between the ages of 45 and 50 years. When CIN is detected by Papanicolaou (Pap) smear in the early stages, treatment outcomes usually are favorable (Peel, 1995; Richart & Wright, 1993). However, the occurrence of CIN in HIV-infected women has been noted to be (1) more rapidly progressive, (2) more advanced, (3) more likely to occur between the ages of 16 and 48 years, (4) less responsive to standard treatments, and (5) given a poorer prognosis than in uninfected women (Maimon et al., 1990, 1993; Schwartz et al., 1991).

Multifactorial risk factors for CIN and cervical cancer include the following (CDC, 1990; Feingold et al., 1990; Franco, 1991; Peel, 1995; Reeves et al., 1989; Richart & Wright, 1993; Rubin & Lauver, 1990):

1. Early age at first intercourse
2. Multiple sex partners
3. Sex with men with multiple sex partners
4. Cigarette smoking
5. Dietary deficiencies
6. Use of oral contraceptives
7. Immunosuppression
8. Low socioeconomic status
9. Lack of access to health care
10. Exposure to diethylstilbestrol in utero
11. A history of sexually transmitted diseases, especially infection with human papillomavirus (HPV)

There appears to be a higher incidence of AIDS-defining cervical cancer in women who are injecting drug users, black, live in the south, average 33 years of age, and have a higher mean CD4+ cell count than in women with other AIDS-defining illnesses (Klevens et al., 1996). There is a strong correlation between HPV, HIV, and cervical dysplasia. According to Borysiewicz and colleagues (1997), HPV is detected in more than 95% of all cervical cancers. There also appears to be an increase in oncogenic HPV types, as well as an increased prevalence and severity of cervical dysplasia as immunosuppression becomes more severe, e.g., CD4+ cell count of less than 500/mm^3 (Abdieb et al., 1997; Cheung et al., 1996; Fruchter et al., 1997; Shah et al., 1996; Six, 1996; Watts et al., 1996).

Cervical cancer is considered a preventable cancer when adequate screening is provided and cervical dysplasia is treated, halting neoplastic progression. It is recommended that women with HIV infection have a Pap smear twice in the first year after diagnosis. If both of these are negative, then yearly Pap smears are recommended. If, however, a woman has a history of abnormal Pap smears or has an abnormal Pap smear after HIV diagnosis, she should be referred for a colposcopic examination with appropriate treatment and follow-up (CDC, 1997d; Denenberg, 1997). According to Denenberg (1997), there is controversy regarding the follow-up for atypical cells of undetermined significance (ACUS). CDC (1997d) recommends that Pap findings of ACUS, without a qualifying statement indicating suspicion of a neoplastic process, can be followed up with a Pap smear without a colposcopic examination. However, most practitioners refer any HIV-infected woman with a Pap smear finding of ACUS for a colposcopic examination (Denenberg, 1997).

Klevens and associates (1996) found an underdiagnosis of cervical cancer among women who are infected with HIV. The reasons vary but include limited access to health care (particularly for women of color), fragmentation of health care services, and the tendency to overlook routine gynecologic care and screening when faced with more immediate life-threatening opportunistic illnesses (Fruchter et al., 1996; Klevens et al., 1996; Lai, 1996; Larsen, 1996). Given the prevalence of undiagnosed HIV infection in women, HIV counseling and testing should be offered to all women in whom CIN has been diagnosed.

PATHOGENESIS. The early stages of cervical disease involve microinvasion of the lesions into the basement membrane. In early stromal invasion, small fingerlike processes extend into the stroma and, if they are left undetected, measurable lesions that increase in size develop and extend into the endometrium and to adjacent areas (Peel, 1995).

Richart and Wright (1993) described CIN and carcinoma of the cervix as a continuum, progressing from mild dysplasia (grade I), to moderate dysplasia (grade II), to severe dysplasia and carcinoma in situ (grade III). The frequency and severity of cervical dysplasia have been correlated with the degree of immunosuppression as measured by CD4+ cell counts, as well as with coinfection with HPV (Cheung et al., 1996; Fruchter et al., 1997; Shah et al., 1996; Six, 1996).

CLINICAL PRESENTATION. The early stages of CIN are clinically asymptomatic and are usually discovered on Pap smears. Among HIV-infected women, 30% to 35% have abnormal Pap test results, which is five to eight times higher than usual (Anderson et al., 1996). Anderson and colleagues (1996) found that abnormal Pap smears correlated well with abnormal biopsy findings and there was no benefit from routine colposcopic examinations as opposed to routine Pap smears.

Vaginal bleeding, usually presenting as postcoital bleeding, is the most common symptom of cervical cancer. Metrorrhagia and a malodorous, blood-tinged vaginal discharge may also be present. As disease progresses, there may be abdominal, pelvic, back, or leg pain, anorexia, weight loss, anemia as a result of vaginal bleeding, and leg edema caused by obstruction of the lymph nodes. In cases of advanced disease, there may be hematuria or rectal bleeding because of involvement of the bowel, bladder, or both (Hatch & Fu, 1996).

DIAGNOSIS. The Pap smear is the primary screening tool to determine the presence of abnormal cells, visible lesions, or both. Women with abnormal Pap results are referred for colposcopic examination and cervical biopsy, which can be used to determine the presence of both HPV infection and CIN (Peel, 1995). If the client is not pregnant, an endocervical curettage will be performed to obtain cervical cells. If the lesion extends into the cervical canal and cannot be evaluated by colposcopy, conization is indicated. Conization, or cone biopsy, is both a diagnostic and a treatment tool; it not only establishes the severity of CIN but also can remove a cone-shaped wedge of abnormal tissue (Bobak et al., 1993).

If the biopsy reveals invasive cervical cancer, examination with the patient under anesthesia will be necessary to stage the disease and to determine the spread of disease beyond the cervix (Peel, 1995). Cervical cancer is staged according to the standards of the International Federation of Gynecology and Obstetrics, with staging sequences ranging from 0 to IV, depending on the extent of tissue or organ involvement. A complete diagnostic study should be performed by a gynecologic oncologist and a radiation oncologist so that an individualized treatment plan can be developed.

TREATMENT. Treatment of CIN and cervical carcinoma in situ includes carbon dioxide (CO_2) laser therapy, conization, cryosurgery, electrocautery, and simple hysterectomy. The loop electrocautery excision procedure is the newest procedure available. Treatment of invasive cervical cancer depends on the stage of the disease. Treatment may include single or combination strategies, including surgery, radiation, or chemotherapy. Because cervical cancer is usually squamous cell carcinoma, chemotherapy has been found to be less effective (Peel, 1995). However, protocols that include cisplatin along with methotrexate, bleomycin, and Adriamycin have demonstrated response rates up to 70% (Peel, 1995).

PREVENTION. Invasive cervical cancer is preventable if cervical dysplasia is diagnosed and treated promptly (CDC, 1992a). Health care providers need to be aware of the relationship between CIN and HIV infection so that they can educate women regarding their risk. Health care providers also have the responsibility to keep track of when the next Pap smear is due for any HIV-infected woman under their care. This is especially important for HIV-infected women who have tenuous living arrangements and may change primary care providers often. In addition, Maimon and colleagues (1993) suggest that all women less than 50 years of age who are given a diagnosis of invasive cervical cancer should receive counseling and testing for HIV.

COCCIDIOIDOMYCOSIS

EPIDEMIOLOGY. *Coccidioides immitis* is a fungus that was originally identified in the United States as the etiologic agent of San Joaquin Valley fever, or valley fever, a self-limited respiratory illness seen frequently in California. *C. immitis* is endemic to desert areas of the American Southwest and parts of California. Studies show that the incidence of coccidioidomycosis in HIV-infected persons ranges from 1.55% to 3.5% in southern California to 24.6% in Arizona (Ampel et al., 1993; Barrett et al., 1996). Risk factors that have been implicated in the development of coccidioidomycosis in HIV-infected persons include a CD4+ T-cell count of less than $250/mm^3$ and injection drug use (Ampel et al., 1993; Barrett et al., 1996; Jones et al., 1995).

PATHOGENESIS. Infection is acquired by inhalation of spores that cause pulmonary disease. Skin testing reveals that the rate of infection with *C. immitis* is as high as 30% but that immunocompetent persons have a very low rate of symptomatic disease (Ampel et al., 1993). In patients with HIV infection, particularly those with clinical AIDS or CD4+ cell counts of less than $250/mm^3$, clinically apparent disease is much more common. In the acute phase, there may be purulent pulmonary infection, followed by lesion fibrosis. As in tuberculosis, caseation can occur (Stevens, 1995). AIDS-related coccidioidomycosis has been shown to occur both by reactivation of a latent infection and by rapid progression of a newly acquired infection (Ampel et al., 1993).

CLINICAL PRESENTATION. The lungs are the primary focus of infection associated with AIDS-related coccidioidomycosis occurring in up to 80% of HIV-infected patients (Singh et al., 1996). Although pulmonary disease may be either focal or diffuse, patients with focal pneumonia have a better prognosis (Ampel et al., 1993; Singh et al., 1996). In addition to pulmonary disease, meningeal involvement has been observed in approximately 15% of the patients (Singh et al., 1996). Patients generally present with fever, chills, weight loss, and fatigue. Comorbid symptoms, indicating both pulmonary and meningeal disease, may include mucopurulent cough, headache, and impaired cognition (Sarosi & Davies, 1996; Singh et al., 1996).

DIAGNOSIS. Outside endemic areas, clinicians may miss the diagnosis of coccidioidomycosis because of a low index of suspicion. A good travel history is essential, and travel to or prior residence in an endemic area should alert clinicians to the possibility of coccidioidomycosis in patients with pulmonary infiltrates or meningitis (Sarosi & Davies, 1996). The definitive diagnosis of coccidioidomycosis is established by culture or by direct visualization of the organism in blood, tissue fluid, or biopsy specimens. The diagnostic yield of sputum examination is low, and fiberoptic bronchoscopy with bronchoalveolar lavage (BAL) or transbronchial biopsy may be required (Sarosi & Davies, 1996). DiTomasso and colleagues (1994) reported that cytologic examination was diagnostic in only 42% of patients with AIDS-related coccidioidomycosis compared with fungal cultures obtained by BAL, which were positive in all such cases. Transbronchial biopsy was also diagnostic in all patients on whom this procedure was performed. The authors point out that although cultures are more sensitive than cytologic examination, cultures take much more time. The median time to diagnosis by fungal cultures was 25 days, compared with 3.5 days for cytologic examination.

TREATMENT. The initial treatment of AIDS-related coccidioidomycosis consists of systemic amphotericin B, followed by lifelong suppressive therapy with oral fluconazole (Sarosi & Davies, 1996). Ampel and colleagues (1993) report success with fluconazole as initial treatment for some patients with mild focal pulmonary disease. Success with fluconazole as primary therapy has also been demonstrated for some patients with AIDS-related coccidioidal meningitis (Gagliani et al., 1993). Other oral azoles, such as itraconazole and ketoconazole, have been used for treatment of coccidioidomycosis, although these treatment options have not been well studied in AIDS patients (Sarosi & Davies, 1996).

PREVENTION. Primary prophylaxis with antifungal agents is not recommended. People living in areas endemic for coccidioidomycosis should be advised to avoid extensive exposure to disturbed soil, such as might occur during dust storms or at building excavation sites (CDC, 1997c). After an initial episode of coccidioidomycosis, secondary prophylaxis or lifelong suppressive therapy is required to prevent relapse (see Table 6–1).

CRYPTOCOCCOSIS

EPIDEMIOLOGY. *Cryptococcus neoformans* is a yeastlike fungus with a worldwide distribution. This ubiquitous organism is found in soil and bird droppings and is aerosolized and inhaled. There is no evidence of either person-to-person or animal-to-person transmission. Although clinical illness can occur occasionally in immunocompetent persons, the majority of patients with severe cryptococcal disease have underlying defects in cellular immunity, such as HIV infection, extensive corticosteroid use, organ transplantation, leukemia, lymphoma, or sarcoidosis. (Mitchell & Perfect, 1995).

Cryptococcosis is the most common life-threatening fungal infection associated with AIDS and the third most common cause of CNS disease, after HIV encephalopathy and toxoplasmosis (Saag, 1993). It is estimated that in industrialized countries life-threatening cryptococcosis will develop in between 5% and 13% of HIV-infected persons (Coker et al., 1993; Powderly, 1993). AIDS-related cryptococcal meningitis carries a very high mortality rate. Between 10% and 25% of patients will die during initial therapy, and between 30% and 60% will die within 1 year of diagnosis (Mitchell and Perfect, 1995).

PATHOGENESIS. The lungs are the portal of entry for *C. neoformans*. Yeast cells are inhaled and settle in the lung. In persons with intact cell-mediated immunity, the initial infection is usually contained by pulmonary macrophages. Dormant cryptococcal infections may reactivate at later stages of immunosuppression (Chernoff & Sande, 1990). In immunocompromised patients, the initial pulmonary infection, rather than being contained, may disseminate rapidly to the meninges and other organs such as skin, bone, and the urinary tract (Mitchell and Perfect, 1995). Although fulminant cryptococcal pneumonia may develop in some patients, the initial pulmonary infection is often asymptomatic, even in immunocompromised patients, and 85% to 95% of patients with AIDS-related cryptococcal meningitis show no evidence of pneumonitis (Saag, 1997).

CLINICAL MANIFESTATIONS. Meningitis is the most common clinical manifestation of AIDS-related cryptococcosis. Patients will typically present with headache, fever, lethargy, and confusion. These symptoms usually develop over a 2- to 4-week period, although in some cases the symptoms may increase in severity within a few days (Mitchell & Perfect, 1995). Neck stiffness and photophobia may occur, but are less common than with bacterial meningitis. Cranial nerve palsies can also occur. Increased intracranial pressure and papilledema may cause decreased vision and can lead to blindness (Johnston et al., 1992).

Patients may have concurrent cryptococcal pneumonia and may present with dyspnea, cough, and infiltrates on chest radiographs. Isolated pulmonary cryptococcosis is rare, and in 94% of patients with AIDS-related cryptococcal pneumonia there is dissemination to the meninges or blood (Mitchell and Perfect, 1995). Infection can also disseminate to numerous other sites, including the bone marrow, kidneys, liver, spleen, lymph nodes, heart, oral cavity, and prostate (Daar & Meyer, 1992). Cutaneous involvement can occur in 10% to 15% of patients and can be confused with other HIV-associated skin lesions, such as molluscum contagiosum, Kaposi's sarcoma, or herpes simplex (Durden & Elewski, 1994). Rare cases of cryptococcal arthritis, adrenalitis, and thyroiditis have been reported (Daar & Meyer, 1992).

DIAGNOSIS. The diagnosis of cryptococcal meningitis is made by examination of cerebrospinal fluid (CSF), which usually reveals increased cellularity with a predominance of mononuclear cells. Some patients may not demonstrate CSF leukocytosis because of a decreased ability to mount an inflammatory response. Other forms of meningitis, such as those caused by viruses, *Mycobacterium tuberculosis,* and lymphoma may present similar abnormalities in the CSF, and the definitive diagnosis is made by detection of *C. neoformans* in the CSF. The organism may be directly visualized by an India ink stain of CSF. Although fungal cultures of CSF offer a reliable way to diagnose cryptococcal meningitis, the diagnosis can be delayed while one waits for cultures to grow. Serologic testing of CSF for cryptococcal antigen can lead to a rapid diagnosis. The test for cryptococcal antigen employs rabbit anti-*C. neoformans* antiserum to de-

tect cryptococcal polysaccharide in CSF, blood, or other body fluids (Mitchell & Perfect, 1995).

Cryptococcal infection of extrameningeal sites can be diagnosed by India ink examination and culture of tissue specimens, urine, sputum, or fluid aspirates. Cryptococcal antigen testing of bronchoalveolar lavage fluid is a reliable method of confirming the diagnosis of cryptococcal pneumonia (Mitchell & Perfect, 1995). Radiologic testing may also be helpful in diagnosis. Patients with cryptococcal meningitis should undergo brain imaging by either magnetic resonance imaging (MRI) or computed tomography (CT) to look for possible cryptococcoma. Radiographs of the chest will show diffuse or focal interstitial infiltrates, with or without hilar and mediastinal adenopathy (Mitchell & Perfect, 1995).

TREATMENT. Primary therapy for the initial cryptococcal infection usually employs amphotericin B, with or without flucytosine, or fluconazole. For the past 35 years, amphotericin B has been the mainstay of therapy for cryptococcal meningitis in immunocompetent persons. Studies of immunosuppressed patients show a slightly less favorable response. Persons who have HIV infection and cryptococcal meningitis and are treated with amphotericin B have a mortality rate in the acute stage of 10% to 40% (Powderly, 1992). Controversy exists over the effectiveness of amphotericin B and flucytosine (Powderly, 1992). Saag and colleagues (1992) found that mild cases of cryptococcal meningitis responded as well to fluconazole as to amphotericin B, but the optimal therapy for patients with moderate to severe cryptococcal disease was inconclusive. Feinberg (1993) recommends high-dose amphotericin B for the first 2 weeks of therapy.

Amphotericin B therapy may be limited by its toxic effects, which include renal impairment, bone marrow suppression, and electrolyte abnormalities. Lipid formulations, such as liposomal amphotericin B, amphotericin B lipid complex, and amphotericin B colloidal dispersion, may reduce toxicity, improve delivery to infected sites, and allow higher doses (Mitchell & Perfect, 1995). High-dose fluconazole combined with flucytosine has been used successfully to treat cryptococcal meningitis in a clinical trial involving 89 patients with AIDS (Milefchik et al., 1997).

Itraconazole, despite its poor penetration of the CSF, may be effective in some cases of cryptococcosis (Mitchell & Perfect, 1995). Parisi and colleagues (1996) report successful treatment with 15 days of amphotericin and flucytosine followed by itraconazole in nine patients with AIDS-related cryptococcosis. Subcutaneous injections of recombinant human granulocyte colony-stimulating factor (GCSF) have been shown to increase the antifungicidal activity of polymorphonuclear leukocytes in patients with AIDS and, therefore, may be useful for the adjunctive treatment of cryptococcal meningitis (Vecchiarelli et al., 1995).

Cryptococcosis may be complicated by increased intracranial pressure, which may lead to papilledema and blindness. Serial lumbar puncture may be used to reduce intracranial pressure, and some patients may benefit from the placement of a ventriculoperitoneal or lumbar-peritoneal shunt (Bach & Tally, 1996). Acetazolamide, which decreases the production of CSF, may also be used to decrease intracranial pressure in patients with cryptococcal meningitis (Johnston et al., 1992).

PREVENTION. Although *Cryptococcus neoformans* is ubiquitous in the environment and avoidance of environmental exposure is difficult, areas with high concentrations of bird droppings, such as pigeon roosts and warehouses, are associated with an increased risk of cryptococcal infection and should be avoided by HIV-positive patients (CDC, 1997c; Hajjeh et al., 1996). Although clinical trials have shown that both itraconazole and fluconazole can reduce the incidence of cryptococcosis in patients with severe immunodeficiency, the use of these antifungal drugs for primary prophylaxis of cryptococcal disease is not recommended by most experts (CDC, 1997c). The rationale for withholding primary prophylaxis relates to the relatively low incidence of cryptococcal disease, the lack of data indicating that such prophylaxis prolongs survival, the cost of such treatment, and the potential for increasing the risk of emergence of resistant strains of more common fungal pathogens such as *Candida* species (CDC, 1997c).

As with many of the OIs associated with AIDS, initial treatment of the acute infection does not cure the patient and secondary prophylaxis or lifetime suppressive therapy is necessary (see Table 6–1). Powderly and colleagues (1992) documented the superiority of daily oral fluconazole over weekly infusions of amphotericin B in longterm suppression of cryptococcal meningitis.

CRYPTOSPORIDIOSIS

EPIDEMIOLOGY. Cryptosporidiosis was not identified in humans until 1976, and until 1982 only seven cases were reported in the literature (CDC, 1984). However, the identification of *Cryptosporidium* as a cause of infection in HIV-infected persons has resulted in further study of this parasite; it is now recognized as an important human pathogen and a frequent cause of diarrhea in both immunocompetent and immunosuppressed populations (McGowan et al., 1993). In 1993 a large outbreak of cryptosporidiosis occurred in Milwaukee, Wisconsin, where approximately 403,000 residents experienced diarrheal disease after drinking municipal water contaminated with this organism (MacKenzie et al., 1994). Although the illness was self-limited in most immunocompetent persons, a number of HIV-seropositive persons affected by this outbreak went on to have chronic cryptosporidiosis and biliary involvement (Vakil et al., 1996). Persons with CD4+ cell counts of less than 50/mm^3 were especially at risk of biliary symptoms and decreased survival at 1 year.

Although the Milwaukee outbreak provides direct evidence that AIDS-related cryptosporidiosis can be acquired through contaminated water supplies, other epidemiologic studies do not support the idea that unfiltered municipal drinking water is a significant factor in cryptosporidium infection in HIV-seropositive persons (Ciesielski et al., 1995; Sorvillo et al., 1994a). Person-to-person spread probably plays a large role in the transmission of cryptosporidium to HIV-infected persons. Epidemiologic studies have shown that AIDS-related cryptosporidiosis occurs more frequently in men who have sex with men than in injection drug users, persons with CD4+ severe immunodeficiency (CD4+ T-cell counts of less than 50/mm^3), heterosexuals, Latinos, older persons, and foreign-born persons (Ciesielski et al., 1995; Colford et al., 1996; Guerrero et al., 1995; Hu et al., 1994; Pedersen et al., 1996; Sorvillo et al., 1994b).

Intestinal cryptosporidiosis has been shown to be a factor in AIDS-related diarrhea in both industrialized and developing countries. The prevalence of cryptosporidium in the stool, as reported in various studies of populations of HIV-positive persons around the world, varies from 19% to 23% in symptom-free patients (Kamel et al., 1994; Sauda et al., 1993) and from 8% to 37.3% in patients with diarrhea (Brandonisio et al., 1993; Cotte et al., 1993; Guerrero et al., 1995; Moolasart et al., 1995).

PATHOGENESIS. Diarrheal disease due to *Cryptosporidium* is most commonly the result of infection of the small intestine, although in immunocompromised persons cryptosporidia have been found throughout the gastrointestinal tract as well as in the respiratory tract (Ma et al., 1984). Clayton and colleagues (1994) described different patterns of disease in patients with AIDS, which correlated with the anatomic site of infection. Whereas small-bowel infection was associated with severe diarrhea, malabsorption, nutritional depletion, and shorter survival, large-bowel involvement was associated with less severe illness.

Immunocompetent persons, including HIV-seropositive persons with higher CD4+ counts, can frequently become free of cryptosporidial infection without specific treatment. It is unclear why severely immunocompromised persons cannot clear the organism. The intestinal mucosa of persons with AIDS-related cryptosporidiosis secretes large amounts of anticryptosporidial IgA, but these antibodies seem ineffective in neutralizing cryptosporidium (Benhamou et al., 1995). The exact mechanism of diarrhea and malabsorption of nutrients is not well understood, but cytokine-mediated inflammation does not appear to play a large role (Snijders et al., 1995). Sciaretta and colleagues (1994) demonstrated significant malabsorption of bile salts in patients with AIDS who had diarrhea caused by cryptosporidiosis.

CLINICAL PRESENTATION. The hallmark of intestinal cryptosporidiosis is profuse, watery diarrhea which, in severely immunocompromised persons, can measure from 1 to 25 L, resulting in weight loss, electrolyte imbalance, and dehydration (Soave & Sepkowitz, 1992). The severity of cryptosporidiosis can be variable. Some patients have unrelenting diarrhea whereas others have a brief period of diarrhea and then become free of symptoms (McGowan et al., 1993). Nausea, vomiting, myalgia, and fever may be present but are less common (Gellin & Soave, 1992).

Biliary tree involvement, presenting as biliary obstruction or cholecystitis, with or without sclerosing cholangitis, occurs in a substantial number of cases (Hashmey et al., 1997; McGowan et al., 1993). Patients with biliary involvement manifest right upper quadrant pain, nausea, vomiting, and fever and may have abnormal liver enzymes. Narrowing of the antrum of the stomach and antral strictures have been reported as consequences of cryptosporidiosis in patients with AIDS (Cersosimo et al., 1992; Forester et al., 1994). Pulmonary cryptosporidiosis, a rare complication of intestinal cryptosporidiosis, may present with cough, dyspnea, fever, and thoracic pain (Clavel et al., 1996; Meynard et al., 1996).

DIAGNOSIS. Intestinal infection with *Cryptosporidium* can be diagnosed by microscopic examination of stool specimens treated by special staining techniques. Many hospital and commercial laboratories do not include staining for *Cryptosporidium* in routine stool examination for ova and parasites, and clinicians must specifically request such staining when cryptosporidiosis is suspected. Individual stool samples may be unrevealing in more than 50% of cases of intestinal cryptosporidiosis, although the sensitivity of stool examination may increase to more than 70% if multiple specimens are submitted for examination (Greenberg et al., 1996). Microscopic examination of intestinal tissue obtained endoscopically may be required for diagnosis. Greenberg and colleagues (1996) performed upper and lower gastrointestinal endoscopic examinations and performed biopsies at multiple sites within the gastrointestinal (GI) tract. The diagnostic sensitivities based on the site of biopsy are 11% in the stomach, 53% in the duodenum, 91% in the terminal ileum, and 50% in the colon.

TREATMENT. Restoration of the immune system has been shown to be effective in treating cryptosporidiosis. Carr and associates (1998) demonstrated that combination antiretroviral therapy that included an HIV protease inhibitor produced complete and sustained clinical, microbiological, and histological resolution of HIV-related microsporidiosis and cryptosporidiosis. Although many antimicrobial agents show potential activity against *Cryptosporidium,* there is currently no proven agent specific for this organism. Treatment of patients with cryptosporidisosis traditionally consisted of treating diarrhea with antimotility agents and replacing lost fluids, electrolytes, and nutrients with oral or parenteral feeding solutions. Intestinal peptide hormones, such as somatostatin and octreotide, can decrease intestinal motility and have shown some usefulness in patients whose diarrhea cannot be controlled with standard antimotility agents (Liberti et al., 1992; Moroni et al., 1993). In the presence of ensuing debilitation, a physical therapy consult should be requested to assess functional mobility and physical limitations in order to develop a plan of care to maintain mobility, strength, skin integrity, and self-management and to prevent complications (American Physical Therapy Association, 1997; McDowell, 1992).

Paromomycin, an oral antiparasitic agent, has been studied extensively and was shown to be somewhat effective in a double-blind, placebo-controlled trial (White et al., 1994). Another promising agent is nitazoxanide (NTZ). Feregrino and colleagues (1996) report almost complete clinical and microbiologic responses in all of 15 patients with refractory cryptosporidiosis who received NTZ through a compassionate-use protocol. Other potentially useful antiparasitic agents include aminosidine, letrazuril, and roxithromycin (Drake et al., 1992; Loeb et al., 1995; Lupo et al., 1992; Sprinz et al., 1996).

In addition to antimicrobial therapy, mechanical intervention may be necessary to relieve biliary obstruction due to cryptosporidiosis. Cholecystectomy, sphincterotomy, and placement of a biliary stent have been shown to reverse symptoms caused by biliary involvement with *Cryptosporidium* (Amiel et al., 1993; Hashmey et al., 1997).

PREVENTION. Prevention of cryptosporidiosis depends on avoidance of inadvertent ingestion of cryptosoporidial cysts. The usual modes of transmission include contact with feces from infected adults and diaper-age children, contact with infected animals, and drinking of contaminated water (CDC, 1997c). Patients should be advised to avoid sexual activities that may result in oral

contact with stool and should refrain from oral-anal contact. Proper attention to hygiene during and after anal intercourse is advisable, and some experts advise avoidance of anal sex (CDC, 1997c). Hands should be washed after changing diapers or handling animals, and only healthy animals that are free of diarrhea should be brought into the home as pets.

Outbreaks of cryptosporidiosis due to contaminated municipal water supplies have been documented, and special precautions should be taken when drinking tap water. Boiling water for 1 minute effectively eliminates the risk of cryptosporidiosis (CDC, 1997c). Water filters may be helpful, but only filters that are capable of removing particles of 1 μm are effective for cyst removal. It should not be assumed that bottled water is safe, as methods of disinfecting bottled water vary (CDC, 1997c). Water that is accidently ingested during recreational activities poses a threat of infection with cryptosporidiosis. Patients ought not drink from rivers or lakes and should avoid swimming in water that is likely to be contaminated with *Cryptosporidium* (CDC, 1997c).

There is evidence that clarithromycin or rifabutin, when prescribed for chemoprophylaxis or treatment of *Mycobacterium avium* complex, decreases the rate of cryptosporidiosis in HIV-infected individuals. Holmberg and colleagues (1998) found that both clarithromycin and rifabutin were highly effective in preventing the development of cryptosporidiosis in immunosuppressed HIV-infected persons.

CYTOMEGALOVIRUS DISEASE

EPIDEMIOLOGY. Infection with cytomegalovirus (CMV), a human herpesvirus, is ubiquitous throughout the world, and most adults demonstrate serologic evidence of CMV infection (Adler, 1992). An increased potential for infection exists during two periods: the perinatal period through the preschool years and later during sexually active years (Ho, 1995). In the first period, CMV can be acquired as an intrauterine or congenital infection, from vaginal delivery through a contaminated cervix, from human milk by breast-feeding or from banked milk, by transmission from child to child in nurseries or day care centers, or among children within a family. The prevalence of CMV antibody increases rapidly between the ages of 15 and 35, when the virus is transmitted primarily through kissing and sexual activity (Drew & Jacobson, 1994).

According to Collier and colleagues (1987), the prevalence rate of CMV infection appears to be higher among homosexual men than among the general adult population, and receptive anal intercourse is associated with an increased risk of CMV seropositivity (Collier et al., 1987). Leach and colleagues (1993) found a CMV seroprevalence rate of 100% among 234 HIV-positive homosexual men. In addition, CMV was recovered from the semen of 45% of these men. Shepp and colleagues (1996) examined a cohort of HIV-positive persons in a large group of demographically diverse persons and reported an incidence of clinical CMV disease of 35.6% among homosexual men, 33.3% among persons acquiring HIV infection through heterosexual contact, and 4.3% among injection drug users. No persons seronegative for CMV antibody developed CMV disease.

The risk of clinical CMV disease increases with decreasing CD4+ lymphocyte count. Kuppermann and associates (1993b) prospectively examined a group of HIV-positive persons and found that CMV retinitis occurred in 30% of those with CD4+ counts of less than $50/mm^3$ and in none of those with CD4+ cell counts above this level. The incidence of CMV disease in AIDS has risen in recent years as patients survive longer with depressed CD4+ counts. In one large cohort of HIV-positive homosexual men, the incidence of CMV disease rose from 24.8% to 44.9% after the introduction in the late 1980s of prophylaxis against *Pneumocystis carinii* pneumonia (Hoover et al., 1993).

PATHOGENESIS. Acute infection with CMV rarely causes significant illness in immunocompetent persons, except for in utero infection, which may result in disseminated CMV disease and congenital abnormalities. In young adults acute CMV may cause a mononucleosis-like syndrome (Ho, 1995). Severe clinical CMV disease in persons with HIV infection most probably occurs as the result of reactivation of latent infection. Although the site of latency is not precisely known, it probably includes leukocytes (Ho, 1995). In immunologically normal adults CMV is not detectable except in cervical secretions of some women and semen of some men (Ho, 1995).

With increasing depletion of cellular immunity in advanced HIV disease, reactivated CMV can cause significant clinical disease by directly destroying tissue in such organs as the retina, brain, lungs, liver, and mucosa of the gastrointestinal tract (Strauss, 1995). Although dissemination of CMV to such organs as the lung and the adrenal glands may not be recognized before the patient's death, postmortem examination reveals that a very high percentage of patients have CMV disease at these sites (Dore et al., 1995).

CLINICAL PRESENTATION. Retinitis is the most commonly recognized clinical complication of CMV in AIDS and, left untreated, can rapidly progress to blindness. Patients may present with visual loss, loss of visual fields, or floaters (Drew et al., 1997). Other ocular manifestations of CMV infection include optic neuritis, uveitis, and conjunctivitis (Mansor & Li, 1995).

Gastrointestinal disease is fairly common and may involve virtually all parts of the gastrointestinal tract, from the oral cavity to the perianal area. Esophageal ulcers present as odynophagia and may be accompanied by painful oral ulcers (Epstein et al., 1993; Wilcox et al., 1994). There are case reports of sialoadenitis and salivary gland dysfunction due to CMV (Greenberg et al., 1997; Wax et al., 1994). CMV can cause ulcerative or inflammatory colitis (Mentec et al., 1994) or ileitis (Lai et al., 1996). Rare cases of mass lesions of the stomach, esophagus, and colon have also been reported (Laguna et al., 1993; Rich et al., 1992). Gallbladder involvement with CMV may present as acalculus cholecystitis (Keshavjee et al., 1993).

The two most commonly reported neurologic manifestations of CMV in AIDS are encephalitis and polyradiculopathy. Patients with CMV encephalitis may manifest cognitive dysfunction, memory impairment, and personality changes (Wiley & Nelson, 1988). CMV polyradiculopathy presents as ascending flaccid paralysis, areflexia, bowel incontinence, bladder dysfunction, and sensory impairment (Cohen et al., 1993; Kim & Hollander, 1993; Meier et al., 1996).

Pulmonary involvement with CMV generally causes diffuse pneumonitis or focal pneumonia, and patients present with fever, dyspnea, cough, and hypoxemia (Salomon et al., 1997; Waxman et al., 1997). Pulmonary nodules, focal lung masses, and alveolar hemorrhage have also been reported as manifestations of pulmonary CMV (Fishman & Batt, 1996; Herry et al., 1996; Northfelt et al., 1993).

DIAGNOSIS. CMV retinitis is diagnosed by visualization of characteristic retinal lesions on ophthalmoscopic examination of a dilated fundus. In other sites, such as the lung and the gastointestinal tract, the diagnosis of CMV disease is made when CMV inclusion bodies are seen on microscopic examination of tissue biopsy specimens. Wilcox and colleagues (1994) suggest that as many as 10 biopsies may be needed for the diagnosis of CMV esophagitis in some patients.

The diagnosis of neurologic disease often remains elusive. Encephalitis due to CMV may be confused with or may coexist with the AIDS-dementia complex. Although MRI of the brain may show changes in the periventricular white matter, these findings are often absent in proven cases of CMV encephalitis (Clifford et al., 1996). In patients with advanced AIDS and a flaccid paralysis, electromyographic and nerve conduction studies may show findings consistent with polyradiculopathy, but these findings do not definitively prove that CMV is the etiologic agent. Likewise, contrast-enhanced MRI scans of the lumbar spine that demonstrate a thickened cauda equina suggest but do not prove CMV poyradiculopathy (Whiteman et al., 1994). The diagnosis of CMV encephalitis still frequently depends on clinical presentation and response to therapy directed against CMV. Examination of CSF with DNA probes and the polymerase chain reaction for CMV are being studied and may soon lead to advances in the diagnosis of neurologic disease that is due to CMV (Gozlan et al., 1992; Musiani et al., 1994).

TREATMENT. Treatment of AIDS-related CMV retinitis has historically consisted of an induction phase with high-dose ganciclovir or foscarnet, followed by lifelong daily intravenous infusions with maintenance doses of one of these two medications, usually through an implanted central venous catheter. Although the treatment of CMV retinitis with foscarnet appears to offer a survival advantage, the drug is less well tolerated than ganciclovir (Studies of Ocular Complications of AIDS Research Group, 1992). In addition, the

two drugs appear to have equal efficacy in controlling the progression of CMV retinitis and preserving vision (Studies of Ocular Complications of AIDS Research Group, 1994). Ganciclovir is associated with significant bone marrow suppression, manifested as anemia and neutropenia, and concurrent treatment with GCSF may be required. Foscarnet can be nephrotoxic, and careful attention to renal function is necessary during treatment with this agent. Foscarnet has been shown to be effective as salvage therapy for patients with CMV retinitis or gastrointestinal disease who are either refractory to or intolerant of ganciclovir (Dieterich et al., 1993b; Jacobson et al., 1994). Some studies suggest that for patients in whom CMV disease recurs on monotherapy with either ganciclovir or foscarnet, combination therapy with the two drugs offers a better clinical result than does continued monotherapy (Dieterich et al., 1993c; Kupperman et al., 1993a; Studies of Ocular Complications of AIDS Research Group, 1996; Weinberg et al., 1994).

Oral ganciclovir is approved for maintenance therapy after intravenous induction for CMV retinitis. Although slightly shorter times to progression of retinitis are seen with oral ganciclovir than with intravenous ganciclovir, oral administration is safer and more convenient (Drew et al., 1995; Oral Ganciclovir European and Australian Cooperative Study Group, 1995). Cidofovir, a nucleotide analogue, offers another alternative for the systemic treatment of CMV retinitis. Although the drug is administered intravenously, its pharmacokinetics allow it to be given only once a week during the treatment phase and every other week during the maintenance phase, thus obviating the need for indwelling venous catheters. Although highly efficacious, cidofovir is associated with significant nephrotoxicity and must be administered with probenicid and proper hydration (Lalezari et al., 1997; Studies of Ocular Complications of AIDS Research Group, 1997). See Table 6–1 for secondary prophylaxis reccommendations.

In addition to their association with bone marrow and renal toxicity, systemic treatments may fail to achieve therapeutic intravitreal drug concentrations (Kupperman et al., 1993c). Local therapy with implanted devices that release ganciclovir in a sustained fashion have been shown to provide high drug levels and to be safe and effective for treatment of CMV retinitis (Anand et al., 1993; Martin et al., 1994; Marx et al., 1996). Local therapy also reduces the potential for systemic toxicity. Musch and associates (1997) noted that sustained-release ganciclovir implants were more effective than systemic ganciclovir in treating CMV retinitis. The limitations of ganciclovir implants include retinal detachment, CMV retinitis in the contralateral eye, and extraocular CMV. Intravitreal injections of ganciclovir, foscarnet, combination ganciclovir and foscarnet, and cidofovir have shown promise in the treatment of CMV retinitis (Baudouin et al., 1996; Desatnik et al., 1996; Diaz-Llopis et al., 1994; Hodge et al., 1996; Kirsch et al., 1995; Rahhal et al., 1996).

For patients with significant loss of vision or blindness, an occupational therapy consult should be included in the plan of care. The therapist can evaluate the patient's ability to participate in activities of daily living and safely maneuver the environment, as well determine the need and amount of training and modifications necessary to help the client achieve maximal function (McReynolds & Galantino, 1995; Reed, 1991). In addition, the patient can be referred to community-based agencies that address the special needs of the visually impaired.

Intravenous ganciclovir has also been shown to be effective in the treatment of colitis and esophagitis due to CMV (Dieterich et al., 1993a; Walter et al., 1993). Esophageal CMV lesions are usually associated with odynophagia, which leads to decreased food and fluid intake and weight loss. Symptom management requires an established pain control program (as opposed to medication only as needed) during the acute-treatment phase to maintain adequate nutrition and hydration. For severe weight loss associated with these symptoms, it is advisable to request a speech-language-pathology consult to teach the patient how to swallow and how to modify the diet to minimize pain while maintaining adequate nutrition (American Speech-Language-Hearing Association, 1996).

PREVENTION. HIV-positive persons should be evaluated for prior exposure to CMV by testing for IgG antibodies to CMV. Persons who are seronegative for CMV should be advised to always use latex condoms during sexual contact to

avoid any possible exposure to CMV (CDC, 1997c). The risk of acquiring CMV through caring for children can be reduced by hand-washing and careful attention to hygiene (CDC, 1997c).

Early detection of CMV retinitis followed by prompt initiation of therapy can prevent visual loss. Patients should be educated to promptly report "floaters" or any disturbances in their vision. Regular fundoscopic examinations should be performed on all patients with CD4+ lymphocyte counts below $100/mm^3$ (CDC, 1997c).

Persons who are infected with CMV, as evidenced by positive CMV antibodies, may be candidates for chemoprophylaxis against CMV disease. Two recent large, randomized, multicenter clinical trials have examined the use of oral ganciclovir for primary prevention of CMV retinitis in patients with CD4+ cell counts below $100/mm^3$. Although one study found a significant reduction in CMV retinitis with oral ganciclovir, a similar study failed to show such a benefit (Brosgart et al., 1996; Spector et al., 1996). Neither study showed a statistically significant survival benefit with administration of prophylactic oral ganciclovir. The drawbacks of prophylactic oral ganciclovir include neutropenia, inconvenience, and high monetary costs associated with this therapy.

HIV-RELATED ENCEPHALOPATHY

EPIDEMIOLOGY. HIV encephalopathy is also referred to as AIDS-dementia complex (ADC), HIV-1 associated dementia (HIVD), HIV-1-associated cognitive/motor deficit, and HIV or AIDS dementia. ADC is a neurobehavioral deficit that occurs in late-stage HIV infection with severe immununosuppression (Price, 1996). More recently the term *HIV-1-associated mild neurocognitive disorder* has been applied to HIV disease with subtle or mild cognitive impairment that has not yet progressed to full-blown ADC (Grant et al., 1995). It is estimated that approximately 50% of persons with AIDS are affected by this mild disorder. It is unclear whether the presence of this mild form of dementia will progress to ADC (Dal Pan & McArthur, 1996). As standardized criteria for defining ADC have been developed, the prevalence of ADC appears to be from 7% to 14% (Dal Pan et al., 1996; Grant et al., 1995).

PATHOGENESIS. HIV invades the CNS in the early stages of infection and remains there until death. A host immune response within the brain results from HIV CNS infection (Price, 1996). It is assumed, although not documented, that CNS microglia and astrocyte cells become infected through infected macrophages or monocytes that cross the blood-brain barrier (Power & Johnson, 1995). HIV dementia is a subcortical dementia, and neuropathologic features include diffuse myelin pallor, neocortical neuronal dropout, multinucleated giant cells, microglial nodules, and HIV antigens and genome. There is also a loss of synaptic contacts and a vacuolar change in neurons in both the deep gray matter and the cortex (Power & Johnson, 1995). The majority of patients with CNS infection experience little or no neurologic illness (Johnson et al., 1996). There is a striking lack of correlation between the severity of dementia and the pathologic changes that occur in the CNS (Power & Johnson, 1995).

Two factors seem to relate to the development of ADC: the degree of immunosuppression and the level and genetic variation of HIV (Johnson et al., 1996; Price, 1996). Johnson and associates (1996) found large amounts of virus in nondemented patients and low viral levels in some demented patients and concluded that qualitative differences in virus versus quantitative differences induce the development of dementia. They also found different HIV strains in demented and nondemented patients.

CLINICAL PRESENTATION. HIV-1-associated mild neurocognitive disorder leads to mild interference in daily functioning. Patients complain of difficulty with concentration and mental agility. They report a need to keep lists, a tendency to forget what they were saying in midsentence, and an inability to concentrate while reading or watching television (Grant et al., 1995; Price, 1996).

In HIV dementia, cognitive impairment is more severe and affects several domains, such as memory and attention (Grant et al., 1995). Patients may have difficulty in the learning of new information or a slowing in the processing of this information and more difficulty with attention and concentration. This leads to a marked interference with activities of daily living. There are also diffuse motor abnormalities that lead to motor impairment, such as difficulty in walking (Price, 1996). Cognitive and motor impairment may progress to complete mutism and paraparesis with urinary and fecal incontinence.

DIAGNOSIS. Diagnosis of ADC initially may be overlooked, especially in an acute-care setting where examination of the mental status of a person with AIDS is not a priority, given the plethora of physical problems that require attention. In addition, a differential diagnosis is required to distinguish ADC from OIs or neoplasms of the CNS, metabolic abnormalities, and psychiatric illnesses. The American Academy of Neurology developed diagnostic criteria for HIV dementia, which includes (1) HIV seropositivity, (2) a history of progressive cognitive and behavioral decline, (3) neurologic or neuropsychological evaluation consistent with a decline from premorbid baseline, and (4) CNS opportunistic processes excluded by CT or MR imaging and CSF analysis (Power & Johnson, 1995). CT and MRI reveal cerebral atrophy and white-matter abnormalities. CSF analysis can show elevated protein levels and pleocytosis, as well as an absence of other infections or neoplasms (Power & Johnson, 1995). The Mini-Mental State Examination (MMSE), the HIV Dementia Scale, and the HIV Dementia Screening Instrument are quick and easy psychomotor tests that help to determine the level of impairment (McLaulin et al., 1996; Power & Johnson, 1995).

TREATMENT. Several studies have suggested that zidovudine has a therapeutic and prophylactic value in the treatment and prevention of ADC (Evers et al., 1998; Powers & Johnson, 1995; Price, 1996). There have been many anecdotal reports of improvement in ADC with zidovudine therapy, and providers have reported a decreased incidence in ADC that is presumed to be secondary to zidovudine therapy. In the only prospective controlled study of zidovudine in persons with symptomatic ADC, high doses of zidovudine (1000 mg/d and 2000 mg/d) resulted in clinical improvement (Price, 1996). However, no study has determined the lowest effective dose of zidovudine, the length of time it is effective, and the time to development of resistant virus. Ongoing studies are evaluating the efficacy of other nonnucleoside reverse transcriptase inhibitors, protease inhibitors, calcium channel blockers, and inhibitors of tumor necrosis factor (TNF)-alpha synthesis.

Breitbart and colleagues (1996) evaluated the efficacy of haloperidol, chlorpromazine, and lorazepam in the treatment of delirium that frequently occurs in HIV-infected patients who are hospitalized. They found improvement within 24 hours with lower than standard doses of haloperidol and chlorpromazine. In several studies in men with late-stage HIV disease and decreased memory and attention span, diminished concentration, apathy, and slowing, methylphenidate has shown good results in improving both affective and cognitive symptoms (Brown, 1995).

The progressive motor impairment seen in ADC should be treated aggressively with physical therapy to maintain independence and safety. Initially, the therapist should evaluate the motor abilities of the patient and the need for instruction in compensation strategies. In addition, periodic follow-up visits should be scheduled to monitor disease progression and the potential need for assist devices. Maintaining or adapting the motor skills of the patient with ADC will also enhance his or her ability to maintain some degree of socialization and stimulate cognitive functioning (Galantino, 1987; Reed, 1991).

PREVENTION. Currently, there is no preventive treatment available. However, with the increasing use of combination antiretroviral therapies, the incidence of ADC may decrease.

HERPES VIRUS DISEASE

Most people think of *herpes* as a synonym for a cold sore or a genital lesion. The name, however, is derived from a family of viruses called Herpesviridae, which has several members including (1) herpes simplex virus type 1 (HSV-1), which causes cold sores and eye infections; (2) herpes simplex virus type 2 (HSV-2), which causes genital herpes; (3) varicella-zoster virus (VZV), the cause of chickenpox and shingles (herpes zoster); (4) Epstein-Barr virus (EBV), the cause of infectious mononucleosis; (5) cytomegalovirus (CMV), which causes mononucleosis; (6) human herpesvirus types 6 and 7, the cause of roseola; (7) simian herpes B virus, which causes skin lesions or brain infection; and (8) the newly identified human herpesvirus 8 (HHV-8), which has been implicated in the development of Kaposi's sarcoma and possibly other malignancies (Moore & Chaisson, 1996; Straus, 1995).

A major biologic feature of the herpesviruses is the phenomenon of latency and reactivation. After initial or primary infection in humans with any herpesviruses, there remain lifelong latent viruses that have the potential to reactivate, producing recurrent or secondary infections. Sites of latency include sensory nerve ganglia for HSV-1, HSV-2, VZV, and herpes B virus; lymphocytes and possibly monocytes and neutrophils for CMV; B lymphocytes and salivary glands for EBV; and lymphocytes for human herpesvirus type 6 (Straus, 1995).

Herpes Simplex Viruses

EPIDEMIOLOGY. Herpes simplex viruses are ubiquitous and have a worldwide distribution. Humans appear to be the only natural hosts. The primary mode of transmission is direct contact with oral secretions (HSV-1) or genital secretions (HSV-2). Transmission of HSV-1 can occur in the genital area through oral sexual contact or autoinoculation (i.e., touching a cold sore and then touching the genital area), and HSV-2 can be transmitted orally by similar modes. Although transmission is facilitated during contact with a person with active infection (lesions present), it can also occur as a result of contact with symptom-free excreters (Hirsch, 1995). It is estimated that the seroprevalence of HSV-1 in the United States is greater than 80% and that of HSV-2 is between 20% and 30%. In men who have sex with men and in injecting drug users, the incidence may be as high as 95% (Stewart et al., 1995).

Serologic studies indicate that exposure to HSV-1 commonly occurs in early childhood and that infection is highest in lower socioeconomic groups (Hirsch, 1995). A different pattern of infection occurs with HSV-2. Exposure usually occurs after puberty and between the ages of 14 and 44 years and is related to sexual transmission (Hirsch, 1995). The frequency varies with the number of sexual contacts. A mother with an active lesion can transmit HSV-2 to her neonate during delivery. Anal and perianal lesions are common among men who have sex with men. Women are at greater risk of heterosexual transmission (Hirsch, 1995). Although latent HSV may reactivate in persons with HIV disease, causing severe recurrent disease, Safrin and colleagues (1991) did not find an increase in the frequency or severity of HSV infection in this population, despite severe immunosuppression.

HSV that is resistant to acyclovir is being diagnosed with increasing frequency, possibly because of the escalating use of acyclovir prophylaxis for HSV (Cockerell, 1993). Current estimates of acyclovir-resistant HSV in HIV-infected persons are not available.

PATHOGENESIS. Primary exposure to HSV at mucosal surfaces or abraded skin permits entry of the virus, initiation of replication, and transport along nerve pathways. Although uncommon in immunocompetent persons, the finding of multiple strains of the same HSV subtype in an immunocompromised person suggests that exogenous infection with different strains of the same subtype is possible (Corey & Spear, 1986).

After resolution of the primary infection, HSV becomes latent within sensory nerve ganglia, usually the trigeminal, sacral, and vagal ganglia. Once latency is established, the virus may be reactivated at any time and may replicate and travel along sensory epithelial surfaces, resulting in acute HSV infection (Hirsch, 1995).

CLINICAL PRESENTATION. Primary HSV-1 infection occurs most commonly in childhood and presents with gingivostomatitis and pharyngitis. Orolabial HSV infection seen in adults with HIV disease usually represents reactivation of a previously acquired infection rather than a primary infection. Infection is noted by the appearance of painful vesicular lesions that rapidly coalesce and rupture, producing ulcers on the lips, tongue, pharynx, or buccal mucosa (Drew et al., 1992). Fever, pharyngitis, and cervical lymphadenopathy may be present. Primary HSV-2 genital infection usually appears in the form of vesicular lesions on an erythematous base. Pain, fever, malaise, anorexia, and tender bilateral inguinal adenopathy are frequent accompanying symptoms (Hirsch, 1995).

Recurrent herpes infections are frequently preceded by prodromal symptoms of pain, burning, tingling, or itching in the affected area. Within 6 to 48 hours vesicular lesions, which may be quite painful, appear. The vesicles progress to become an ulcer and then a crusted lesion within 48 hours. Symptoms usually resolve within several weeks.

Perianal and anorectal HSV infection and HSV proctitis may also be seen in HIV-infected persons. The result can be localized pain, itching, pain on defecation, tenesmus, constipation, sacral radiculopathy, impotence, and neurogenic bladder (Hirsch, 1995).

HSV esophagitis can occur in the absence of oropharyngeal HSV lesions, and in HIV-positive persons it is estimated to be the cause of 4% to 16% of esophageal symptoms (Genereau et al., 1996). Initial presentation may include dysphagia, which, if untreated, can result in odynophagia and retrosternal pain.

Although rare, HSV encephalitis can occur as a life-threatening complication in HIV disease. HSV encephalitis presents as an acute encephalitis with headache, fever, altered mentation, and frequently focal neurologic signs (Safrin, 1994).

DIAGNOSIS. The optimal method of laboratory diagnosis of HSV is direct culture of material from the suspected lesion. The highest yield of HSV is from cultures of vesicles or cultures taken at the base of an ulcer. If a vesicle is present, it should be unroofed with an 18-gauge needle and the area swabbed with a cotton-tipped or Dacron swab. An ulcerative lesion should be swabbed vigorously over the base of the ulcer. The swab should be immediately placed in a transport medium, which must be kept cold until it reaches the laboratory. Some settings may not have access to HSV cultures, or there may be a high false-negative rate. In that case, empiric therapy with acyclovir is indicated.

TREATMENT. Acyclovir, which is available in intravenous, oral, and topical preparations, is used in primary therapy for HSV infection. Intravenously administered acyclovir is used for severe HSV infections and is specifically indicated for HSV encephalitis. Orally administered acyclovir, in suspension or capsules, may be used for either acute HSV infection or long-term suppressive therapy. Topical acyclovir ointment is used to relieve subjective symptoms of skin lesions and to reduce viral shedding. Acyclovir-resistant strains of HSV that cause significant clinical disease in immunocompromised patients are being isolated with increasing frequency (Kessler et al., 1996; Pottage & Kessler, 1995). Foscarnet has been used successfully for treatment of acyclovir-resistant HSV-2 infection (Erlich et al., 1989; Safrin et al., 1991). Cidofovir topical gel was recently approved for the treatment of herpes, and studies have shown it to be effective against acyclovir-resistant HSV (Lalezari et al., 1996). Kessler and colleagues (1996) found that 1% ophthalmic trifluridine solution was effective for the treatment of chronic mucocutaneous HSV that was unresponsive to acyclovir.

Esophageal HSV lesions are usually associated with odynophagia, which leads to decreased food and fluid intake and weight loss. Symptom management requires an established pain control program (as opposed to medication only as needed) during the acute treatment phase to maintain adequate nutrition and hydration. For severe weight loss associated with these symptoms, it is advisable to request a speech-language-pathology consult to teach the patient how to swallow and how to modify the diet to minimize the pain while maintaining adequate nutrition (American Speech-Language-Hearing Association, 1996; DeBolt et al., 1996).

PREVENTION. Prophylaxis of initial episodes of HSV disease is not recommended. Table 6–1 contains the recommendations for secondary prophylaxis in certain instances.

The health history of an HIV-infected person is important to determine the potential for recurrent HSV infection. The person's knowledge of HSV transmission, as well as prevention related to specific sexual behaviors such as condom use and oral sex, should be assessed. The practice of safer sex should be reviewed with all HIV-infected persons to prevent transmission or acquisition of sexually transmitted diseases. HIV-infected clients sometimes assume that if they have sex with another HIV-infected person, they no longer need to practice safer sex. Health teaching should stress that the rate of HSV infection is high in HIV-infected persons and that, even if no HSV lesions are visible, symptom-free excreters can pass on the virus (Hirsch, 1995).

The risk of nosocomial transmission of HSV from infected patients, most often causing herpetic whitlow, is well documented (Hirsch 1995). Health care providers should wear gloves during physical examination of a new client because they cannot predict what types of mucocutaneous lesion may be present. Gloves should also be worn for any procedures that involve oral or genital secretions, such as mouth care, suctioning, urinary catheter procedures, or vaginal care. Meticulous hand-washing should be performed, and skin-to-lesion contact should be avoided as much as possible.

HISTOPLASMOSIS

EPIDEMIOLOGY. *Histoplasma capsulatum* is a fungus that exists in the soil and on bird and bat droppings. The major endemic regions in the United States are the Middle, Central, and South Central states. In HIV-infected persons living outside endemic areas, sporadic outbreaks of progressive disseminated histoplasmosis (PDH) may be seen as a result of reactivation of latent infection (Sarosi & Davies, 1996). Immigrants from the Caribbean, South America, and Central America are also at risk of PDH due to reactivation of infection acquired in an endemic area. In endemic areas of the United States, the incidence of PDH in patients with AIDS may be as high as 27% (Sarosi & Davies, 1996).

PATHOGENESIS. Infection begins with inhalation of *H. capsulatum* spores into the alveoli, where they germinate into the yeast form. This is followed by hematogenous spread of the yeast to regional lymph nodes and the reticuloendothelial system, including bone marrow, liver, and spleen. The organisms are ingested by macrophages and, in immunocompetent persons, the organisms are contained within granulomas and cell-mediated immunity to the fungus develops 1 to 3 weeks after infection (Lee & Tauber, 1994). Patients with HIV infection may fail to mount an adequate immune response to infection and PDH may develop, resulting in disseminated infection involving multiple organs. In patients with HIV infection PDH may develop as the result of an old infection or by activation of a latent infection.

CLINICAL MANIFESTATIONS. Patients with PDH present with symptoms of a persistent disseminated infection. The reported incidence of symptoms observed in persons with AIDS and PDH are (1) fever in 75% to 100%, (2) weight loss in 48% to 100%, (3) hepatosplenomegaly in 52% to 100%, and (4) mouth ulcers, primarily of the palate, in 65% (Alves et al., 1996; Liliana et al., 1997; Neubauer & Bodensteiner, 1992; Segura et al., 1996). Bone marrow involvement leads to anemia, thrombocytopenia, leukopenia, or even pancytopenia in a large proportion of patients.

Patients may also manifest signs and symptoms of particular organ system involvement. Pulmonary involvement may present as cough or dyspnea, with interstitial infiltrates evident on chest radiographs (Stansell, 1993). Additional manifestations of *H. capsulatum* infection in patients with AIDS include (1) cutaneous lesions, (2) gastrointestinal obstruction and perforation, (3) prosthetic abscess, and (4) optic neuritis (Cimponeriu et al., 1994; Cirillo-Hyland & Gross, 1995; Heneghan et al., 1993; Myers & Kamino, 1996; Spivak et al., 1996; Yau et al., 1996; Zighelboim et al., 1992).

DIAGNOSIS. The diagnosis of disseminated histoplasmosis is made by direct visualization or culture of the organism from blood, bone marrow, or other involved tissue. Although visualization of the organism on a peripheral blood smear provided the diagnosis in 32% of cases, microscopic examination of bone marrow biopsies stained for fungus confirmed the diagnosis in 75% to 86% of cases (Neubauer & Bodensteiner, 1992; Zarabi et al., 1992). The most reliable method of identifying *H. capsulatum* is by culture of bone marrow or blood, which has established a diagnosis in 70% to 90% of cases. Culture and microscopic examination of biopsy specimens of lung, skin, pleura, esophagus, colon, sputum, CSF, and peritoneal or pleural fluid occasionally leads to a diagnosis (Zarabi et al., 1992). Although culture and histochemical examination of tissue are equally reliable, Zarabi and colleagues (1992) point out that direct microscopic examination provided a diagnosis in less than 48 hours, allowing more rapid initiation of therapy.

Serologic testing of tissue fluid may prove to be useful in the diagnosis of histoplasmosis. The detection of *H. capsulatum* polysaccharide antigen (HPA) in lavage specimens obtained bronchoscopically was 70% sensitive in the diagnosis of pulmonary histoplasmosis in one series (Wheat et al., 1992). The same authors report that HPA could be detected in urine in 92.6% of cases and in serum in 88.5% of cases.

TREATMENT. Historically, the response to treatment with amphotericin B or ketoconazole has been poor (Stevens, 1994), prompting interest in the newer oral azoles such as fluconazole and intraconazole. Sharkey-Mathis and colleagues (1993) reported modest success with itraconazole but less impressive results with fluconazole. A recent open-label, nonrandomized study of oral itraconazole reported an 85% response rate when itraconazole was used in the primary therapy for disseminated histoplasmosis (Wheat et al., 1995).

PREVENTION. HIV-positive persons who live in areas endemic for histoplasmosis should avoid activities associated with exposure to *H. capsulatum*. Such activities include cleaning chicken coops, disturbing soil beneath bird-roosting sites, and cave exploration (CDC, 1997c). Patients who have CD4 counts of less than $100/mm^3$ and who live in areas endemic for H. capsulatum may benefit from primary chemoprophylaxis (see Chapter 5, Table 5–14). After initial treatment of acute disease, lifetime suppressive therapy should be instituted (see Table 6–1 for recommendations).

ISOSPORIASIS

EPIDEMIOLOGY. *Isospora belli* is a coccidian parasite that is widely distributed throughout the animal kingdom and is endemic to parts of Chile, Africa, and Southeast Asia (Soave & Gellin, 1992). The mode of transmission is thought to be direct contact with infected animals or persons or with contaminated water (Gellin & Soave, 1992). The prevalence of clinically diagnosed isosporiasis among persons with HIV/AIDS ranges between 0.2% and 1% (Hu et al., 1994; Sorvillo et al., 1995). However, when the infection rate is measured by prospective examination of stool specimens, the rate of infection with *I. belli* has been shown to be as high as 10% (Esfandiari et al., 1995).

Latinos and foreign-born persons are found to be at greater risk of isosporiasis than white persons born in the United States. Likewise, persons who report either homosexual or heterosexual sex as their HIV transmission risk factor are at greater risk than those who report injection drug use (Hu et al., 1994). Interestingly, Sorvillo and colleagues (1995) found that a prior history of *Pneumocystis carinii* pneumonia was associated with a decreased incidence of isosporiasis, most likely because trimethoprim-sulfamethoxazole, which is used to treat and prevent PCP, is effective against *I. belli.*

PATHOGENESIS. Oocysts from *I. belli* are shed in the stool of human or animal hosts. Infection occurs through the ingestion of contaminated food or water or by accidental oral-fecal contact (Lindsay et al., 1997). Although infection is normally confined to the intestine in immunocompetent persons, in immunocompromised persons the organism causes chronic intestinal infection and in some instances results in disseminated extraintestinal infection (Heyworth, 1996; Lindsay et al., 1997).

CLINICAL MANIFESTATIONS. Clinical presentation of isosporiasis includes profuse, watery diarrhea, with the stool output usually averaging 8 to 10 bowel movements per day, steatorrhea, headache, fever, malaise, abdominal pain, vomiting, dehydration, and weight loss (Lindsay et al., 1997; Peterson & Wofsy, 1994). Acalculous cholecystitis and reactive arthritis have been reported as complications of AIDS-related isosporiasis (Benator et al., 1994; Gonzales-Dominguez et al., 1994).

DIAGNOSIS. Diagnosis of isosporiasis is made by identification of the oocysts in fecal specimens. Several specimens, as well as specimen-concentration techniques, may be required for diagnosis, since *Isospora* oocysts may be shed only intermittently and in small numbers (Sears, 1995). Pape and colleagues (1989) recommend that a minimum of four stool examinations be performed for patients with AIDS and chronic diarrhea. A rapid autoflourescence technique shows promise as a means of making a more rapid and reliable diagnosis of isosporiasis (Berlin et al., 1996).

TREATMENT. The effective treatment of isosporiasis in people with HIV is a 7- to 10-day course of trimethoprim-sulfamethoxazole (TMP-SMZ) (Gellin & Soave, 1992; Pape et al., 1989). For prevention of relapse, chronic suppressive therapy with TMP-SMZ or sulfadoxine-pyrimethamine can be prescribed; pyrimethamine can be prescribed for persons who are allergic to sulfonamides (Gellin & Soave, 1992; Pape et al., 1989). Other agents that have been used to treat isosporiasis include pyrimethamine plus sulfadiazine, albendazole plus ornidazole, roxithromycin, metronidazole, quinacrine, and nitrofurantoin (Dionisio et al., 1996; Ebrahimzadeh & Bottone, 1996; Gellin & Soave, 1992).

PREVENTION. Chemoprophylaxis for isosporiasis is not recommended. The illness is relatively rare in persons with AIDS and is easily treated. Although no specific water or food precautions are recommended by the United States Public Health Service, it is reasonable to recommend avoidance of sexual practices that may lead to ingestion of fecal matter. Proper hand-washing and the use of gloves during activities that involve contact with human or animal feces are advisable for prevention of isosporiasis as well as other intestinal parasitic infections.

KAPOSI'S SARCOMA

EPIDEMIOLOGY. Variations in the epidemiologic patterns, clinical manifestation, and course of Kaposi's sarcoma (KS) are classified as four types: (1) classic, or non-HIV-related, KS; (2) African, or endemic, KS; (3) KS associated with iatrogenic immunosuppression, sometimes referred to as renal transplant KS; and (4) epidemic, or HIV-related, KS (Friedman-Kien et al., 1989). The most notable characteristics that distinguish epidemic, or HIV-related, KS from the other three types are its fulminant, widely disseminated course and shorter survival. The histopathologic features of KS are essentially the same for all four variations (Friedman-Kien et al., 1989). The following discussion is limited to the HIV-related, or epidemic, form of KS.

Kaposi's sarcoma is the most common cancer, occurring in about 10% of patients with AIDS (Cooley et al., 1996). In more recent years a decrease in the number of cases of KS among HIV-infected patients has been noted (Safai & Dias, 1994). Safer sexual practices, a change in environmental cofactors, and improved antiretroviral therapy may account for the decline in KS. Factors that contribute to longer survival of patients with KS include KS as the only manifestation of

AIDS, male gender, younger age, homosexuality, bisexuality, and white race (Safai & Dias, 1994). KS is reported to occur in only 1% or fewer of American women. However, in a study of women who attended clinic at a Boston city hospital, Cooley and colleagues (1996) found an incidence of KS of 3.6% among women. In addition, 42% had a risk behavior of sexual contact with bisexual men, which has been noted as a strong correlation between KS and women. However, a significant number were foreign-born women. Although women presented with more advanced KS than men, they were comparable to men in tumor response rates to therapy and toxicity profiles.

PATHOGENESIS. In 1994 Chang and colleagues reported the discovery of a new human herpesvirus that they found present in AIDS-associated KS lesions. The virus has been termed Kaposi's sarcoma-associated herpesvirus (KSHV) and human herpesvirus-8 (HHV-8). KSHV/HHV-8 belongs to the subfamily Gammaherpesvirinae, which also includes Epstein-Barr virus and herpesvirus saimiri, two lymphotropic herpesviruses (Monini et al., 1996). More recent studies focus on the incidence of KSHV/HHV-8 in both the HIV-infected and the noninfected populations and in patients with KS.

Multiple studies identify the presence of KSHV/HHV-8 in all four epidemiologic forms of KS (Boshoff et al., 1997; Friedman-Kien et al., 1996; Ganem, 1997; Huang et al., 1997; Williams et al., 1997). Lennette and colleagues (1996) conducted an extensive serosurvey and determined that HHV-8 infects the general population worldwide with an infectivity profile similar to herpes simplex virus type 2. Seroprevalence rates were 2% to 8% in children, which is consistent with the cases of KS in African and European children. They found that 20% to 30% of adults were infected with HHV-8. The highest rate of infection was in HIV-seropositive men. The presence of HHV-8 in children suggests a nonsexual route of transmission.

Several studies have determined that in most patients with KS, seroconversion to positivity for antibodies against KSHV/HHV-8–related nuclear antigens occurs before the clinical appearance of KS, suggesting a viral reactivation from a primary infection (Gao et al., 1996; Kedes &

Ganen, 1997; Monini et al., 1996). A number of factors may contribute to reactivation: immunostimulation, immunosuppression, contact with other infectious agents, and genetic, behavioral, or environmental conditions.

KSHV/HHV-8 has been shown to infect vasoformative spindle cells and mononuclear cells, resulting in the formation of intranuclear inclusions (Kedes & Ganen, 1997; Orenstein et al., 1997). Histologically, KS tumors include interweaving bands of spindle cells and vascular structures embedded in a network of collagen and reticular fibers (Safai & Dias, 1994).

CLINICAL PRESENTATION. KS is generally manifested with single or multiple pink, red, or violaceous macular papules or nodules that are nonblanching, painless, nonpruritic, and palpable (Heyer et al., 1990; Safai & Dias, 1994). Discrete patch-stage lesions appear early in some persons and may be mistaken for bruises, purpura, or diffuse cutaneous hemorrhages (Friedman-Kien et al., 1989). The patches can then form plaques and eventually coalesce and form nodular tumors. New multifocal lesions may appear at any time, and characteristic sites include the tip of the nose, eyelid, hard palate, posterior pharynx, glans penis, thigh, and sole of the foot (Heyer et al., 1990). Although rare, the skin over the tumors can break down, with bleeding, necrosis, and pain. Lymphatic involvement can lead to lymphatic obstruction, resulting in lymphedema of the face, penis, scrotum, and lower extremities. The fluid collected is usually firm and nonpitting (Heyer et al., 1990).

AIDS-KS frequently involves extracutaneous sites, such as the mucous membranes, GI tract, lung, liver, spleen, adrenal gland, pancreas, and testis (Safai & Dias, 1994). The most common extracutaneous site is the GI tract, although it is often clinically inapparent. Pulmonary KS may present with dyspnea, hemoptysis, or both and may be difficult to distinguish clinically and radiologically from *P. carinii* pneumonia.

DIAGNOSIS. Many clinicians state that KS lesions are readily recognized and the CDC revised definition of AIDS in 1987 included the presumptive diagnosis of KS (based on the characteristic gross appearance of any erythematous or violaceous plaquelike lesion on skin or mucous membrane). However, numerous mucocutaneous lesions that are manifestations of other conditions can be easily confused with epidemic KS. The CDC (1987, 1992a) has cautioned clinicians against making a presumptive diagnosis if they have seen only a few cases of epidemic KS. In addition, a presumptive diagnosis should be made only when laboratory evidence supports the diagnosis of HIV infection, because KS in homosexual men who are at risk of HIV infection but who are HIV-seronegative has been reported (Bowden et al., 1991; Friedman-Kien et al., 1989). Definitive diagnosis is by punch biopsy of an accessible cutaneous lesion that can establish a histologic diagnosis. A definitive diagnosis is usually required before treatment with chemotherapeutic agents or radiation is started.

In 1989 the Oncology Subcommittee of the AIDS Clinical Trials Group, sponsored by the National Institutes of Health, proposed a staging classification based on tumor bulk, immune function, and the presence of systemic illness (Krown et al., 1989). This system essentially predicts a favorable prognosis for persons with (1) tumors confined to skin or lymph nodes or with minimal oral disease, (2) CD4+ T-cell counts of more than $200/mm^3$, (3) no history of thrush, OI, or constitutional symptoms, and (4) a Karnofsky performance status score of 70 or higher. Poor prognosis is associated with (1) tumor-related edema or extensive ulceration of the viscera, (2) a CD4+ cell count of less than $200/mm^3$, (3) a history of thrush, OIs, or neurologic or constitutional disease, and (4) a Karnofsky performances status score of less than 70. Krown and colleagues (1997) have recently reevaluated this staging system and find it valid with the modification of CD4+ cell count of $150/mm^3$. Additional changes may be required by the inclusion of other variables such as viral load, markers of immune activation, or more specific poor-risk tumor features.

TREATMENT. When treatment options are evaluated, many factors must be considered, including the extent and location of lesions, the presence of KS-related symptoms (pain, edema, cough, GI tract bleeding), and the stage of HIV infection. Patients with a CD4+ cell count greater than $200/mm^3$ and no HIV-related symptoms have a better prognosis.

Cosmetically unacceptable small lesions can be treated with localized radiation, cryotherapy, laser therapy, and intralesional therapy with vinblastine or interferon alfa. Radiation therapy is also used to alleviate pain and edema from obstructive tumors.

For persons with rapidly progressive disease or advanced, widespread symptomatic disease, systemic therapy with antineoplastic agents may be appropriate. Single or combination agents used for systemic therapy include bleomycin, doxorubicin, etoposide, vinblastine, vincristine, and mitoxantrone. Numerous studies have evaluated the effectiveness of liposomal doxorubicin in the treatment of KS and have found the drug to be effective in the long-term, single-agent treatment of AIDS-related KS (Esser et al., 1996; Girard et al., 1996; Masood et al., 1996; Medve et al., 1997; Northfelt et al., 1997).

Physical therapy should be considered for persons who manifest mobility problems related to KS of the lower extremities. Patients with pedal lesions, especially on the sole of the foot, will limit weight-bearing activity and may benefit from such assist devices as a cane, crutches, or a walker (Galantino & Levy, 1988; LeCocq, 1995). Skin lesions surrounding joints may limit physical activity and result in contractures, edema, and loss of independence in performing activities of daily living (McDowell, 1992). In some instances, this may be due to fear of moving a joint over which KS lesions have developed. Maintaining mobility in the person with KS on the extremities can also decrease dependence in personal care.

With strong evidence supporting the role of KSHV/HHV8 as the etiologic agent for KS, researchers are evaluating the effectiveness of antiherpesvirus therapy and the risk of developing KS. Mocroft and colleagues (1996) studied patients receiving foscarnet, ganciclovir, and acyclovir and determined that both foscarnet and ganciclovir might have some activity in preventing KS, whereas acyclovir was of no benefit. With the advent of protease inhibitors and combination therapy for HIV infection, indications are that there may be regression of KS after significant increases in CD4+ counts (Little et al., 1997; Routy et al., 1997; Workman et al., 1996).

PREVENTION. With increasing evidence that KS may be associated with an oncogenic virus that may be sexually transmitted, it is advisable to re-inforce safer sex practices to prevent transmission.

NON-HODGKIN'S LYMPHOMA

EPIDEMIOLOGY.

Although non-Hodgkin's lymphoma (NHL) may develop in persons with and without HIV infection, the incidence of NHL among those with AIDS is much higher than in the general population. Ragni and colleagues (1993) showed a 29-fold increase in the risk of NHL among hemophiliac patients with AIDS compared with hemophiliac patients without HIV infection. NHL is frequently the initial AIDS-defining diagnosis, and the incidence appears similar in several epidemiologic studies. NHL was the initial AIDS-defining illness in 3.5% of patients with AIDS in a European series and 3.7% among persons with AIDS in the United States (Pedersen et al., 1995; Ward & Fleming, 1993). NHL may develop after patients present with another AIDS-defining illness, and in one study the rate of NHL among persons with AIDS was 2.4 per 100 patient-years (Ward & Fleming, 1993).

NHL occurs in all populations of persons with AIDS, regardless of the mode of HIV transmission. Several studies, however, have suggested a modest increase in incidence among men who have sex with men compared with other persons with HIV/AIDS (Cote et al., 1996; Serraino et al., 1992; Ward & Fleming, 1993). In contrast, Pedersen and colleagues (1995) found a slightly higher incidence of NHL among injecting drug users than among men who have sex with men. White race and increasing age have also been associated with increased risk of developing AIDS-related NHL (Cote et al., 1996; Pedersen et al., 1995; Ragni et al., 1993; Serriano et al., 1992; Ward & Fleming, 1993).

PATHOGENESIS.

Lymphomas are cancers of the immune system and begin with abnormal growth of lymph tissue cells, which spreads to other organs. Although AIDS-related NHL can originate as a malignancy of T cells, the vast majority occur as B lymphocyte malignant neoplasms. The NHLs are a heterogeneous group of malignancies that range from indolent to fulminant in their course (Jacobsen, 1997). Pathologic and morphologic characteristics are used to classify NHLs as low-grade, intermediate-grade, and high-grade lymphomas.

The brain is a common site of involvement, and in one series cerebral lymphoma represented 43% of all AIDS-related lymphomas (Schlacht et al., 1994). In persons with HIV disease, 80% to 90% of the NHL is extranodal, making lymph node–based NHL tumors uncommon. Extranodal disease commonly occurs in the GI tract, the liver, and the bone marrow (Levine, 1992). Other sites of NHL in persons with AIDS include the gallbladder, orbit, jaw, rectum, earlobe, popliteal fossa, heart, lung, skin, pancreas, subcutaneous and soft tissue, epidural spaces, appendix, gingiva, parotid gland, and paranasal sinuses (Levine, 1992).

Two herpesviruses, EBV and HHV-8, potentially play a role in the pathogenesis of AIDS-related NHL. Several investigators have examined pathologic tissue from patients with AIDS-related NHL for the presence of EBV DNA. Morgello (1992) found EBV DNA in 50% of cases of AIDS-related NHL. Levine and colleagues (1992) found EBV DNA in 68% of AIDS-related NHL but only in 15% on non-HIV lymphoma. HHV8 is associated with a particular form of lymphoma, body cavity–based lymphoma (BCBL), which presents as lymphomatous effusions without evidence of a solid tumor. Several studies have found that a high proportion of BCBL cells contain HHV8 DNA (Biberfeld et al., 1996; Carbone et al., 1996; Gessain et al., 1997; Nador et al., 1996).

CLINICAL PRESENTATION.

Approximately 74% of patients with AIDS-related NHL present with nonspecific symptoms of unexplained fever, weight loss, and drenching night sweats (Levine, 1992). Elevations in the serum lactate dehydrogenase level are also common. Depending on the location of the tumor, patients may present with localizing symptoms. NHL of the brain commonly presents with focal neurologic deficits such as hemiparesis, mental status changes, seizures, or headache (Hazard et al., 1996; Rubio et al., 1996). Lymphoma of the GI tract presents with abdominal pain or tenderness, weight loss, or gastrointestinal bleeding (Beck et al., 1996; Capell & Bostros, 1994). Unusual manifestations of small-bowel lymphoma include obstructive jaundice and small-bowel intussusception (Danin et al.,

1992; Schoeppner et al., 1995). The lungs and pleura are also common sites of NHL.

DIAGNOSIS. The definitive diagnosis of NHL is established with the pathologic examination of biopsy specimens or resected tissue or the cytologic examination of tissue fluid. Noninvasive radiographic imaging is helpful in localizing lymphomatous masses and guiding diagnostic biopsies. Abdominal CT scans of the abdomen commonly show enlargement of abdominal lymph nodes or extranodal masses (Radin et al., 1993). With thoracic lymphoma, CT scans of the chest may show pleural effusions, lung nodules, axillary adenopathy, or interstitial lung disease (Sider & Melany, 1993). On CT scan, brain lymphomas appear as low-density, contrast-enhancing mass lesions, usually with surrounding edema (Rubio et al., 1996).

Lymphoma must be differentiated from infection, since infectious processes often present as tissue masses or effusions. Methods of obtaining specimens to establish a diagnosis include surgical biopsy or needle aspiration of tissue fluid. For cerebral lymphoma, stereotactic biopsies reveal the cause of brain masses in a high percentage of cases (Iacoangeli et al., 1994). Because of reluctance to subject patients to a brain biopsy, a 2-week trial of empiric antitoxoplasmosis therapy is often attempted and brain biopsy is reserved for patients whose lesions do not decrease in size with therapy for toxoplasmosis. The search for noninvasive methods to differentiate CNS lymphoma from infection has led to the investigation of nuclear scanning techniques. Both single-positron emission computed tomography (SPECT) and positron emission tomography (PET) have shown a high degree of sensitivity and specificity for the diagnosis of cerebral malignant lesions in persons with AIDS (Hoffman et al., 1993; Lorberboym et al., 1996; O'Malley et al., 1994; Pierce et al., 1995; Ruiz et al., 1994).

TREATMENT. CNS lymphoma is generally treated with radiation. Although the tumors often respond, survival is poor, with a mean length of survival of only 3 months (Ling et al., 1994). Combined-modality treatment of CNS lymphoma with both systemic chemotherapy and radiotherapy is being studied for its potential to improve survival in AIDS-related NHL of the CNS (Forsyth et al., 1994; Levine et al; 1996a). Chamberlain and Dirr (1993) report limited success in treating lymphomatous meningitis with combined radiotherapy and intraventricular chemotherapy administered through an Ommaya reservoir.

Disease outside the CNS is generally treated with combination chemotherapy. Although published clinical trials of various chemotherapeutic regimens have reported some degree of success, there currently is no standard treatment regimen. Chemotherapy may be detrimental to the immune system and may accelerate the course of HIV disease (Gisselbrecht et al., 1993; Sawka et al., 1992; Schuman et al., 1995; Sparano et al., 1994). Sparano and colleagues (1996) showed that chemotherapy for AIDS-related NHL was associated with a progressive decline in the CD4+ cell count and a twofold increase in the incidence of OIs.

Neutropenia due to chemotherapy increases the risk of bacterial and fungal infections. Administration of colony-stimulating factors (CSFs), such as G-CSF and granulocyte-macrophage colony-stimulating factor (GM-CSF), which increase the number of circulating neutrophils, along with chemotherapy has shown some effectiveness in reducing complications related to chemotherapy-induced neutropenia (Newell et al., 1996; Tirelli et al., 1993; Walsh et al., 1993). Another approach to decreasing chemotherapy neutropenia is the use of agents that have a less suppressive effect on the bone marrow. Mitoguazone (MGBG) is effective against NHL and may be less myelosuppressive than other agents (Levine et al., 1997).

Antiretroviral agents may enhance the clinical response to chemotherapy and may have some antineoplastic activity. Both zidovudine and zalcitabine have shown promise as adjuvant agents when combined with chemotherapy (Levine et al., 1996b; Tirelli et al., 1992; Tosi et al., 1997). Successful treatment with combined chemotherapy, antiretroviral therapy, and G-CSF has also been reported (Gabarre et al., 1995; Sparano et al., 1996).

PREVENTION. There are currently no recommendations that can be made regarding primary prevention of NHL in HIV-infected persons, and the key to improved outcome remains early diagnosis. Neurologic changes or unexplained abdominal pain should prompt imaging studies such as CT or MRI scanning. Rapid enlargement of a peripheral lymph node should be evaluated by means of tissue biopsy. Fever of unknown origin or an unexplained elevation in the serum lactate dehydrogenase level should raise the clinical suspicion of occult lymphoma.

MYCOBACTERIUM AVIUM-INTRACELLULARE COMPLEX DISEASE

EPIDEMIOLOGY. *Mycobacterium avium-intracellulare* complex (MAC) disease is caused by two closely related organisms, *Mycobacterium avium* and *Mycobacterium intracellulare* (Peloquin, 1993). These organisms are classified as "atypical" mycobacteria, which often must be distinguished from *Mycobacterium tuberculosis* (TB). Like other atypical mycobacteria and like TB, MAC stains positively with acid-fast preparations, and is therefore grouped with the acid-fast bacilli (AFB). The organisms exist in soil, water, and foodstuffs such as eggs and unpasteurized dairy products. Infection is acquired from the environment, and person-to-person transmission most likely does not occur (Havlir & Ellner, 1995). Von Reyn and colleagues (1994) have implicated contamination of drinking water systems as a source of MAC infection.

Before the AIDS epidemic, *M. avium* was recognized as a cause of pulmonary infection, primarily in persons with preexisting chronic lung disease (Peloquin, 1993). Disseminated disease due to MAC is a frequent cause of mortality and morbidity in persons with advanced AIDS, and the incidence of disseminated MAC (dMAC) in persons with AIDS has increased since the late 1980s, presumably as a result of longer survival of patients who are given prophylaxis against *Pneumocystis carinii* pneumonia (PCP). Studies have shown a doubling in the incidence of dMAC since the introduction of PCP prophylaxis (Dore et al., 1996; Hoover et al., 1993). The risk of dMAC rises sharply with decreasing cell-mediated immunity, and the disease is rare in patients with CD4+ T-cell counts above 100/mm^3 (Horsburgh, 1991). Gastric hypochlorhydria has been implicated as a risk factor for the development of dMAC (Koch et al., 1996).

PATHOGENESIS. MAC is acquired orally or inhaled, resulting in local colonization of the GI or respiratory tract. Although colonization with MAC is often asymptomatic, local involvement may be clinically apparent; e.g., intestinal involvement may be a cause of diarrhea or pneumonia as a manifestation of pulmonary infection (Ruf et al., 1990). Although the clinical significance of asymptomatic colonization with MAC may be debated, rapid dissemination after local colonization has been reported (Gori et al., 1996). Disseminated disease usually involves the blood and the reticuloendothelial system, including the lymph nodes, spleen, liver, and bone marrow (Horsburgh, 1991). There have been reported cases of MAC infection in the eye, brain, meninges, skin, tongue, heart, stomach, thyroid, breast, parathyroid, adrenal glands, kidney, pancreas, prostate gland, testis, and urinary tract (Horsburgh, 1991; Klatt et al., 1987; Pitchenik & Fertel, 1992; Wallace & Hannah, 1988).

CLINICAL MANIFESTATIONS. Patients with dMAC usually present with constitutional signs and symptoms that include a high, unremitting fever without any obvious sign of local infection, night sweats, weight loss, and debilitation (Chaisson et al., 1992; Hawkins et al., 1986; Modilevsky et al., 1989; Wallace & Hannah, 1988). In persons with HIV infection with a fever of unknown origin and low CD4+ T-cell counts, dMAC should always be included in the differential diagnosis. Bone marrow involvement may cause anemia, neutropenia, or pancytopenia. Intestinal malabsorption and diarrhea can occur as a consequence of intestinal involvement, and abdominal lymph node infection may be manifest as abdominal pain. Rarer manifestations of local involvement with MAC include pneumonia, arthritis, skin lesions, pericarditis, meningitis, endophthalmitis, and osteomyelitis (Pitchenik & Fertel, 1992).

DIAGNOSIS. The diagnosis of dMAC is made by culturing the organism from normally sterile sites, such as blood, bone marrow, or lymph nodes (CDC, 1992a; Klatt et al., 1987; Wallace & Hannah, 1988). *M. avium* does not grow in ordinary blood culture media, and special culture media and techniques must be used. Blood cultures are at least as sensitive as bone marrow cultures, but morphologic examination of bone marrow biopsy specimens can provide an earlier diagnosis by demonstrating granulomas or acid-fast organisms (Rademacher et al., 1995). When organisms first grow, they initially can be determined only to be "acid-fast." Further biochemical testing to distinguish MAC from TB or other acid-fast organisms can take between 3 and 12 weeks (Bull & Shanson, 1992). Gene probe techniques, which are now becoming widely used, can reduce this time significantly. Bull and Shanson (1992) report that a chemiluminescent gene probe, which can distinguish accurately between TB and MAC, can be performed in 1 hour.

TREATMENT. Before the recent introduction of macrolide agents (clarithromycin and azithromycin), the response to therapy for dMAC was poor, although some success was reported with regimens containing rifampin, clofazimine, ethambutol, or rifampin plus either ciprofloxacin or amikacin (Chiu et al., 1990; Kemper et al., 1992). The introduction of the macrolides has greatly improved survival of patients with dMAC (Ives et al., 1995). Clarithromycin is highly effective at decreasing MAC bacteremia, but resistant organisms emerge when this agent is used for monotherapy, and multidrug therapy is required for ongoing success (Chaisson et al., 1994).

CDC recommendations for the treatment of AIDS-related dMAC include either clarithromycin or azithromycin plus one to three other agents, such as ethambutol, rifabutin, ciprofloxacin, clofazimine, or amikacin (CDC, 1993a). Recent large multicenter trials have focused on determining the best regimen for dMAC. The combination of ethambutol and clarithromycin has been shown to be more effective than a triple combination of ethambutol, clarithromycin, and clofazimine (the use of clofazimine was associated with increased mortality) (Chaisson et al., 1996, 1997). A multicenter Canadian trial compared a three-drug regimen of clarythromycin, ethambutol, and rifabutin with a four-drug regimen of rifampin, ethambutol, clofazimine, and ciprofloxacin and noted an improved clearance of bacteremia and prolonged survival with the three-drug combination (Shafran et al., 1996).

Some patients with dMAC may continue to experience progressive weight loss and fevers despite antimycobacterial treatment. In two small, uncontrolled studies, the use of adjunctive corticosteroids was associated with decreased fever and increased body weight in patients with dMAC re-

fractory to antimicrobial therapy (Dorman & Sax, 1996; Wormser et al., 1994).

The hallmark of dMAC is profound fatigue, which is present in all patients. Management of the symptom of fatigue, which can have an enormous negative effect on the patient's activity level and often on his or her quality of life, unfortunately is overlooked by many clinicians. Primary care providers should consider requesting a physical therapy consult to teach the patient energy-conserving strategies and how to develop a graduated program of energy-enhancing activities to increase endurance (DeBolt et al., 1996).

PREVENTION. Because of its ubiquitous presence in the environment, it is not possible to prevent exposure to the organism, and primary chemoprophylaxis is the principal means of preventing disease caused by MAC. (See Chapter 5, Table 5–7, for primary prophylaxis and Table 6–1 for secondary prophylaxis recommendations.)

Clinicians should be aware that a significant drug interaction exists between protease inhibitors and rifabutin. If a patient requires concurrent treatment with both a protease inhibitor and rifabutin, the drug of choice is nelfinavir or indinavir, and the dose of rifabutin should be reduced by one half (CDC, 1997c).

MYCOBACTERIAL TUBERCULOSIS

EPIDEMIOLOGY. An estimated 1.7 billion persons, one third of the world's population, are infected with *Mycobacterium tuberculosis,* resulting in 8 million new cases of tuberculosis (TB) and 2.9 million deaths annually (Barnes & Barrows, 1993; Pablos-Méndez et al., 1996). The number of cases of TB reported annually in the United States decreased steadily from 1954 to 1983; then the trend reversed dramatically, with the incidence increasing to an annual incidence of 8.7 per 100,000 persons in 1995 (Barnes & Barrows, 1993; Markowitz et al., 1997). However, a decrease in TB cases was reported for 1993 and 1994 as a result of enhanced TB control measures (Jones et al., 1996). The increase in cases of TB correlates with minority racial/ethnic groups, the 25- to 44-year age group, and large urban areas. The increase in persons 25 to 44 years of age is believed to be attributable to the high incidence of HIV infection in this age group (Jones et al.,

1996). TB is not evenly distributed throughout all segments of the United States. Although New York City represents 3% of the nation's population, it accounts for the highest incidence of TB in the United States (Jones et al., 1996; Markowitz et al., 1997).

HIV infection has contributed to the resurgence of TB. Persons with HIV infection are susceptible to reactivation of latent TB infection and progressive primary TB infection (Barnes & Barrows, 1993; Jones et al., 1996; Markowitz et al., 1997). Additional factors that have contributed to the resurgence of TB in the United States include poverty, homelessness, crowded living conditions, immigration from countries with a high incidence of TB infection, injecting drug use, and the dismantling of the national TB control program (Jones et al., 1996; Pablos-Méndez et al., 1996).

With the increasing number of tuberculosis cases, large outbreaks of multiple-drug-resistant TB (MDR TB) have been reported (Edlin et al., 1992; Fischl et al., 1992; Frieden et al., 1993; Pearsen et al., 1992). The principal causes of MDR TB are thought to be attributed to the ingestion of single antituberculosis agents for prolonged periods or to erratic compliance with therapy (Barnes & Barrows, 1993). The majority of patients reported with MDR TB are infected with HIV, and nearly all of the patients have organisms that are resistant to both isoniazid and rifampin. An outbreak of MDR TB in New York City involved one strain that was resistant to at least six and usually seven antituberculosis agents (Frieden et al., 1996). Many of the outbreaks of MDR TB have been associated with nosocomial transmission, affecting health care workers as well as patients. Factors contributing to these outbreaks include (1) delayed diagnosis of TB, (2) delayed recognition that the TB was in fact MDR TB, with resultant prolonged ineffective therapy and prolonged periods of infectiousness, (3) delayed initiation and adequate duration of TB isolation, (4) inadequate ventilation in TB isolation rooms, (5) lapses in TB isolation practices, and (6) inadequate precautions for cough-inducing procedures (Barnes & Barrows, 1993; Barnes et al., 1996). Carey and colleagues (1996) found that MDR TB was more prevalent in men, injecting drug users, and prisoners. The resurgence of TB has prompted federal, state, and local governments to redevelop effective tuberculosis-control programs. As a result of new programs, including directly observed therapy, New York City saw a decline of 21% in the number of new cases of TB and a 60% decline in multidrug isolates from 1992 to 1994 (Pablos-Méndez et al., 1996).

PATHOGENESIS. TB is caused by inhalation of droplet nuclei of infectious particles that are aerosolized by coughing, sneezing, or talking. The droplet nuclei dry while airborne and can remain suspended in the air for long periods of time (Haas & Des Prez, 1995). Although the source of these infectious particles is usually pulmonary infection, cases of aerosolized transmission to health care workers during dressing changes of cutaneous lesions have been reported. Without adequate ventilation, particles may remain in a room even when the infected person is out of the room.

Infection occurs when a susceptible person inhales the droplet nuclei and they reach the alveoli of the lungs. Once in the alveoli, the organisms spread throughout the body. Usually within 2 to 10 weeks after initial infection, the immune response limits the multiplication and spread of the tubercle bacilli. However, some of the bacilli remain dormant and viable for many years. This is referred to as latent TB infection, and affected persons have positive results on a purified protein derivative (PPD) skin test. They have no symptoms of active TB (disease) and are not infectious. Among these persons, the estimated lifetime risk of the development of active TB is approximately 5% to 10% (Barnes et al., 1991; Shafer, 1994). Progressive primary TB occurs when mycobacterial replication cannot be controlled by the body's immune system. In approximately 5% of persons who are HIV-negative and infected with TB, clinical disease will develop within the first 2 years after exposure (Shafer, 1994).

Persons infected with HIV are particularly susceptible to reactivation of latent TB infection and progressive primary TB infection. In some HIV-seropositive populations it is estimated that there is a 1000-fold higher rate of TB than in the general population (Markowitz et al., 1997). Extrapulmonary TB develops in as many as 70% of HIV-infected persons. It is estimated that in 37% of HIV-infected persons primary TB develops within 5 months of exposure (Barnes & Barrows, 1993). Other studies support the finding that in one third to two thirds of HIV-infected persons primary TB develops rather than reactivation of latent TB (Barnes et al., 1996; Carey et al., 1996; Frieden et al., 1996). In addition, 10% of those HIV-infected persons with a positive tuberculin skin test from a previous exposure will develop TB.

TB in persons with HIV infection depresses the CD4+ T-cell count and raises the viral load. It has been shown that in patients with TB, the HIV RNA copies per cubic millimeter of plasma increase up to 160-fold during the acute stage of TB (Ellner, 1997; Goletti et al., 1996). Ellner and colleagues (1997) found that TB in persons with HIV infection was associated with shortened survival. Death was not attributable to TB but to advancing immunodeficiency despite antituberculosis treatment. The CD4+ lymphocyte count, which is the best predictor of disease progression, remained suppressed while TB was being treated.

CLINICAL PRESENTATION. Clinically apparent TB can precede, coincide with, or follow a diagnosis of AIDS. Consistent with the nature of clinical problems associated with HIV disease, the clinical features vary with the degree of immunosuppression; the more severe the CD4+ lymphopenia, the more atypical the clinical presentation (Haas & Des Prez, 1995).

Fever, weight loss, night sweats, and fatigue may be the initial complaints, but these symptoms, along with lymphadenopathy, are present in other diseases associated with HIV disease. Whereas dyspnea, chills, hemoptysis, and chest pain may occur with pulmonary TB infection, extrapulmonary disease occurs in 40% to 75% of persons with a dual diagnosis of HIV disease and TB (Barnes & Barrows, 1993; Haas & Des Prez, 1995; Shafer, 1994). It is common for persons with HIV infection to have both pulmonary and extrapulmonary TB (Haas & Des Prez, 1995; Shafer, 1994). Extrapulmonary sites or fluids that may show evidence of TB in HIV-infected persons include lymph nodes, bones, joints, bone marrow, liver, spleen, cerebrospinal fluid, skin, gastrointestinal mucosa, CNS, mass lesions (tuberculoma), urine, and blood or TB bacteremia (Jacobson, 1992).

DIAGNOSIS. Persons with HIV infection may have suppressed reactions to tuberculin skin test-ing because of anergy, especially with low CD4+ T-cell counts. In the presence of anergy, they will have a negative tuberculin skin test result, regardless of whether they are infected with *M. tuberculosis*. It is no longer recommended that anergy testing be done in conjunction with PPD testing (CDC, 1997d). According to current CDC recommendations, any person with HIV infection who has a PPD test result of 5 mm or more induration is considered to have a positive PPD and should be evaluated for tuberculosis (CDC, 1989; CDC, 1997c, 1997d). If there is no history of prior positive PPD and treatment, and no evidence of active TB, 12 months of preventive therapy with isoniazid should be instituted.

TB should be suspected in any person with HIV infection who presents with unexplained fever, cough, pulmonary infiltrates, lymphadenopathy, meningitis, brain abscess, pericarditis, pleural effusions, or intraabdominal, musculoskeletal, or cutaneous abscesses (Shafer, 1994). The chest radiograph may show a classic reactivation TB pattern, an atypical pattern, or evidence of past TB infection.

Acid-fast smears and culture examination of three sputum specimens collected on different days are the main diagnostic tests for pulmonary TB. Sputum smears that fail to demonstrate acid-fast bacilli do not exclude the diagnosis of TB. In HIV-infected persons with pulmonary TB, the sensitivity of sputum examination is 40% to 67% and specimens grow *M. tuberculosis* in 74% to 95% of HIV-infected patients with TB (Shafer, 1994). With advanced HIV disease, sputum specimens for acid-fast bacilli may be negative more frequently because of severe immunosuppression resulting in a decrease of pulmonary cavitation.

Mycobacterial growth is tested with a liquid medium, Bactec. Bactec detects growth approximately 10 days before it would be seen on a solid medium (Haas & Des Prez, 1995; Shafer, 1994). After mycobacterium is grown from Bactec, a nucleic acid hybridization assay can determine the species within 1 day. Polymerase chain reaction (PCR), which can detect *M. tuberculosis* in clinical specimens more rapidly than the procedures currently being used, is being standardized and evaluated clinically (Haas & Des Prez, 1995; Losso et al., 1996; Shafer, 1994). With the increase in MDR TB, it is necessary to determine drug susceptibility. Bactec tests for susceptibility to isoniazid, rifampin, pyrazinamide, ethambutol, and streptomycin. It is also possible to identify individual strains of *M. tuberculosis* by molecular DNA fingerprinting techniques that allow for the tracking of TB outbreaks and the identification of the index case.

TREATMENT. Currently the CDC (1993b) recommends that a four-drug regimen with isoniazid, rifampin, pyrazinamide, and either streptomycin or ethambutol be used for initial empiric treatment of TB. When adherence with the regimen is assured, as with directly observed therapy (DOT), the four-drug regimen usually results in effective treatment and a rapid sputum conversion. The four-drug regimen can also be administered in a DOT program, either three times a week from the beginning of therapy or twice a week after a 2-week induction phase of daily therapy (CDC, 1993b). Patients who are treated with the four-drug regimen but who default on therapy are more likely to be cured without relapse than patients treated with a three-drug regimen (CDC, 1993b). Institutions, such as health care and correctional facilities, that have had outbreaks of MDR TB, or that are resuming treatment of a person with a prior history of anti-TB therapy, may need to use five- or six-drug regimens as initial therapy. With an alternative regimen in areas where the resistance to isoniazid occurs in fewer than 4% of the TB cases, the initial therapy may be limited to isoniazid, rifampin, and pyrazinamide (CDC, 1993b).

Drug-susceptibility testing should be performed on the first isolate of all persons with TB from whom *M. tuberculosis* has been isolated, and the results should be reported to the local health department. Drug-susceptibility testing will provide the basis for determination of the continuation phase of therapy and identify drug resistance. The treatment of patients with MDR TB should be determined in consultation with physicians who are experienced specialists in the treatment of MDR TB. Second-line medications that may be prescribed for treatment include ciprofloxacin, ofloxacin, kanamycin, amikacin, capreomycin, ethionamide, cycloserine, para-aminosalicylic acid, and clofazimine. Several studies have evaluated the effectiveness of a four- to five-drug regimen with the addition of levofloxacin in sus-

pected cases of MDR TB (El-Sadr et al., 1996; Telzak et al., 1997).

Treatment of HIV-infected persons should continue for a total of 9 months and for at least 6 months after sputum conversion (CDC, 1989). Regimens used for pulmonary TB and extrapulmonary TB are similar. However, therapy may be extended in cases of disseminated disease, miliary disease, disease involving the bones or joints, or tuberculous lymphadenitis. Treatment regimens for pregnant women should be adjusted because streptomycin may cause congenital deafness and because pyrazinamide teratogenicity has not been determined. Second-line medications that may not be safe during pregnancy include kanamycin, amikacin, capreomycin, ciprofloxacin, ofloxacin, ethionamide, cycloserine, pyrazinamide, and clofazimine (New York City Department of Health, 1996).

Mahmoudi and Iseman (1993) studied the records of 35 patients with MDR TB to identify medical mismanagement practices that deviated from established guidelines and determine the impact of these practices on the development of MDR TB and adverse medical sequelae. Medical mismanagement was detected in 80% of the cases, with an average of 3.93 errors noted per patient record. The most common errors were the addition of a single drug to a failing regimen, failure to identify preexisting or acquired drug resistance, initiation of an inadequate primary regimen, failure to identify and address noncompliance, and inappropriate isoniazid preventive therapy.

Special consideration should be given to the impact of HIV protease inhibitors on the treatment of HIV-infected patients with TB. For HIV-infected patients with drug-susceptible TB for whom protease-inhibitor therapy is being considered but has not been started, the suggested strategy is to complete TB treatment with a regimen containing rifampin before starting protease-inhibitor therapy (CDC, 1997e). There are three options for managing HIV-infected patients with TB who have already started protease-inhibitor therapy:

1. Discontinue protease-inhibitor therapy and complete a short course of TB treatment (minimum 6 months) and include rifampin.
2. Stop the protease inhibitor and use a four-drug regimen including rifampin (i.e., daily isoni-

azid, pyrazinamide, rifampin, and ethambutol or streptomycin) for a minimum of 2 months and until bacteriologic response is achieved; then continue with a modified regimen of isoniazid and ethambutol for 16 months and restart protease-inhibitor therapy.

3. Continue protease-inhibitor therapy with indinavir and substitute rifabutin for rifampin (CDC, 1997e).

PREVENTION. Chemoprophylaxis to prevent the development of active TB should be provided for HIV-infected persons or those likely to be at risk of HIV infection who refuse testing, who have a tuberculin skin test lesion at least 5 mm in diameter, who are close contacts of patients with infectious TB, who were untreated previously after a positive PPD test result, and whose chest x-ray films suggest previous untreated TB (CDC, 1997c,d). Preventive chemotherapy for this group consists of 12 months of INH. Chemoprophylaxis for persons exposed to MDR TB is a complex issue that should be determined by an expert medical consult; it will usually involve identification of the source patient so that the drug-susceptibility pattern can be evaluated.

Bacille Calmette-Guérin (BCG) is not routinely recommended for use in the United States. Although limited data suggest that the vaccine may be safe for use in HIV-infected, symptom-free children, it is not recommended for HIV-infected adults (CDC, 1997c).

PNEUMOCYSTOSIS

EPIDEMIOLOGY. *Pneumocystis carinii* is a ubiquitous organism that was originally classified as a protozoan, but new data suggest that *P. carinii* is more closely related to fungi (Sattler, 1994; Walzer, 1995). Studies have shown that *P. carinii* is probably transmitted by the airborne route and is possibly communicable (Walzer, 1995). Support for the communicability of *P. carinii* comes from reports of outbreaks among immunosuppressed patients who have had prolonged contact with each other. Questions exist as to whether *P. carinii* infections represent reactivations of latent infection or reinfection in an immunocompromised host (Keely et al., 1996; Wakefield, 1997; Walzer, 1995). Seroepidemiologic studies have indicated that the most healthy children have ac-

quired *P. carinii* infection at an early age (Sattler, 1994; Walzer, 1995).

P. carinii pneumonia (PCP) remains the most common AIDS-defining OI despite dramatic results of prophylaxis (Cohn et al., 1996; Huang et al., 1997). Since 1987 the incidence of PCP has decreased significantly. The decrease has been attributed to the introduction of antiretroviral therapy and the initiation of standard prophylactic strategies to prevent PCP. It is estimated that, without PCP prophylaxis, 75% of persons with HIV infection will have PCP during the course of their illness (Phair et al., 1990).

PATHOGENESIS. *P. carinii* is inhaled, escapes the defenses of the upper respiratory tract, and is deposited in the alveoli, where it maintains an extracellular existence. In an immunocompetent person, infection is suppressed by the normal host defense mechanisms and causes no observable damage. In immunocompromised persons, *P. carinii* proliferates and gradually fills the alveolar lumina. Eventually air sacs become completely filled with organisms. Increasing evidence suggests that alterations in pulmonary surfactant are linked to the pathophysiology of *P. carinii* infection, resulting in increased alveolar-arterial oxygen gradient and respiratory alkalosis (Sattler, 1994; Walzer, 1995). Persons with HIV infection are at greatest risk of *P. carinii* infection when they have a CD4+ lymphocyte count of less than $200/mm^3$, unexplained fever for 2 weeks or longer, or a history of oropharyngeal candidiasis (CDC, 1992a).

Extrapulmonary pneumocystosis, uncommon in the pre-AIDS era, is estimated to occur in 0.5% to 3% of patients with AIDS (Sattler, 1994; Walzer, 1995). Prophylaxis with aerosolized pentamidine and late stage of AIDS contribute to the development of extrapulmonary pneumocystosis. Reported sites of infection are the lymph nodes, spleen, liver, bone marrow, gastrointestinal tract, eyes, thyroid, adrenal, and kidneys (Walzer, 1995).

CLINICAL PRESENTATION. PCP develops over a period of 1 to 2 weeks, with shortness of breath, fever, and a nonproductive cough being the cardinal symptoms (Sattler, 1994; Walzer, 1995). Fever may be present for a shorter period of time than the cough or shortness of breath (Sattler, 1994). Left untreated, the cough may become productive, shortness of breath may be noted at rest, and chest tightness may be reported. Tachypnea and tachycardia are noted in patients who have more severe pneumonia. Rales are present in 30% to 40% of patients (Sattler, 1994). Signs indicative of severe immunocompromise, such as weight loss, fatigue, and candidiasis, may be present.

DIAGNOSIS. Radiographic findings usually reveal diffuse interstitial or alveolar infiltrates, or both, but atypical findings range from normal chest films to the presence of a localized infiltrate, nodule, cavity, or pneumothorax (Weinberger, 1993). Arterial blood gas studies may reveal hypoxemia, hypocapnia, and an increase in the alveolar-arterial oxygen gradient, especially with exercise (Sattler, 1994).

Definitive diagnosis of PCP is established with identification of *P. carinii* on microscopic examination. Specimens are usually obtained by induced sputum procedures or by bronchoscopy with bronchoalveolar lavage. Presumptive diagnosis can be made on the basis of

1. A history of dyspnea on exertion or a nonproductive cough of recent onset (within the past 3 months)
2. Chest x-ray evidence of diffuse bilateral interstitial infiltrates or gallium scan evidence of diffuse bilateral pulmonary disease
3. Arterial blood gas analysis showing an arterial oxygen tension of less than 70 mm Hg or a low respiratory diffusing capacity (less than 80% of predicted values)
4. No evidence of bacterial pneumonia (CDC, 1992a)

TREATMENT. The drug of choice for the treatment of PCP is either TMP-SMZ or pentamidine isethionate (Walzer, 1995). Other drug regimens are used when patients are intolerant of TMP-SMZ. Dapsone-trimethoprim, clindamycin-primaquine, and atovaquone have been studied and are used for the treatment of mild to moderate PCP (Safrin et al., 1996; Walzer, 1995; Wu et al., 1996) Trimetrexate glucuronate, which has antineoplastic and antifolate as well as antiprotozoal activities, is used to treat moderate to severe PCP (Voelker, 1994; Walzer, 1995).

Despite treatment, some patients experience a deterioration of their blood oxygenation. As a re-

sult of several studies, many clinicians recommend the use of corticosteroids during the first 72 hours of treatment for moderate to severe PCP. The severity of PCP is determined by an arterial pressure of <70 mm Hg or an alveolar-arterial gradient of >35 mm Hg (Walzer, 1995). Generally, the patient is given prednisone, 40 mg twice daily, and the dose is gradually tapered over a period of 20 days. There has been concern that the use of corticosteroids will increase the risk of tuberculosis or other AIDS-related diseases. However, Martos and colleagues (1995) determined that the short duration of corticosteroid therapy for PCP did not increase the risk of TB or other AIDS-related diseases.

PCP destroys lung tissue. Repeated bouts of PCP often leave the patient with a decrease in functioning lung surface area and mechanical problems in mobilizing secretions. This can be further intensified if there is some degree of obstructive lung disease (common in smokers). In addition to expectorants and bronchodilators, a physical therapy consult may benefit the patient. Chest physical therapy and teaching the patient how to perform postural drainage procedures can enhance removal of secretions as well as minimize the spread of pulmonary infiltrates (American Physical Therapy Association, 1997).

PREVENTION. Primary prophylaxis (to prevent an initial episode of PCP) is indicated for HIV-infected patients if there is a CD4+ cell count of less than 200/mm³, unexplained fever (>100° F) for 2 or more weeks, or a history of oropharyngeal candidiasis (see Chapter 5, Table 5–14). The CDC recommends TMP-SMZ as the preferred prophylactic agent. Studies have shown that TMP-SMZ provides the most effective protection against PCP, particularly in persons with a CD4+ cell count of less than 50/mm³ (Powderly, 1996). It is estimated that up to 80% to 90% of patients develop adverse reactions to TMP-SMZ. The reactions include fever, rash, neutropenia, thrombocytopenia, and hepatitis (Walzer, 1995). Because of the superior effectiveness of TMP-SMZ, studies have evaluated the effectiveness of TMP-SMZ desensitization (Beardsell et al., 1996; Kelly et al., 1996; Para et al., 1997). Protocols vary from beginning TMP-SMZ at very low doses and increasing the dose over varying lengths of time until full strength is reached to desensitizing only those persons who have reactions to full-dose TMP-SMZ therapy. In the event a patient is intolerant of TMP-SMZ, alternative therapies include dapsone, dapsone plus pyremethamine plus leucovorin, and aerolosized pentamidine administered by the Respirgard II nebulizer. The CDC does not recommend aerosolized pentamidine administered by other nebulization devices currently available, intermittently administered parenteral pentamidine, oral pyrimethamine/sulfadoxine, oral clindamycin plus primaquine, oral atovaquone, or intravenous trimetrexate. Secondary prophylaxis is an absolute necessity for patients with a history of PCP (see Table 6–1).

RECURRENT PNEUMONIA

EPIDEMIOLOGY. Selwyn and colleagues (1988) conducted the first prospective study of HIV-infected persons without AIDS. They studied a group of injecting drug users who were enrolled in a methadone treatment program and found a markedly increased incidence of bacterial pneumonia associated with HIV infection in injection drug users without AIDS. More recent studies support Selwyn's findings of a higher incidence of bacterial pneumonia in injecting drug users (Davenny et al., 1996; Hirschtick et al., 1995; Miller et al., 1994; Mitchell & Miller, 1995). It is believed that needle sharing, environmental conditions associated with exposure to respiratory pathogens, and cofactors such as heavy alcohol use and inadequate nutrition may predispose patients to bacterial pneumonia (Farizo et al., 1992).

Streptococcus pneumoniae and *Haemophilus influenzae* are the most common causes of bacterial pneumonia in persons with HIV infection (Baril et al., 1996; CDC, 1997c, Miller, 1994). These organisms are also the most frequent causes of community-acquired pneumonia in immunocompetent persons. Other causes of bacterial pneumonia in HIV-infected persons include *Moraxella catarrhalis, Klebsiella pneumoniae, Neisseria meningitidis, Rhodococcus, Escherichia coli, Escherichia faecium,* and *Chlamydia* species (Baril et al., 1996; Mitchell & Miller, 1995). *Staphylococcus aureus* is associated with a higher mortality rate in more immunosuppressed persons. Patients with AIDS and low CD4+ T-cell counts have been noted to have a pulmonary *Pseudomonas aeruginosa* infection that is indolent and relapsing

and resembles bronchopulmonary *P. aeruginosa* infection in patients with cystic fibrosis (Mitchell & Miller, 1995).

The AIDS Surveillance Data Project found that persons with a CD4+ T-cell count of less than 200/mm^3 had a five times greater chance of having one episode of bacterial pneumonia in a 12-month period than an HIV-infected person with a CD4+ T-cell count of more than 200/mm^3 (CDC, 1992a). In addition, the risk of having multiple episodes of bacterial pneumonia in a 12-month period is 20 times higher in the group with a lower CD4+ T-cell count (CDC, 1992a). Recurrent bacterial pneumonia as an AIDS-defining disease is defined as two or more episodes of bacterial pneumonia within 1 year, regardless of the CD4+ T-cell count.

PATHOGENESIS. Microorganisms that cause bacterial pneumonia reach the lungs by (1) direct inhalation of the organism, (2) aspiration of secretions from the mouth and nasopharynx, (3) spread by the blood to the lungs from another site, and (4) penetration of the lung tissue (Reynolds, 1991). As HIV infection progresses, it has an adverse effect on humoral immunity and B-cell function. Defects in B-cell function lead to failure to mount an effective antibody response to invading pathogens and can result in repeated episodes of bacterial pneumonia in the HIV-infected person. Community-acquired pneumonia generally occurs earlier in the course of HIV infection, and nosocomial infections are associated with higher morbidity and mortality rates.

CLINICAL PRESENTATION. The presentation of bacterial pneumonia in the person with HIV infection may differ from that in the immunocompetent person. There may be a more abrupt onset with fever, cough with purulent sputum, and systemic toxic effects. With pneumococcal pneumonia and a significantly decreased CD4+ cell count, there may be more bacteremia and empyema and a higher mortality rate. It is common to see concurrent bacterial pneumonia and PCP. Bacterial pneumonia may also be difficult to differentiate from PCP (Magnenat et al., 1991; Selwyn et al., 1992).

DIAGNOSIS. The chest radiograph is the first diagnostic procedure performed. In an immunocompetent person the chest radiograph frequently shows dense segmental or lobar consolidation. Chest radiographs are frequently atypical in patients with HIV infection and bacterial pneumonia. Atypical changes that may be seen are nodular patterns, consolidation, upper or lower lobe changes, cavities, or diffuse interstitial infiltrates (Mitchell & Miller, 1995).

Microscopic examination and culture of respiratory secretions continue to be used for the laboratory evaluation of pneumonia, despite questions about their sensitivity and specificity (American Thoracic Society, 1993; Donowitz & Mandell, 1995). If sputum is to be used for culture and sensitivity, the specimen should be obtained before antimicrobial therapy is instituted. More invasive procedures (e.g., sputum induction, bronchoscopy with bronchial-alveolar lavage) should be considered if

1. No sputum is produced.
2. There is no clear predominance of a potential pathogen on Gram stain or culture of sputum.
3. There has been a poor response to antibiotics chosen on the basis of expectorated sputum.
4. Gram-negative rods or yeast forms are found in the sputum.
5. There is a possibility of superinfection (Donowitz & Mandell, 1995).

TREATMENT. Empiric antimicrobial therapy should be started while the results of laboratory studies are pending. If a community-acquired organism is suspected, a drug active against *Streptococcus pneumoniae* and *Haemophilus influenzae* should be used. It may be possible to treat this type of pneumonia with oral antibiotic therapy on an outpatient basis.

A pneumonia that develops during hospitalization is probably caused by a gram-negative bacillus or *Staphylococcus aureus*. A broad-spectrum antibiotic should be given until the organism is identified. When results of cultures and sensitivity tests are available, the treatment can be changed to an antimicrobial agent appropriate for the identified organism. Additional treatment measures include fluids, antipyretic drugs, airway suction or postural drainage, and bronchodilators for bronchospasm (Reynolds, 1991).

Patients who have recurrent episodes of pneumonia may have problems mobilizing secretions,

especially if there is some degree of obstructive lung disease (common in smokers). In addition to expectorants and bronchodilators, a physical therapy consult may benefit the patient. Chest physical therapy, and teaching the patient how to sequence postural drainage procedures can enhance secretion removal as well as minimize the spread of pulmonary infiltrates (American Physical Therapy Association, 1997).

PREVENTION. Pneumococcal vaccination is recommended by the CDC for all adults as soon as possible after diagnosis of HIV infection (CDC, 1997c). Immunization appears to be beneficial regardless of CD4+ T-cell count (Currier & Feinberg, 1996). Since the incidence of *H. influenzae* type B infection in adults is low, the administration of *H. influenzae* type B vaccine is not generally recommended (CDC, 1997c). Studies have demonstrated the reduced incidence of community-acquired bacterial pneumonia among patients receiving TMP-SMZ prophylaxis for PCP (Hirschtick et al., 1995; Rimland et al., 1996; Tacconelli et al., 1997). The CDC (1997c) recommends that the added benefit of preventing bacterial pneumonia with TMP-SMZ be considered when the prophylactic agent for PCP is selected. In addition, the use of clarithromycin daily or azithromycin weekly for prophylaxis of MAC disease may also prevent bacterial pneumonia (CDC, 1997c).

PROGRESSIVE MULTIFOCAL LEUKOENCEPHALOPATHY

EPIDEMIOLOGY. The Papovaviridae is a family of DNA viruses that is named from the prefixes of papillomavirus, polyomavirus, and vacuolating virus. Papillomavirus, which is associated with infection of surface epithelia, produces benign tumors or warts. Polyomaviruses include three types: the JC virus (JCV), the BK virus (BKV) (both labeled with the initials of the names of the patients from whom they were first isolated), and simian virus 40 (SV40). JCV is associated with progressive multifocal leukoencephalopathy (PML), and BKV causes hemorrhagic cystitis in immunocompromised persons (Chaisson & Griffin, 1990). The SV40 virus, which causes asymptomatic latent infection in Asiatic macaques, was accidentally introduced into large numbers of persons immunized against the poliovirus between 1955 and 1961 but did not cause any identified diseases (Hansen et al., 1996).

Both JCV and BKV have a worldwide distribution and cause childhood infection without a recognized disease syndrome. By the age of 5 years, 10% of children have antibodies to JCV, which increases to between 69% and 90% in late adulthood. The incidence of BKV antibodies in adults is between 69% and 80% (Hansen et al., 1996). Before AIDS, PML was associated primarily with chronic lymphocytic leukemia and Hodgkin's disease; however, today it is most closely associated with HIV disease. It is estimated that approximately 4% of persons with AIDS have PML (Hansen et al., 1996).

PATHOGENESIS. The pathogenesis of PML is unknown, but several theories propose that PML results from (1) late primary infection, (2) reactivation of latent JCV in the brain, and (3) spread in relation to reactivated kidney infection (Hansen et al., 1996). The most widely supported theory is that after primary infection, the virus establishes a latent stage in the kidneys. With immunosuppression the JCV reactivates and is carried by lymphocytes to the CNS (Hansen et al., 1996). Autopsy studies using PCR have detected JCV-DNA in normal brain tissue in 30% to 68% of persons without PML. Other studies have found JCV-DNA in the peripheral blood of HIV-infected persons who do not exhibit symptoms of PML (Dubois et al., 1996; Dutronc et al., 1997). These results suggest there may be two JCV strains—one that establishes itself in the kidneys and a PML type in the brain (Hansen et al., 1996).

PML is a subacute demyelinating disease of the CNS that affects the subcortical white matter of the cerebrum, the gray matter, the deep layers of the cortex, and the corticomedullary transitional zone. The disease progresses rapidly and often leads to dementia, blindness, and paralysis; in most cases, it results in death within 4 to 6 months (Fong et al., 1995; Moreno et al., 1996).

CLINICAL PRESENTATION. Symptoms of confirmed PML include mental deficits, visual defects, motor weakness, lack of motor coordination, speech deficits, sensory deficits, headaches, vertigo, and seizures (Hansen et al., 1996).

Hansen and colleagues (1996) found hemiparesis to be the most frequent symptom at onset, followed by cognitive impairment, dysarthria, gait imbalance, headache, limb dystaxia, and quadrantanopia. The mean CD4+ T-cell count at the time of diagnosis of PML was found to be less than 90/mm^3 (Fong et al., 1995). For those patients with a CD4+ cell count of 90/mm^3 or more, survival was significantly longer.

DIAGNOSIS. Until recently, the diagnosis of PML was made by excluding other causes of focal brain lesions by means of CT scans and MRI that revealed diffuse lesions in the white matter without edema, contrast enhancement, or mass effect. The lesions may be multifocal or confluent. In some instances, the findings on CT scan may not be recognized or may show only moderate changes when the clinical symptoms are more extreme, and MRI may demonstrate variable findings with atypical features. A definitive diagnosis of PML was made by means of a brain biopsy, which revealed multiple patches of demyelination with numerous enlarged bizarre astrocytes (Kasner et al., 1997).

The development of the PCR has given clinicians the opportunity to diagnose PML on the basis of a positive JCV-DNA result in the CSF. Antinori and colleagues (1997) recommend a PCR for PML-DNA when a typical MRI pattern for PML is present. Other diagnostic strategies include magnetization transfer imaging (MTI), a technique that enables evaluation of the structural integrity of macromolecular structures. According to Kasner and associates (1997), MTI may aid in subcategorizing white matter abnormalities and may be of potential diagnostic benefit when applied to the demyelinating patches characteristic of PML.

If all tests are negative for PML, a brain biopsy should be considered. A small study found that brain biopsies entail little risk when performed by experienced neurosurgeons (Petit et al., 1996). Another retrospective study determined that CT-guided stereotactic brain biopsies are safe and diagnostically useful in HIV-infected persons (MacArthur et al., 1996).

TREATMENT. No form of therapy for PML has been efficacious. Attempted therapies have included vidarabine (adenine arabinoside), acyclovir, foscarnet, antiretrovirals, interferon-alfa, and cytarabine (Hansen et al., 1996; Moreno et al., 1996). Moreno and colleagues (1996) evaluated the effectiveness of cytarabine therapy for PML and concluded that, since the drug had no significant toxicity and clinical and radiologic signs of improvement had been observed in a some patients, cytarabine may be considered for patients with AIDS and PML. More recently there have been reports of clinical remissions in patients with PML who are receiving antiretroviral combination therapy that includes a protease inhibitor (Elliot et al., 1996; Henry et al., 1997; Power et al., 1997). The authors of those reports conclude that clinical improvement is a result of suppression of HIV replication, resulting in improved immune function.

In the presence of a progressively debilitating disease such as PML, physical therapy can teach formal and informal caregivers how to maintain functional activities and how to prevent complications. In the case of PML, loss of both motor and sensory functions can lead not only to contractures, decubiti, and pneumonia but also to preventable accidents (American Physical Therapy Association, 1997; Obbens & Galantino, 1992). The initial case assessment should be followed up with periodic visits to assess the progressive losses and determine the increasing need to teach care strategies and order assist devices.

PREVENTION. With the advent of antiretroviral therapy and protease inhibitors, the prognosis for persons with PML may improve. Currently, however, there are no recommended preventive measures for PML.

SALMONELLOSIS

EPIDEMIOLOGY. Salmonellae are gram-negative bacteria that can be pathogenic to both animals and humans. Salmonellae may be divided into typhoid and nontyphoid species. *Salmonella typhi,* which causes typhoid fever, is associated with waterborne outbreaks or contamination of food by infected food handlers who may be carriers (Miller et al., 1995). Humans are the only known hosts for *S. typhi.* Outbreaks of typhoid fever are more common in developing countries than in industrialized nations, and there have been no reported associations between HIV infection and

typhoid fever. Nontyphoid *Salmonella* species, such as *S. enteritidis, S. typhimurium,* and others cause significant clinical disease in patients with AIDS as well as in the general population. *Salmonella* infections occur in an estimated 2 to 4 million persons in the United States annually (CDC, 1997b). Although nontyphoidal salmonellae may be transmitted from person to person by the oral-fecal route, infection in animals is the principal source of nontyphoidal *Salmonella* in humans. *Salmonella* has been found in chickens, turkeys, ducks, cows, pigs, turtles, cats, dogs, mice, guinea pigs, hamsters, doves, pigeons, parrots, starlings, sparrows, cowbirds, sheep, seals, donkeys, lizards, and snakes (Miller et al., 1995). Outbreaks of *Salmonella* gastroenteritis generally occur as a result of exposure to infected pets, such as turtles, chicks, or ducklings, or from consumption of animal-derived foodstuffs, such as undercooked beef and pork, raw and powdered milk, and undercooked poultry and eggs. Transmission of *Salmonella arizonae* has occurred by ingestion of rattlesnake preparations sold as Mexican folk remedies (Riley et al., 1988).

HIV-positive patients are at particular risk of disease related to *Salmonella* and particularly to *Salmonella* bacteremia with or without clinical signs of gastrointestinal disease. Levine and colleagues (1991) found an increased risk of salmonellosis among HIV-positive persons who were residents of the Northeast, had a history of injection drug use, or were African-American or Hispanic.

PATHOGENESIS. The development of disease after *Salmonella* infection is related to the virulence of the organism, the size of the inoculum, and the host defenses. In HIV-infected persons with severe cell-mediated immunodeficiency, infection can become disseminated. *Salmonella* passes through the stomach and begins multiplying in the small intestine. Small inocula of *Salmonella* may be inactivated by gastric pH, but larger inocula may survive and cause infection (Miller et al., 1995). Salmonellae can then pass through the intestinal mucosa to the large lymphatic vessels and, through hematogenous spread, can infect virtually any organ.

Disruption of the intestinal mucosa by infectious pathogens may play a role in the development of *Salmonella* bacteremia in persons with

AIDS (Miller et al., 1995). A retrospective chart review by DeAgostini and colleagues (1994) demonstrated frequent intestinal disease due to cytomegalovirus in patients in whom *Salmonella* bacteremia had been diagnosed.

CLINICAL MANIFESTATIONS. Patients with AIDS-related salmonellosis often have bacteremia without signs of localizing infection and manifest nonspecific signs and symptoms of septicemia, such as fever and rigors. Bacteremia in patients is frequently recurrent, possibly because of hidden foci of infection. Recurrences due to prostatic foci and psoas abscesses have been documented (Decazes et al., 1992). Bacteremia can be complicated by endocarditis or by infection of abdominal aortic aneurysms (Bestetti et al., 1991; Dupont et al., 1989; Gouny et al., 1992; Mestres et al., 1990).

Patients can present with signs of gastroenteritis, including diarrhea or abdominal pain (Martin et al., 1991). A multitude of localized *Salmonella* infections have been reported in HIV-infected persons; these include osteomyelitis, septic arthritis, pyomyositis, meningitis, parotitis, and chorioamnionitis (Decazes et al., 1992; Fraimow et al., 1990; Hatcher & Schranz, 1996; Hedriana et al., 1995; Medina et al., 1995; Stein et al., 1993).

DIAGNOSIS. The diagnosis of bacteremia of salmonellosis is made by bacterial culture. Routine blood cultures, done as part of an evaluation for unexplained fever, often yield the diagnosis of *Salmonella* bacteremia. *Salmonella* enteritis is diagnosed by positive stool cultures. Other localized infections are diagnosed by culture of CSF, aspirated joint fluid, or pus aspirated from an abscess.

TREATMENT. Effective treatment has been reported with ampicillin, trimethoprim-sulfamethoxazole, quinolones, and third-generation cephalosporins to treat AIDS-related salmonellosis (Decazes et al., 1992; Martin et al., 1991). Antibiotic resistance can develop, and therapy should be tailored to the individual susceptibility profile of cultured organisms. Therapy begun before the completion of susceptibility testing should include a third-generation cephalosporin because of the high incidence of antimicrobial resistance (Miller et al., 1995). Recurrence of infection as a result of reactivation from subclinical foci is common, and the role of chronic suppressive therapy has been examined (Detruchis et al., 1990). Miller and colleagues (1995) recommend that HIV-positive patients with *Salmonella* bacteremia be treated with a 1- to 2-week course of intravenous therapy followed by 4 weeks of an oral quinolone. Heseltine and colleagues (1988) demonstrated eradication of organisms when a 30-day course of norfloxacin was given to patients with multiple recurrences of salmonellosis.

PREVENTION. *Salmonella* is transmitted primarily by animals or contaminated foodstuffs (see Appendix I, Health Teaching for the Client with HIV Infection). Recommendations for secondary prophylaxis are contained in Table 6–1.

TOXOPLASMOSIS

EPIDEMIOLOGY. *Toxoplasma gondii* is an obligate protozoan that causes toxoplasmosis in humans and domestic animals. Infection with *T. gondii* occurs worldwide, and the organism infects herbivorous, carnivorous, and omnivorous animals. Although the definitive hosts of *Toxoplasma* are members of the cat family, not all cats are infected. Beaman and colleagues (1995) noted that excretion of *Toxoplasma* oocysts has been reported in approximately 1% of the cats in diverse parts of the world. Although cats are considered of primary importance in transmission of the infection, toxoplasmosis has been found in locales without cats, and a low prevalence of infection has been reported in areas with cats (Beaman et al., 1995). Wallace and associates (1993) studied 723 HIV-infected adults to determine whether cat ownership contributed to the risk of toxoplasmosis and found that cat ownership or exposure did not appear to be a risk factor for seroconversion.

The incidence of seropositivity for antibody to *Toxoplasma* is between 3% and 70% in healthy adults in the United States. The major means of transmission of *Toxoplasma* to humans is through ingestion of meats and vegetables containing oocysts (Beaman et al., 1995). The prevalence of *Toxoplasma* tissue cysts in meat consumed by humans is high. Although tissue cysts are rarely found in beef, as many as 25% of lamb and pork samples tested have been shown to contain the cysts (Beaman et al., 1995). Eggs, vegetables, and other food products contaminated with *Toxoplasma* cysts account for seropositivity in vegetarians (Beaman et al., 1995). The only human-to-human transmission appears to be from mother to fetus when the mother has acquired infection during pregnancy. Rarer documented sources of infection include accidental self-inoculation by laboratory workers, transfusion of infected whole blood or white blood cells, and organ transplantation (Beaman et al., 1995).

The seroprevalence of *Toxoplasma* among HIV-infected patients in the United States is estimated at 15% to 40%, and toxoplasmic encephalitis has been reported in 1% to 5% of patients with AIDS (Beaman et al., 1995; Jones et al., 1996; Wong and Remington, 1994). Within the United States, however, there are geographic differences in the incidence of toxoplasmosis, with a higher incidence in Florida and in persons from Haiti.

PATHOGENESIS. After primary infection, *Toxoplasma* cysts remain in the tissues and may reactivate in immunosuppressed persons in the form of pneumonia, disseminated disease, or toxoplasmic encephalitis (Jones et al., 1996). In patients with HIV infection, the risk of reactivation of *Toxoplasma* infection increases with a decreasing CD4+ T-cell count. It is greatest when the CD4+ count falls below $100/mm^3$. *Toxoplasma* infection may be acquired after acquisition of HIV; however, toxoplasmic encephalitis is usually a result of reactivation of latent infection (Beaman et al., 1995). Local reactivation in the brain may result from intermittent cyst disruption combined with impaired immune responses. Initial reactivation may also occur outside the central nervous system and may be spread hematogenously to the brain (Beaman et al., 1995).

Toxoplasmic encephalitis in patients with AIDS produces brain abscesses with (1) an avascular area, centrally located and surrounded by an intermediate hyperemic area with a prominent inflammatory infiltrate, (2) perivascular cuffing by lymphocytes, plasma cells, and macrophages, and (3) an outer peripheral zone containing *Toxoplasma* cysts. Edema, vasculitis, hemorrhage, and cerebral infection may be evident. Without treatment, the clinical course is one of rapid progression and death (Beaman et al., 1995).

T. gondii infection of the lungs has been increasingly recognized in patients with AIDS (Wong and Remington, 1994). Pulmonary infection with *T. gondii* reveals, on histologic examination, interstitial pneumonitis, necrotizing pneumonitis, and areas of consolidation (Wong and Remington, 1994). *T. gondii* can infect the eye, causing toxoplasmic retinochoroiditis. Histopathologic findings reveal segmental panophthalmitis with areas of coagulative necrosis involving all layers of the retina (Wong and Remington, 1994).

CLINICAL PRESENTATION. Toxoplasmic encephalitis frequently causes multifocal involvement of the CNS, resulting in a wide array of clinical findings. Alteration of mental status, seizures, motor weakness, cranial nerve disturbances, sensory abnormalities, cerebellar signs, meningismus, movement disorders, and neuropsychiatric manifestations may be evident. Characteristically, toxoplasmosis has a subacute onset with focal neurologic abnormalities in 58% to 89% of patients (Wong and Remington, 1994). Between 15% and 25% of cases may present more abruptly with seizures. However, hemiparesis and abnormalities of speech are the most common focal neurologic manifestations of toxoplasmic encephalitis. Patients may also exhibit disorientation, decrease in mentation, lethargy, and coma. More uncommon presentations of toxoplasmic encephalitis include parkinsonism, focal dystonia, rubral tremors, hemichorea-hemiballismus, panhypopituitarism, diabetes insipidus, and the syndrome of inappropriate antidiuretic hormone secretion.

DIAGNOSIS. In the presence of HIV disease, the appearance of neurologic symptoms can suggest any number of OIs and neoplastic processes. The health care provider must direct the clinical diagnosis not only toward establishing the presence of toxoplasmosis but also toward clearly ruling out other infections, such as cryptococcal meningitis, progressive multifocal leukoencephalopathy, herpes simplex encephalitis, mycobacterial encephalitis, HIV disease of the CNS, and neoplasms, such as primary lymphoma of the brain and Kaposi's sarcoma.

In most cases, toxoplasmosis in clients with laboratory-confirmed HIV disease is diagnosed presumptively according to guidelines suggested by the CDC (1987). These guidelines include

1. Recent onset of a focal neurologic abnormality consistent with intracranial disease or a reduced level of consciousness

2. Brain-imaging evidence of a lesion with a mass effect (on CT or nuclear MRI) or with a radiographic appearance that is enhanced by injection of contrast medium
3. Serum antibody to *Toxoplasma* or successful response to therapy for toxoplasmosis (CDC, 1987, 1992a)

More recently, PCR amplification for detection of *T. gondii* DNA in brain tissue, CSF, BAL, and blood has proved useful in the diagnosis of toxoplasmosis and, with increased availability, may alter the methods for diagnosis of toxoplasmosis (Beaman et al., 1995; Roberts & Storch, 1996; Rodriguez et al., 1996).

TREATMENT. The mainstay of therapy for toxoplasmosis in persons with HIV has been the combination of pyrimethamine and sulfadiazine (or trisulfapyrimidines). Symptoms usually diminish within 7 to 14 days, and abnormalities seen on CT scans resolve between the first and fourth weeks of therapy (Reinis-Lucey et al., 1990; Wong and Remington, 1994). Adjunctive therapy may include dexamethasone for abscesses associated with a severe mass effect, phenytoin for infection-induced seizure, and folinic acid to ameliorate the bone marrow toxicity of pyrimethamine (Wong and Remington, 1994).

An appropriate algorithm for the treatment of patients with HIV infection and CNS signs and symptoms is to obtain *Toxoplasma* IgG antibody and a CT or MRI with contrast and, if the IgG antibody is positive and there are multiple lesions on CT or MRI, begin empiric treatment for toxoplasmic encephalitis. If there is no improvement within 10 to 14 days, a brain biopsy should be considered. If there is clinical improvement by 7 days, then treatment should be continued for 3 to 6 weeks, followed by maintenance therapy (Wong and Remington, 1994).

AIDS patients who take sulfadiazine and pyrimethamine for toxoplasmosis have a high incidence of adverse reactions. Up to 40% of patients will have side effects severe enough to necessitate discontinuation of therapy. An alternative is pyrimethamine with clindamycin. However, this combination is also known to have significant adverse reactions. Other drugs that may be used in combination with pyrimethamine and folinic acid include TMP-SMZ, clar-

ithromycin, azithromycin, atovaquone, and dapsone (Wong and Remington, 1994). Alternative regimens include cessation of sulfadiazine and continuation of pyrimethamine alone or with the addition of clindamycin.

With treatment, the clinical manifestations of an acute episode of toxoplasmosis, such as hemiparesis, motor apraxia, and aphasia, will begin to resolve. Although full recovery is unlikely, rehabilitation services (physical and occupational therapies and speech-language-pathology consult) can help the patient obtain optimum function in the presence of residual motor deficits (Rogers, 1992; Westmoreland, 1994). Shared care management using rehabilitation services is crucial to reduction of complications in the hemiparetic patient. Physical therapy commonly focuses on teaching the patient movement patterns to maximize his or her function in transfers, ambulatory status, and other daily mobility tasks (American Physical Therapy Association, 1997). Devices such as canes, walkers, and foot splints may be used to improve the patient's functional status and reduce his or her dependence on others. Occupational therapy often provides help to increase the patient's self-care in dressing, bathing, and completing daily activities important to the patient's daily regimen (Reed, 1991). A speech-language-pathology consult is commonly used to improve communication (as in expressive or receptive aphasias) and swallowing in the hemiparetic client (American Speech-Language-Hearing Association, 1996). Other CNS involvement, such as seizures or confusion or cognitive impairment, may focus the rehabilitation program on instruction to caregivers in how to monitor and manage deficits that are not controllable by the patient.

PREVENTION. Increasing emphasis is being placed on prophylaxis of toxoplasmosis. To prevent exposure, all HIV-infected persons should be tested for IgG antibody to *Toxoplasma* to detect latent infection. All patients who lack IgG antibody to *Toxoplasma* should be taught proper hand-washing, food safety, and pet care (see Appendix I). To prevent toxoplasmosis in *Toxoplasma*-seropositive patients with a CD4+ lymphocyte count of less than 100/μl, prophylaxis should be instituted (see Chapter 5, Table 5–7).

Approximately 50% to 80% of patients with toxoplasmic encephalitis will experience a relapse within several months after therapy is discontinued (Wong & Remington, 1994). To prevent relapse, it is necessary to continue patients on lifelong maintenance therapy (see Table 6–1).

WASTING SYNDROME CAUSED BY HIV

EPIDEMIOLOGY. HIV wasting is the AIDS-defining illness in 11% to 47% of patients and is diagnosed more frequently in women, blacks, Puerto Ricans, injection drug users, and persons in the hemophilia/transfusion risk group (Kotler & Grunfeld, 1996). Precise estimates of the incidence of HIV wasting may be difficult to determine. Nahlen and colleagues (1993), in a study of 26,251 persons with AIDS reported to the CDC between 1987 and 1991, found that persons at risk of being injection drug users were more likely to be reported with wasting syndrome. However, careful analysis revealed that the identification of HIV wasting in persons with AIDS was probably related to geographic variations in diagnostic and reporting practices and to differences in access to medical care. Kotler and Grunfeld (1996) maintain that malnutrition influences functional status and course of illness independent of CD4+ T-cell count.

PATHOGENESIS. There are multifactorial causes of weight loss that include the underlying HIV infection, tissue cytokines, intercurrent infections, and inadequate caloric intake. Mechanisms of weight loss and malnutrition seen in HIV disease can be related to decreases in nutrient intake, decreased nutrient absorption, and metabolic disturbances (Kotler & Grunfeld, 1996). Factors related to reduced food intake include anorexia, oral or esophageal lesions, nausea or vomiting, diarrhea, neurologic or psychiatric conditions, fatigue, inadequate finances, lack of facilities to store and prepare food, lack of knowledge about nutrition, disinterest in diet and weight loss, and side effects of medications.

Decreased nutrient absorption is a result of malabsorption and is related to injury to the small intestine and, in some instances, disease of the digestive organs. Kotler (1992) identified three categories of intestinal disease: primary infection of the enterocytes (e.g., cryptosporidiosis, isosporiasis), secondary involvement from systemic or disseminated disorders (e.g., cytomegalovirus infec-

tion or Kaposi's sarcoma), and inflammatory bowel disease (e.g., intestinal infection caused by HIV).

Metabolic changes may be related to alterations in cytokine activities as a result of HIV or other infections (Kotler, 1992). Cytokines, the hormones that mediate the immune and inflammatory response, are responsible for the metabolic disturbances and anorexia. Several cytokines have been implicated: tumor necrosis factor (TNF), interleukin-1 (IL-1), leukemia-inhibitory factor (LIF), and interferons (IFN) alpha, beta, and gamma (Kotler & Grunfeld, 1996). However, no single cytokine can be linked to AIDS-related wasting.

Recent work has shown that body weight may not be an accurate measure of nutritional status in clinically ill patients, as weight may change without actually affecting the underlying nutritional status. Body cell mass, the nonadipose cellular mass, is a more relevant measure of the amount of functional protoplasm (Kotler & Grunfeld, 1996). The muscle and viscera are the major components of body cell mass. In patients with AIDS there is greater depletion of body cell mass than loss of body weight. Body cell mass is a more accurate predictor of death than weight. At death, body cell mass is 54% of normal, whereas body weight is 66% of ideal (Kotler & Grunfeld, 1996).

CLINICAL PRESENTATION. Lethargy and fatigue are associated with AIDS-related wasting. Both result in decreased activity, which helps to maintain weight in the presence of increased resting energy expenditure and normal caloric intake. However, decreased activity leads to loss of muscle mass, which is the most important component of body cell mass (Grunfeld & Schambelan, 1994). Muscle atrophy results from inactivity that leads to a decreased ability to perform activities of daily living. In addition, anorexia, diarrhea, nausea or vomiting, oral lesions, dysphagia, changes in taste or smell, physical limitations, neuropsychiatric symptoms including HIV encephalopathy, medication interactions or side effects, and allergies or intolerance may contribute to weight loss, and their underlying causes should be investigated and treated (Newman, 1992). Patients who present with a rapid weight loss (>4 kg in <4 months) should be evaluated for infection. Patients with a slow weight loss (>4 kg in >4 months) should be evaluated for a treatable gastrointestinal disease (Kotler & Grunfeld, 1996). Treatment of any underlying cause of wasting may reverse the wasting.

DIAGNOSIS. Diagnosis of HIV wasting syndrome is made only with a definitive diagnosis of HIV infection based on laboratory confirmation. The criteria for the diagnosis of HIV wasting syndrome include profound involuntary weight loss of 10% of baseline body weight plus either chronic diarrhea (at least two loose stools per day for ≥30 days) or chronic weakness and documented fever (for ≥30 days, intermittent or constant) in the absence of a concurrent illness or condition other than HIV infection that could explain the findings (e.g., neoplasm, tuberculosis, enteritis) (CDC, 1992). See Chapter 5 for a detailed discussion of nutritional assessment.

TREATMENT. Nutritional support through alimentation, therapy for anorexia, and anabolic therapies are part of the treatment of AIDS-related wasting. Alimentation is indicated for patients with a treatable gastrointestinal disease that prevents adequate oral intake. Alimentation increases caloric intake, leading to increased body cell mass (Grunfeld & Schambelan, 1994). Nutritional supplementation with a formula containing peptides, medium-chain triglycerides, fish oil, and fiber in early stages of HIV infection may lead to significant weight gain (Kotler & Grunfeld, 1996). Oral supplements most frequently used for treatment of weight loss include Ensure, Sustacal, and Resource (Cimoch, 1992). For patients with fat malabsorption, Lipisorb and Isosource may be prescribed. Chlebowski and colleagues (1993) demonstrated the benefits of nutritional support by prescribing an enterotropic peptide-based formula (a nutritional supplement known as Advera) instead of standard enteral formulas in the treatment of HIV-infected patients. In addition to maintaining weight, the patients who received this supplement had significantly fewer hospitalizations.

One study evaluated the effectiveness of total parenteral nutrition (TPN) in a group of malnourished and severely immunodepressed patients with AIDS (Melchior et al., 1996). The authors found that 2 months of TPN administered

at home improved the nutritional and functional status of the study participants; however, there was no improvement in complications of HIV or overall survival.

Anorexia is a common symptom in patients with HIV infection. Currently there are two FDA-approved drugs for the treatment of anorexia. Dronabinol is a synthetic form of the active ingredient tetrahydrocannabinol (THC) in marijuana. Kotler and Grunfeld (1996) report that study results have been mixed, with subjective improvement but nonsignificant weight gain. Megestrol acetate, a drug that has been used to stimulate appetite and increase weight during breast cancer therapy, has demonstrated effectiveness in increasing weight in patients with AIDS and significant weight loss (Kotler & Grunfeld, 1996). Although patients report increased appetite and a feeling of well-being, bioelectrical impedance analysis revealed that most of the weight gain represented fat rather than lean muscle mass.

Anabolic therapies that increase body cell mass are of particular interest because of the relationship between body cell mass and function or survival. Studies are evaluating the effectiveness of human growth hormone, oxandrolone, and nandrolone decanoate (Berger et al., 1996; Fisher & Abbaticola, 1997; Gold et al., 1996; Poles et al., 1997; Schambelan et al., 1996; Waters et al., 1996). Thalidomide, which selectively inhibits the production of tumor necrosis factor-alpha, has been used in the treatment of AIDS-related wasting. Reyes-Terán and colleagues (1996) found thalidomide to reverse the wasting syndrome.

There may be a role for exercise in the treatment of wasting. Exercise can increase strength and exercise tolerance and develop muscle mass. However, the role of and the long-term effect of exercise in the prevention and treatment of wasting require further study.

PREVENTION. Nutrition counseling and education should be provided as soon as HIV disease is diagnosed (see Chapter 5). Although weight loss is a common occurrence in HIV disease, it should not be casually accepted as a consequence of the disease process. Strategies to maximize food intake include substituting calorie-containing and nutrient-dense foods and beverages for low- or no-calorie foods and beverages; increasing the number and size of feedings daily; fortifying foods with calorie- and protein-containing ingredients; using calorie-containing condiments; modifying the diet according to tolerance; and adding nutritional supplements as indicated (Newman, 1992)

SUMMARY

With the use of primary prophylaxis for more OIs and more effective antiretroviral therapy, the incidence of AIDS-defining diseases has decreased. As a result, providers are seeing fewer acutely ill patients. There is a risk of losing the experience of diagnosing and treating OIs. Therefore it is incumbent on anyone caring for persons with HIV infection to always consider the possibility of an OI in a person with HIV infection who is severely immunocompromised and to keep abreast of the most current diagnostic and treatment recommendations for OIs.

REFERENCES

Abdieb, L., Muñoz, A., Cohn, S., et al. (1997). *HIV infection and associated immunosuppression accelerates progression of HPV related cervical neoplasia in injection drug using women.* Presented at National AIDS Malignancy Conference, Bethesda, Maryland.

Adler, S. (1992). Hospital transmission of cytomegalovirus. *Infectious Agents and Disease, 1*(1), 43–49.

Alves, K., DelNegro, G.B., Melhem, M.S., et al. (1996). *Disseminated histoplasmosis in HIV patients with mucocutaneous lesions: A prospective study in São Paulo, Brazil.* Presented at XI International Conference on AIDS, abstract PubB1053, Vancouver, British Columbia.

American Physical Therapy Association. (1997). Guide to physical therapist practice. *Physical Therapy, 77*(11), 1395–1405, 1461–1471.

American Speech-Language-Hearing Association. (1996). Preferred practice patterns for the professions of speech-language pathology and audiology. *Asha Practice, 40*(92), 28–33.

American Thoracic Society. (1993). Guidelines for the initial management of adults with community-acquired pneumonia: Diagnosis, assessment of severity, and initial antimicrobial therapy. *American Review of Respiratory Disease, 148,* 1418–1426.

Amiel, C., May, T., Mansuy, L., et al. (1993). *Cryptosporidium cholangitis treated by celioscopic cholecystectomy and sphincerotomy.* Presented at IX International Conference on AIDS, abstract PoB10-1460, Berlin, Germany.

Ampel, N.M., Dols, C.L., Galgiani, J.N. (1993). Coccidioidomycosis during human immunodeficiency virus infection: Results of a prospective study in a coccidioidal endemic area. *The American Journal of Medicine, 94*(3), 235–240.

Anand, R., Nightengale, S.D., Fish, R.H., et al. (1993). Control of cytomegalovirus retinitis using sustained release of intraocular ganciclovir. *Archives of Ophthalmology, 111*(2), 223–227.

Anderson, J., Cohen, S., Kelly, W., et al. (1996). *Results of routine colposcopic examinations (colpo) in women enrolled in the HIV epidemiology research study (HERS).* Presented at XI International Conference on AIDS, abstract TuB2255, Vancouver, British Columbia.

Antinori, A., Ammassari, A., DeLuca, A., et al. (1997). Diagnosis of AIDS-related focal brain lesions: A decision-making analysis based on clinical and neuroradiologic characteristics combined with polymerase chain reaction assays in CSF. *Neurology, 48,* 687–694.

Bach, M.C., Tally, P.S. (1996). *Ventricular shunting in patients with cryptococcal meningitis and uncontrollable intracranial hypertension.* Presented at XI International Conference on AIDS, abstract MoB1231, Vancouver, British Columbia.

Barbaro, G., Giesorio, B., Calderon, W., et al. (1996). *A long-term randomized controlled clinical trial comparing fluconazole and itraconazole in the treatment of AIDS patients with Candida esophagitis.* Presented at XI International Conference on AIDS, abstract MoB111, Vancouver, British Columbia.

Baril, L., Astagneu, P., Mengual, X., et al. (1996). *Bacterial pneumonia in HIV-infected patients: Clinical and epidemiologic study.* Presented at XI International Conference on AIDS, abstract MoB1216, Vancouver, British Columbia.

Barnes, P.F., Barrows, S.A. (1993). Tuberculosis in the 1990s. *Annals of Internal Medicine, 119*(5), 400–410.

Barnes, P.F., Block, A.B., Davidson, P.T., Snider, D.E. (1991). Tuberculosis in patients with human immunodeficiency virus infection. *The New England Journal of Medicine, 324*(23), 1645–1650.

Barnes, P.F., El-Hajj, H., Preston-Martin, S., et al. (1996). Transmission of tuberculosis among the urban homeless. *JAMA, 275*(4), 305–307.

Barrett, M.F., Rutherford, G.W., Sun, R.K., et al. (1996). *Epidemiology of AIDS-related coccidioidomycosis in California.* Presented at XI International Conference on AIDS, abstract MoC1407, Vancouver, British Columbia.

Baudouin, C., Chassain, C., Caujolle, C., et al. (1996). Treatment of cytomegalovirus retinitis in AIDS patients using intravitreal injections of highly concentrated ganciclovir. *Ophthalmologica, 210*(6), 329–335.

Beaman, M.H., McCabe, R.E., Wong, S., Remington, J.S. (1995). Toxoplasmosis *gondii.* In G.L. Mandell, J.E. Bennett, R. Dolin (Eds.), *Principles and practice of infectious diseases* (4th ed., pp. 2455–2474). New York: Churchill Livingstone.

Beardsell, A.D., Coker, K., Woodfall, B. (1996). *Cotrimoxazole (TMP-SMX) desensitization using adjunctive steroid therapy in HIV/AIDS patients.* Presented at XI International Conference on AIDS, abstract TuB414, Vancouver, British Columbia.

Beck, P.L., Gill, M.J., Sutherland, L.R. (1996). HIV-associated non-Hodgkins lymphoma of the gastrointestinal tract. *American Journal of Gastroenterology, 91*(11), 2377–2381.

Benator, D.A., French, A.L., Beaudet, L.M, et al. (1994). *Isospora belli* infection associated with acalculous cholecystitis in a patient with AIDS. *Annals of Internal Medicine, 121*(9), 663–664.

Benhamou, Y., Kapel, N., Hoang, C., et al. (1995). Inefficacy of intestinal secretory immune response to *Cryptosporidium* in acquired immunodeficiency syndrome. *Gastroenterology, 108*(3), 627–635.

Berlin, O.G., Conteas, C.N., Sowerby, T.M. (1996). Detection of *Isospora* in the stools of AIDS patients using a new rapid autofluorescence technique. *AIDS, 10*(4), 442–443.

Berger, J.R., Pall, L., Hall, C.D., et al. (1996). Oxandrolone in AIDS-wasting myopathy. *AIDS, 10,* 1657–1662.

Bestetti, R.B., Figueiridio, J.F., DaCosta, J.D. (1991). *Salmonella* tricuspid endocarditis in an intravenous drug abuser with human immunodeficiency virus infection. *International Journal of Cardiology, 30*(3), 361–362.

Biberfeld, P., Elkman, M., Kaaya, E.E., et al. (1996). *HHV8 and other herpes virus in AIDS related and endemic Kaposi's sarcoma and malignant lymphoma.* Presented at XI International Conference on AIDS, abstract ThA272, Vancouver, British Columbia.

Bobak, I.M., Jensen, M.D., Lowdemilk, D.L. (1993). *Maternity and gynecologic care* (5th ed.). St. Louis: Mosby–Year Book.

Boshoff, C., Whitby, S., Matthews, S.J., et al. (1997). *Kaposi's sarcoma–associated herpesvirus.* Presented at 4th Conference on Retroviruses and Opportunistic Infections, Washington, D.C.

Borysiewicz, L.K., Nimako, M., Evans, E., et al. (1997). *Papillomavirus vaccines as therapy for cervical cancer.* Presented at 4th Conference on Retroviruses and Opportunistic Infections, Washington, D.C.

Bowden, F.J., McPhee, D.A., Deacon, N.J., et al. (1991). Antibodies to gp41 and nef in an otherwise HIV-negative homosexual man with Kaposi's sarcoma. *The Lancet, 337*(8753), 1313–1314.

Brandonisio, O., Maggi, P., Panaro, M.A., et al. (1993). Prevalance of cryptosporidiosis in HIV-infected patients with diarrhoeal illness. *European Journal of Epidemiology, 9*(2), 190–194.

Breitbart, W., Marotta, R., Platt, M.M., et al. (1996). A double-blind trial of haloperidol, chlorpromazine, and lorazepam in the treatment of delirium in hospitalized AIDS patients. *American Journal of Psychiatry, 153*(2), 231–237.

Brew, B.J., Dunbar, N., Druett, J.A., et al. (1996). Pilot study of the efficacy of ativerdine in the treatment of AIDS dementia complex. *AIDS, 10*(12), 1357–1360.

Brosgart, C., Craig, C., Hillman, D., et al. (1996). *Final results from a randomized, placebo controlled trial of the safety and efficacy of oral ganciclovir for prophylaxis of CMV retinal and gastrointestinal disease.* Presented at XI International Conference on AIDS, abstract ThB301, Vancouver British Columbia.

Brown, G.R. (1995). The use of methylphenidate for cognitive decline associated with HIV disease. *International Journal of Psychiatry in Medicine, 25*(1), 21–37.

Bull, T.J., Shanson, D.C. (1992). Evaluation of a commercial chemiluminescent gene probe system "AccuProbe" for the rapid differentiation of mycobacteria, including 'MAICX,' isolated from blood and other sites, from patients with AIDS. *Journal of Hospital Infection, 21*(2), 143–149.

Cappell, M.S., Botros, N. (1994). Predominantly gastrointestinal symptoms and signs in 11 consecutive AIDS patients with gastrointestinal lymphoma. *American Journal of Gastroenterology, 89*(4), 545–549.

Carbone, A., Gloghini, A., Vaccher, E., et al. (1996). Kaposi's sarcoma-associated herpesvirus DNA sequences in AIDS-related and AIDS-unrelated lymphomatous effusions. *British Journal of Haematology, 94*(3), 533–543.

Carey, J., Chopra, A., Sepkowitz, K., et al. (1996). *Epidemiologic and clinical characteristics of HIV positive patients with MDRTB.* Presented at XI International Conference on AIDS, abstract TuB2361, Vancouver, British Columbia.

Carpenter, C.C., Mayer, K.H., Stein, M.D., et al. (1991). Human immunodeficiency virus infection in North American women: Experience with 200 cases and a review of the literature. *Medicine, 70*(5), 307–325.

Carr, A., Marriott, D., Field, A., et al. (1998). Treatment of HIV-1-associated microsporidiosis and cryptosporidiosis with combination antiretroviral therapy. *Lancet, 351*(9098), 256–261.

Cartledge, J.D., Midgley, J., Gazzard, B.G. (1997). Itraconazole cyclodextrin solution: The role of in vitro susceptibility testing in predicting succeesful treatment of HIV-related fluconazole-resistant and fluconazole-susceptible oral candidiasis. *AIDS, 11*(2), 163–168.

Cello, J.P. (1992). Gastrointestinal tract manifestations of HIV infection. In M.A. Sande, P.A. Volberding (Eds.), *The medical management of AIDS* (3rd ed., pp. 176–192). Philadelphia: Saunders.

Centers for Disease Control. (1984). Update: Treatment

of cryptosporidosis in pateints with acquired immun-odeficiency sydrome (AIDS). *Morbidity and Mortality Weekly Report, 33*(9), 117–119.

Centers for Disease Control. (1987). Revision of the CDC surveillance case definition for acquired immu-nodeficiency syndrome. *Morbidity and Mortality Weekly Report, 36*(No. 1S), 3S–15S.

Centers for Disease Control. (1989). Tuberculosis and human immunodeficiency virus infection: Recom-mendations of the Advisory Committee for the Elimi-nation of Tuberculosis (ACET). *Morbidity and Mor-tality Weekly Report, 38*(14), 236–238, 243–250.

Centers for Disease Control. (1990). Risk for cervical dis-ease in HIV infected women. *Morbidity and Mortality Weekly Report, 39*(47), 846–849.

Centers for Disease Control. (1991). Purified protien de-rivative (PPD)-turberculin anergy and HIV infection: Guidelines for anergy testing and management of an-ergic persons at risk of tuberculosis. *Morbidity and Mortality Weekly, 40*(RR-5), 27–33.

Centers for Disease Control and Prevention. (1992a). 1993 Revised classification system for HIV infection and expanded surveillance case definition for AIDS among adolescents and adults. *Morbidity and Mortal-ity Weekly Report, 41*(RR-17), 1–19.

Centers for Disease Control and Prevention. (1992b, Oc-tober). *Addendum to the prososed expansion of the AIDS surveillance case definition.* Atlanta, Georgia: CDC.

Centers for Disease Control and Prevention. (1993a). Recommendations on prophylaxis and therapy for dis-seminated *Mycobacterium avium* complex for adults and adolescents infected with human immunodefi-ciency virus. *Morbidity and Mortality Weekly Report, 42*(RR-9), 14–20.

Centers for Disease Control and Prevention. (1993b). Initial therapy for tuberculosis in the era of multidrug resistance. *Morbidity and Mortality Weekly Report, 42*(RR-7), 1–8.

Centers for Disease Control and Prevention. (1995). Guidelines for the prevention of opportunistic infec-tions in persons infected with HIV: A summary. *Morbidity and Mortality Weekly Report, 44*(RR-8), 1–34.

Centers for Disease Control and Prevention. (1997a). Update: Trends in AIDS incidence, deaths, and preva-lence—United States, 1996. *Morbidity and Mortality Weekly Report, 46*(8), 165–173.

Centers for Disease Control and Prevention. (1997b). *Salmonella* serotype *montevideo* infections associated with chicks—Idaho, Washington, and Oregon, spring 1995 and 1996. *Morbidity and Mortality Weekly Report, 46*(11), 237–239.

Centers for Disease Control and Prevention. (1997c). 1997 USPHS/IDSA guidelines for the prevention of opportunistic infections in persons infected with human immunodeficiency virus. *Morbidity and Mor-tality Weekly Report, 46*(RR-12), 1–13.

Centers for Disease Control and Prevention. (1997d). Anergy skin testing and preventive therapy for HIV-in-fected persons: Revised recommendations. *Morbidity and Mortality Weekly Report, 46*(RR-15), 1–12.

Cersosimo, E., Wilkowske, C.J., Rosenblatt, J.E. (1992). Isolated antral narrowing associated with gastrointesti-nal cryptosporidiosis in acquired immunodeficiency syndrome. *Mayo Clinic Proceedings, 67*(6), 553–556.

Chaisson, M.A., Kelley, K.F., Williams, R., et al. (1996). *Invasive cervical cancer (ICC) in HIV+ women in New York City (NYC).* Presented at XI International Con-ference on AIDS, abstract WeC3412, Vancouver, British Columbia.

Chaisson, R.E., Benson, C.A., Dube, M.P., et al. (1994). Clarithromycin therapy for bacteremic *Mycobacterium avium* complex disease: A randomized, double-blind, dose-ranging study in patients with AIDS. *The Annals of Internal Medicine, 121*(12), 905–911.

Chaisson, R.E., Griffin, D.E. (1990). Progressive multi-focal leukoencephalopathy in AIDS. *Journal of the American Medical Association, 264*(1), 79–82.

Chaisson, R.E., Keser, P., Pierce, M., et al. (1997). Clar-ithromycin and ethambutol with or without clofaz-imine for the treatment of bacteremic *Mycobacterium avium* complex disease in patients with HIV infection. *AIDS, 11,* 311–317.

Chaisson, R. E., Keiser, P., Pierce, M., et al. (1996). *A controlled trial of clarithromycin/ethambutol with or without clofazimine for* Mycobacterium avium *complex bacteremia in AIDS.* Presented at The 3rd Conference on Retroviruses and Opportunistic Infections, Wash-ington, DC.

Chaisson, R.E., Moore, R.D., Richman, D.D., et al. (1992). Incidence and natural history of *Mycobac-terium avium* complex in patients with advanced human immunodeficiency virus disease treated with zi-dovudine: The Zidovudine Epidemiology Study Group. *American Review of Respiratory Disease, 146*(2), 285–289.

Chamberlain, M.C., Dirr, L. (1993). Involved-field ra-diotherapy and intra-Omaya methotrexate/cytarabine in patients with AIDS-related lymphomatous menin-gitis. *Journal of Clinical Oncology, 11*(10), 1978–1984.

Chang, Y., Ceasarman, E., Pessin, M.S., et al. (1994). Identification of herpesvirus-like DNA sequences in AIDS-associated Kaposi's sarcoma. *Science, 266,* 1865–1869.

Chernoff, D., Sande, M.A. (1990). Candidiasis. In P.T. Cohen, M.A. Sande, P.A. Volberding (Eds.), *The AIDS knowledge base* (pp. 632.1–632.6). Waltham, MA: Medical Publishing Group.

Cheung, T.W., Cohen, S., Gurtman, A., et al. (1996). *Cervical dysplasia in HIV-infected women in an inner city population.* Presented at XI International Conference on AIDS, abstract WeB3279, Vancouver, British Columbia.

Chiu, J., Nussbaum, J., Bozzette, S., et al. (1990). Treatment of disseminated *Mycobacterium avium* complex infection in AIDS with amikacin, ethambutol, rifampin, and ciprofloxacin. *The Annals of Internal Medicine, 113*(5), 358–361.

Chlebowski, R.T., Beal, G., Grosvenor, M., et al. (1993). Long-term effects of early nutritional support with new enterotropic peptide-based formula versus standard enteral formula in HIV-infected patients: Randomized prospective trial. *Nutrition, 9*(6), 507–512.

Ciesielski, C., Kaplan, J., Mays, M., et al. (1995). *Cryptosporidiosis in AIDS patients in the United States—relationship to municipal water supplies?* Presented at The II National Conference on Human Retroviruses and Related Infections, Washington, D.C.

Cimoch, P. (1992). Current agents for the management of wasting and malnutrition in HIV/AIDS. In G. Nary (Ed.), *Nutrition and HIV/AIDS* (vol. 1, pp. 27–32). Chicago: PAAC Publishing.

Cimponeriu, D., LoPresti, P., Lavelanet, M., et al. (1994). Gastrointestinal histoplasmosis in HIV infection: Two cases of colonic psuedocancer and review of the literature. *American Journal of Gastroenterology, 89*(1), 129–131.

Cirillo-Hyland, V.A., Gross, P. (1995). Disseminated histoplasmosis in a patient with acquired immunodeficiency syndrome. *Cutis, 55*(3), 161–164.

Clavel, A., Arnal, A.C., Sanchez, E.C., et al. (1996). Respiratory cryptosporidiosis: Case series and review of the literature. *Infection, 24*(5), 341–346.

Clayton, F., Heller, T., Kotler, D.P. (1994). Variation in the enteric distribution of cryptosporidia in acquired immunodeficiency syndrome. *American Journal of Clinical Pathology, 102*(4), 420–425.

Clifford, D.B., Arribas, J.R., Storch, G.A., et al. (1996). Magnetic resonance brain imaging lacks sensitivity for AIDS-associated cytomegalovirus encephalitis. *Journal of Neurovirology, 2*(6), 397–403.

Cockerell, C.J. (1993). Update on cutaneous manifestations of HIV infection. *AIDS, 7*(Suppl. 1), S213–S218.

Coe, M.C., Grossman, M.E. (1995). Disseminated histoplamosis presenting as tongue nodules in a patient infected with human immunodeficiency virus. *Cutis, 55*(2), 104–106.

Cohen, B.A., McArthur, J.C., Grohman, S., et al. (1993). Neurologic prognosis of cytomegalovirus polyradiculomyelopathy in AIDS. *Neurology, 43*(3 pt. 1), 493–499.

Cohn, D.L., Benson, C.A., Williams, P., et al. (1996). *A prospective, randomized, double-blind, comparative study of the safety and efficacy of clarithromycin (CLA) vs ri-fabutin (RBT) vs the combination for the prevention of Mycobacterium avium complex (MAC) bacteremia or disseminated MAC disease (DMAC) in HIV-infected patients (pts) with CD4 counts less than or equal to 100 cells/mm³.* Presented at XI International Conference on AIDS, abstract WeB421, Vancouver, British Columbia.

Coker, R.J., Vivani, M., Gazzard, B.G., et al. (1993). Treatment of cryptococcosis with liposomal amphotericin B (AmBisome) in 23 patients with AIDS. *AIDS, 7*(6), 829–835.

Cole, M.C., Grossman, M.E. (1995). Disseminated histoplasmosis presenting as tongue nodules in a patient infected with human immunodeficiency virus. *Cutis, 55*(2), 104–106.

Coleman, D.C., Sullivan, D.J., Bennett, D.E., et al. (1997). Candidiasis: The emergence of a novel species, *Candida dubliniensis. AIDS, 11*(5), 557–567.

Colford, J.M., Jr., Tager, I.B., Hirozawa, A.M., et al. (1996). Cryptosporidiosis among patients infected with human immunodeficiency virus: Factors related to symptomatic infection and survival. *American Journal of Epidemiology, 144*(9), 807–816.

Collier, A.C., Meyers, J.D., Corey, L., et al. (1987). Cytomegalovirus infection in homosexual men: Relationship to sexual practices, antibody to human immunodeficiency virus, and cell mediated immunity. *American Journal of Medicine, 82*(3), 593–601.

Cooley, T.P., Hirschhorn, L.R., O'Keane, J.C. (1996). Kaposi's sarcoma in women with AIDS. *AIDS, 10*(11), 1221–1225.

Corey, L., Spear, P.G. (1986). Infection with herpes simplex viruses. *New England Journal of Medicine, 314*(11), 686–691.

Cote, T.R., Manns, A., Hardy, C.R., et al. (1996). Epidemiology of brain lymphoma among people with or without acquired immunodeficiency syndrome: AIDS/Cancer Study Group. *Journal of the National Cancer Institute, 88*(10), 675–679.

Cotte, L., Rabodonirina, M., Piens, M.A., et al. (1993). Prevalence of intestinal protozoans in French patients infected with HIV. *Journal of Acquired Immunodeficiency Syndromes, 6*(9), 1024–1029.

Currier, J.S., Feinberg, J. (1996). Bacterial infections in HIV disease. In P. Volberding, M.A. Jacobson (Eds.), *AIDS clinical review 1995/1996* (pp. 131–152). New York: Marcel Dekker, Inc.

Daar, E.S., Meyer, R.D. (1992). Bacterial and fungal infections. *The Medical Clinics of North America, 76*(1), 173–203.

Dal Pan, G.J., McArthur, J.C. (1996). Neuroepidemiology of HIV infection. *Neurologic Clinics, 14*(2), 359–382.

Dalsgaard Hansen, N.J., Madsen, C., Stinager, E. (1996). Progressive multifocal leucoencephalopathy. *The Italian Journal of Neurological Sciences, 17,* 393–399.

Danin, J.D., McCarty, M., Coker, R. (1992). Case report: Lymphoma causing small bowel intussusception in a patient with the acquired immune deficiency syndrome. *Clinical Radiology, 46*(5), 350–351.

Darouiche, R.O., Graybill, J.R., Vazquez, J., et al. (1996). *Itraconazole oral solution for the treatment of oropharyngeal candidiasis: Results of two randomized, blinded studies.* Presented at XI International Conference on AIDS, abstract MoB117, Vancouver, British Columbia.

Davenny, K., Smeriglio, V., Coales, P., et al. (1996). *Research of HIV disease progression at the National Institute of Drug Abuse (NIDA), National Institutes of Health.* Presented at XI International Conference on AIDS, abstract WeC3424, Vancouver, British Columbia.

DeAgostini, M., Lipani, F., Sinicco, A. (1994). *CMV gastrointestinal disease and* Salmonella *sepsis in AIDS.* Presented at The X International Conference on AIDS, abstract PB0174, Yokohama, Japan.

DeBolt, S., Bell, A., Ovitt, D. (1996). *Nutrition and HIV disease: Rehabilitation implications.* Presented at American Physical Therapy Association Combined Sections Meeting, abstract J114-65AB, Atlanta, GA.

Decazes, J.M., Welker, Y., Csin, I., et al. (1992). Salmonella *infection in 15 HIV-infected patients: Clinical and therapeutic aspects.* Presented at VIII International Conference on AIDS, abstract PoB3136, Amsterdam, Netherlands.

Denenberg, R. (1997). Cervical cancer and women with HIV. *GMHC: Treatment Issues, 11*(7/8), 10–18.

Desatnik, H.R., Foster, R.E., Lowder, C.Y. (1996). Treatment of clinically resistant cytomegalovirus retinitis with combined intravitreal infections of ganciclovir and foscarnet. *American Journal of Ophthalmology, 122*(1), 121–123.

Detruchis, P., Jaccard, A., Salmon, D., et al. (1990). *Outcome and prevention of relapses on non-typhoidal* Salmonella *bacteremia in 55 AIDS patients.* Presented at VI International Conference on AIDS, abstract ThB532, San Francisco, California.

DeWit, S., Weerts, D., Goosens, H., Clumeck, N. (1989). Comparison of fluconazole and ketaconazole for oropharyngeal candidiasis in AIDS. *The Lancet, 1*(8641), 746–748.

Diaz-Llopis, M., Espana, E., Munoz, G., et al. (1994). High dose intravitreal foscarnet in the treatment of cytomegalovirus retinitis in AIDS. *British Journal of Ophthalmology, 78*(2), 120–124.

Dieterich, D.T., Kotler, D.P., Busch, D.F., et al. (1993a). Ganciclovir treatment of cytomegalovirus colitis in AIDS: A randomized, double-blind, placebo controlled multicenter study. *Journal of Infectious Diseases, 167*(2), 278–282.

Dieterich, D.T., Poles, M.A., Dicker, M., et al. (1993b). Foscarnet treatment of cytomegalovirus gastrointestinal infections in acquired immunodeficiency syndrome patients who have failed ganciclovir induction. *American Journal of Gastroenterology, 88*(4), 542–548.

Dieterich, D.T., Poles, M.A., Lew, E.A., et al. (1993c). Concurrent use of ganciclovir and foscarnet to treat cytomegalovirus infection in AIDS patients. *The Journal of Infectious Diseases, 167*(5), 1184–1188.

Dionisio, D., Sterrantino, G., Meli, M., et al. (1996). Treatment of isosporiasis with combined albendazole and ornidazole in patients with AIDS. *AIDS, 10*(11), 1301–1302.

DiTomasso, J.P., Ampel, N.M., Sobonya, R., et al. (1994). Bronchoscopic diagnosis of pulmonary coccidioidomycosis: Comparison of cytology, culture, and transbronchial biopsy. *Diagnostic Microbiology and Infectious Disease, 18*(20), 83–87.

Donowitz, G.R., Mandell, G.L. (1995). Acute pneumonia. In Mandell, G.L., Bennett, J.E., Dolin, R. (Eds.), *Principles and practice of infectious diseases* (4th ed., pp. 619–637). New York: Churchill Livingstone.

Dore, G., Kaldor, J., Hoy, J. (1996). *Trends in AIDS-related illness in Australia: The Australian AIDS cohort.* Presented at XI International Conference on AIDS, abstract TuB2236, Vancouver, British Columbia.

Dore, G.J., Marriott, D.J., Duflou, J.A. (1995). Clinicopathological study of cytomegalovirus (CMV) in AIDS autopsies: Under-recognition of CMV pneumonitis and CMV adrenalitis. *Australia and New Zealand Journal of Medicine, 25*(5), 503–506.

Dorman, S.E., Sax, P.E. (1996). *Salvage adjunctive corticosteroid therapy for disseminated* Mycobacterium avium *complex infection in patients with AIDS.* Presented at XI International Conference on AIDS, abstract WeB3366, Vancouver, British Columbia.

Drake, J., Cattarall, L., Olliaro, P., et al. (1992). *Aminosidine for the treatment of cryptosporidial diarrhoea in AIDS.* Presented at VIII International Conference on AIDS, abstract PoB3229, Amsterdam, Netherlands.

Drew, W.L., Bukles, W., Erlich, K.S. (1992). Management of herpesvirus infections (CMV, HSV, VZV). In M.A. Sande, P.A. Volberding (Eds.), *The medical management of AIDS* (3rd ed., pp. 359–382). Philadelphia: Saunders.

Drew, W.L., Erlich, K.S. (1990). Cytomegalovirus epidemiology. In P.T. Cohen, M.A. Sande, P.A. Volberding (Eds.), *The AIDS knowledge base* (pp. 644.1–644.2). Waltham, MA: Medical Publishing Group.

Drew, W.L., Ives, D., Lalezri, J.P., et al. (1995). Oral ganciclovir as maintenance treatment for cytomegalovirus retinitis in patients with AIDS. *New England Journal of Medicine, 333*(10), 615–620.

Drew, W.L., Jacobson, M.A. (1994). Cytomegalovirus. In P.T. Cohen, M.A. Sande, P.A. Volberding (Eds.), *The AIDS knowledge base* (2nd ed., pp.6.13-1–6.13-12). Boston: Little, Brown.

Drew, W.L., Stempien, M.J., W., Erlich, K.S. (1997). Management of herpesvirus infections (CMV, HSV, VZV). In M.S. Sande, P.A. Volberding (Eds.), *The medical management of AIDS* (5th ed., pp. 359–382). Philadelphia: Saunders.

Dubois, V.L., Lafon, M.E., Ragnaud, J.M., et al. (1996). *JC virus mRNA in the peripheral blood of JC-positive HIV-infected patients.* Presented at XI International Conference on AIDS, abstract ThA4054, Vancouver, British Columbia.

Dupont, J.R., Bonavita, J.A., DiGiovanni, R.J., et al. (1989). Acquired immunodeficiency syndrome and mycotic abdominal aortic aneurysm: A new challenge? *Journal of Vascular Surgery, 10*(3), 254–257.

Durden, F.M., Elewski, B. (1994). Cutaneous involvement with *Cryptococcus neoformans* in AIDS. *Journal of the American Academy of Dermatology, 30*(5 pt. 2), 844–848.

Dutronc, H., Dubois, V., Lafron, M.E., et al. (1997). *Latency and reactivation of JCV at different sites in AIDS.* Presented at 4th Conference on Retroviruses and Opportunistic Infections, Washington, D.C.

Ebrahimzadeh, A., Bottone, E.J. (1996). Persistent diarrhea caused by *Isospora belli:* Therapeutic response to pyrimethamine and sulfadiazine. *Diagnostic Microbiology and Infectious Diseases, 26*(2), 87–89.

Edlin, B.R., Tokars, J.I., Grieco, M.H., et al. (1992). An outbreak of multidrug-resistant tuberculosis among hospitalized patients with acquired immunodeficiency syndrome. *New England Journal of Medicine, 326*(23), 1514–1521.

Edwards, J.E. (1995). Candida species. In G.L. Mandell, J.E. Bennett, R. Dolin (Eds.), *Principles and practice of infectious diseases* (4th ed., pp. 2289–2301). New York: Churchill Livingstone.

Eisner, M.D., Kaplan, L.D., Herdier, B., et al. (1996). The pulmonary manifestations of AIDS-related non-Hodgkin's lymphoma. *Chest, 110*(3), 729–736.

Elliot, B.C., Aromin, I., Flanigan, T.P., et al. (1996). *Prolonged remission of AIDS-associated progressive multifocal leucoencephalopathy with combined antiretroviral therapy.* Presented at XI International Conference on AIDS, abstract ThB183, Vancouver, British Columbia.

Ellner, J.J. (1997). *The interaction between HIV and My-cobacterium tuberculosis.* Presented at 4th Conference on Retroviruses and Opportunistic Infections, abstract S21, Washington, D.C.

El-Sadr, W.F., Perlman, D.C., Matts, J.P., et al. (1996). *Outcome of an induction regimen for the treatment of HIV-related tuberculosis (TB): Evaluation of the addition of a quinolone.* Presented at XI International Conference on AIDS, abstract TuB2358, Vancouver, British Columbia.

Epstein, J.B., Sherlock, C.H., Wolber, R.A. (1993). Oral manifestations of cytomegalovirus infection. *Oral Surgery, Oral Medicine, and Oral Pathology, 75*(4), 443–451.

Erlich, K.S., Jacobson, M.S., Koehler, J.E., et al. (1989). Foscarnet therapy for severe acyclovir-resistant herpes simplex virus type-2 infections in patients with the acquired immunodeficiency syndrome (AIDS). *Annals of Internal Medicine, 110*(9), 710–713.

Esfandiari, A., Jordan, W.C., Brown, C.P. (1995). Prevalence of enteric parasitic infection among HIV-infected attendees of an inner city AIDS clinic. *Cellular and Molecular Biology, 41*(Suppl. 1), S19–S23.

Esser., S., Bleil, N., Reimann, G., et al. (1996). *Long term treatment with liposomal doxorubicin in patients with AIDS-related Kaposi's sarcoma.* Presented at XI International Conference on AIDS, abstract ThA4077, Vancouver, British Columbia.

Evers, S., Grotemeyer, K.H., Reichelt, D., et al. (1998). *Journal of Acquired Immune Deficiency Syndromes and Human Retrovirology, 17*(2), 143–148.

Farizo, K.M., Buehler, J.W., Chamberland, M.E., et al. (1992). Spectrum of disease in persons with human immunodeficiency infection in the United States. *Journal of the American Medical Association, 267*(13), 1798–1805.

Feinberg, J. (1993) Fluconazole versus amphotericin B for acute cryptococcal meningitis: The pendulum swings back. *AIDS Clinical Care, 5*(5), 39–43.

Feingold, A.R., Vermund, S.H., Burk, R.D., et al. (1990). Cervical cytologic abnormalities and papillomavirus in women infected with human immunodeficiency virus. *Journal of Acquired Immune Deficiency Syndromes, 3*(9), 896–903.

Feregrino, G.M., Higuera, R.F., Rossignol, J.F., et al. (1996). *Extraordinary potency of the nitoxanida: A new antiparasitary against the* Cryptosporidium parvum *infections in advanced AIDS.* Presented at XI International Conference on AIDS, abstract ThB4213, Vancouver, British Columbia.

Fichtenbaum, C., Yiannoutsos, C., Holland, F., et al. (1997). *Clinical factors associated with recurrent oral candidiasis in HIV infection.* Presented at 4th Conference in Retroviruses and Opportunistic Infections, Washington, D.C.

Fischl, M.A., Uttamchardani, R.B., Daikos, G.G., et al. (1992). An outbreak of tuberculosis caused by multiple-drug resistant tubercle bacilli among patients with HIV infection. *Annals of Internal Medicine, 117*(3), 177–183.

Fisher, A., Abbaticola, M. (1997). *Effects of onandrolone and L-glutamine on body weight, body cell mass, and body fat in patients with HIV infection-preliminary analysis.* Presented at 4th Conference on Retroviruses and Opportunistic Infections, Washington, D.C.

Fishman, J.E., Batt, H.D. (1996). Cytomegalovirus pneumonia manifesting as a focal mass in acquired immunodeficiency syndrome. *Southern Medical Journal,* 89(11), 1121–1122.

Folkers, G. (August 1, 1996). TB increases HIV replication in HIV-infected people. *NIAID News.*

Fong, I.W., Toma, E., Canadian PML Study Group. (1995). The natural history of progressive multifocal leukoencephalopathy in patients with AIDS. *Clinical Infectious Diseases, 20,* 1305–1310.

Forester, G., Sidhom, O., Nahass, R. (1994). AIDS-associated cryptosporidiosis with gastric stricture and a therapeutic response to paramomycin. *American Journal of Gastroenterology, 89*(7), 1096–1098.

Forsyth, P.A., Yahoalom, J., DeAngelis, L.M. (1994). Combined-modality therapy in the treatment of primary central nervous system lymphoma in AIDS. *Neurology, 44*(88), 1473–1479.

Fraimow, H.S., Wormser, G.P., Coburn, K.D., et al. (1990). *Salmonella* meningitis and infection with HIV. *AIDS, 4*(12), 1271–1273.

Franco, E.L. (1991). Viral etiology of cerical cancer: A critique of the evidence. *Review of Infectious Diseases, 13*(6), 1195–1206.

French, A.L., Benator, D.A., Beaudet, L.M., et al. (1993). *Acalculous cholecystitis caused by* Isospora belli *in a patient with AIDS.* Presented at First National Conference on Human Retroviruses and Related Infections, abstract 99, Washington, D.C.

Frieden, T.R., Sherman, L.F., Maw, K.L., et al. (1996). A multi-institutional outbreak of highly drug-resistant tuberculosis. *JAMA, 276*(15), 1229–1235.

Frieden, T.R., Sterling, T., Pablos-Méndez, A., et al. (1993). The emergence of drug-resistant tuberculosis in New York City. *The New England Journal of Medicine, 328*(8), 521–526.

Friedman-Kien, A.E., Li, J.J., Jensen, P., Huang, Y.Q. (1996). *Herpes-like virus (HHV-8) DNA sequences in various types of immunocompromised patients with Kaposi's sarcoma.* Presented at XI International Conference on AIDS, abstract WeA167, Vancouver, British Columbia.

Friedman-Kien, A.E., Ostreicher, R., Saltzman, B. (1989). Clinical manifestations of classical, endemic African, and epidemic AIDS-associated Kaposi's sarcoma. In A.E. Friedman-Kien (Ed.), *Color atlas of AIDS* (pp. 11–48). Philadelphia: Saunders.

Fruchter, R.G., Maiman, M., Chapman, J., et al. (1996). *Is HIV infection a risk factor for advanced cervical cancer?* Presented at XI International Conference of AIDS, abstract ThB4139, Vancouver, British Columbia.

Fruchter, R.G., Polefsky, J., Riester, K.A., et al. (1997). *Abnormal cervical cytology in HIV infected women.* Presented at National AIDS Malignancy Conference, Bethesda, Maryland.

Gabarre, J., Lepage, E., Thyss, A., et al. (1995). Chemotherapy combined with zidovudine and GM-CSF in human immunodeficiency virus-related non-Hodgkin's lymphoma. *Annals of Oncology, 6*(10), 1025–1032.

Gagliani, J.N., Catanzaro, A., Cloud, G.A., et al. (1993). Fluconazole therapy for coccidioidal meningitis: The NAIAD-Mycosis Study Group. *Annals of Internal Medicine, 119*(1), 28–35.

Galantino, M.L. (1987). An overview of the AIDS patient. *Clinical Management in Physical Therapy, 7*(2), 12–13.

Galantino, M.L., Levy, J.K. (1988). Neurological implications for rehabilitation. *Clinical Management in Physical Therapy, 8*(1), 6–13.

Ganem, D. (1997). *KSHV/HHV8 and Kaposi's sarcoma.* Presented at 4th Conference on Retroviruses and Opportunistic Infections, Washington, D.C.

Gao, S.J., Kingsley, L., Hoover, D.R., et al. (1996). Seroconversion to antibodies against Kaposi's sarcoma-associated herpesvirus-related latent nuclear antigens before the development of Kaposi's sarcoma. *The New England Journal of Medicine, 335*(4), 233–241.

Gates, E.J., Maiman, M., Fruchter, R.G., et al. (1997). *Cervical cancer as an AIDS-defining illness.* Presented at National AIDS Malignancy Conference, Bethesda, Maryland.

Gellin, B., Soave, R. (1992). Coccidian infections in AIDS: Toxoplasmosis, cryptosporidiosis, and isosporiasis. *The Medical Clinics of North America, 3*(4), 205–234.

Genereau, T., Lortholary, G., Bouchaud, O., et al. (1996). Herpes simplex esophagitis in patients with AIDS: Report of 34 cases. *Clinical Infectious Diseases, 22*(6), 926–931.

Gessain, A., Briere, J., Angelin-Duclos, C., et al. (1997). Human herpes virus 8 (Kaposi's sarcoma herpes virus) and malignant proliferations in France: A molecular study of 250 cases including two AIDS-associated body cavity lymphomas. *Leukemia, 11*(2), 266–272.

Giraldo, P.C., Daniel-Ribeiro, A.F., Simons, J.A., et al. (1996). *Vaginal flora of HIV infected women.* Presented at XI International Conference on AIDS, abstract MoC1637, Vancouver, British Columbia.

Girard, P.M., Bouchaud, O., Goetschel, A., et al. (1996). Phase II study of liposomal encapsulated daunorubicin in the treatment of AIDS-associated mucocutaneous Kaposi's sarcoma. *AIDS, 10*(7), 753–757.

Gisselbrecht, C., Oksenhendler, E., Tirelli, U., et al. (1993). Human immunodeficiency virus-related lymphoma treatment with intensive combination chemotherapy: French-Italian Cooperative Group. *Annals of Internal Medicine, 95*(2), 188–196.

Glatt, A.E., Chirgwin, K., Landesman, S.H. (1988). Treatment of infections with human immunodeficiency virus. *The New England Journal of Medicine, 318*(22), 1439–1448.

Goetz, M.B. (1995). Relationship between fluconazole dosage regimens and the emergence of fluconazole-resistant Candida albicans. *AIDS, 10*(3), 335–336.

Gold, J., High, H.A., Li, Y., et al. (1996). Safety and efficacy of nandrolone decanoate for treatment of wasting in patients with HIV infection. *AIDS, 10,* 745–752.

Goletti, D., Weissman, D., Jackson, R.W., et al. (1996). Effect of *Mycobacterium tuberculosis* on HIV replication: Role of immune activation. *Journal of Immunology, 157*(3), 1271–1278.

Gonzales-Dominguez, J., Roldan, R., Villanueva, J.L., et al. (1994). *Isospora belli* reactive arthritis in a patient with AIDS. *Annals of Rheumatic Disease, 53*(9), 618–619.

Gori, A., Rossi, M.C., Vezzoli, S., et al. (1996). *Evaluation of frequency of* Mycobacterium avium *complex (MAC) colonization and correlation with the development of disseminated disease in HIV-positive adult and pediatric patients.* Presented at XI International Conference of AIDS, abstract MoB1247, Vancouver, British Columbia.

Gouny, P., Valverde, A., Vincent, D., et al. (1992). Human immunodeficiency virus and infected aneurysm of the abdominal aorta: Report of three cases. *Annals of Vascular Surgery, 6*(3), 239–243.

Gozlan, J., Salord, J.M., Roullet, E., et al. (1992). Rapid detection of cytomegalovirus DNA in cerebrospinal fluid of AIDS patients with neurologic disorders. *Journal of Infectious Diseases, 166*(6), 1416–1421.

Grant, I., Heaton, R.K., Atkinson, J.H., et al. (1995). Neurocognitive disorders in HIV-1 infection. In M.B.A. Oldstone, L.Vitkovi (Eds.), *Current Topics in Microbiology and Immunology, 202,* 11–32.

Greenberg, M.S., Glick, M., Nghiem, L., et al. (1997). Relationship of cytomegalovirus to salivary gland dysfunction in HIV-infected patients. *Oral Surgery, Oral Medicine, Oral Pathology, and Oral Radiology and Endodontics, 83*(3), 334–339.

Greenberg, P.D., Koch, J., Cello, J.P. (1996). Diagnosis of *Cryptosporidium parvum* with severe diarrhea and AIDS. *Digestive Disease and Science, 41*(11), 2286–2290.

Greenspan, D., Greenspan, J.S. (1996). HIV-related oral disease. *The Lancet, 348*(Sept. 14), 729–733.

Grunfeld, C., Schambelan, M. (1994). The wasting syndrome: Pathophysiology and treatment. In S. Broder., Merigan, T.C., Bolognesi, D. (Eds.), *Textbook of AIDS medicine* (pp. 637–649). Baltimore: Wilkins & Wilkins.

Guerrero, A., Moreira, V., Villanueva, R. (1995). Intestinal and extraintestinal cryptosporidiosis in AIDS patients. *European Journal of Clinical Microbiology and Infectious Disease, 14*(8), 677–681.

Haas, D.W., Des Prez, R.M. (1995). *Mycobacterium tuberculosis.* In G.L. Mandell, J.E. Bennett, R. Dolin (Eds.), *Principles and practice of infectious diseases* (4th ed., pp. 2213–2243). New York: Churchill Livingstone.

Hajjeh, R., Stephens, D., Baughman, W., et al. (1996). *A case-controlled study of risk factors for cryptococcosis in HIV infected persons.* Presented at XI International Conference on AIDS, abstract TuB186, Vancouver, British Columbia.

Hansen, D., Madsen, C., Stenager, E. (1996). Progressive multifocal leucoencephalopathy. *The Italian Journal of Neurological Sciences, 17,* 393–396.

Hashmey, R., Smith, N.H., Cron, S., et al. (1997). Cryptosporidiosis in Houston, Texas: A report of 95 cases. *Medicine, 76*(2), 118–139.

Hatch, K.D., Fu, Y.S. (1996). Cervical and vaginal cancer. In J.S. Berek, E.Y. Adashi, P.A. Hillard (Eds.), *Novak's gynecology* (12th ed., pp. 1111–1122). Baltimore: Williams & Wilkins.

Hatcher, J., Schranz, J. (1996). Salmonella *group D parotitis in an HIV infected individual.* Presented at XI International Conference on AIDS, abstract MoB1217, Vancouver, British Columbia.

Havlir, D.V., Dube, M.P., Sattler, F.R., et al. (1996). Prophylaxis against disseminated *Mycobacterium avium* complex with weekly azithromycin, daily ruifabutin, or both. *The New England Jounal of Medicine, 335*(6), 392–398.

Havlir, D.V., Ellner, J.J. (1995). *Mycobacerium avium* complex. In G.L. Mandell, J.E. Bennet, R. Dolin (Eds.), *Principles and practices of infectious diseases* (4th ed., pp. 2250–2264). New York: Churchill Livingstone.

Hawkins, C.C., Gold, J.W., Whimbey, E., et al. (1986). *Mycobacterium avium* complex infections in patients with the acquired immunodeficiency syndrome. *Annals of Internal Medicine, 105*(2), 184–188.

Hazard, S., Bissuel, F., Henry-Feugeas, M.C. (1996). *Primary cerebral lymphoma: Clinical and radiological findings in 16 patients with AIDS.* Presented at XI International Conference on AIDS, abstract ThB4228, Vancouver, British Columbia.

Heald, G.E., Cox, G.M., Schell, W.A., et al. (1996). Oropharyngeal yeast flora and fluconazole resistance in HIV-infected patients receiving long-term continuous versus intermittent fluconazole therapy. *AIDS, 10*(3), 263–268.

Hedrian, H.L., Mitchell, J.L., Williams, S.B. (1995). *Salmonella typhi* chorioamnionitis in a human immunodeficiency virus infected preganat woman: A case report. *Journal of Reproductive Medicine, 40*(2), 157–159.

Heneghan, S.J., Li, J., Petrossian, E., et al. (1993). Gastrointestinal involvement with histoplasmosis in patients with the acquired immunodefiency syndrome: Case report and review of the literature. *Archives of Surgery, 128*(4), 464–466.

Henry, K., Worley, J., Sullivan, C., et al. (1997). *Documented improvement in late stage manifestations of AIDS after starting ritonavir in combination with two reverse transcriptase inhibitors.* Presented at 4th Conference on Retroviruses and Opportunistic Infections, Washington, D.C.

Herry, I., Cadranel, J., Antoine, M., et al. (1996). Cytomegalovirus-induced alveolar hemorrhage in patients with AIDS: A new clinical entity? *Clinical Infectious Disease, 22*(4), 616–620.

Heseltine, P.N., Causey, D.M., Appleman, M.D., et al. (1988). Norfloxacin in the eradication of enteric infections in AIDS patients. *European Journal of Cancer and Clinical Oncology, 24*(Suppl. 1), S25–S28.

Heyer, D.M., Kahn, J.O., Volberding, P.A. (1990). HIV-related Kaposi's sarcoma. In P.T. Cohen, M.A.. Sande, P.A. Volberding (Eds.), *The AIDS knowledge base* (pp. 713.1–713.19). Waltham, MA: The Medical Publishing Group.

Heyworth, M.F. (1996). Parasitic diseases in immunocompromised hosts: Cryptosporidiosis, isosporiasis, and strongyloidiasis. *Gastroenterology Clinics of North America, 25*(3), 691–707.

Hilton, E., Isenberg, H.D., Alperstein, P., et al. (1992). Ingestion of yogurt containing *Lactobacillus acidophilus* as prophylaxis for Candida vaginitis. *Annals of Internal Medicine, 116*(5), 353–357.

Hirsch, M.S. (1995). Herpes simplex virus. In G.L. Mandell, J.E. Bennett, R. Dolin (Eds.), *Principles and practice of infectious diseases* (4th ed., pp. 1336–1345). New York: Churchill Livingstone.

Hirschtick, R.E., Glassroth, J., Jordan, M.C., et al. (1995). Bacterial pneumonia in persons infected with the human immunodeficiency virus. *The New England Journal of Medicine, 33*(13), 845–851.

HIV Hotline. (1997). Rethinking resistance in candidiasis, 7(1), 1–6.

Ho, M. (1995). Cytomegalovirus. In G.L. Mandell, J.E. Bennet, R. Dolin (Eds.), *Principles and practices of infectious diseases* (4th ed., pp. 1351–1364). New York: Churchill Livingstone.

Hodge, W.G., Lalonde, R.G., Sampalis, J., et al. (1996). Once-weekly intraocular injections of ganciclovir for maintenance therapy of cytomegalovirus retinitis: Clinical and ocular outcome. *Journal of Infectious Diseases, 174*(2), 393–396.

Hoffman, J.M., Waskin, H.A., Schifter, T., et al. (1993). FDG-PET in differentiating lymphoma from nonmalignant central nervous system lesions in patients with AIDS. *Journal of Nuclear Medicine, 34*(4), 567–575.

Hogg, R.S., Heath, K.V., Yip, V., et al. (1998). Improved survival among HIV-infected individuals following initiation of antiretroviral therapy. *Journal of the American Medical Association, 279*(6), 450–454.

Holmberg, S.D., Moorman, A.C., Von Bargen, J.C., et al. (1998). Possible effectiveness of clarithromycin and rifabutin for cryptosporidiosis chemoprophylaxis in HIV disease. HIV Outpatient Study (HOPS) Investigators. *Journal of the American Medical Association, 279*(5), 384–386.

Hoover, D.R., Saah, A.J., Bacellar, H. (1993). Clinical manifestations of AIDS in the era of pneumoscystis prophylaxis: Multicenter AIDS Cohort Study. *New England Journal of Medicine, 329*(26), 1922–1926.

Horsburgh, C.R. (1991). *Mycobacterium avium* complex infection in the acquired immunodeficiency syndrome. *The New England Journal of Medidine, 324*(19), 1332–1338.

Hu, D.J., Fleming, P.L., Jones, J.L., Word, J.W. (1994). *Epidemiology of protozoal opportunistic infections (POI) among persons with AIDS in the United States.* Program Abstracts of the Interscience Conference on Antimicrobial Agents and Chemotherapy, abstract 168, Orlando, Florida.

Huang, Y.Q., Li, J.J., Poiesz, B.J., et al. (1997). Detection of the herpesvirus-like DNA sequences in matched specimens of semen and blood from patients with AIDS-related Kaposi's sarcoma by polymerase chain reaction in situ hybridization. *American Journal of Pathology, 150*(1), 147–153.

Iacoangeli, M., Roselli, R., Antinor, A., et al. (1994). Experience with brain biopsy in acquired immune deficiency syndrome-related focal lesions of the central nervous system. *British Journal of Surgery, 81*(10), 1508–1510.

Ives, D.V., Davis, R.B., Currier, J.S. (1995). The impact of clarithromycin and azithromycin on patterns of treatment and survival among AIDS patients with disseminated *Mycobacterium avium* complex. *AIDS, 9*(3), 261–266.

Jacobson, M.A. (1992). Mycobacterial diseases: Tuberculosis and disseminated *Mycobacterium avium* complex infection. In M.A. Sande, P.A. Volberding (Eds.), *The medical management of AIDS* (3rd ed., pp. 284–296). Philadelphia: Saunders.

Jacobson, M.A. (1997). Disseminated *Mycobacterium avium* complex and other bacterial infections. In M.A. Sande, P.A. Volberding (Eds.), *The medical management of AIDS* (5th ed., pp. 301–310). Philadelphia: Saunders.

Jacobson, M.A., Wulfsohn, M., Feinberg, J.E., et al. (1994). Phase II dose-ranging trial of foscarnet salvage therapy for cytomegalovirus retinitis in AIDS patients intolerant of or resistant to ganciclovir (ACTG protocol 093). *AIDS, 8*(4), 451–459.

Johnson, R.T., Glass, J.D., McArthur, J.C., Chesebro, B.W. (1996). Quantitation of human immunodeficiency virus in brains of demented and nondemented patients with acquired immunodeficiency syndrome. *Annals of Neurology, 39*(3), 392–395.

Johnston, S.R., Corvett, E.L., Foster, O., et al. (1992). Raised intracranial pressure and visual complications in AIDS patients with cryptococcal meningitis. *Journal of Infection, 2*(4), 185–189.

Jones, J.L., Burwen, D.L., Fleming, P.L., et al. (1996). Tuberculosis among AIDS patients in the United States, 1993. *Journal of Acquired Immune Deficiency Syndromes and Human Retrovirology, 12*(3), 293–297.

Jones, J.L., Fleming, P.L., Ciesielski, C.A., et al. (1995). Coccidioodomycosis among persons with AIDS in the United States. *Journal of Infectious Diseases, 171*(4), 961–966.

Jones, J.L., Hanson, D.L., Chu, S.Y., et al. (1996). Toxoplasmic encephalitis in HIV-infected persons: Risk factors and trends. *AIDS, 10*(12), 1393–1399.

Kamel, A.G., Maning, N., Arulmainathan, S., et al. (1994). Cryptosporidiosis among HIV positive intravenous drug users in Malaysia. *Southeast Asian Journal of Tropical Medicine and Public Health, 25*(4), 650–653.

Kaplan, L.D., Northfelt, D.W. (1997). Malignancies associated with AIDS. In M.A. Sande, P.A. Volberding (Eds.), *The medical management of AIDS* (5th ed., pp. 413–439). Philadelphia: Saunders.

Kasner, S.E., Galetta, S.L., McGowan, J.C., et al. (1997). Magnetization transfer imaging in progressive multifocal leukoencephalopathy. *Neurology, 48,* 534–536.

Kedes, D.H., Ganem, D. (1997). *Susceptibiliity of KSHV (HHV8) to antiviral drugs in culture.* Presented at 4th Conference on Retroviruses and Opportunistic Infections, Washington, D.C.

Keely, S.P., Baughman, R.P., Smulian, A.G., et al. (1996). Source of *Pneumocystis carinii* in recurrent episodes of pneumonia in AIDS patients. *AIDS, 10*(8), 881–888.

Kelly, M., Carr, A., Furner, V., et al. (1996). *Outpatient trimethoprim-sulphamethoxazole (TMP-SMX) desensitisation is safe and effective.* Presented at XI International Conference on AIDS, abstract TuB2287, Vancouver, British Columbia.

Kelly, S.L., Lamb, D.C., Kelly, D.E., et al. (1996). Resistance to fluconazole and amphotericin Candida albicans from AIDS patients. *Lancet, 348,* 1523–1524.

Kemper, C.A., Meng, T.C., Nussbaum, J., et al. (1992). Treatment of *Mycobacterium avium* complex bacteremia in AIDS with a four-drug oral regimen. *The Annals of Internal Medicine, 116*(6), 466–472.

Keshavjee, S.H., Magee, L.A., Mullen, L.A., et al. (1993). Acalculous cholecystitis associated with cytomegalovirus and sclerosing cholangitis in a patient with acquired immunodeficiency syndrome. *Canadian Journal of Surgery, 36*(4), 321–325.

Kessler, H.A., Hurivitz, S., Farthing, C., et al. (1996). Pilot study of topical trifluridine for the treatment of acyclovir-resistant mucocutaneous herpes simplex disease in patients with AIDS. *Journal of Acquired Immune Deficiency and Human Retrovirology, 12*(2), 147–152.

Kim, Y.S., Hollander, H. (1993). Polyradiculopathy due to cytomegalovirus: Report of two cases in which improvement occurred after prolonged therapy and review of the literature. *Clinical Infectious Disease, 17*(1), 32–37.

Kirsch, L.S., Arevelo, J.F., DeClerq, E., et al. (1995). Phase I/II study of intravitreal cidofovir for the treatment of cytomegalovirus retinitis in patients with the acquired immunodeficiency syndrome. *American Journal of Ophthalmology, 119*(4), 466–476.

Kirschtick, R.E., Glasseroth, J., Jordan, M.C., et al. (1995). Bacterial pneumonia in persons infected with the human immunodeficiency virus. *New England Journal of Medicine, 333*(13), 845–851.

Klatt, C., Jensen, D.F., Meyer, P.R. (1987). Pathology of *Mycobacterium avium-intracellulare* infection in acquired immunodeficiency syndrome. *Human Pathology, 18*(7), 709–714.

Klevens, M.R., Fleming, P.L., Mays, M.A., et al. (1996). Characteristics of women with AIDS and invasive cervical cancer. *Obstetrics and Gynecology, 88*(2), 269–273.

Koch, J., Scott, M.K., Morgan, D., et al. (1996). *Gastric hypochlorydria is associated with* Mycobacterium avium *infection in patients with HIV/AIDS.* Presented at XI International Conference of AIDS, abstract MoB118, Vancouver, British Columbia.

Kotler, D. (1992). Causes and consequences of malnutrition in HIV/AIDS. In G. Nary (Ed.), *Nutrition and HIV/AIDS* (Vol. 1, pp. 5–8). Chicago: PAAC Publishing.

Kotler, D.P., Grunfeld, C. (1996). Pathophysiology and treatment of the AIDS wasting syndrome. In P. Volberding, M.A. Jacobson (Eds.), *AIDS clinical review 1995/1996* (pp. 229–275). New York: Marcel Dekker, Inc.

Krouse, J.H. (1985). A psychological model of adjustment in gynecologic cancer patients. *Oncology Nursing Forum, 12*(6), 45–49.

Krown, S.E., Huang, J., Testa, M., et al. (1997). *Validation and refinement of the ACTG staging systme for AIDS-associated Kaposi's sarcoma (KS).* Presented at National AIDS Malignancy Conference, abstract 19, Bethesda, Maryland.

Krown, S.E., Metroka, C., Wernz, J.C. (1989). Kaposi's sarcoma in the acquired immunodeficiency syndrome: A proposal for uniform evaluation, response, and staging criteria. *Journal of Clinical Oncology, 7*(9), 1201–1207.

Kuppermann, B.D., Flores-Aguilar, M., Quiceno, J.I., et al. (1993a). Combination ganciclovir and foscarnet in the treatment of clinically resistant retinitis in patients with acquired immunodeficiency syndrome. *Archives of Ophthalmology, 111*(10), 1359–1366.

Kupperman, B.D., Petty, J.G., Richman, D.D., et al. (1993b). Correlation between CD4+ counts and prevalence of cytomegalovirus retinitis and human immunodeficiency virus-related noninfectious retinal vasculopathy in patients with acquired immunodeficiency syndrome. *Journal of Ophthalmology, 115*(5), 575–582.

Kupperman, B.D., Quiceno, J.I., Flores-Aguilar, M., et al. (1993c). Intravitreal ganciclovir concentration after retinitis: Implications for therapy. *Journal of Infectious Diseases, 168*(6), 1506–1509.

Laguna, F., Garcia-Samaniego, J., Alonso, M.J., et al. (1993). Pseudotomoral appearance of cytomegalovirus esophagitis and gastritis in AIDS patients. *American Journal of Gastroenterology, 88*(7), 1108–1011.

Lai, I.R., Chen, K.M., Shun, C.T., et al. (1996). Cytomegalovirus enteritis causing massive bleeding in a patient with AIDS. *Hepatogastroenterology, 43*(10), 987–991.

Lai, K.K. (1996). *Incidence of cervical dysplasia and human papilloma virus infection among HIV-infected women.* Presented at XI International Conference on AIDS, abstract WeC3405, Vancouver, British Columbia.

Laine, L., Dretler, R.H., Conteas, C.N., et al. (1992). Fluconazole compared with ketoconazole for the treatment of Candida esophagitis in AIDS. *Annals of Internal Medicine, 117*(8), 665–660.

Lalezari, J., Schacker, T., Feinberg, J., et al. (1996). *A randomized, double-blinded, placebo-controlled study of cidofovir topical gel for acyclovir-resistant herpes simplex virus infections in patients with AIDS.* Presented at XI International Conference on AIDS, abstract TuB184, Vancouver, British Columbia.

Lalezari, J.P., Stagg, R.J., Kupperman, B.D., et al. (1997). Intravenous cidofovir for peripheral cytomegalovirus retinitis in patients with AIDS: A randomized, controlled trial. *Annals of Internal Medicine, 126*(4), 257–263.

Lange, J.M., Tapper, M.L. (1993). Clinical treatment. *AIDS, 7*(Suppl.), S171–S172.

Larsen, C. (1996). *Pap smear screening for squamous intraepithelial lesion in HIV infected women.* Presented at XI International Conference on AIDS, abstract WeB542, Vancouver, British Columbia.

Leach, C.T., Cherry, J.D., English, P.A., et al. (1993). The relationship between T-cell levels and CMV infection in asymptomatic HIV-1 antibody-positive homosexual men. *Journal of the Acquired Immunodeficiency Syndromes, 6*(4), 407–413.

LeCocq, L., Bonck, J., MacRae, A. (1995). The role of rehabilitation after human immunodeficiency virus (HIV) infection. In D.A. Umphred (Ed.), *Neurological rehabilitation* (3rd ed., pp. 558–566). St. Louis: Mosby–Year Book.

Lee, B.L., Tauber, M.G. (1994). Histoplasmosis. In P.T. Cohen, M.A. Sande, P.A. Volberding (Eds.), *The AIDS knowledge base* (2nd ed., pp. 6.9-1–6.9-7). Boston: Little, Brown.

Lennette, E.T., Blackbourn, D.J., Levy, J.A. (1996). Antibodies to human herpesvirus type 8 in the general population and in Kaposi's sarcoma patients. *The Lancet, 348,* 858–861.

Levine, A. (1992). AIDS-associated malignant lymphoma. *Medical Clinics of North America, 71*(1), 253–268.

Levine, A.M., Shibata, D., Sullivan-Hurley, J., et al. (1992). Epidemiological and biological study of acquired immunodeficiency syndrome-related lymphoma in the County of Los Angeles: Preliminary results. *Cancer Research, 52*(Suppl. 19), 5482s–5484s.

Levine, A., Tulpule, A., Espina, B.M., et al. (1996a). *Mitoguazone (MGBG) with radiation therapy in AIDS-related primary CNS lymphoma.* Presented at XI International Conference on AIDS, abstract ThB184, Vancouver, British Columbia.

Levine, A.M., Tulpule, A., Espina, B., et al. (1996b). Low dose methotrexate, bleomycin, doxorubicin, cyclophosphamide, vincristine, and dexamethasone with zalcitabine in patients with acquired immunodeficiency syndrome-related lymphoma: Effect on human immunodeficiency virus and serum interleukin-6 levels over time. *Cancer, 78*(3), 517–526.

Levine, A.M., Tulpule, A., Tessman, D., et al. (1997). Mitoguazone therapy in patients with refractory or relapsed AIDS-related lymphoma: Results from a multicenter phase II trial. *Journal of Clinical Oncology, 15*(3), 1094–1003.

Levine, W.C., Buehler, J.W., Bean, N.H., et al. (1991). Epidemiology of non-typhoidal *Salmonella* bacteremia during the human immunodeficiency virus epidemic. *Journal of Infectious Diseases, 164*(1), 81–87.

Liberti, A., Biscogno, A., Izzo, E. (1992). Octreotide treatment in secretory and cryptosporidial diarrhea in patients with acquired immunodeficiency syndrome (AIDS): Clinical evaluation. *Journal of Chemotherapy, 4*(5), 303–305.

Liliana, P., Sforza, R., Benetucci, J., et al. (1997). *Disseminated histoplasmosis: Oral lesions in HIV patients in Argentina.* Presented at 4th Conference on Retroviruses and Opportunistic Infections, Washington, D.C.

Lindsay, D.S., Dubay, J.P., Blagburn, B.L. (1997). Biology of *Isospora* spp. from humans, nonhuman primates, and domestic animals. *Clinical Micriobiology Reviews, 10*(1), 19–34.

Ling, S.M., Roach, M. 3rd, Larson, D.A., et al. (1994). Radiotherapy of primary central nervous system lymphoma in patients with and without human immunodeficiency virus: Ten years of treatment experience at the University of Californa San Francisco. *Cancer, 73*(10), 2570–2582.

Little, S., Haubrich, R., Hwang, J., et al., (1997). *Protease inhibitors are associated with favorable response to topical treatment of Kaposi's sarcoma.* Presented at 4th Conference on Retroviruses and Opportunistic Infections, Washington, D.C.

Loeb, M., Walach, C., Phillips, J., et al. (1995). Treatment with letrazuril of refractory cryptosporidial diarrhea complicating AIDS. *Journal of Acquired Immunodeficiency Syndromes and Human Retrovirology, 10*(1), 48–53.

Lorberboym, M., Estok, L., Machac, J., et al. (1996). Rapid differential diagnosis of cerebral toxoplasmosis and primary central nervous system lymphoma by thallium-201 SPECT. *Journal of Nuclear Medicine, 37*(7), 1150–1154.

Losso, M., Fischer, N., Kalina, M., et al. (1996). *Early diagnosis of tuberculosis (TB) in HIV patients by standard methods and polymerase chain reaction (PCR).* Presented at XI International Conference on AIDS, abstract MoB1355, Vancouver, British Columbia.

Lupo, S., Fernandez, A., Bortolozzi, R., et al. (1992). *First experiences with roxithromycin in the AIDS related cryptosporidiosis treatment in Argentina.* Presented at VIII International Conference on AIDS, abstract PoB3209, Amsterdam, Netherlands.

Ma, P., Villanueva, T.G., Kaufman, D., et al. (1984). Respiratory cryptosporidiosis in acquired immune deficiency syndrome. *Journal of the American Medical Association, 252*(10), 1298–1301.

MacArthur, R.D., Nandi, P., McMillen, L., et al. (1996). *CT guided brain biopsy finding in HIV-infected persons: A retrospective review of 44 cases at an urban medical center.* Presented at XI International Conference on AIDS, abstract WeB3286, Vancouver, British Columbia.

MacKenzie, W.R., Hoxie, M.S., Proctor, M.E., et al. (1994). A massive outbreak in Milwaukee of *Cryptosporidium* infection transmitted through the public water supply. *The New England Journal of Medicine, 331*, 161–167.

Maenza, J.R., Keruly, J.C., Moore, R.D., et al. (1996). Risk factors for fluconazole-resistant candidiasis in human immunodeficiency virus-infected patients. *Journal of Infectious Diseases, 173*(1), 219–225.

Magnenat, J., Nicod, L.P., Auckenthaler, R. (1991). Mode of presentation and diagnosis of bacterial pneumonia in human immunodeficiency virus-infected patients. *American Review of Respiratory Disease, 144*(4), 917–922.

Mahmoudi, A., Iseman, M.D. (1993). Pitfalls in the care of patients with tuberculosis: Common errors and their association with the acquisition of drug resistance. *Journal of the American Medical Association, 270*(1), 65–68.

Maiello, A., Sciandro, M., Calvo, M.M. (1996). *Fungal infections: Prevalence in HIV infection.* Presented at XI International Conference on AIDS, abstract TuB2194, Vancouver, British Columbia.

Maimon, M., Fruchter, R.G., Guy, L., et al. (1993). Human immunodeficiency virus infection and invasive cervical carcinoma. *Cancer, 71*(2), 402–406.

Maimon, M., Fruchter, R.G., Serur, E., et al. (1990). Human immunodeficiency virus infection and ceervical neoplsia. *Gynecologic Oncology, 38*, 377–382.

Malnza, J.R., Keruly, J.C., Moore, R.D., et al. (1996). Risk factors for fluconazole-resistant candidiasis in human immunodeficiency virus-infected patients. *Journal of Infectious Diseases, 173*(1), 219–225.

Mansor, A.M., Li, H.D. (1995). Cytomegalovirus optic neuritis: Characteristics, therapy, and survival. *Ophthalmologica, 209*(5), 260–266.

Markowitz, N., Hansen, N.I., Hopewell, P.C., et al. (1997). Incidence of tuberculosis in the United States among HIV-infected persons. *Annals of Internal Medicine, 126*(2), 123–132.

Martin, A., Castillo, R., Dupla, M., et al. (1991). *Nontyphoidal salmonellosis in HIV-infection: A report of 17 patients in Madrid.* Presented at VIII International Conference on AIDS, abstract WB2313, Amsterdam, Netherlands.

Martin, D.F., Parks, D.J., Mellow, S.D., et al. (1994). Treatment of cytomegalovirus retinitis with an intraocular sustained-release ganciclovir implant: A randomized controlled clinical trial. *Archives of Ophthalmology, 112*(12), 1531–1539.

Martos, A., Podzamczer, D., Martinez-Lacasa, J., et al. (1995). Steroids do not enhance the risk of developing tuberculosis or other AIDS-related diseases in HIV-infected patients treated for *Pneumocystis carinii* pneumonia. *AIDS, 9*(9), 1037–1041.

Marx, J.L., Kapusta, M.A., Patel, S.S., et al. (1996). Use of the ganciclovir implant in the treatment of recurrent cytomegalovirus retinitis. *Archives of Ophthalmology, 114*(7), 815–820.

Masood, R., Lee, M.J.A., Espina, B.M., et al. (1996). *Liposomal daunorubicin (daunoxome) has enhanced cytotoxicity in an AIDS-related Kaposi's sarcoma cell line.* Presented at XI International Conference on AIDS, abstract MoB1256, Vancouver, British Columbia.

McCreary, C.E., Bennett, D., Sullivan, D., et al. (1996). *A prospective study of oral Candida species displacement in AIDS patients with recurrent oral candidiasis.* Presented at XI International Conference on AIDS, Abstract ThB4207, Vancouver, British Columbia.

McDowell, D. (1992). The patient in the home setting. In M.L. Galantino (Ed.), *Clinical assessment and treatment of HIV* (pp. 175–190). Thorofare, NJ: SLACK.

McGowan, I., Hawkins, A.S., Weller, I.V. (1993). The natural history of cryptosporidial diarrhoea in HIV-infected patients. *AIDS, 7*(3), 349–354.

McLaulin, J.B., Rosenberg, D., Bennett, M., et al. (1996). *Diagnosing patterns for HIV dementia in a primary care setting and the development of an HIV dementia screening instrument.* Presented at XI International Conference on AIDS, abstract TuB2265, Vancouver, British Columbia.

McMullin, M. (1992). Holistic care of the patient with cervical cancer. *Nursing Clinics of North America, 27*(4), 847–858.

McReynolds, M.A., Galantino, M.L. (1995, June). Physical therapy management of HIV disease: A retrospective study. *Journal of the International Association of Physicians in AIDS Care, 1*(5), 15–18.

Medina, F., Fuentes, M., Jara, L.J., et al. (1995). *Salmonella* pyomyositis in patients with the human immunodeficiency virus. *British Journal of Rheumatology, 34*(6), 568–571.

Medve, M., Manegold, C., Häussinger, D., et al. (1997). *Long term experience with liposomal doxorubicin as treatment for AIDS-related Kaposi's sarcoma.* Presented at 4th Conference on Retroviruses and Opportunistic Infections, Washington, D.C.

Meier, P.A., Stephan, K.T., Blatt, S.P. (1996). Cytomegalovirus polyradiculopathy in HIV-infected patients. *Journal of General Internal Medicine, 11*(1), 47–49.

Melchior, J.C., Chastang, C., Gelas, P., et al. (1996). Efficacy of 2-month total parenteral nutrition in AIDS patients: A controlled randomized prospective trial. *AIDS, 10,* 379–384.

Mentec, H., Leport, C., Leport, J., et al. (1994). Cytomegalovirus colitis in HIV-1 infected patients: A prospective research in 55 patients. *AIDS, 8*(4), 461–467.

Mestres, C.A., Ninot, S., de Lacy, A.M., et al. (1990). AIDS and *Salmonella*-infected abdominal aortic aneurysm. *Australia and New Zealand Journal of Surgery, 60*(3), 225–226.

Meynard, J.L., Meyohas, M.C., Binet, D., et al. (1996). Pulmonary cryptosporidiosis in the acquired immunodeficiency syndrome. *Infection, 24*(4), 328–331.

Milefchik, E., Leal, M., Haubrich, R., et al. (1997). *A phase II dose escalation trial of high dose fluconazole with and without flucytosine for AIDS associated cryptococcal meningitis.* Presented at IV Conference on Retroviruses and Opportunistic Infections, Washington, D.C.

Miller, R. (1996). HIV-associated respiratory diseases. *Lancet, 348,* 307–312.

Miller, R.F., Foley, N.M., Kessel, D., Jeffrey, A.A. (1994). Community acquired lobar pneumonia in patients with HIV infection and AIDS. *Thorax, 49*(4), 367–368.

Miller, S.I., Hohman, E.L., Pegues, D.A. (1995). *Salmonella.* In G.L. Mandell, J.E. Bennet, R.D. Dolin (Eds.), *Principles and practice of infectious diseases* (5th ed., pp. 2013–2033). New York: Churchill Livingstone.

Milliken, S., Boyle, J. (1993). Update on HIV and neoplastic disease. *AIDS, 7*(Suppl.), S203–S209.

Mitchell, D.M., Miller, R.F. (1995). New developments in the pulmonary diseases affecting HIV infected individuals. *Thorax, 50,* 294–302.

Mitchell, T.G., Perfect, J.R. (1995). Cryptococcosis in the era of AIDS—100 years after the discovery of *Cryptococcus neoformans. Clinical Microbiology Reviews, 8*(4), 525–548.

Mocroft, A., Youle, M., Gazzard, B., et al. (1996). Antiherpesvirus treatment and risk of Kaposi's sarcoma in HIV infection. *AIDS, 10*(10), 1101–1105.

Modilevsky, T., Sattler, F.R., Barnes, P.F. (1989). Mycobacterial diseases in patients with acquired immunodeficiency virus infection. *Archives of Internal Medicine, 149*(10), 2201–2205.

Monini, P., DeLillis, L., Fabris, M., et al. (1996). Kaposi's sarcoma-associated herpesvirus DNA sequences in prostate tissue and human semen. *The New England Journal of Medicine, 334*(18), 1168–1172.

Moolasart, P., Eampokalap, B., Ratanasrithong, M., et al. (1995). Cryptosporidiosis in HIV infected patients in Thailand. *Southeast Asian Journal of Tropical Medicine and Public Health, 26*(2), 335–338.

Moore, R.D., Chaisson, R.E. (1995). Survival analysis of two controlled trials of rifabutin prophylaxis against *Mycobacterium avium* complex in AIDS. *AIDS, 9*(12), 1337–1342.

Moreno, S., Miralles, M.D., Diaz, J., et al. (1996). Cytarabine therapy for progressive multifocal leukoencephalopathy in patients with AIDS. *Clinical Infectious Diseases, 23,* 1066–1068.

Morgello, S. (1992). Epstein-Barr and human immunodeficiency viruses in acquired immunodeficiency syndrome-related primary central nervous system lymphoma. *American Journal of Pathology, 141*(2), 441–450.

Moroni, M., Esposito, R., Cernuschi, M., et al. (1993). Treatment of AIDS-related refractory diarrhoea with octreotide. *Digestion, 54*(Suppl. 1), 30–32.

Moskovitz, B.L., Wilcox, C.M., Darouiche, R., et al. (1996). *Itraconazole oral solution compared with fluconazole for treatment of esophageal candidiasis.* Presented at XI International Conference on AIDS, abstract MoB116, Vancouver, British Columbia.

Musch, D.C., Martin, D.F., Gordon, J.F., et al. (1997). Treatment of cytomegalovirus retinitis with a sustained-release ganciclovir implant. *The New England Journal of Medicine, 337*(20), 83–90.

Musiani, M., Zerbini, M., Venturoli, S., et al. (1994). Rapid diagnosis of cytomegalovirus encephalitis in patients with AIDS using in situ hybridisation. *Journal of Clinical Pathology, 47*(10), 886–891.

Myers, S.A., Kamino, H. (1996). Cutaneous cryptococcosis and histoplasmosis co-infection in a patient with AIDS. *Journal of the American Academy of Dermatology, 34*(5 part 2), 898–900.

Nador, R.G., Cesarman, E., Chadburn, A., et al. (1996). Primary effusion lymphoma: A distinct clincopathologic entity associated with the Kaposi's sarcoma-associated herpes virus. *Blood, 88*(2), 645–656.

Nahlen, B.L., Chu, S.Y., Nwanyanwu, C., et al. (1993). HIV wasting syndrome in the United States. *AIDS, 7*(2), 183–188.

National Institute of Allergy and Infectious Diseases. (1990, May). *HIV associated opportunistic infections: NIAID-supported clinical research. OI Backgrounder.* Bethesda, MD: The Institute.

Neubauer, M.A., Bodensteiner, D.C. (1992). Disseminated histosplasmosis in patients with AIDS. *Southern Medical Journal, 85*(12), 1166–1170.

Newell, M., Goldstein, D., Milliken, S., et al. (1996). Phase I/II trial of filgrastim (r-metHuG-CSF), CEOP chemotherapy and antiretroviral therapy in HIV-related non-Hodgkin's lymphoma. *Annals of Oncology, 7*(10), 1029–1036.

Newman, C.F. (1992). The role of nutritional assessments and nutritional plans in the management of HIV/AIDS. In G. Nary (Ed.), *Nutrition and HIV/AIDS* (Vol. 1, pp. 57–106). Chicago: PAAC Publishing.

New York City Department of Health. (1996). Tuberculosis treatment. *CHI: City Health Information, 15*(S1), 1–4.

Northfelt, D.W., Sollitto, R.A., Miller, T.R., et al. (1993). Cytomegalovirus pneumonitis: An unusual cause of pulmonary nodules in a patient with AIDS. *Chest, 103*(6), 1918–1920.

Northfelt, D., Stewart, S. (1997). *Doxil (pegylated liposomal doxorubicin) as first-line therapy of AIDS-related Kaposi's sarcoma (KS): Integrated efficacy and safety results from two comparative trials.* Presented at 4th Conference on Retroviruses and Opportunistic Infections, Washington, D.C.

Obbens, E., Galantino, M. (1992). Rehabilitation perspectives for neurologic complications of HIV. In M.L. Galantino (Ed.), *Clinical assessment and treatment of HIV* (pp. 87–99). Thorofare, NJ: SLACK.

O'Malley, J.P., Ziessman, H.A., Kuman, P.N., et al. (1994). Diagnosis of intracranial lymphoma in patients with AIDS: Value of 201Tl single-photon emission computed tomography. *American Journal of Roentgenology, 163*(2), 417–421.

Oral Ganciclovir European and Australian Cooperative Study Group. (1995). Intravenous versus oral ganciclovir: European/Australian comparative study of efficacy and safety in the preventions of cytomegalovirus retinitis recurrence in patients with AIDS. *AIDS, 9*(5), 471–477.

Orenstein, J.M., Alkan, S., Blauvelt, A., et al. (1997). *Appearance of human herpesvirus type 8 in Kaposi's sarcoma.* Presented at 4th Conference on Retroviruses and Opportunistic Infections, Washington, D.C.

Pablos-Méndez, A., Sterling, T.R., Frieden, T.R. (1996). The relationship between delayed or incomplete treatment and all-cause mortality in patients with tuberculosis. *JAMA, 276*(15), 1223–1228.

Palella, F.J. Jr., Delaney, K.M., Moorman, A.C., et al. (1998). Declining morbidity and mortality among patients with advanced human immunodeficiency virus infection. HIV Outpatient Study investigators. *New England Journal of Medicine, 338*(13), 853–860.

Palmieri, P.J., Southern, P., Haley, R., et al. (1996). *Fluconazole resistant oropharyngeal candidiasis in a large urban HIV clinic.* Presented at XI International Conference on AIDS, abstract TuB2197, Vancouver, British Columbia.

Pape, J.W., Verdier, R.I., Johnston, W.D., Jr. (1989). Treatment and prophylaxis of *Isospora belli* infection in patients with the acquired immunodeficiency syndrome. *The New England Journal of Medicine, 320*(16), 1044–1047.

Para, M.F., Dohn, M., Frame, P., et al. (1997). *Gradual initiation of trimethoprim/sulfamethoxazole (T/S) as primary prophylaxis for* Pneumocystis carinii *pneumonia (PCP).* Presented at 4th Conference on Retroviruses and Opportunistic Infections, Washington, D.C.

Parisi, A., Calderon, W., Capellini, R., et al. (1996). *Cryptococcosis in AIDS: Current prospects of therapy.* Presented at XI International Conference on AIDS, abstract ThA4062, Vancouver, British Columbia.

Pearsen, M.L., Jereb, J.A., Frieden, T.R., et al. (1992). Nosocomial transmission of multidrug-resistant *Mycobacterium tuberculosis. Annals of Internal Medicine, 117*(3), 191–196.

Pedersen, C., Barton, S.E., Cjiesi, A., et al. (1995). HIV-related non-Hodgkin's lymphoma among European AIDS patients: AIDS in Europe Study Group. *European Journal of Haemotology, 55*(4), 245–250.

Pedersen, C., Danner, S., Lazzarin, A., et al. (1996). Epidemiology of cryptosporidiosis among European AIDS patients. *Genitourinary Medicine, 72*(2), 128–131.

Peel, K.R. (1995). Premalignant and malignant disease of the cervix. In C.R. Whitefield (Ed.), *Dewhurst's textbook of obstetrics and gynecology for postgraduates* (5th ed., pp. 717–737). London: Blackwell Scientific.

Peloquin, C.A. (1993). Controversies in the management of *Mycobacterium avium* complex infection in AIDS patients. *Annals of Pharmacotherapy, 27*(7-8), 928–937.

Peterson, C., Wofsy, C.B. (1994). Cytomegalovirus. In P.T. Cohen, M.A. Sande, P.A. Volberding (Eds.), *The AIDS knowledge base* (2nd ed., pp. 6.20-1–6.20-5). Boston: Little, Brown, & Company.

Petit, N., Heuberger, L., Drougoal, M.P., et al. (1996). *Brain biopsies: Usefulness and side-effects in HIV-positive patients with brain tumors.* Presented at XI International Conference on AIDS, abstract ThB4256, Vancouver, British Columbia.

Phair, J., Munoz, A., Detels, R., et al. (1990). The risk of *Pneumocystis carinii* pneumonia among men infected with human immunodeficiency virus type 1. Multicenter AIDS cohort study group. *New England Journal of Medicine, 322*(3), 161–165.

Pierce, M., Crampton, S., Henry, D., et al. (1996). A randomized trial of clarithromycin as prophylaxis against disseminated *Mycobacterium avium* complex infection in patients with advanced acquired immunodeficiency syndrome. *The New England Journal of Medicine, 335*(6), 384–389.

Pierce, M.A., Johnson, M.D., Maciunas, R.J., et al. (1995). Evaluating contrast-enhancing brain lesions in patients with AIDS by using positron emission tomography. *Annals of Internal Medicine, 123*(8), 594–598.

Pindborg, J.J. (1994). The use of the term "thrush" (letter). *Journal of Acquired Immune Deficiency Syndromes, 7*(10), 98.

Pitchenik, A.E., Fertel, D. (1992). Medical management of AIDS patients. Tuberculosis and nontuberculous mycobacterial disease. *Medical Clinics of North America, 76*(1), 121–171.

Poles, M.A., Meller, J.A., Lin, A., et al. (1997). *Oxandrolone as a treatment for AIDS-related weight loss and wasting.* Presented at 4th Conference on Retroviruses and Opportunistic Infections, Washington, D.C.

Pottage, J.C., Kessler, H.A. (1995). Herpes simplex virus resistance to acyclovir: Clinical relevance. *Infectious Agents and Diseases, 4*(3), 115–124.

Powderly, W.G. (1992). Therapy for cryptococcal meningitis in patients with AIDS. *Clinical Infectious Diseases, 14*(Suppl. 1), S27–S58

Powderly, W.G. (1993). Cryptococcal meningitis and AIDS. *Clinical Infectious Diseases, 17,* 837–842.

Powderly, W.G. (1996). Recent advances in opportunistic infection prophylaxis. Presented at XI International Conference on AIDS, abstract TuB532, Vancouver, British Columbia.

Powderly, W.G., Saag, M.S., Cloud, G.A., et al. (1992). Controlled trial of amphotericin B to prevent relapse of cryptococcal meningitis in patients with acquired immunodeficiency syndrome. *The New England Journal of Medicine, 326*(12), 793–798.

Power, C., Johnson, R.T. (1995). HIV-1 associated dementia: Clinical features and pathogenesis. *Canadian Journal of Neurological Science, 22*(2), 92–100.

Power, C., North, A., Aoki, F.Y., et al. (1997). Remission of progressive multifocal leukoencephalopathy following splenectomy and antiretroviral therapy in a patient with HIV infection. *New England Journal of Medicine, 336*(9), 661–662.

Price, R.W. (1996). Neurological complications of HIV infection. *The Lancet, 348,* 445–452.

Rademacher, S., Keiser, P., Skiest, D., et al. (1995). *Bone marrow culture for the diagnosis of infections in AIDS.* Presented at the II National Conference on Human Retroviruses and Related Infections, abstract 573, Washington, D.C.

Radin, D.R., Esplin, J.A., Levine, A.M., et al. (1993). AIDS-related non-Hodgkin's lymphoma: Abdominal CT findings in 112 patients. *American Journal of Roentgenology, 160*(5), 1133–1139.

Ragni, M.V., Belle, S.H., Jaffee, R.A., et al. (1993). Acquired immunodeficiency syndrome-associated non-Hodgkin's lymphomas and other malignancies in patients with hemophilia. *Blood, 81*(7), 1889–1897.

Rahhal, F.M., Arevato, J.M., Chavez de la Paz, E., et al. (1996). Treatment of cytomegalovirus retinitis with intravitreous cidofovir in patients with AIDS: A preliminary report. *Annals of Internal Medicine, 125*(2), 98–103.

Raza, J., Harris, M.T., Bauer, J.J. (1996). Gastrointestinal histoplasmosis in a patient with acquired immunodeficiency syndrome. *The Mount Sinai Journal of Medicine, 63*(2), 136–140.

Reed, K. (1991). *Quick reference to occupational therapy* (pp. 366–369). Gaithersburg, MD: Aspen.

Reef, S.E., Mayer, K.H. (1995). Opportunistic candidal infections in patients infected with human immunodeficiency virus: Prevention issues and priorities. *Clinical Infectious Disease, 21*(Suppl. 1), 599–602.

Reeves, W.C., Rawls, W.E., Brintan, L.A. (1989). Epidemiology of genital papillomavirus and cervical cancer. *Reviews of Infectious Diseases, 11*(3), 426–439.

Reinis-Lucey, C., Sande, M.A., Gerberding, J.L. (1990). Toxoplasmosis. In P.T. Cohen, M.A. Sande, P.A. Volberding (Eds.), *The AIDS knowledge base* (pp. 656.1–656-15). Waltham, MA: Medical Publishing Group.

Restrepo, C., Macher, A.M., Radnay, E.H. (1987). Disseminated extraintestinal isosporiasis in a patient with acquired immune deficiency syndrome. *American Journal of Clinical Pathology, 87*(4), 536–542.

Reyes-Terán, G., Sierra-Madero, J.G., del Cerro, V.M., et al. (1996). Effects of thalidomide on HIV-associated wasting syndrome: A randomized, double-blind, placebo-controlled clinical trial. *AIDS, 10,* 1501–1507.

Reynods, H.Y. (1991). Pneumonia and lung abscess. In J.D. Wilson, I. Braunwald, K.J. Isselbacher, et al. (Eds.), *Harrison's principles of internal medicine* (12th ed., pp. 1064–1069). New York: McGraw-Hill.

Rich, J.D., Crawford, J.M., Kazanjian, S.N., et al. (1992). Discrete gastrointestinal mass lesions caused by cytomegalovirus in patients with AIDS: Report of three cases and review. *Clinical Infectious Disease, 15*(4), 609–614.

Richart, R.M., Wright, T.C. (1993). Controversies in the management of low-grade cervical intraepithelial neoplasia. *Cancer 71*(Suppl. 4), 1413–1421.

Riley, K.B., Antoniskis, D., Maris, R., et al. (1988). Rattlesnake capsule-associated *Salmonella arizona* infections. *Archives of Internal Medicine, 148*(5), 1207–1210.

Rimland, D., Navin, T.R., Lennox, J., et al. (1996). *Prospective study of etiologic agents of community-acquired pneumonia in patients with HIV infection.* Presented at XI International Conference on AIDS, abstract WeB3319, Vancouver, British Columbia.

Roberts, T.C., Storch, G.A. (1996). *Multiplex polymerase chain reaction for diagnosis of AIDS-related central nervous system lymphoma and toxoplasmosis.* Presented at XI International Conference on AIDS, abstract TuA154, Vancouver, British Columbia.

Rodriguez, J.C., Mora, A., Blazquez, J.C., et al. (1996). *Sensitivity of poymerase chain reaction (PCR) in cerebrospinal fluid in the diagnosis of cerebral toxoplasmosis.* Presented at XI International Conference on AIDS, abstract ThB181, Vancouver, British Columbia.

Rogers, E.A. (1992). The interdisciplinary HIV team. *Clinical Management, 12*(6), 38–41.

Rolston, K.V. (1993). Candidiasis. *PAAC Notes, 5*(2), 54–56.

Routy, J.P., Urbanek, A., MacLeod,J., et al. (1997). *Significant regression of Kaposi's sarcoma following initiation of an effective antiretroviral combination treatment.* Presented at National AIDS Malignancy Conference, abstract 23, Bethesda, Maryland.

Rubin, M.M., Lauver, D. (1991). Assessment and management of cervical intraepithelial neoplasia. *Nurse Practitioner, 15*(9), 23–31.

Rubio, R., Rubio, M., Grauss, F., et al. (1996). *Primary central nervous system lymphoma (PCNSL) in AIDS: A multicentric clinical study.* Presented at XI International Conference on AIDS, abstract ThB4232, Vancouver, British Columbia.

Ruf, B., Jautzke, G., Schumann, D., et al. (1990). Clinical aspects and pathology of mycobacterial infections in AIDS: Pulmonary and extrapulmonary manifestations. *Pneumonologie, 44*(Suppl. 1), 502–503.

Ruiz, A., Gans, W.I., Post, M.J., et al. (1994). Use of thallium-201 brain SPECT to differentiate cerebral lymphoma from *Toxoplasma* encephalitis in AIDS patients. *American Journal of Neuroradiology, 15*(10), 1885–1894.

Saag, M.S. (1993). Cryptococcal meningitis. *PAAC-NOTES, 5*(1), 34–37.

Saag, M.S., Powderly, W.G., Cloud, G.A., et al. (1992). Comparison of amphotericin B with fluconazone in the treatment of acute AIDS-associated cryptococcal meningitis. *The New England Journal of Medicine, 326*(2), 83–89.

Safai, B., Dias, B.M. (1994). Kaposi's sarcoma and cloacogenic carcinoma associated with AIDS. In S. Broder, T.C. Merigan, D. Bolognesi (Eds.), *Textbook of AIDS medicine* (pp. 401–415). Baltimore: Williams & Wilkins.

Safrin, S. (1994). Herpes simplex and varicella-zoster virus infections in HIV-infected individuals. In S.

Broder, T.C. Merigan, D. Bodognesi (Eds.), *Textbook of AIDS medicine* (pp. 373–385). Baltimore: Williams & Wilkins.

Safrin, S., Crumpacher, C., Chatis, P., et al. (1991). A controlled trial comparing foscarnet with vidarabine for acyclovir-resistant mucocutaneous herpes simplex in the acquired immunodeficiency syndrome. *New England Journal of Medicine, 325*(8), 551–555.

Safrin, S., Finkelstein, D.M., Feinberg, J., et al. (1996). Comparison of three regimens for treatment of mild to moderate *Pneumocystis carinii* pneumonia in patients with AIDS. *Annals of Internal Medicine, 124*(9), 792–802.

Salomon, N., Gomez, T., Perlman, D.C., et al. (1997). Clinical features and outcomes of HIV-related cytomegalovirus pneumonia. *AIDS, 11*(3), 319–324.

Sarosi, G.A., Davies, S.F. (1996). Endemic mycosis complicated human immunodeficiency virus infection. *Western Journal of Medicine, 164*(4), 335–340.

Sattler, F.R. (1994). *Pneumocystis carinii* pneumonia. In S. Broder, T.C. Merigan, D. Bolognesi (Eds.), *Textbook of AIDS medicine* (pp. 193–223). Baltimore: Williams & Wilkins.

Sauda, F.C., Zamarioli, L.A., Ebner, F.W., et al. (1993). Prevalence of *Cryptosporium* sp. and *Isospora belli* among AIDS patients attending Santos Reference Center for AIDS, Sao Paulo, Brazil. *Journal of Parisitology, 79*(3), 454–456.

Sawka, C.A., Shepherd, F.A., Brandwein, J., et al. (1992). Treatment of AIDS-related non-Hodgkin's lymphoma with a twelve week chemotherapy regimen. *Leukemia and Lymphoma, 8*(3), 213–220.

Schambelan, M., Mulligan, K., Grunfeld, C., et al. (1996). Recombinant human growth hormone in patients with HIV-associated wasting. *Annals of Internal Medicine, 125*(11), 873–882.

Schlacht, I., Landonio, G., Nosar, A.M., et al. (1994). *HIV-related lymphomas (NHL): Report of 53 cases.* Presented at X International Conference on AIDS, abstract PB0129, Yokohama, Japan.

Schoeppner, H.L., Wong, D.K., Bresalier, R.S. (1995). Primary small bowel lymphoma manifested as obstructive jaundice in a patient with AIDS. *Southern Medical Journal, 88*(5), 583–585.

Schuman, P., Vazquez, J., Sobel, J.D., et al. (1996). *A randomized trial comparing fluconazole with placebo for prophylaxis of mucosal candidiasis in women with human immunodeficiency virus infection.* Presented at XI International Conference on AIDS, abstract TuB411, Vancouver, British Columbia.

Schurmann, D., Grunewald, T., Weiss, R., et al. (1995). Intensive treatment of AIDS-related non-Hodgkin's lymphomas with the MACOP-B protocol. *European Journal of Haematology, 54*(2), 73–77.

Schwartz, L.B., Carcangiu, M.L., Bradham, L., Schwartz,

D.E. (1991). Rapidly progressive squamous cell carcinoma of the cervix coexisting with human immunodeficiency virus infection: Clinical opinion. *Gynecologic Oncology, 41,* 255–258.

Sciaretta, G., Bonazzi, L., Monti, M., et al. (1994). Bile acid malabsorption in AIDS-associated diarrhea: A prospective one year study. *American Journal of Gastroenterology, 89*(3), 379–381.

Sears, C.L. (1995). "*Isospora belli, Sarcocystis* species, *Balantidium coli, Bastocystis hominis,* and *Cyclospora.* In G.L. Mandell, J.E. Bennet, R. Dolin (Eds.), *Principles and practices of infectious diseases* (4th ed., pp. 2510–2522). New York: Churchill Livingstone.

Segura, L., Rojas, M., Klaskala, W., et al. (1996). *Disseminated histoplasmosis in AIDS patients in Guatemala.* Presented at XI International Conference on AIDS, abstract PubB1054, Vancouver, British Columbia.

Selwyn, P.A., Alcalus, P., Hartel, D., et al. (1992). Clinical manifestations and predictors of disease progression in drug users with human immunodeficiency virus infection. *The New England Journal of Medicine, 237*(24), 1697–1703.

Selwyn, P.A., Feingold, A.R., Hartel, D., et al. (1988). Increased risk of bacterial pneumonia in HIV-infected intravenous drug users without AIDS. *AIDS, 2*(4), 267–272.

Serriano, D., Salamina, G., Francheschi, S., et al. The epidemiology of AIDS-associated non-Hodgkin's lymphoma in the World Health Organization European Region. *British Journal of Cancer, 66*(5), 912–916.

Shafer, R.W. (1994). Tuberculosis. In S. Broder, T.C. Merigan, E. Bolognesi (Eds.), *Textbook of AIDS medicine* (pp. 259–282). Baltimore: Williams & Wilkins.

Shafran, S.D., Singer, J.S., Zarowny, D.P., et al. (1996). A comparison of two regimens for the treatment of *Mycobacterium avium* complex bacteremia in AIDS: Rifabutin, ethambutol, and clarithromycin versus rifampin, ethambutol, clofazimine, and ciprofloxacin. *New England Journal of Medicine, 335*(6), 337–398.

Shah, K.V., Muñoz, A., Klein, R.S., et al. (1996). *Prolonged persistence of genital human papillomavirus infecions in HIV-infected women.* Presented at XI International Conference on AIDS, abstract TuC2466, Vancouver, British Columbia.

Sharkey-Mathis, P.K., Velez, J., Fetchick, R., et al. (1993). Histoplasmosis in the acquired immunodeficiency syndrome (AIDS): Treatment with itraconazole and fluconazole. *Journal of Acquired Immune Deficiency Syndromes, 6*(7), 809–819.

Shepp, D.H., Moses, J.E., Kaplan, M.H. (1996). Seroepidemiology of cytomegalovirus in patients with advanced HIV disease: Influence on disease expression and survival. *Journal of Acquired Immunodeficiency Syndromes and Human Retrovirology, 11*(5), 460–468.

Sider, L., Melany, M. (1993). Thoracic AIDS-related lymphoma: CT apperance and CD4 counts. *American Journal of Roentgenology, 160*(Suppl. 4), 97.

Singh, V.R., Smith, D.K., Lawrence, J., et al. (1996). Coccidioidomycosis in patients infected with immunodeficiency virus: Review of 91 cases at one institution. *Clinical Infectious Disease, 23*(3), 563–568.

Six, C. (1996). *Comparative prevalence, incidence and short-term prognosis of squamous intraepithelial lesions (SIL) among HIV (+) and HIV (–) women.* Presented at XI International Conference on AIDS, abstract WeB543, Vancouver, British Columbia.

Smith, P.D., Janoff, E.N. (1988). Infectious diarrhea in human immunodeficiency virus infection. *Gastroenterology Clinics of North America, 17*(3), 587–598.

Snijders, F., van Deventer, S.J., Bartelsman, J.F. (1995). Diarrhoea in HIV-infected patients: No evidence of cytokine-mediated inflammation in jejunal mucosa. *AIDS, 9*(4), 367–373.

Soave, R., Sepkowitz, K.A. (1992). *Cryptosporidium, Isospora, Dientamoeba.* In S.L. Gorbach, J.G. Bartlett, N.R. Blackow (Eds.), *Infectious diseases* (pp. 2122–2130). New York: Churchill Livingstone.

Soave, R., Weikel, C.A. (1990). *Cryptosporidium* and other protozoa including *Isospora, Sarcocystis, Balantidium coli,* and *Blastocystis.* In G.L. Mandell, R.G. Douglas, Jr., J.E. Bennett (Eds.), *Principles and practice of infectious diseases* (3rd ed., pp. 2122–2130). New York: Churchill Livingstone.

Sobel, J.D., Schuman, P., Mayer, K., et al. (1996). *Candida colonization and mucosal candidiasis in women with or at risk for HIV infection.* Presented at XI International Conference on AIDS, abstract WeC3408, Vancouver, British Columbia.

Sorvillo, F., Lieb, L.E., Nahlen, B., et al. (1994a). Municipal drinking water and cryptosporidiosis among persons with AIDS in Los Angeles County. *Epidemiology of Infection, 113*(2), 313–320.

Sorvillo, F.J., Lieb, L.E., Kerndt, P.R., Ash, L.R. (1994b). Epidemiology of cryptosporidiosis among persons with acquired immunodeficiency syndrome in Los Angeles County. *American Journal of Tropical Medicine and Hygiene, 51*(3), 326–331.

Sorvillo, F.J., Lieb, L.E., Seidel, J. (1995). Epidemiology of isosporiasis among persons with acquired immunodeficiency syndrome in Los Angeles County. *American Journal of Tropical Medicine and Hygiene, 53*(6), 656–659.

Sparano, J.A., Wiernik, P.H., Hu, S., et al. (1996). Pilot trial of infusional cyclophosphamide, doxorubicin, and etoposide plus didanosine and filgrastim in patients with non-Hodgkin's lymphoma. *Journal of Clinical Oncology, 14*(11), 3026–3035.

Sparano, J.A., Wiernik, P.H., Strack, M., et al. (1994). Infusional cyclophosphamide, doxorubicin, and etoposide in HIV-related non-Hodgkin's lymphoma: A follow-up report of a highly active regimen. *Leukemia and Lymphoma, 14*(3-4), 263–271.

Spector, S.A., McKinley, G.F., Lalezari, J.P., et al. (1996). Oral ganciclovir for the prevention of cytomegalovirus disease in persons with AIDS. Roche Cooperative Oral Ganciclovir Study Group. *New England Journal of Medicine, 334*(23), 1491–1497.

Spivak, H., Schlasinger, M.H., Tabanda-Lichauco, R., et al. Small bowel obstruction from gastrointesinal histoplasmosis in acquired immunodeficiency syndrome. *American Surgeon, 62*(5), 369–372.

Sprinz, E., Barcellow, S., Bem, D.D., et al. (1996). *A phase II trial with roxithromycin in AIDS-related* Cryptosporidium *diarrhea.* Presented at XI International Conference on AIDS, abstract ThB4211, Vancouver, British Columbia.

Stansell, J.D. (1993). Pulmonary fungal infections in HIV-infected persons. *Seminars in Respiratory Infections, 8*(2), 116–153.

Stein, M., Houston, S., Pozniak, A., et al. (1993). HIV infection and *Salmonella* septic arthritis. *Clinical and Experimental Rheumatology, 11*(2), 187–189.

Stevens, D.A. (1994). Management of systemic manifestations of fungal disease in patients with AIDS. *Journal of the American Academy of Dermatology, 31*(3, part 2), S64–S67.

Stevens, D.A. (1995). *Coccidioides immitis.* In G.L. Mandell, J.E. Bennet, R. Dolin (Eds.), *Principles and practices of infectious diseases* (4th ed., pp. 2365–2374). New York: Churchill Livingstone.

Stewart, J.A., Reef, S.E., Pellett, P.E., et al. (1995). Herpesvirus infections in persons with human immunodeficiency virus. *Clinical Infectious Diseases, 21*(Suppl. 1), S114–120.

Strauss, S.S. (1995). Introduction to herpesviridae. In G.L. Mandell, J.E. Bennet, R. Dolin (Eds.), *Principles and practices of infectious diseases* (4th ed., pp. 1330–1336). New York: Churchill Livingstone.

Studies of the Ocular Complications of AIDS Research Group. (1992). Mortality in patients with the acquired immunodeficiency syndrome treated with either foscarnet or ganciclovir for cytomegalovirus retinitis. *The New England Journal of Medicine, 326*(4), 213–219.

Studies of the Ocular Complications of AIDS Research Group. (1994). Foscarnet-ganciclovir cytomegalovirus retinitis trial 4: Visual outcomes. *Ophthalmology, 101*(7), 1250–1261.

Studies of the Ocular Complications of AIDS Research Group. (1996). Combination foscarnet and ganciclovir versus monotherapy for the treatment of relapsed cytomegalovirus retinitis in patients with AIDS. *Archives of Ophthalmology, 114*(1), 23–33.

Studies of the Ocular Complications of AIDS Research Group. (1997). Parenteral Cidofovir for cytomegalovirus retinitis in patients with AIDS: The HPMPC peripheral cytomegalovirus retinitis trial: A randomized, controlled trial. *Annals of Internal Medicine, 126*(4), 264–274.

Sullivan, D., Harringtton, J., McCreary, C., et al. (1996). *Candida dubliniensis: A new species associated with oral candidiasis in HIV-infected individuals.* Presented at XI International Conference on AIDS, abstract ThA4057, Vancouver, British Columbia.

Sullivan, D.J., Westerneng, T.J., Haynes, K.A., et al. (1995). Candida dubliniensis species now: Phenotypic and molecular characterization of a novel species associated with oral candidosis in HIV-infected individuals. *Microbiology, 141*(Pt 7), 1507–1521.

Tacconelli, E., Tumbarello, M., Cauda, R., et al. (1997). *PCP prophylaxis and bacterial pneumonia (BP).* Presented at 4th Conference on Retroviruses and Opportunistic Infections, Washington, D.C.

Talezari, J., Schacker, T., Feinberg, J., et al. (1996). *A randomized, double-blinded palacebo-controlled study of Cidofovir topical gel for acyclovir-resistant herpes simplex virus infections in patients with AIDS.* Presented at XI International Conference on AIDS, abstract TuB184, Vancouver, British Columbia.

Telzak, E.E., Chirgiven, K., Nelson, E., et al. (1997). *Predictors for multi-drug resistant tuberculosis (MDRTB) among HIV-infected patients and response to specific MDRTB drug regimens.* Presented at 4th Conference on Retroviruses and Opportunistic Infections, Washington, D.C.

Tirelli, U., Errante, D., Oskenhendler, E., et al. (1992). Prospective study with combined low-dose chemotherapy and zidovudine in 37 patients with poor-prognosis AIDS-related non-Hodgkin's lymphoma: French-Italian Cooperative Study Group. *Annals of Oncology, 3*(10), 843–847.

Tirelli, U., Errante, D., Tavio, M., et al. (1993). *Treatment of HIV-related non-Hodgkin's lymphoma (NHL) with chemotherapy (CT) and granulocyte-colony stimulating factor (G-CSF), reduction of toxicity and days of hospitalization with concomitant overall reduction of the cost.* Presented at IX International Conference on AIDS, abstract WS-B16-2, Berlin, Germany.

Tobin, M.J. (1995). Vulvovaginal candidiasis: Topical vs oral therapy. *American Family Physician, 51*(7), 1715–1720.

Torres, G. (1993). Opportunistic infections over-view. *Treatment Issues, 7*(8), 1–5.

Tosi, P., Gherlinzoni, F., Mazza, P., et al. (1997). 3'-Azido 3'-deoxythymidine plus methotrexate as a novel antineoplastic combination in the treatment of human immunodeficiency virus-related non-Hodgkin's lymphoma. *Blood, 89*(2), 419–425.

U.S. Public Health Service Task Force on Antipneumocystis Prophylaxis in Patients with Human Immunodeficiency Virus Infection. (1993). Recommendations for prophylaxis against *Pneumocystis carinii* pneumonia for persons with human immunodeficiency virus. *Journal of Acquired Immune Deficiency Syndromes, 6*(1), 46–55.

Vakil, N.B., Schwartz, S.M., Buggy, B.P., et al. (1996). Biliary cryptosporidiosis in HIV-infected people after the waterborne outbreak of cryptosporidiosis in Milwaukee. *The New England Journal of Medicine, 334*(1), 19–23.

Vecchiarelli, A., Monari, C., Baldelli, F., et al. (1995). Beneficial effect of recombinant human granulocyte colony-stimulating factor on fungicidal activity of polymorphonuclear leukocytes from patients with AIDS. *Journal of Infectious Diseases, 171*(6), 1448–1454.

Voelker, R. (1994). More choices for treating AIDS-related pneumonia. *Journal of the American Medical Association, 271*(3), 176–177.

von Reyn, C.F., Maslow, J.N., Barber, T.W., et al. (1994). Persistent colonisation of potable water as a source of *Mycobacterium avium* infection in AIDS. *The Lancet, 343*(8906), 1137–1141.

Wakefield, A. (1997). *Molecular biological insights into the epidemiology of Pneumocystis carinii pneumonia.* Presented at 4th Conference on Retroviruses and Opportunistic Infections, Washington D.C.

Wallace, J.M., Hannah, J. (1988). *Mycobacterium avium* complex infection in patients with acquired immunodeficiency syndrome: Findings in an autopsy series. *Chest, 93*(5), 198–203.

Wallace, M.R., Rossetti, R.J., Olson, P.E. (1993). Cats and toxoplasmosis risk in HIV-infected adults. *Journal of the American Medical Association, 269*(1), 76–77.

Walsh, C., Wernz, J.C., Levine, A., et al. (1993). Phase I trial of m-BACOD and granulocyte macrophage colony stimulating factor in HIV-associated non-Hodgkin's lymphoma. *Journal of Acquired Immunodeficiency Syndromes, 6*(3), 265–271.

Walter, H., Nehm, K., Skorde, J., et al. (1993). *Ganciclovir in CMV gastrointestinal disease: A randomised double blind study of two dose regimens in acute therapy.* Presented at IX International Conference of AIDS, abstract PoB191837, Berlin, Germany.

Walzer, P.D. (1995). *Pneumocystis carinii.* In G.L. Mandell, J.E. Bennett, R. Dolin (Eds.), *Principles and practice of infectious diseases* (4th ed., pp. 2475–2487). New York: Churchill Livingstone.

Ward, J.W., Fleming, P. (1993). *The epidemiology of AIDS-related lymphomas (ARL), United States.* Presented at IX International Conference on AIDS, abstract WS-B16-1, Berlin, Germany.

Waters, D., Danska, J., Hardy, K., et al. (1996). Recombinant human growth hormone, insulin-like growth factor 1, and combination therapy in AIDS-associated wasting. *Annals of Internal Medicine, 125*(11), 865–872.

Watts, D.H., Spino, C., Benson, C., et al. (1996). *A comparison of gynecologic findings in HIV positive women with CD4 lymphocyte counts 200 to 500/cc and 100/cc.* Presented at XI International Conference on AIDS, abstract ThB4137, Vancouver, British Columbia.

Wax, T.D., Layfield, L.J., Zaleski, S., et al. (1994). Cytomegalovirus sialadenitis in patients with the acquired immunodeficiency syndrome: A potential diagnostic pitfall with fine-needle aspiration cytology. *Diagnostic Cytopathology, 10*(2), 169–172.

Waxman, A.B., Goldie, S.J., Brett-Smith, H., et al. (1997). Cytomegalovirus as a primary pulmonary pathogen in AIDS. *Chest, 111*(1), 128–134.

Weber, J.T., Sidhu, J.S. (1997). *Prevalence of TB, invasive cervical cancer, and recurrent pneumonia among HIV infected hospital patients, 1994–1995.* Presented at 4th Conference on Retroviruses and Opportunistic Infections, Washington, D.C.

Weinberg, D.V., Murphy, R., Naughton, K. (1994). Combined daily therapy with intravenous ganciclovir and foscarnet for patients with recurrent cytomegalovirus retinitis. *American Journal of Ophthalmology, 117*(6), 776–782.

Weinberger, S.E. (1993). Recent advances in pulmonary medicine [second of two parts]. *New England Journal of Medicine, 328*(2), 1462–1470.

Westmoreland, B.F. (1994). *Medical neurosciences: An approach to anatomy, pathology and physiology by systems and level* (3rd ed., pp. 71–75). Rochester, MN: Mayo Foundation.

Wheat, J., Connolly-Stringfield, P., Williams, B., et al. (1992). Diagnosis of histoplasmosis in patients with the acquired immunodeficiency syndrome by detection of *Histoplasma capsulatum* polysaccharide antigen in bronchoalveolar lavage fluid. *American Review of Respiratory Disease, 145*(6), 1421–1424.

Wheat, J., Hafner, R., Korzun, A.H., et al. (1995). Itraconazole treatment of disseminated histoplasmosis in patients with the acquired immunodeficiency syndrome. *American Journal of Medicine, 98*(4), 336–342.

White, A.C., Jr., Chappell, C.L., Hayat, C.S., et al. (1994). Paromomycin for cryptosporidiosis in AIDS: A prospective, double-blind trial. *Journal of Infectious Disease, 170*(2), 419–424.

White, M.H. (1996). Is vulvo-vaginal candidiasis an AIDS-related illness? *Clinical Infectious Disease, 22*(Suppl. 2), S124–S127.

Whiteman, M.L., Dandapani, D.K., Shebert, R.T., et al. (1994). MRI of AIDS-related polyradiculomyelitis. *Journal of Computer Assisted Tomography, 18*(8), 7–11.

Wilcox, C.M., Schwartz, D.A. (1996). Endoscopic-pathologic correlates of candida esophagitis in acquired immunodeficiency syndrome. *Digestive Diseases and Sciences, 41*(7), 1337–1345.

Wilcox, C.M., Straub, R.F., Schwartz, D.A. (1994).

Prospective endoscopic characterization of cytomegalovirus esophagitis in AIDS. *Gastrointestinal Endoscopy, 40*(4), 481–484.

Wiley, C.A., Nelson, J.A. (1998). Role of human immunodeficiency virus and cytomegalovirus in AIDS encephalitis. *American Journal of Pathology, 133*(1), 73–81.

Williams, S., Strussenberg, J., Nelson, J. (1997). *HHV8/KSHV specifically infects human microvascular but not macrovascular endothelial cells.* Presented at 4th Conference on Retroviruses and Opportunistic Infections, Washington, D.C.

Wong, S., Remington, J.S. (1994). Toxoplasmosis in the setting of AIDS. In S. Broder, T.C. Merigan, D. Bolognesi (Eds.), *Textbook of AIDS medicine* (pp. 223–259). Baltimore: Williams & Wilkins.

Workman, C., Lewis, C., Smith, D.O., et al. (1996). *Resolution of Kaposi's sarcoma associated with saquinavir therapy: Case report.* Presented at XI International Conference on AIDS, abstract TuB2217, Vancouver, British Columbia.

Wormser, G.P., Horowitz, H., Dworkin, B. (1994). Low-dose dexamethasone as adjunctive therapy for disseminated *Mycobacterium avium* complex infections in AIDS patients. *Antimicrobial Agents and Chemotherapy, 38*(9), 2215–2217.

Wu, A.W., Gray, S., Brookmeyer, R., et al. (1996). *Quality of life in a double-blind randomized trial of 3 oral regimens for mild-to-moderate* Pneumocystis carinii *pneumonia in AIDS (ACTG 108).* Presented at XI International Conference on AIDS, abstract TuB112, Vancouver, British Columbia.

Yau, T.H., Rivera-Velazquez, P.M., Mark, A.S., et al. (1996). Unilateral optic neuritis caused by *Histoplasma capsulatum* in a patient with the acquired immunodeficiency syndrome. *American Journal of Ophthalmology, 121*(3), 324–326.

Zarabi, C.M., Thomas, R., Adesokan, A. (1992). Diagnosis of systemic histoplasmosis in patients with AIDS. *Southern Medical Journal, 8*(12), 1171–1175.

Zighelboim, J., Goldfarb, R.A., Mody, D., et al. (1992). Prostatic abscess due to *Histoplasma capsulatum* in a patient with the acquired immunodeficiency syndrome. *Journal of Urology, 147*(1), 166–168.

Zingman, B.S. (1996). Resolution of refractory AIDS-related mucosal candidiasis after initiation of didanosine plus saquinavir. *The New England Journal of Medicine, 334*(25), 1674–1675.

7

Psychosocial and Neuropsychiatric Dysfunction

JACQUELYN HAAK FLASKERUD ■ ERIC N. MILLER

HIV disease generates a unique series of stresses for infected persons, sexual partners, family members, and health care professionals. It creates serious social and psychologic problems for everyone with whom the infected person has close contacts, including friends and employers. It causes distress in HIV-infected healthy persons, in those with clinical disease, in the worried well, and in the general public.

HIV disease may also represent comorbidity in populations with preexisting mental illness. In these populations the prevalence of risk factors may be especially high. Hypersexuality and the practice of unsafe sex may be a particular risk, as may drug use and trading sex for drugs. HIV disease also may exacerbate preexisting mental illnesses, such as major affective disorders and schizophrenia. Finally, HIV disease is associated with neuropsychiatric dysfunctions. These may create extreme distress and burden for persons living with HIV disease (PLWH) and their loved ones. They also may produce a variety of psychiatric symptoms, such as anxiety syndromes, mania, hallucinations, and paranoia. Whether because of stress, previous mental illness, or the viral infection itself, HIV disease produces psychosocial and neuropsychiatric consequences that often require the intervention and support of health care givers.

UNIQUE FEATURES OF THE AIDS EPIDEMIC

As the HIV epidemic matures, different aspects emerge as requiring more attention from one time period to the next. Currently several features of the epidemic have become apparent and require added emphasis. First, there is an increasing concern for persons with serious mental illness and their risks of HIV. These persons may also be homeless, they may use injection drugs, and they may engage in high-risk sexual practices with multiple partners (Coverdale, 1996; Herman et al., 1994; Kalichman et al., 1995, 1996).

A second and related concern is the recognition that injecting drug users (IDUs) have high rates of psychopathology (in psychiatry known as dual diagnoses), most commonly major depression, dysthymia, anxiety/panic disorders, and personality disorders. These may or may not be superimposed on the neuropsychiatric disorders that accompany HIV disease (Cabaj, 1996; Camacho et al., 1996; Rabkin et al., 1997; Snyder et al., 1996). Which of these diagnoses is considered primary probably depends on the health professionals present and the services offered in a particular setting. In this chapter psychopathology and treatment are the focus.

Third, the advent of improved medication management of HIV disease brings with it a new set of psychologic problems. Combination therapy, protease inhibitors, and interleukin-2 immunomodulating therapy hold out promise to PLWH of a chronic disease as opposed to a terminal disease. Psychologic reactions range from renewed hope, to regret over choices made with intense consequences, to extreme disappointment that comes to some when the new therapies do not work for them (Enger et al., 1996; Wells,

1997a, 1997b). Finally, with the advances in research on brain function and dysfunction, neurochemical changes, and hormonal processes have come advances in psychopharmacology that have an impact on HIV clinical practice (Cole & Kemeny, 1997; Kemeny et al., 1994; Leiphart, 1997; McEnany et al., 1996). Each of these features is given added emphasis in this edition.

The spectrum of disease caused by HIV infection includes a constellation of unique characteristics that make it a public health problem without contemporary counterpart. HIV disease is a relatively new communicable, sexually transmitted, frequently fatal disease. It was first identified and occurs most often in socially stigmatized or marginalized groups: men who have sex with men (MSM), IDUs, women, children, and ethnic people of color. The diagnosis of HIV/AIDS is a traumatic event because the disease is known to have a progressive course, no curative treatment, and a poor prognosis. The complexity and multiplicity of problems confronting people with HIV infection and the psychologic fear it engenders affect every aspect of a person's life. Specific features of the AIDS epidemic contribute to the unique psychologic, social, and psychiatric aspects of the disease (Amaro, 1995; Enger et al., 1996; Grossman, 1994, 1995; McKirnan et al., 1996):

1. Persons with HIV disease are generally young. About 18% are in their twenties, 45% are in their thirties, and 25% are in their forties.
2. HIV disease is incurable, requires lifelong changes in behavior, and threatens a person's most intimate relationships.
3. The diagnosis of HIV infection may force the person's identification as a likely member of a stigmatized minority.
4. The social stigma and fear associated with the contagious aspect of the disease can cause others, even family members, to avoid social and physical contact with the infected person.
5. Because of moral disapproval and negative societal attitudes, there is a tendency to blame the infected person for the disease if he or she was exposed to the disease through sexual or drug use practices.
6. The entire continuum of HIV disease, from exposure through infection to diagnosis, is characterized by extreme uncertainty, resulting in marked psychologic distress.
7. Persons with HIV disease are vulnerable to feelings of guilt, self-hatred, rejection, and ostracism, as well as to the commonly recognized feelings of fear, anxiety, depression, and anger that accompany other life-threatening illnesses.
8. There is a dynamic relationship between HIV disease and mental illness: HIV disease may exacerbate mental illness, and mental illness may perpetuate behaviors that facilitate transmission.
9. HIV disease is associated with the highest incidence of neurologic and neuropsychiatric morbidity of any serious common illness that is not primary to the nervous system.
10. AIDS is associated with severe chronic physical disability that may leave persons debilitated and disfigured.
11. Health care professionals and the current treatment system for PLWH are severely taxed and often overwhelmed by the complexity and multiplicity of problems associated with care of PLWH. This situation is likely to worsen as the numbers of patients increase. In addition, fear and a lack of knowledge and sensitivity among health care workers are detrimental to patient care.
12. HIV disease has had a highly visible social and political impact. It has attracted a barrage of media attention that is not always accurate, is often stressful to PLWH, aggravates public fears, and leads to attempts at repressive measures such as quarantines or mandatory HIV testing.

Because of these characteristics of both the disease and the epidemic, the care of PLWH requires special attention to the psychologic, social, and psychiatric aspects of their disease. Also of concern to health care professionals is the distress experienced by the worried well, by symptom-free seropositive persons, and by the sexual partners and families of PLWH. The distress that health care professionals themselves experience in giving care to PLWH is a further consideration.

PSYCHOLOGIC RESPONSES TO HIV AMONG UNINFECTED PERSONS

HIV disease is occurring in a society that disapproves of homosexuality, drug use, and sexual promiscuity. This disapproval is accompanied by fear of contagion, prejudice, discrimination, stigmatization, and, in extreme cases, hatred and violence. It is within this social context that psychologic responses to HIV infection occur (Grossman, 1994, 1995; Hamburg, 1996; Merson, 1996).

Psychologic responses to HIV occur in both persons who are infected and persons who are not infected. Many persons who are not infected also are not worried about being infected. The major psychologic responses of this group are denial and dissociation (Alonzo & Reynolds, 1995). Some heterosexuals practice denial by underestimating their vulnerability to infection. Although they are very much aware of HIV disease, they do not consider it a threat to themselves. This underestimation of vulnerability is evidenced in the lack of behavioral change among heterosexual adolescents and young adults. In these groups the use of condoms has shifted, with African-American men and women using condoms with primary partners more frequently than Hispanic or white men and women but not using condoms with casual partners (Choi & Catania, 1996; Choi et al., 1994; Norris et al., 1996). However, the number of sexual partners does not appear to have changed, and rates of infection continue to rise among heterosexuals (Choi & Catania, 1996; Choi et al., 1994; Singleton et al., 1996). Risk-reduction practices appear to be limited also among women (Choi & Catania, 1996; Singleton et al., 1996). Some women may not be aware of a sexual partner's risk behaviors and do not consider themselves at risk. Consequently, they do not practice risk reduction (Neal et al., 1997; Norris et al., 1996). Other investigators have found that, even when women are aware of their risk behaviors and have been counseled about them, they continue to practice these behaviors (Sikkema et al., 1996; Solomon et al., 1996; Wells & Mayer, 1997).

Dissociation from HIV disease occurs among heterosexuals both by a physical separation of themselves from the so-called risk groups and by a psychologic dissociation with sexually transmitted diseases (STDs), drug use, and male-to-male sexual contact. Many people think that these conditions are so morally reprehensible that they would consider it an extreme insult to question a sexual partner about a history of sexually transmitted diseases, drug use, and sexual practices.

Because of these two psychologic responses—dissociation and denial of HIV risk—some heterosexuals might be characterized as unworried but also as not vigilant and therefore vulnerable to HIV infection. These persons rarely seek HIV antibody testing or psychologic and social support related to their affective responses to AIDS (Phillips & Thomas, 1996).

Denial and dissociation may occur in homosexuals also. Several studies on both the East and West Coasts have reported that homosexual men have significantly changed their sexual behavior in response to the threat of AIDS (CDC, 1997; Singleton et al., 1996; Torian et al., 1996). However, other investigators have found that some gay men had misperceptions of risky behaviors and only a weak perception of their own vulnerability to HIV disease (Grossman, 1995). Furthermore, some men might be engaging in risky behaviors because they believe the protease inhibitors (as part of an anti-HIV drug cocktail) can be used as a "morning-after pill" (Gorman, 1997; Katz & Gerberding, 1997). Young gay men also may not be practicing safer sexual behaviors because they perceive the disease to be that of an older generation of gays (Boxall, 1995; Grossman, 1994). These groups might also be characterized as using psychologic responses of denial and dissociation from any perception of personal vulnerability.

Among gay and bisexual African-American men, risk practices also continue; however, according to some investigators, they were aware of their risk (Brashers et al., 1998; McKirnan et al., 1996). Other psychologic responses, e.g., certain cognitive and affective responses among gay men and IDUs, may be influencing their unwillingness to change their behavior (McKirnan et al., 1996). The value that gay men place on freedom of sexual expression may conflict with the sexual behavior change demanded by the AIDS epidemic. In the same way, among IDUs the value placed on sharing, closeness, and interaction with their sharing network may conflict with required changes in needle-sharing behaviors (Latkin et al., 1996; Neaigus et al., 1994). This may be especially true among women who, because of gender role relationships, believe that they should share with a partner. Persons with these beliefs may choose not to change their risk behaviors (Erickson, 1997; Neaigus et al., 1994). Several investigators have reported that, although IDUs are willing to use bleach and syringe-exchange programs, they do not change their sexual risk behaviors (CDC, February 23, 1996; Sikkema et al., 1996; Solomon et al., 1996). Psychologic responses to the HIV epidemic may occur in these persons, who, although they are aware that their behaviors put them at risk, do not choose to change them. The psychologic responses of these persons may be based on anxiety (Alonzo & Reynolds, 1995). Their responses may include generalized anxiety and panic attacks, obsessive-compulsive behavior, hypochondriasis, and anxiety-based physical symptoms related to perceptions of risk. These persons often have a long history of multiple HIV testings.

Finally, a variety of other responses may occur in persons who are seronegative for HIV antibody. Such persons may have a false sense of security that could foster continued high-risk behaviors (Grossman, 1994, 1995). Some persons believe that they are immune to the virus. Other seronegative persons involved in high-risk behaviors have ongoing anxiety related to uncertainty regarding their HIV antibody status. Still others vacillate between periods of hope and despair over their HIV status (Alonzo & Reynolds, 1995). Persons who are not infected but are engaged in high-risk behaviors may require ongoing intervention and repeated HIV testing (Irwin et al., 1996). This intervention should include counseling, education, and strategies for changes in behavior.

PSYCHOSOCIAL STRESSES ON PERSONS WITH THE SPECTRUM OF HIV DISEASE

Persons who are infected with HIV have a variety of psychologic and social stresses that may differ in degree of severity, depending on stage of illness and whether or not symptoms have appeared. As noted earlier, the stresses associated with HIV disease are compounded by the age of the population affected; the high mortality rate and accompanying anxiety and depression; the social stigma, fear, ostracism, and discrimination associated with diagnosis of the disease; the debilitation, disfigurement, and symptoms of the disease; and its contagious nature.

Psychosocial Assessment

Gathering information about persons across the spectrum of HIV infection in various cate-

gories of psychosocial adjustment can help the health care professional anticipate reactions, needs, and vulnerability to psychologic dysfunction and aid in designing an appropriate psychosocial intervention plan (Alonzo & Reynolds, 1995; Capaldini, 1997; Cole et al., in press; Grimes & Grimes, 1995; Grossman, 1994, 1995; Levy & Fernandez, 1997). Psychosocial assessment should be conducted frequently with persons who have HIV infection, especially at the various crisis points in the disease spectrum.

SOCIAL AND PSYCHIATRIC HISTORY. The person's history of interpersonal relationships, education, and career can provide insight into vulnerability to psychologic dysfunction. Use of nonprescribed drugs and alcohol, prior psychiatric care, and preexisting mental illness are other indicators of possible psychologic dysfunction. Psychologically healthy persons usually have stable jobs and stable interpersonal relationships. Psychologically vulnerable HIV-infected persons may have preillness behaviors that include drug use and multiple sexual contacts. The presence of a personality disorder or of a previous depressive, anxiety, or thought disorder is more likely to result in severe psychologic symptoms and a maladaptive response to the stresses of illness (see Box, below).

CURRENT DISTRESS AND CRISIS. What specific threats and losses is the person experiencing currently? What aspect of the illness is the most distressing and bothersome to the person at the present time? The person's level of anxiety, fear, and behavioral disorganization will change from time to time and will be related to the duration, intensity, and precipitant of the current crisis.

■ **PSYCHOSOCIAL ASSESSMENT** ■

1. Psychosocial history
2. Current distress and crisis
3. Past and current coping
4. Social support needed and available
5. Life-cycle phase
6. Illness phase
7. Individual identity
8. Experience with loss and grief

COPING. The person who is facing HIV disease will call into action previous patterns of understanding problems and methods of resolving them. Knowing which approaches have been successful for this person in the past and which approaches are currently being tried will give an indication of how he or she will attempt to cope with the illness and how successful that attempt might be. It will also give direction for providing support to the person's coping responses.

SOCIAL SUPPORT. What sources of support are available to the person: family, spouse, lover, friends, and social groups? What is the person's social identity? To which cultural groups does he or she belong? What are the possibilities for support within this social identity? Gender, age, ethnicity, and route of exposure all affect the amount and kind of social support available and needed by PLWH. Fewer organized resources are available for women, African-Americans and Latinos, and IDUs. Furthermore, the needs of these groups differ from one another and from those of gay white men. The following questions should be asked: What types of support and assistance do PLWH need? Practical assistance? Social interaction? Emotional support? How can that assistance be provided?

LIFE-CYCLE PHASE. People have different goals, resources, skills, and social roles, depending on their age. The majority of PLWH are in their twenties, thirties, and forties. Young adults are not developmentally prepared to confront their mortality. Those in their twenties have fewer resources and skills than those in their forties. The former are involved in the psychosocial tasks of establishing independence, autonomy, and adult identity. At times of illness this age group typically becomes intensely reinvolved, emotionally and financially, with the family of origin. Older persons (those in their thirties and forties) have more resources (money, housing, insurance) and have established independent adult roles. At times of illness they are more likely to depend on a spouse or lover and friends for support.

ILLNESS PHASE. People's needs for psychosocial support differ according to the phase of their illness. Stresses on the person are different in the HIV testing, AIDS diagnosis, treatment, and after-treatment phases. They also differ according to the person's clinical syndrome—an opportunistic infection (OI), a neoplasm, or a central nervous system (CNS) disease. PLWH fear CNS disease more than other clinical syndromes; the associated memory loss and mood changes result in depression, anger, and strain on their social network. Emotional reactions and methods of coping differ in response to the illness phase and the clinical syndrome.

INDIVIDUAL IDENTITY. A person's personal identity also affects his or her reaction to a life-threatening illness. Sources of self-esteem, valued achievements, and future goals make up that person's identity. These and his or her orientation to living and search for meaning all play a role in determining how the person perceives and combats the illness.

LOSS AND GRIEF. The losses that the person has had, is currently having, and anticipates having as a result of the illness determine the kind of psychosocial support needed. Persons may be currently grieving a loss and going through the grief process. They may have had previous experiences with loss and grief and feel some recognition and equanimity toward the process, or they may have had no previous experience and are anxious and fearful about anticipated losses and the grieving process.

An assessment in these various areas will provide the health care professional with the information needed to design a psychosocial intervention plan for the person with HIV disease. This plan can be individualized to meet the specific needs of persons as they move through the various phases of the disease spectrum and of their emotional and social responses to the illness. The common psychosocial crises that occur in PLWH have been identified, and intervention strategies have been designed to support them during these crises.

Psychologic Stresses

The major psychologic stress on PLWH is the knowledge that they have a fatal disease with the potential for a rapid decline to death. Most frequently, psychologic reactions are those of fear, anxiety, and depression, which are compounded by the uncertainty of the course of the disease. Social stresses on PLWH include exposure, stigma, rejection, abandonment, and isolation. Common psychologic reactions are guilt, fear, anger, and suspicion (Alonzo & Reynolds, 1995; Brashers et al., 1998; Capaldini, 1997; Grimes & Grimes, 1995; Grossman, 1994, 1995; Levy & Fernandez, 1997). In different studies of gay men and substance abusers, psychologic reactions have been reported to reach levels of clinical psychopathology in 30% of subjects (Grossman, 1994, 1995; Levy & Fernandez, 1997; Lyketsos & Federman, 1995; Snyder et al., 1996).

CRISIS POINTS. Certain crisis points in the course of the disease precipitate intense anxiety, fear, and depression (Alonzo & Reynolds, 1995; Brashers et al., 1998; Grimes & Grimes, 1995; Levy & Fernandez, 1997). The initial intense crisis is at the time of confirmation of HIV seropositivity. Risks, benefits, and the components of comprehensive pretest and posttest HIV counseling are addressed in depth in Chapter 2. Psychologic responses are described here. For symptom-free persons who are seropositive, significant adverse reactions in the form of depression, anxiety, and preoccupation with AIDS are commonly reported (Grimes & Grimes, 1995). Suicide risk has been reported to be higher in persons recently infected with HIV than in the general population (Dannenberg et al., 1996; van Haastrecht et al., 1994). The devastating effects of seropositive test results may include feelings of panic, depression, and hopelessness.

Interpersonal and social responses may also be devastating. Many persons lose their sexual partners because of disclosure of seropositive test results. In addition, discrimination in employment and housing, loss of insurance benefits, and social ostracism may occur. Persons who receive HIV-positive test results may require prolonged counseling; they also need a variety of social, medical, and psychiatric support services. Counseling during the HIV testing process provides an opportunity to identify those most at risk of psychopathologic abnormalities: those with a history of current depression, anxiety, cognitive symptoms, and drug use (Dannenberg et al., 1996; Irwin et al., 1996; Stall et al., 1996).

During the long asymptomatic phase of HIV infection, many persons do not experience severe distress but, instead, become actively involved in managing their illness and engaging in health promotion activities. Those who do experience sustained psychopathologic problems have been identified as those who, at the time of HIV testing, demonstrated depression, anxiety, and cognitive symptoms within clinical ranges and as those who use drugs (Levy & Fernandez, 1997; Snyder et al., 1996). In general, during the asymptomatic phase, most persons live with a degree of hope and an absence of anxiety (Wells, 1997a). These findings represent a change from earlier times in the epidemic and are thought to be related to a greater understanding of the difference between HIV infection and AIDS, to the renewed hope engendered by the effective new treatments, and to the knowledge that HIV disease involves a long asymptomatic stage (Wells, 1997a).

When HIV-infected people begin having symptoms of disease, they may experience all the psychologic and social stresses associated with AIDS (Alonzo & Reynolds, 1995; Bindels et al., 1996; Brasher et al., 1998; Grimes & Grimes, 1995). Each development (for instance, the appearance of symptoms) that signals to the person further deterioration toward AIDS and eventually death has the potential of stimulating a psychologic crisis (Capaldini, 1997). The same existential issues that accompany a diagnosis of other life-threatening illnesses occur with AIDS. One set of responses to an AIDS diagnosis is characterized by denial, followed by anger, turmoil, disruptive anxiety, a feeling of being already dead, and depressive symptoms (Alonzo & Reynolds, 1995; Capaldini, 1997). Another coping response may be a period of problem solving during which PLWH focus on adhering to a medication regimen and on health-promoting lifestyle changes (Grimes & Grimes, 1995; Keet et al., 1994).

The treatment phase may be accompanied by weakness, depression, alienation, and dysphoria. Patients fear disfigurement, debilitation, and pain (Alonzo & Reynolds, 1995; Brasher et al., 1998). Treatment may include isolation procedures that make patients feel alienated and socially abandoned. The termination of treatment often brings on increased anxiety and fears of renewed disease progression. Hypervigilance about body functions and the appearance of new symptoms can result in hypochondriasis, demanding behavior toward medical personnel, and excessive dependence on caregivers.

Recurrence or relapse of disease is often accompanied by feelings of hopelessness, helplessness, sadness, low self-esteem, discouragement, loss of control, dependence, isolation, and suicidal ideation. Patients fear being abandoned by loved ones and caregivers who might decide that continued treatment is futile. At this point, some persons may seek medically assisted suicide (Bindels et al., 1996). This stage may be accompanied by cognitive impairment because of CNS disease. The terminal phase of illness is marked by deterioration and decline and can be accompanied by ambivalence, dependence, disinterest, or resolution (Grimes & Grimes, 1995).

SUICIDE ASSESSMENT. The potential for suicide has been recognized at several crisis points in HIV infection and disease. Increased risk of suicide is associated with any aspect of HIV disease that may cause psychologic distress. HIV antibody testing and learning of a seropositive status, appearance of an AIDS-indicator disease, a drop in CD4+ cell count or an increase in viral load, pain, treatment regimens, and dementia (Capaldini, 1997; Grimes & Grimes, 1995; Levy & Fernandez, 1997; McEnany et al., 1996; Valente & Saunders, 1997). The relative risk of suicide may be high. In a survey of 370 ambulatory PLWH, 55% reported that they were considering physician-assisted suicide for themselves (Breitbart et al., 1996). This consideration was related to high levels of psychologic distress, depression, and hopelessness and not to pain, symptoms, or progression of HIV disease.

PLWH who are more likely to take their own lives are those with previous depressive episodes, adjustment disorders, personality disorders, alcohol abuse, high levels of environmental stress, inadequate counseling before and after the HIV antibody test, and poor support networks (Levy & Fernandez, 1997; Snyder et al., 1996; van Haastrecht et al., 1994). Several groups whose behavior puts them at risk of acquiring HIV infection are also at greater risk of committing suicide. IDUs frequently have preexisting personality or affective disorders (Snyder et al., 1996). Gay men and lesbians have been reported to attempt suicide two to three times as often as their heterosexual counterparts; racial stigma also has been linked with suicide (Grossman, 1994; Perkins et al., 1994).

Suicide risk should be assessed at any of the transition points in the HIV disease spectrum. Assessment should include the following suicide risk factors (Cabaj, 1996; Depression Guideline Panel, 1993; Valente & Saunders, 1997):

History
1. Prior suicide attempt(s)
2. Mental illness, especially affective disorders
3. Substance abuse
4. Family (or significant other) history of suicide or suicide attempts
5. Family history of substance abuse
6. Family history of mental illness

Current Illness Conditions
1. Pain, disability, or both
2. Comorbid medical illness
3. Comorbid mental illness
4. Comorbid substance abuse

Psychosocial Conditions
1. Socioeconomic problems (housing, employment, insurance)
2. Loss or lack of spirituality, meaning, purpose
3. Extent, availability, and supportiveness of social network
4. A plan and method for suicide, lethality of plan, and potential for death
5. Age, gender, ethnicity

PLWH contemplating suicide may have made suicide pacts with friends and loved ones, and they may be grieving the loss of friends who died of AIDS. They may be experiencing the loss of independent functioning accompanied by a loss of self-esteem. They may also be facing an existential crisis in which life has ceased to have meaning. Any or all of these factors may be motivation for suicide. Persons who are male, white, advanced in age, and living alone are more likely to commit suicide (Depression Guideline Panel, 1993).

CRISIS INTERVENTION AND SUPPORT. During transitional points in their disease trajectory, PLWH need a full range of psychosocial interventions, including immediate crisis intervention, individual therapy, or both, to deal with feelings of extreme anxiety, fear, and anger and with impulsive behavior and suicidal thoughts and behaviors. Persons with HIV disease should be encouraged to express their anxiety, fear, sadness, and anger and to grieve with the understanding that grief can be a healing process. Pharmacotherapy should be used for intense anxiety, depression, hopelessness, and insomnia. Clients also need ongoing psychosocial support in the form of support groups to dispel self-blame and guilt, provide reassurance, share information and experiences, and reduce feelings of isolation and loneliness (Alonzo & Reynolds, 1995).

Infected persons need education regarding the disease and its treatment, liaison with community resources to help them resolve practical problems, and instruction in techniques of reducing stress and anxiety, such as relaxation. They also need supportive intervention from a social network that includes family, friends, health care professionals, volunteers, an attorney, and clergy. These people can offer encouragement, comfort, concern, compassion, affection, and legal and spiritual assistance.

All these interventions play a role in the treatment of PLWH during crisis points in their disease. Which will take priority at any given time depends on individual response and can be determined by psychosocial assessment of the person at various points. Given the heterogeneity of the population of HIV-infected persons, no single therapeutic strategy is likely to be universally efficacious. If possible, the HIV-infected person should be assigned a primary caregiver or case manager who will coordinate service needs and provide a central and familiar person the client can see to ensure continuity of care throughout the course of the illness, hospitalizations, community care, and referrals.

PSYCHOLOGIC CONFLICTS. People with HIV disease are subjected to an unusual number of psychologic or internal conflicts. Some of these conflicts revolve around transmission of the disease—from whom the person got it or to whom he or she might have transmitted it. People may also experience guilt over their previous lifestyles, especially if they have had a number of anonymous sexual partners or have used injection drugs or other recreational substances. Strong feelings of guilt and self-blame among PLWH may cause them to internalize society's prejudicial attitudes toward the group(s) to which they belong and lead them, in turn, to stigmatize others (Grossman, 1994, 1995). Among homosexuals, this is called internalized homophobia, but it may

happen in any group toward whom society expresses disapproval, such as drug users, commerical sex workers, and persons with multiple sexual partners.

Finally, many conflicts occur over continuing personal relationships, especially those that have a sexual focus. Fears of social abandonment, isolation, and loneliness accompany the giving up of intimate sexual relationships. This is especially true if sexual relationships were used to provide interpersonal contacts (McKirnan et al., 1996). Certain sexual practices (e.g., anal intercourse among gay men and social network needle-sharing among IDUs) may have functioned to integrate the person into the homosexual or drug-using community (Latkin et al., 1996; McKirnan et al., 1996; Tabet et al., 1996). Giving up these practices and making major lifestyle changes may cause an emotional crisis. Restraints on sexual or drug-use behavior may demand new social skills for negotiation, limit setting, or partner rejection, as well as new psychologic skills for tolerating frustration, managing anxiety, and creating or enhancing self-reassurance and self-control.

Some of the psychologic conflicts experienced by PLWH can be resolved through individual or group education that focuses on transmission and protection from infection by means of an intervention that involves training in cognitive-behavioral skills (Capaldini, 1997). Others can be resolved through support groups and finding reassurance, shared experiences, and intimacy among persons with the same concerns (Alonzo & Reynolds, 1995). Support groups can also help prevent loneliness and isolation and can identify ways for members to reach out to family and friends. Community resources can help people build social networks and develop sustained relationships that are not predicated on sex or drug use and sharing. The use of anxiety-reduction and stress-reduction techniques, such as relaxation or other behavioral techniques, can help persons deal with their fears and anxieties.

More recently, psychologic problems have come from an unexpected source. The advent of effective treatments for HIV has resulted in increased hopefulness for many people. This renewed hope has led many to initiate lifestyle changes such as improved diet and exercise and attempts to eliminate substance abuse (Wells, 1997a). There also has been an increased need for counseling concerning a return to school, careers, and training. Some other PLWH have had more negative experiences. Many persons have used their illness as a way of avoiding the past and painful emotional issues and relationships. With a better prognosis, these relationships and issues may now have to be revisited. Others are experiencing what has come to be known as a "Lazarus syndrome." Thinking they would die, they have abandoned careers, used up their assets, sold their life insurance, run up debts, and engaged in health-compromising behaviors (Holzemer, 1997). For them, the changing prognosis has resulted in intense regrets and many losses. Counselors working with these clients should encourage corrective actions, keeping a focus on the future, and establishing workable goals that are possible to achieve.

Another group of PLWH have not experienced benefit from the new antiretroviral treatments (Wells, 1997b). Several situations contribute to the lack of benefit, including viral resistance and intolerable side effects. Others occur because of health system constraints, poverty, and lack of access. Still others are the result of clients' inabilities to make lifestyle changes, such as discontinuation of substance abuse. Because of side effects or distrust of the medical establishment, it may be difficult for some persons to participate in treatment regimens. PLWH who do not experience benefits from the new treatments may feel disappointed and angry and may blame themselves for the treatment failure. There are several ways that counselors can help PLWH who do not benefit from treatment. For those who experience medical treatment failure, it is important to maintain hope for new antiretroviral drugs and for participation in clinical trials. These clients should be encouraged to use prophylactic treatments available and to maintain a health-promoting lifestyle.

For clients who do not have access to new treatments, counselors can act as advocates, especially with drug companies. All HCWS involved in HIV care can work at a legislative level to get state AIDS drug assistance programs (ADAP) to cover protease inhibitors. For PLWH who are not able (i.e., substance abusers, homeless) or willing (those who distrust medical professionals or have other priority survival issues) to attend to their health care needs, counselors can remind them that effective treatment for HIV is available. Counselors should refrain from judgment, as these clients have a right and a responsibility to make their own choices.

Social Stresses

Persons with HIV disease are subject to an unusual number of social and societal stresses (Alonzo & Reynolds, 1995; Peterson et al., 1995). The first of these may involve public identification as a member of a highly stigmatized group (Grossman, 1994, 1995). Social stigmatization is attached to both of the largest transmission groups for HIV infection: men who have sex with men and IDUs. Persons who have considered their sexuality or drug use to be private matters are now subject to exposure and possible rejection by family and friends (Alonzo & Reynolds, 1995). At a time when people most need social support, comfort, compassion, and closeness, they might be left alone and isolated.

Persons with asymptomatic disease are faced with a dilemma as to whether to confide in friends, family, and health care providers, because stigmatization and social rejection are likely to result from divulging this information (Alonzo & Reynolds, 1995; Grossman, 1996). Peterson and colleagues (1995) found that gay and bisexual African-American men sought help from peers and professionals and not from parents and siblings or clergy or spiritual advisors because of the stigma of homosexuality in the African-American culture and the desire to avoid disclosure. Similar findings have been reported for gay white men.

PLWH have been confronted with a variety of problems involving employment and insurance. Some have been fired from their jobs because employers and coworkers feared they would contract AIDS. In some cases, this discrimination has extended to the families of PLWH. Others have had to leave jobs because of physical disability. In many instances, health insurance is lost when the job is lost. Many PLWH are without financial security, material resources, and insurance. Community resources that they might need include ADAP, Social Security Disability Insurance, Supplemental Security Income, and Medicaid. These should be applied for immediately, and arrangements should also be made for legal assistance.

Finally, many PLWH may have limited social support networks (Peterson et al., 1995, 1996;

Williams et al., 1997). The family may not be involved with the person or may live in distant places. The reason could be alienation from the family because of lifestyle or relocation by the PLWH to a large urban area, such as New York, San Francisco, or Los Angeles, that is far from where the family lives. Some families abandon a relative with HIV infection when they learn of the diagnosis (Flaskerud & Tabora, 1998). This action could be the result of a desire to avoid social stigma, fear of contagion, or a belief that the disease is a just retribution for homosexuality, drug use, or having multiple sexual partners. Such a situation leaves the infected person without a family network to assist with basic physical needs and to provide emotional support at a crucial time, and it forces greater dependence on a single family member, lovers, or friends, and sometimes children (Williams et al., 1997).

Community resources can help meet basic physical needs of PLWH at home through practical services, such as shopping and housekeeping. Some clergy and churches help visiting parents and siblings find places to stay when they come from out of town. The gay community and gay service agencies in large cities have organized a variety of supportive services for persons with limited or distant social support networks. These services include case management, which provides social services, nursing service, insurance counseling, client advocacy, and emotional and physical support through a "buddy" system.

Political and social organizations that offer specialized services are less commonly available to drug users who have AIDS, women and children with AIDS, and persons with hemophilia and other blood transfusion recipients (Anastasio et al., 1995; Regan-Kubinski & Sharts-Hopko, 1995). The social network and support resources of drug users usually consist of other drug users and family; there is little organized community support (Latkin et al., 1996; Neaigus et al., 1994). Close liaison with drug rehabilitation programs, mental health services, and self-help groups of former addicts may provide some supportive service for IDUs with AIDS (CDC, February 23, 1996). Women with AIDS are often IDUs or the sexual partners of IDUs. Specialized AIDS services for women are extremely limited, but supportive services are sometimes provided through other women's organizations that focus

on domestic violence, rape, homelessness, and other infectious diseases and through reproductive, pediatric, and family planning clinics (CDC, September 27, 1996; Regan-Kubinski & Sharts-Hopko, 1995; Rose & Clark-Alexander, 1996). Children with HIV/AIDS most frequently have parents with AIDS and a very limited support network (Rose & Clark-Alexander, 1996). Studies of HIV-positive women have shown that their children are central forces in their lives and, in some cases, their primary source of support (Rose & Clark-Alexander, 1996; Williams et al., 1997). Community resources that treat children and their mothers together, such as pediatric AIDS clinics and inpatient units as well as family-planning clinics, are most useful.

Persons with hemophilia have supportive medical and social resources to deal with their hemophilia, and these resources might be mobilized to assist with problems associated with AIDS, but there are few hemophilia-specialized AIDS services (Bussing & Burket, 1993; Stewart et al., 1995). Persons with hemophilia and HIV may have difficulty coping with the physical and emotional symptoms and the social consequences of their diseases, and they may require both clinical intervention and social support (Steward et al., 1995). Blood transfusion recipients have extremely limited AIDS support services and have been reported to have high rates of depression (Cleary et al., 1993). In addition, both persons with hemophilia and other blood transfusion/blood product recipients may feel betrayed by the medical system because of the means of their infection with HIV (Steward et al., 1995).

As can be noted from the foregoing discussion, the psychosocial stresses on persons with AIDS are overwhelming and result in psychologic reactions that may vary in severity. These stresses call for a range of psychologic, social, economic, and legal interventions, and at any given time in the course of a person's disease they may call for all the interventions and services discussed in this section.

PSYCHIATRIC DISORDERS AND HIV

Psychiatric morbidity in HIV occurs through a variety of mechanisms. The foregoing discussion of psychologic and social stresses notes that persons may have severe psychologic reactions to a

diagnosis of HIV and to the societal consequences of the disease. Reactive depression or
anxiety disorders and adjustment disorders may
occur in response to crisis points in the illness or
to stresses engendered by it (Capaldini, 1997;
McEnany et al., 1996). These reactive disorders
may be transitory and may respond to crisis intervention, focused psychoeducational interventions, and pharmacotherapy. Short-term cognitive-behavioral therapy may be especially useful
in relieving the PLWH's psychologic distress in a
cost-efficient manner without in-depth psychiatric treatment (Capaldini, 1997; Lovejoy &
Matteis, 1997). Techniques within this model include reframing, role reversal, clarifying the
meaning of the HIV disease situation, relax-
ation/distraction, biofeedback, and graded task
management. Successful therapy is evidenced in
the PLWH's ability to demonstrate self-promot-
ing behaviors and constructive thought patterns
(Capaldini, 1997; Lovejoy & Matteis, 1997).

HIV disease can occur also in persons with
preexisting mental illness and may represent a situation of comorbidity (Camacho et al., 1996;
Coverdale, 1996; Kalichman et al., 1996; Rabkin
et al., 1997). Persons with substance abuse disorders, schizophrenic disorders, major depression,
and bipolar disorders who also have HIV disease
exemplify instances of comorbidity. Several investigators have found that PLWH who have preexisting mental disorders are also those who have
the most severe and pathologic reactions to their
HIV disease (Coverdale, 1996; Kalichman et al.,
1996; Rabkin et al., 1997). In addition, currently
existing mental illness may facilitate the behaviors
involved in transmission of HIV; injection drug
use, hypersexuality, and the practice of unsafe sex
may be high in mentally ill persons (Camacho et
al., 1996; Lilleleht & Leiblum, 1993). Unprotected sexual activity with multiple partners who
are chosen casually is frequent (Susser et al.,
1996). Impulsive and hypersexual behaviors, especially among persons with bipolar and schizophrenic disorders and those who use recreational
drugs, may be high. Finally, the existence of mental disorders in PLWH complicates the diagnosis
of reactive disorders and neuropsychiatric disorders associated with HIV. It also complicates
treatment. Psychoeducational interventions are
appropriate for this group of PLWH but are considerably more difficult to implement (Herman et

al., 1994; Kalichman et al., 1995). Pharmacologic
treatments are also indicated.

Depression

Depression is extremely common in patients
with chronic medical disorders, life-threatening
diseases, and diseases affecting the central nervous
system, all characteristics of HIV disease (Cabaj,
1996; Capaldini, 1997). Persons with depression
are commonly seen in primary care situations (up
to 30% of primary care patients have depressive
disorders) and often present with somatic complaints, memory and concentration problems, insomnia, and low energy (Zung et al., 1993).
Among PLWH, the prevalence of depression has
been estimated at 10% to 25% (Atkinson &
Grant, 1994). Among HIV-negative and HIV-
positive gay men, the lifetime prevalence of depression has been estimated at 29% and 45%, respectively (Perkins et al., 1994).

Depression is a psychobiologic illness that is
quite treatable if diagnosed accurately. A person
who is suffering from the diagnosable disease of
depression will experience depressed mood, low
energy, sleep disturbance, anhedonia, inability to
concentrate, loss of libido, weight changes, and
possible menstrual irregularities (McEnany et al.,
1996). The major risk factor for depression is a
history of depression, substance abuse, or both
and a family history of the same (Cabaj, 1996;
Levy & Fernandez, 1997).

The most common types of depression are displayed in the Box on pages 266 and 267. These
disorders are based on criteria from the *Diagnostic
and Statistical Manual of Mental Disorders,* fourth
edition, *Primary Care,* published by the American
Psychiatric Association (APA) (1995). Forms of
depression other than those displayed in the Box
include seasonal affective disorder and postpartum
depression, which may also affect PLWH.

It is important to note the frequency with
which depression accompanies the use of drugs,
such as alcohol, opioids, and cocaine (Cabaj,
1996; Camacho et al., 1996; Rabkin et al., 1997).
Rabkin and colleagues (1997) found that 15% of
HIV-negative IDUs and 33% of HIV-positive
IDUs had diagnosable major depression or dysthymia, regardless of gender. These high rates of
psychopathy indicate a need for neuropsychiatric
treatment among substance abusers. Other investigators have noted high rates of recreational drug

---

▪ DEPRESSED MOOD ALGORITHM ▪

Presenting symptoms might include the following:
  Decreased energy
  Insomnia
  Weight loss
  Unexplained general medical complaint (e.g., chronic pain, gastrointestinal distress, dizziness)

STEP I. Consider the role of **a general medical condition or substance use** and whether the depressed mood is better accounted for by **another mental disorder.**
  A. Mood disorder due to a general medical condition
      1. Depressed mood or markedly diminished interest or pleasure in all or almost all activities causes clinically significant impairment in social or occupational functioning or causes marked distress.
      2. A general medical condition is judged to be etiologically related by a direct pathophysiologic mechanism to the depressed mood.
  B. Substance-induced mood disorder (including medication)
      1. Depressed mood or markedly diminished interest or pleasure in all or almost all activities causes clinically significant impairment in social or almost all activities causes marked distress.
      2. There is evidence from the history, physical examination, or laboratory findings of a substance intoxication or withdrawal, and the symptoms developed during or within a month of significant substance intoxication or withdrawal, or it is judged that the depressed mood is etiologically related to the substance use or medication.

STEP II. If depressed mood or loss of interest or pleasure **persists over a 2-week period,** consider
  A. Major depressive episode
      1. At least five of the following symptoms have been present during the same 2-week period, nearly every day, and represent a change from previous functioning. At least one of the symptoms must be either depressed mood or loss of interest or pleasure:
          a. Depressed mood (or, alternatively, an irritable mood in children and adolescents)
          b. Markedly diminished interest or pleasure in all, or almost all, activities
          c. Significant weight loss or weight gain when not dieting
          d. Insomnia or hypersomnia
          e. Psychomotor agitation or retardation
          f. Fatigue or loss of energy
          g. Feelings of worthlessness or excessive or inappropriate guilt
          h. Diminished ability to think or concentrate
          i. Recurrent thoughts of death, recurrent suicidal ideation without a specific plan, or a suicide attempt or a specific plan for committing suicide
      2. Symptoms are not better accounted for by a mood disorder due to a general medical condition, a substance-induced mood disorder, or bereavement (normal reaction to the death of a loved one).
      3. Symptoms are not better accounted for by a psychotic disorder (e.g., schizoaffective disorder).

STEP III. If depressed mood has been present for **most of the past 2 years in adults** or 1 year in children, consider
  A. Dysthymic disorder
      1. Chronic depressed mood more often than not, lasting for at least 2 years (1 year for children and adolescents).
      2. The symptoms are not as severe or disabling as a major depressive disorder and include two or more of the following features: poor appetite or overeating; insomnia or hypersomnia; low energy or fatigue; low self-esteem; poor concentration or difficulty making decisions; and feelings of hopelessness.

■ DEPRESSED MOOD ALGORITHM *Continued* ■

STEP IV. If depressed mood is associated with **the death of a loved one and persists for less than 2 months,** consider
    A. Bereavement
        1. This category can be used when the focus of clinical attention is a reaction to the death of a loved one. As part of their reaction to the loss, some grieving persons present with symptoms characteristic of a major depressive episode (e.g., feelings of sadness and associated symptoms, such as loss of interest or pleasure, insomnia, poor appetite, and difficulty concentrating). The bereaved person typically regards the depressed mood as "normal," although the person may seek professional help for relief of associated symptoms such as insomnia.

STEP V. If depressed mood occurs **in response to an identifiable psychosocial stressor** and does not meet criteria for any of the preceding disorders, consider
    A. Adjustment disorder with depressed mood
    B. Adjustment disorder with mixed anxiety and depressed mood
        1. The development of emotional or behavioral symptoms in response to an identifiable stressor(s), which occur within 3 months of the onset of the stressor(s) (e.g., loss of job, divorce).
        2. These symptoms or behaviors are clinically significant as evidenced by either of the following:
            a. Marked distress that is in excess of what would be expected from exposure to the stressor, or
            b. Significant impairment in social or occupational (academic) functioning preceding mood disorders, or other mental disorders, and is not merely an exacerbation of a preexisting mental disorder or general medical condition
        3. The stress-related disturbance does not meet the criteria for any of the preceding mood disorders, or other mental disorders, and is not merely an exacerbation of a preexisting mental disorder or general medical condition.
        4. Symptoms do not persist longer than 6 months after the cessation of the stressor.

STEP VI. If the depressed mood is clinically significant but the **criteria are not met for any of the previously described disorders,** consider
    A. Depressive disorder not otherwise specified
        1. Minor depressive disorder
        2. Recurrent brief depressive disorder
        3. Mixed anxiety-depressive disorder
            a. Premenstrual dysphoria
            b. Suspected or masked depression

STEP VII. If the clinician has determined that a disorder is not present but wishes to note the presence of **symptoms,** consider
    A. Sadness
    B. Decreased energy
    C. Insomnia

Data from American Psychiatric Association (1995) and Depression Guideline Panel (1993a).

use among MSM, sometimes as a means of self-medication against depression (Grossman, 1994, 1995; McKirnan et al., 1996; Perkins et al., 1994).

The diagnosis and treatment of depression in PLWH are complicated by the constitutional signs and symptoms of HIV itself, by opportunistic infections, by HIV-associated malignant neoplasms, and by HIV CNS disease (Roy-Byrne & Fann, 1997). The medications (e.g., zidovudine, acyclovir, anticonvulsants, corticosteroids, NSAIDs, sulfonamides, H_2 receptor antagonists, and interferon-alfa among others) used to treat HIV disease also may cause depression (Capaldini, 1997). HIV-infected persons may have increased sensitivity to medications and experience more intense side effects (Levy & Fernandez, 1997). A general rule of thumb is to start with a lower dose and to increase the dosage slowly. The pharmacologic agent chosen should target the symptoms manifested by the client. It may take 3 to 6 weeks for the initial effects of pharmacologic agents to appear, and a full 6-month trial should be followed before switching to another agent. The most common antidepressants used with PLWH are listed in Table 7–1 with the recommended dosages, effects, and side effects. Monamine oxidase (MAO) inhibitors are *not* recommended because of dietary restrictions and interactions with the multiple medications required in HIV disease.

Anxiety/Panic Disorder

In persons with HIV disease, the stresses associated with antibody testing, diagnosis, and treatment may cause anxiety. Anxiety may occur also as a complication of medications used in the treatment of HIV-related diseases, such as anticonvulsants, sulfonamides, NSAIDs, corticosteroids, and ganciclovir. In addition, anxiety occurs as a part of withdrawal from substance use and is frequently seen in persons who use alcohol, cocaine, and heroin (Cabaj, 1996; Camacho et al., 1996; Capaldini, 1997; Levy & Fernandez, 1997; Roy-Byrne & Fann, 1997). Finally, withdrawal from selective serotonin reuptake inhibitors (SSRIs) may produce agitation, along with dizziness, malaise, and nausea.

Anxiety disorders are common in primary care

Table 7–1 ▪ Antidepressants

Agent	Starting Dose (mg)	Therapeutic Dose (mg)	Comments
TRICYCLICS: INDICATED FOR ANXIOUS DEPRESSION, INSOMIA, LOW DAYTIME ENERGY, NEUROPATHY PAIN			
Nortriptyline (Aventyl, Pamelor)	25–50 hs	75–200	Low anticholinergic and hypotensive potential
			Analgesic for neuropathy pain
Doxepin (Sinequan)	10–25 hs	150–300	Very sedating, excellent antihistamine
Desipramine (Norpramin)	25–50	150–300	Low anticholinergic
			Analgesic for neuropathy pain
			Least sedating
SELECTIVE SEROTONIN REUPTAKE INHIBITORS (SSRIs)*: INDICATED FOR LETHARGY, HOPELESSNESS, HYPERSOMNIA			
Fluoxetine (Prozac)	20 qAM	20–80	Long half-life
			May take 8 weeks for full effect
			Initial stimulant symptoms
Sertraline (Zoloft)	25–50 qAM	50–200	May cause diarrhea, GI side effects
Paroxetine (Paxil)	10–20 qAM	25–50	May cause daytime drowsiness
Fluvoxamine (Luvox)	25	50–300	Most sedating
			Withdrawal symptoms
STIMULANTS†: INDICATED FOR FATIGUE, HYPERSOMNIA, POOR APPETITE, TO IMPROVE COGNITIVE FUNCTION			
Methylphenidate (Ritalin)	5 qAM and early PM (bid)	10–60	Fast onset of action
			Give early in day
Dextroamphetamine (Dexadrine)	5 qAM	5–40	Contraindicated with anxiety, agitation
UNCLASSIFIED: INDICATED FOR DEPRESSION REFRACTORY TO OTHER MEDICATION			
Venlafaxine (Effexor)	37.5 bid	50–100 bid	Risk of hypertension
			May have stimulant effect

*All SSRIs may cause sexual dysfunction.
†Psychostimulants may be more effective in persons with depression and cognitive impairment or dementia.
Data from Cabaj (1996), Capaldini (1997), Depression Guideline Panel (1993b), Wood (1996), Levine et al. (1993), Levy and Fernandez (1997), and Roy-Byrne and Fann (1997).

Table 7–2 ■ Anxiolytics

Agent	Indication	Starting Dose (mg)	Therapeutic Dose (mg)	Comments
Clonazepam (Klonopin)	Chronic anxiety Pain syndromes Movement disorders	0.5 bid	0.5–2 bid	Excellent, long acting, onset of action slow
Buspirone (Buspar)	Chronic anxiety Useful in substance abuse Antidepressant properties	10 tid	10–15 tid	Long acting, nonaddictive, nonsedating
Alprazolam (Xanax)	Intermittent anxiety Antidepressant properties	0.5–1 q8h prn	0.5–2 q8h prn	Rapid onset, addictive potential, may cause withdrawal syndrome
Lorazepam (Ativan)	Intermittent anxiety Delirium (with Haldol)	0.5–1 q8h prn	0.5–2 q8h prn	Same as above

Data from Cabaj (1996), Capaldini (1997), Levy and Fernandez (1997), Roy-Byrne and Fann (1997), and Wood (1996).

settings and are estimated to have a 1-year prevalence in the general population of 12% to 13% (APA, 1995). Anxiety is common among persons with HIV disease (Camacho et al., 1996). Symptoms involve the autonomic, circulatory, gastrointestinal, musculoskeletal, respiratory, and neurologic systems and are often considered by the client to represent a medical condition. Generalized anxiety disorder is manifested by pervasive worry, trouble falling asleep, impaired concentration, psychomotor agitation, hypersensitivity, hyperarousal, and fatigue (Capaldini, 1997; APA, 1995; Levy & Fernandez, 1997; Roy-Byrne & Fann, 1997). Panic attack or disorder is characterized by sweating, palpitations, and shortness of breath, dizziness, headache, paresthesias, derealization, and depersonalization. Anxiety and panic disorder frequently are accompanied by mood disorders, substance abuse, and posttraumatic stress disorders (Capaldini, 1997; Camacho et al., 1996; APA, 1995). See Box on pages 270 and 271 for diagnostic information.

Pharmacologic treatment of anxiety and panic disorder associated with HIV disease should take into account the nature and severity of the symptoms and the coexistence of other psychiatric syndromes, such as mood disorders or substance abuse. Quick and short-acting medicines (e.g., alprazolam [Xanax], lorazepam [Ativan]) should be considered for intermittent symptoms. For persons with chronic anxiety, long-acting anxiolytics should be used (e.g., buspirone [Buspar], clonazepam [Klonopin]). Long-term treatment of panic disorder may be best achieved with antidepressant tricyclics or SSRIs. The anxiety and insomnia resulting from treatment with zidovudine or steroids or secondary to HIV effects on the CNS may be treated with benzodiazepines, such as lorazepam or alprazolam, for short-term relief and with alprazolam or clonazepam for long-term relief. Finally, anxiety disorders in substance-abusing clients are best treated with buspirone to avoid drug dependence on benzodiazepines (Capaldini, 1997; Levy & Fernandez, 1997; Roy-Byrne & Fann, 1997). See Table 7–2 for dosage and use.

Psychosis

Seriously mentally ill adults with chronic illnesses include persons with various forms of schizophrenia and major affective disorders (Coverdale, 1996; Herman et al., 1994; Kalichman et al., 1995, 1996). Several behaviors associated with these illnesses put people at risk of HIV disease. These behaviors include sex with multiple partners, homosexual and heterosexual anal intercourse, substance use preceding sexual intercourse, injection drug use, coerced sexual activity, failure to use condoms, and chronically and variably impaired autonomy (Coverdale, 1996; Kalichman et al., 1996; Lilleleht & Leiblum, 1993). Persons with HIV disease who have seri-

▨ ANXIETY ALGORITHM ▨

Presenting symptoms might include the following:
    Fear
    Worry
    Repetitive, intrusive, inappropriate thoughts or actions
    Unexplained general medical complaint

STEP I. Consider the role of **a general medical condition or substance use** and whether the anxiety is better accounted for by **another mental disorder.**

  A. Anxiety disorder due to a general medical condition
    1. Prominent anxiety, panic attacks, obsessions, or compulsions cause clinically significant distress or impairment in social, occupational, or other important areas of functioning.
    2. A general medical condition is judged to cause the anxiety symptoms by a direct pathophysiologic mechanism.
  B. Substance-induced (including medication) anxiety disorder
    1. Prominent anxiety, panic attacks, obsessions, or compulsions cause clinically significant distress or impairment in social, occupational, or other important areas of functioning.
    2. There is evidence from the history, physical examination, or laboratory findings of significant substance intoxication or withdrawal, and the symptoms developed during or within a month of this substance intoxication or withdrawal, or it is judged that the anxiety is etiologically related to the substance use or medication.

STEP II. If the presenting symptom is recurrent **panic attacks,** consider
  A. Panic attack
    1. A discrete period of intense fear or discomfort, in which at least four of the following symptoms developed abruptly and reached a peak within 10 minutes:
      a. Cardiopulmonary symptoms
        (1) Chest pain or discomfort
        (2) Sensations of shortness of breath or smothering
        (3) Palpitations, pounding heart, or accelerated heart rate
      b. Autonomic symptoms
        (1) Sweating
        (2) Chills or hot flushes
      c. Gastrointestinal symptoms
        (1) Feeling of choking
        (2) Nausea or abdominal distress
      d. Neurological symptoms
        (1) Trembling or shaking
        (2) Paresthesias (numbness or tingling sensation)
        (3) Feeling dizzy, unsteady, lightheaded, or faint
      e. Psychiatric symptoms
        (1) Derealization (feelings of unreality) or depersonalization (being detached from oneself)
        (2) Fear of losing control or going crazy
        (3) Fear of dying

STEP III. If the presenting symptoms are related to **reexperiencing highly traumatic events,** consider
  A. Posttraumatic stress disorder
    1. The person has been exposed to a highly traumatic event.
    2. The person persistently reexperiences the traumatic event through distressing recollections, dreams, sense of reliving, or psychologic or physiologic reactions when exposed to cues that may represent the event.
    3. The person persistently avoids stimuli associated with the trauma and has a numbing of general responsiveness.

■ ANXIETY ALGORITHM *Continued* ■

STEP III. Continued

   4. The person persistently experiences increased arousal, such as changes in sleep, an enhanced startle response, or hypervigilance.
   5. Symptoms in criteria 3, 4, and 5 persist for at least 1 month, and the disturbance causes clinically significant distress or impairment in social or occupational functioning.

   B. Acute stress disorder
   1. The person has been exposed to a highly traumatic event.
   2. The person experienced at least three of the following symptoms while experiencing or immediately after the event:
      a. Numbing, detachment, or absence of emotional attachment
      b. Reduction in awareness of one's surroundings
      c. Derealization (an alteration in the perception or experience of the external world so that it seems strange or unreal [e.g., people may seem unfamiliar or mechanical])
      d. Depersonalization (an alteration in the perception or experience of the self so that one feels detached from, and as if one is an outside observer of, one's mental processes or body [e.g., feeling like one is in a dream])
      e. Dissociative amnesia
   3. The traumatic event is persistently reexperienced.
   4. There are marked symptoms of anxiety or increased arousal and avoidance of stimuli that arouse recollections of the trauma.
   5. Symptoms last for a minimum of 2 days and a maximum of 4 weeks and occur within 4 weeks of the traumatic event.

STEP IV. If pervasive symptoms of anxiety and worry are associated with a **variety of events or situations** and have persisted for at least **6 months,** consider

   A. Generalized anxiety disorder
   1. Excessive anxiety and worry, for more days than not, that are out of proportion to the likelihood or impact of feared events.
   2. The worry is pervasive and difficult to control.
   3. The worry is associated with symptoms of motor tension (e.g., trembling, muscle tension), autonomic hypersensitivity (e.g., dry mouth, palpitations), or hyperarousal (e.g., exaggerated startle response, insomnia)
   4. The anxiety, worry, or physical symptoms cause clinically significant distress or impairment in social, occupational, or other important areas of functioning.
   5. The condition has lasted for at least 6 months.

Box continued on following page

---

ous, chronic mental illnesses may also suffer from CNS disease associated with HIV.

New-onset psychosis in persons with HIV disease may occur as a complication of medications, as a first manifestation of an opportunistic or systemic illness, as a result of substance use, or as a manifestation of HIV disease itself (APA, 1995; Capaldini, 1997; Levy & Fernandez, 1997). Therefore the clinician should conduct a thorough medical evaluation, medication review, and substance use assessment. Medications that can cause psychosis include anabolic steroids, amphotericin, anticonvulsants, buspirone, ketoconazole, ciprofloxacin, corticosteroids, dapsone, ganciclovir, H_2 receptor antagonists, interferon-alfa, isoniazid, NSAIDs, metronidazole (Flagyl), salicylates, sulfonamides, and zidovudine (*Medical Letter,* 1993). (Please see Appendix II for additional information.) Presenting symptoms might include delusions, hallucinations, disorganized speech or behavior, catatonia, and "negative" symptoms (apathy, avolition, flattened affect, anhedonia) (APA, 1995).

The neuroleptics are commonly used to treat psychosis. Persons with HIV may be more sensitive to neuroleptics. Therefore they are given in as

---

▪ ANXIETY ALGORITHM *Continued* ▪

STEP V.   If the symptoms are in response to a specific, psychosocial stressor, consider
    A. Adjustment disorder with anxiety
      1. The development of nervousness, worry, or jitteriness in response to an identifiable stressor(s) occurring within 3 months of the onset of the stressor(s).
      2. These symptoms are clinically significant as evidenced by either of the following:
        a. Marked distress that is in excess of what would be expected from exposure to the stresssor
        b. Significant impairment in social or occupational (academic) functioning
      3. The stress-related disturbance does not meet the criteria for any of the preceding anxiety disorders or other mental disorders and is not merely an exacerbation of a preexisting mental disorder or general medical condition.
      4. Symptoms do not persist longer than 6 months after cessation of the stressor.
    B. Adjustment disorder with mixed anxiety and depression
      1. Presistent or recurrent dysphoric mood lasting at least 1 month and accompanied by at least 1 month of other depressive and anxiety symptoms (e.g., difficulty concentrating or mind going blank, sleep disturbance, fatigue or low energy, irritability, worry, being easily moved to tears, hypervigilance, anticipating the worst, hopelessness). Symptoms must cause impairment in social, occupational, or other important areas of functioning.
STEP VI.   If clinically significant anxiety is present but **the criteria are not met for any of the previously described disorders,** consider
    A. Anxiety disorder not otherwise specified
STEP VII.   If the clinician has determined that a disorder is not present but wishes to note the presence of symptoms, consider
    A. Anxiety

Adapted from American Psychiatric Association. (1995). *Diagnostic and Statistical Manual of Mental Disorders* (4th ed.). *Primary Care Version.* Washington, DC: Author.

low a dose and for as short a duration as possible to avoid extrapyramidal syndromes, neuroleptic malignant syndrome, and a possible interaction with HIV-related central nervous system (CNS) disease (Capaldini, 1997; Levy & Fernandez, 1997; Roy-Byrne & Fann, 1997; Wood, 1996). Table 7–3 contains information on use and dosage of neuroleptics.

Mania

Acute mania can occur in persons with HIV disease because of premorbid bipolar disorder, right frontal lobe tumor or focus of infection, the first manifestation of an opportunistic or systemic illness, medications, and substance use (APA, 1995; Capaldini, 1997; Levy & Fernandez, 1997; Roy-Byrne & Fann, 1997). Presenting symptoms might include elevated or expansive mood, irritable mood, pressured speech, psychomotor agitation, less need for sleep, grandiosity, and flight of ideas (APA, 1995; Capaldini, 1997). Substance-induced mania may be caused by cocaine, amphetamines, and phencyclidine, among others. Medications that cause mania include zidovudine, metoclopramide, corticosteroids, isoniazid, anticonvulsants, antidepressants, antiparkinsonian medications, sympathomimetics, H_2 receptor antagonists, and others (APA, 1995; Capaldini, 1997; *Medical Letter*, 1993).

Mania occurs late in HIV disease and carries a poor prognosis. It is usually comorbid with cognitive impairment. Treatment of mania in HIV disease is complicated by the problems of advanced HIV disease that may involve dehydration and altered renal function. Treatment should consist of eliminating medications that may precipitate mania. Cautious rapid tranquilization with medium- or high-potency neuroleptics is followed by lithium treatment in patients with a stable volume and renal status. Lithium is given in a starting dose of 300 to 900 mg daily and maintained with a target daily dose of 600 to 400 mg

Table 7–3 ■ Neuroleptics/Antipsychotics

Agent	Indication	Starting Dose (mg)	Therapeutic Dose (mg)	Comments
PHENOTHIAZINES				
Chlorpromazine (Thorazine)	Mixed psychosis Agitation	25–50 q8–12h	50–800 qd	Very anticholinergic, sedating, hypotension
Thioridazine (Mellaril)	Low potency	10–200 qd	150–800 qd	Fewer extrapyramidal side effects (EPSs)
Perphenazine (Trilafon)	Medium potency	4 q8–12h	12–64 qd	Medium anticholinergic, sedating, EPSs
Haloperidol (Haldol)	High potency Delirium	1.2 q6–8h	2–10	Low anticholinergic, sedating, high EPSs, possible neuroleptic malignant syndrome (NMS)
ATYPICALS				
Risperidone (Risperdal)	Manic psychosis	1–2 qd	2–4 qd	Less EPSs, less proconvulsant and sedative
Molindone (Moban)	Mixed psychosis Agitation	15–45 qd	100	Less EPSs, sedation, less NMS
Clozapine (Clozaril)	Not recommended			Agranulocytosis; lowers seizure levels; additive CNS depressant effects

Data from Capaldini (1997), Levy and Fernandez (1997), Physicians Desk Reference (1997), Roy-Byrne and Fann (1997), and Wood (1996).

daily. Blood levels must be monitored to establish a therapeutic response.

Recent anticonvulsants have emerged as a useful alternative for patients with HIV-associated mania whose renal or electrolyte status makes the use of lithium problematic. Table 7–4 contains information on use and dosage of mood stabilizers. Also see Appendix II.

CNS Cognitive/Motor Disorders

HIV-infected persons are at particularly high risk of developing a number of different neuropsychiatric complications secondary to CNS disease (Dal Pan et al., 1997; Lyketsos & Federman, 1995; Zeifert et al., 1995). The most common HIV-associated diseases of the CNS are displayed in the Box on page 274 and reflect a wide variety of etio-

Table 7–4 ■ Mood Stabilizers/Antimania

Agent	Indication	Starting Dose (mg)	Therapeutic Dose (mg)	Comments
Lithium	Mania	300–900 qd	600–1500 qd	Avoid in patients with unstable volume or renal status; do not use with nephrotoxic drugs
Carbamazepine (Tegretol)	Anticonvulsant Trigeminal neuralgia Neuropathic pain	200–600 qd	400–800 qd	Monitor liver function tests (LFTs), complete blood count (CBC) with platelets, drug levels
Valproate (Depakote)	Anticonvulsant Neuropathic pain	250–500 qd	500–750 qd	Monitor LFTs, CBC, drug levels, nausea

Data from Capaldini (1997), Levy and Fernandez (1997), Roy-Byrne and Fann (1997), and Wood (1996).

▪ **HIV AND CENTRAL NERVOUS SYSTEM (CNS) CONDITION** ▪

HIV-associated Disorders
HIV-1-associated cognitive/motor complex
HIV-1-associated dementia complex
HIV-1-associated minor cognitive/motor disorder
HIV-1-associated myleopathy

Infections
Fungal
    Cryptococcal disease
    Coccidioidomycosis
    Candida albicans
    Histoplasma capsulatum
    Nocardia asteroides
Protozoal
    Toxoplasma gondii
Bacterial
    Listeria monocytogenes
    Mycobacterium avium-intracellulare
    Mycobacterium tuberculosis
Viral
    Cytomegalovirus
    Herpesviruses
    Papovavirus (progressive multifocal leukoencephalopathy)
    Adenovirus

Neoplasms
Primary cerebral lymphoma
Metastatic lymphoma
Metastatic Kaposi's sarcoma

Cerebrovascular Disorders
Infarction
Hemorrhage
Vasculitis

Adverse Effects of Treatments

Data from Capaldini (1997), Levy and Fernandez (1997), and Sweeney and Agger (1997).

---

logic factors, including primary HIV brain disease, metabolic derangements, space-occupying lesions such as tumors or abscesses, cerebral infections, and side effects of medication. The clinical manifestations of these disorders are discussed in depth in Chapters 5 and 6. In the neuropsychiatric context, these disorders are associated with mental confusion, paresthesias, diplopia, neuropathies, and cognitive, behavioral, and motor dysfunctions (Sweeney & Agger, 1997).

The most common manifestation of HIV-associated CNS disease is a primary dementia caused by the indirect cytopathic effects of the virus on the CNS. This disorder has been variously termed HIV dementia, the AIDS dementia complex, and HIV encephalopathy. Current nomenclature adopted by the American Academy of Neurology (1991) groups all of this spectrum of HIV-associated neurocognitive disorders under the term *HIV-1-associated cognitive/motor disorder.* The more specific diagnosis of HIV-1-associated dementia (HAD) complex is used to describe clearcut HIV-specific CNS disease that leads to significant changes in quality of life. The diagnostic label of HIV-1-associated minor cognitive/motor disorder (HAMCMD) is used to describe more subtle changes in cognitive or motor functioning (American Academy of Neurology, 1991).

The HIV-1-associated CNS diseases are reported as the initial manifestation of AIDS in 7% to 10% of HIV-infected persons, and are eventually diagnosed in 15% to 20% of persons with AIDS. In addition, a much larger number of persons may show more subtle neurocognitive impairments, and 50% to 75% of HIV-infected persons will show some neuropathologic changes in brain tissue at the time of death (Dal Pan et al., 1997; Janssen, 1997; McArthur et al., 1993). Most of these neurocognitive manifestations occur in late-stage HIV disease, usually around the time of severe immunocompromise, although there are isolated but well-documented cases of early-onset dementia (Heaton et al., 1994; McArthur et al., 1993; Selnes & Miller, 1993). There continues to be considerable disagreement about the relative prevalence of minor cognitive/motor disorders in medically asymptomatic persons (Bornstein et al., 1993; Miller et al., 1994a, 1994b). Most investigators agree that early neurocognitive effects, if they are present, are subtle and difficult to measure and probably do not interfere with normal activities of daily living. Median survival after a diagnosis of full HIV dementia is around 6 months, although these figures may change as new antiretroviral treatments are developed (McArthur et al., 1993). It is worth noting, however, that despite the beneficial systemic effects of triple antiretroviral therapies and protease inhibitors, the extent to which these medications cross the blood-brain barrier and reduce the viral load in the CNS remains unclear.

The cardinal symptoms of HIV-related cognitive impairment remain consistent according to many reports and include apathy, withdrawal, loss of memory and concentration, impaired cognitive flexibility, mental and motor slowing, decreased problem-solving ability, and visual-spatial integration and construction (Baumann, 1993; Levy & Fernandez, 1997; Swanson et al., 1993a, 1993b). The diagnostic symptoms associated with HIV-1-associated minor cognitive/motor disorder are displayed in the Box below. On the basis of neuropathologic studies, functional neuroimaging, and the constellation of symptoms associated with HIV dementia, most of the CNS damage associated with HIV is thought to occur in the subcortical regions of the brain (Aylward et al., 1995; Dal Pan et al., 1997; Hinkin et al., 1995). Late cognitive signs and symptoms of HIV-1-associated dementia complex include se-

vere dementia, confusion, psychologic slowing, aphasia or autism, and disorientation. Behavioral signs and symptoms include psychosis, mania, marked motor abnormalities, severe behavioral inhibition, and incontinence (Levy & Fernandez, 1997).

The differential diagnosis of neuropsychologic disorders, preexisting mental disorders, and reactive disorders is complicated in HIV disease (Baumann, 1993; Capaldini, 1997; Levy & Fernandez, 1997). Many affective, behavioral, cognitive, and somatic symptoms, such as depressed mood, apathy or agitation, loss of concentration, and insomnia, may be etiologically related to a variety of medical or psychologic illnesses or to the adverse effects of complicated medication regimens. Some studies have suggested that persons who complain of neurocognitive symptoms and mild somatic symptoms are more likely to be depressed than they are to show neuropsychologic deficits (Hinkin et al., 1995; Moore et al., 1997; Perkins et al., 1995). Extreme symptoms seen in late stages of brain disease, such as paranoia, hallucinations, or catatonia, may also be confused with severe psychiatric disturbances such as schizophrenia.

Therefore it is vitally important for the clinician to consider all potential etiologic factors and their relative likelihoods. A reliable differential diagnosis requires that the clinician obtain an accurate and detailed history of the onset of symptoms, as well as a full medical diagnostic work-up to rule out OIs of the brain. The clinician also should consider the patient's psychiatric history and current medications, particularly if there have been any recent changes. It is not possible to make an accurate diagnosis in a person who is delirious or showing other acute signs of brain compromise. Any neurologic symptoms with a rapid onset or any unusual signs, such as changes in olfaction, taste, hearing, or vision, require immediate neurologic work-up, often including neuroimaging. It is also important that any mood disorders be treated as soon as practical. Severe depression may masquerade as a dementia syndrome, particularly in older persons or in persons with severe medical illnesses. Even if the mood changes are etiologically related to primary HIV brain disease, they are usually responsive to pharmacologic interventions.

The use of mental status examinations that

> ▪ **HIV-1-ASSOCIATED MINOR COGNITIVE DISORDERS** ▪
>
> **Diagnostic Criteria: American Academy of Neurology**
> The patient must meet all four of the following criteria:
>
> 1. Cognitive/motor/behavioral dysfunction (affects two or more neuropsychologic domains for at least 1 month as documented by neurologic examination or neuropsychologic testing)
>   a. Concentration/attention impairment
>   b. Mental slowing
>   c. Motor slowing
>   d. Loss of coordination
>   e. Personality change, irritability, emotional lability
>   f. Conceptualization and problem-solving difficulties
>   g. Language-comprehension problems
> 2. Increased difficulty with school, work, or activities of daily living
> 3. Level of impairment does not meet criteria for HIV-1-associated dementia complex
> 4. No evidence of another etiologic factor (OI, neoplasm, substance abuse, psychiatric disorder) documented by clinical, laboratory, and radiologic examinations

Data from American Academy of Neurology (1991), Levy and Fernandez (1997), and Mascolini (1996).

the health professional can employ as a quick screening device for cognitive dysfunction has been supported in several studies (Crum et al., 1993; Cummings, 1993; Power et al., 1995). These studies concluded that mental status examinations such as the Mini-Mental State Examination, the HIV Dementia Scale, and the Neurobehavioral Rating Scale are useful for screening or identifying persons with cognitive difficulties but not for making a diagnosis (Baumann, 1993; Crum et al., 1993; Power et al., 1995). The HIV Dementia Scale (Power et al., 1995) provides a more specific index of cognitive dysfunction related to HIV disease than other examinations. Clinicians should consider seriously the addition of a short mental status examination to their assessment of PLWH. One note of caution: The Mini-Mental State Examination is not particularly sensitive to the subcortical psychomotor slowing seen in HIV disease, although it can be useful for documenting other symptoms of dementia, such as impaired orientation or memory.

Treatment of HAMCMD and HAD includes the use of high doses of zidovudine (up to 2000 mg/d) to ameliorate symptoms and attenuate the course of the disease (Levy & Fernandez, 1997; Mascolini, 1996; Roy-Byrne & Fann, 1997). Newer antiretrovirals do not seem to have the same effect. Vitamin supplementation (E, 3000 IU/d; B_6, 50–2000 mg/d; B_{12}, 100 U/d) has been shown to improve cognition (Levy & Fernandez, 1997; Mascolini, 1996). Psychostimulants (methylphenide) also have been found to enhance cognitive functioning, specifically verbal memory, rate of cognitive tracking, and mental set shifting (see Table 7–1, Antidepressants).

Treatment involves also milieu management, adjusting the home environment to maximize the client's autonomy and minimize risk. This includes reality-orientation cues, memory-compensation techniques, communication strategies, and institution of home safety measures. Home-based caregivers will benefit from teaching about the course of the disease, techniques for basic care of the PLWH and problems that can occur, appropriate respite services, and home care services (Capaldini, 1997, Levy & Fernandez, 1997; McKeogh, 1995). Psychosocial treatment and support should include mobilizing family, friends, self-help groups, and financial support networks; regulating stressors and modifying behavior; monitoring personal emotional health and crises; and providing realistic hope and referrals for spiritual care.

DELIRIUM. Delirium represents a disturbance in cognition that is characterized by cognitive and perceptual impairment, clouded consciousness, and reduced ability to focus, sustain, or shift attention. There may be a prodromal phase in which clients complain of difficulty in thinking, restlessness, irritability, or insomnia. A mental status examination during the prodromal stage should focus on arousal, attention, short-term memory, and orientation. Disturbance of consciousness, disorientation, diurnal fluctuations, and involuntary movements, such as multifocal myoclonus and asterixis, are seen in delirium (APA, 1995; Levy & Fernandez, 1997). Causes of delirium in the medically ill person with HIV include systemic infections, metabolic disorders (e.g., hypoxia, hypercarbia, hypoglycemia), fluid or electrolyte imbalance, hepatic or renal disease, thiamine deficiency, focal lesions of the brain, use or withdrawal from benzodiazepines, other sedatives, and recreational drugs (APA, 1995; Capaldini, 1997). HIV medications that can cause delirium include amphotericin, anticonvulsants, ciprofloxacin, corticosteroids, ganciclovir, interferon-alfa, and metoclopramide (*Medical Letter,* 1993). (See Appendix II also.)

Treatment of delirium in persons with HIV disease includes orienting information, minimizing disruption of the sleep-wake cycle, avoiding medications with CNS side effects, and pharmacologic intervention (Capaldini, 1997). Current pharmacologic treatment of delirium with agitation combines intravenous haloperidol (Haldol) in combination with lorazepam (Ativan) (see Tables 7–2 and 7–3). A mean dose as low as 2.8 mg of haloperidol has been show to effect a decrease in delirious symptoms within 24 hours, with minimal extrapyramidal side effects (EPSs) (Levy & Fernandez, 1997). Protection against EPSs and neuroleptic malignant syndrome may be obtained by intravenous administration of haloperidol and the coadministration of lorazepam. For persons who cannot tolerate haloperidol because of EPSs, molindone may be a particularly useful alternative in the management of delirious symptoms.

PSYCHOSOCIAL STRESSES ON PARTNERS, FAMILY, FRIENDS, INFORMAL CAREGIVERS

Partners and Spouses

A diagnosis of HIV disease has widespread consequences that affect the entire social support network of PLWH. Affected most immediately and extensively is the partner or spouse. This person experiences both psychologic and social effects of having a partner with HIV infection, including fears about transmission and social stigma (Alonzo & Reynolds, 1995; Grossman, 1995, 1996). (See Table 7–5.) These issues can be discussed in support groups for the partner or spouse or in couples groups. Through sharing experiences, support groups help members avoid self-blame and guilt. These groups also provide information on contagion and transmission, as well as a safe setting in which members can discuss frankly needed changes in sexual practices.

The psychologic stresses related to the diagnosis of a life-threatening illness and the premature death of a young adult can cause the same existential crisis, anxiety, and depression in the partner or spouse as it does in the infected person. Among gay men especially, the loss of loved ones can occur frequently, sometimes without any time to recuperate from previous losses and sometimes unrelentingly for a long period (Grossman, 1995; Perrault, 1995). Some social networks have been decimated by AIDS, which has led to chronic bereavement in survivors. Often bereavement is accompanied by significant physical and psychologic symptoms (Kemeny et al., 1994; Kemeny & Dean, 1995; Perrault, 1995). Partners and spouses should seek individual counseling to assist them to deal with their crisis as well as with the ongoing sadness, fear, and anxiety that can accompany impending death in a young partner. Support groups can also provide emotional support to spouses and lovers.

Various interpersonal stresses affect the partners or spouses of PLWH. Major stresses may occur because the equilibrium of the relationship is disrupted (Regan-Kubinski & Sharts-Hopko, 1995; Powell-Cope, 1996). A relationship based on interdependence, mutual support, autonomy, and egalitarianism may be severely threatened when one partner becomes emotionally and physically dependent, unable to contribute financially, limited in ability to provide support, and impaired in cognitive functions. Partners and spouses can find themselves involved in activities that drain them physically, emotionally, and financially (Flaskerud & Tabora, 1998; Capaldini, 1997). Caring for the partner with HIV can entail losing time from work, constantly supervising the PLWH, assisting with all aspects of daily living, and providing emotional support, comfort, compassion, and affection. The diagnosis of HIV disease also requires a change in sexual activities, both to prevent transmission of infection and in response to decreased sexual desires because of the illness (Grossman, 1995; Regan-Kubinski & Sharts-Hopko, 1995).

Stresses associated with frequent and prolonged hospitalization of the partner can range from the logistics of visiting, to making sure that the partner's financial and insurance resources re-

Table 7–5 ■ Psychosocial Stresses

Stresses	Interventions
ON PARTNERS	
Anxiety, fear, depression over life-threatening illness	Lover-spouse support groups or couples groups
Disrupted relationship equilibrium	Individual therapy Community resources
Decisions regarding treatment	Attorney, clergy, liaison psychiatry
Conflicts with family and hospital staff	Bereavement groups
Anticipatory and postmortem grief	
ON FAMILIES AND FRIENDS	
Preexisting conflicts	Supportive interventions of consultation-liaison team, clergy, attorney
Revelation of lifestyle	
Fear of social stigma	
Physical, emotional, and financial drain	
Loss and grief	Support groups Community resources
ON INFORMAL CAREGIVERS	
Conflicting demands	Respite care
Financial burden	Financial assistance
Role changes	Social support
Lack of knowledge	Education
Stigma	Emotional support
Fatigue	Psychiatric care
Loss and grief	

main adequate, to making decisions about the partner's medical treatment (Capaldini, 1997; Grossman, 1996). The partner or spouse is often called on to make decisions when the partner's mental status is compromised or when the partner is extremely ill. Decisions about life support and the disposition of property often fall to the spouse or lover. Early in the illness, the PLWH should discuss his or her wishes regarding treatment, life support, funeral, burial, and disposition of property. Unmarried partners must obtain a durable power of attorney to carry out these wishes.

Decisions made by the PLWH and his or her partner can create conflicts with hospital staff and with the extended family and can cause additional stress on the partner or spouse (Alonzo & Reynolds, 1995; Grossman, 1996). Decisions regarding treatment and life support may conflict with the course of action that the hospital staff believes is necessary or indicated. These conflicts can often be resolved with the assistance of the psychiatric consultation-liaison team, the hospital chaplain, and the hospital attorney. These same persons can assist in mediating conflicts between the spouse or partner and the client's family.

Finally, partners and spouses of PLWH must face anticipatory grief over the loss of a partner and postmortem grief when the person dies (Grossman, 1996; Perrault, 1995). Sometimes a bereaved gay partner is denied a rightful place at the funerals or memorial service. There may be disputes over wills and life insurance. HIV support groups in large cities focus specifically on bereavement and the grief process. These groups encourage persons to grieve and to express sadness, fear, loneliness, anger, and guilt with the understanding that grief is a healing process that is important to the recovery of the bereaved.

Families and Friends

The families and friends of PLWH often need supportive care. For gay men, friends may represent a reconstituted family. All the emotional and social reactions that occur with the PLWH, lovers, and spouses also occur with families and friends: shock, denial, anxiety, anger, fear, guilt, and depression (Capaldini, 1997; Grossman, 1995, 1996). Thus families and friends are often viewed as emotionally "coinfected" because they experience similar psychologic and social reac-

tions (Alonzo & Reynolds, 1995). Families experience conflict under the best of circumstances; a chronic, life-threatening illness strains family relationships and requires nurturing of a sick member at a time when families might least expect or be equipped to do so (see Table 7–5).

Preexisting conflicts between the family and the PLWH regarding lifestyle or sexual preference may have resulted in the family's emotional and geographic distance from the client (Grossman, 1996; Peterson et al., 1995; Regan-Kubinski & Sharts-Hopko, 1995). In other cases, the distance is only geographic and results from the person's having relocated to a major metropolitan area. Either situation makes the family's relationship with the PLWH difficult and imposes stress on the family. Anger at the PLWH may be generated by the thought that the person's behavior (i.e., sexual activity or injection drug use) is killing him or her; however, families are often unwilling to express anger toward a family member with a life-threatening illness. Some families have other stresses. The diagnosis of HIV disease may be their first knowledge that their relative is homosexual, abuses drugs, or has had multiple sexual partners. This news is greeted with shock, anger, bewilderment, rejection, and sometimes guilt. In this case, families experience double grieving: for their relative's behavior or identity and for his or her life-threatening illness.

When the PLWH is an IDU, other kinds of family conflict occur. Some families and friends serve as enablers of the person's drug use by providing support, housing, and money (Latkin et al., 1996; Neaigus et al., 1994). Other family members and friends of IDUs may be users themselves. Such family and friend networks may feel guilty that they are responsible for the person's disease. In other cases, the diagnosis of HIV disease reveals to the family that a person is still using drugs. Under these circumstances, families feel hurt, anger, and betrayal.

Mothers who are infected with HIV experience the stresses of caring for children, guilt over eventually abandoning their children, and emotional and physical fatigue from the care of children who may also be infected (Regan-Kubinski & Sharts-Hopko, 1995; Rose & Clark-Alexander, 1996, 1998). When the PLWH is a young child, other stresses and conflicts occur within the family. In families in which parents are also infected, siblings may feel fear and insecurity about who will care for them. They may also feel resentment and anger toward the PLWH because of the lack of attention given the siblings by the family during the PLWH's illness.

In all these situations, families need compassionate, supportive, constructive assistance from clergy, health care providers, and the psychiatric consultation-liaison team to deal with their feelings, work together, help the PLWH cope, and assist in the PLWH's care. They can also use assistance with such practical needs as housing and transportation and can benefit from sharing feelings and experiences in a support group for families. Support groups for children and younger siblings of PLWH can help them cope with their special issues. Recurring themes are fear of transmission, dealing with bereavement and grief, relating positively to children, and coping with discrimination and stigmatization (Anastasio et al., 1995; Grossman, 1996; Regan-Kubinski & Sharts-Hopko, 1995; Williams et al., 1997).

Another social stress that families face is whether to disclose the diagnosis of HIV disease to friends and then which friends to tell (Regan-Kubinski & Sharts-Hopko, 1995). Having a child or sibling with HIV disease subjects the family to the powerful threat of social stigma and rejection by friends, neighbors, coworkers, and schoolmates. Children and adolescents are often kept in the dark about a parent's or sibling's HIV disease in an effort to protect them from social stigma and rejection. They may be confused and distressed about being excluded from a family problem. On the other hand, rejection and taunting by schoolmates and neighbors are real possibilities if the family member's disease becomes known. In addition, adolescents may suffer embarrassment because they are in the process of confronting their own sexuality.

The consequence of social rejection and stigma is that families lack the social support they would normally receive when a family member has a life-threatening illness (Alonzo & Reynolds, 1995; Regan-Kubinski & Sharts-Hopko, 1995). In addition, during their bereavement some of the emotional support that usually accompanies mourning may not be available to them. When the diagnosis is not disclosed to others, pain often becomes intensified and sorrow is prolonged. In some ethnic groups stigmatization is particularly

intense (Grossman, 1996; Peterson et al., 1995). Whether to tell friends can present a major conflict. Because of this situation, support groups become an important part of a family's social network. In addition, clergy can take the lead in establishing an atmosphere of compassion and concern among parishioners so that the traditional social support of religion is available. For many survivors, the grief and healing process is long (Grossman, 1996; Kemeny & Dean, 1995). Sadness, hurt, anger, and guilt can go on for a significant period after the death. Families and friends must deal with the ambivalence of grief and anger, as well as the confusion and pain caused by social rejection. Ongoing involvement in family support groups for as long as 2 years may be beneficial. The services of mental health counselors and clergy can greatly facilitate the grief process.

Informal Caregivers

Persons who provide home care for PLWH are referred to as informal caregivers and include gay partners, friends, mothers, and other relatives. In addition to the stresses on partners, family, and friends addressed earlier, several other burdens are borne by informal caregivers (Clipp et al., 1995; Flaskerud & Tabora, 1998; Powell-Cope, 1996; Rose & Clark-Alexander, 1998; Theis et al., 1997). (See Table 7–5.) As the PLWH develops serious symptoms, more and more of his or her care is transferred to an informal caregiver. Powell-Cope (1996) describes this process as moving from independent to interdependent to dependent symptom management. Informal caregivers deal with personal care (bathing, dressing, walking), providing emotional support, instrumental care (household chores, shopping, transportation), safety associated with cognitive-neuropsychologic declines, and household contagion (Clipp et al., 1995; Flaskerud & Tabora, 1998; Theis et al., 1997).

There are both negative and positive consequences of informal caregiving. The positive rewards of caregiving include increased commitment and love, a feeling of satisfaction in one's ability to provide care even in difficult situations, an increased sense of personal strength and self-esteem, and renewed filial bonding, affection, and nurturance (Clipp et al., 1995; Flaskerud & Tabora, 1998; Powell-Cope, 1996). The burden of caregiving is related often to being overwhelmed by the number of sometimes conflicting demands and tasks, readjusting routines, financial concerns, dealing with loss and grief, fear and helplessness regarding the ability to perform the caregiving role, and providing moral and emotional support to the care recipient (Clipp et al., 1995; Flaskerud & Tabora, 1998; Irving et al., 1995; Pakenham et al., 1995). As the HIV-infected person becomes more symptomatic, the number of hours of care increase and the demands of job and caregiving conflict with one another. Financial burden, fatigue, and isolation can all become problems. The cost of informal care to one PLWH has been estimated at $26,000 per year (Ward & Brown, 1994). Even though this is donated care, it involves sacrifice of other work, social activities, and emotional expression.

There is evidence that caregiving in the context of AIDS differs for men and women, for gay lovers and parents, for various ethnic groups, and for different income groups (Clipp et al., 1995; Flaskerud & Tabora, 1998; Schiller, 1993; Sher, 1993; Smith & Rabkin, 1996; Theis et al., 1997). Women in one study were more concerned than men about balancing caregiving with other aspects of their lives, with lack of AIDS knowledge, making decisions, getting AIDS, and the stigma of AIDS (Theis et al., 1997). Traditionally, women more than men manage multiple roles and role demands and have lower incomes and fewer support services (Flaskerud & Tabora, 1998; Schiller, 1993; Sher, 1993). Especially among AIDS caregivers, there are few support services for women, and most programs for caregivers have targeted male partners of gay men. Stigma concerning AIDS and homosexuality may be especially intense among some ethnic groups, leaving the female caregiver of an adult with HIV disease totally isolated and unsupported, even by family members (Flaskerud & Tabora, 1998). In addition, lower socioeconomic status may contribute to a lack of knowledge of AIDS and fear of household contagion. In contrast to gay male caregivers, female caregivers are often involved with caring for blood relatives, sons, husbands, partners, or daughters, and among these women caregiving is accompanied by the nurture and comfort associated with gender role expectations. Caregiving from this perspective would favor female caregivers for their ability to provide emotional support (Clipp et al., 1995; Flaskerud & Tabora, 1998).

The burden of caregiving is often predicted to result in negative health outcomes in the caregiver, although this is frequently not measured. In a study of predominantly white, middle-income male and female caregivers, Theis and colleagues (1997) found that two thirds considered their health to be good or excellent. On the other hand, in a study of low-income, ethnically diverse women caregivers, it was reported that the women perceived their physical health to be poor to very poor (59%) and were moderately depressed (Flaskerud & Tabora, 1998). The number of symptoms of the PLWH, depression, and anger were the best predictors of poor physical health. Considerable amounts of anger have been found among AIDS caregivers by other investigators also (Phillips & Thomas, 1996; Schiller, 1993).

Programs to support caregivers of PLWH are needed, especially for low-income female caregivers of ethnically diverse backgrounds. Mobilizing the traditional support services of churches is one possibility (Boyle et al., 1997). Caregiver services should address problems of physical care, emotional care, resource provision and respite, knowledge, isolation, and stigma.

SPIRITUAL NEEDS

Throughout the discussion of psychosocial stresses on PLWH and on their partners, families, children, and friends, references have been made to the need for the services of clergy. The spiritual needs of PLWH, their loved ones, and caregivers involve existential concerns about self-identity; the meaning of life, adversity, and individual destiny; the need for love and acceptance; and sometimes the need for reconciliation and forgiveness. Spiritual needs may also have a religious dimension, which focuses on affirming a positive relationship with God or a higher being. Spiritual needs of PLWH may present a special challenge to nursing care, particularly in the face of organized religion's condemnation and rejection of homosexuals, drug users, and sexually promiscuous persons (Andrews et al., 1993; Broadley, 1993; Carson, 1993; Carson & Green, 1992; Cherry & Smith, 1993; Hart, 1993; Pace, 1996; Pace & Stables, 1997; Saunders & Hughes, 1998; Sumner, 1998).

Spirituality, or the spiritual dimension of a person's life, involves questions about the meaning of life, hope, self-identity, and self-worth. It can also embody forgiveness and reconciliation. In contrast to religious practice and organized religion (although these are meant to serve the spiritual needs of their members), spirituality does not involve a particular creed, liturgy, or theism. The spiritual needs of PLWH and their significant others include a profound need for meaning and hope. Most people create a self-identity and a sense of self-worth from their professional and personal relationships and the consequent productivity and satisfaction engendered. These relationships give their lives meaning, a sense of purpose, direction, and value. HIV disease threatens a person's meaning and hope with physical debility, anxiety, loss of personal relationships, social alienation, rejection, and loss of job and productivity. PLWH often must reestablish the sense that their life has value, direction, and purpose. The significant others of PLWH also experience anxiety, personal and social isolation, alienation, and an unacceptable and abrupt death of a loved one from a controversial disease.

Traditionally, people turn to the clergy, religion, and pastoral care to help them meet their spiritual needs. Many PLWH, however, view organized religion and its value system as oppressive and irrelevant. Their experiences with organized religion often have been negative, and they are alienated from the religious community. Many have lived without spiritual comfort and support. When they feel spiritual needs, they may not recognize them as such or they may repress or deny them.

The ultimate spiritual concerns of PLWH include questions of self-identity ("Who am I now?"), questions about the meaning of life ("Is there any value or purpose to this suffering? Is there a reason to go on living?"), questions about adversity ("Is life essentially cruel and unfair?"), questions about destiny ("Why did this happen to me?"), and questions about being or existence ("Has my life made a difference? Have I made a contribution to the world? Will I be remembered?"). PLWH also ask other questions that relate directly to AIDS, its stigma, and social ostracism. Questions about AIDS as a punishment for homosexuality, for using drugs, or for enjoying life can leave PLWH guilt ridden.

Table 7–6 ▪ Spiritual Needs and Care of Persons with AIDS

Spiritual Needs	Spiritual Care
Meaning, value, hope, purpose, direction	Know spiritual concerns and issues
Love, acceptance	Strengthen person's sense of worth, identity, and dignity
Reconciliation with family, church	Provide compassionate, accepting care
Rituals and practices of organized religion	Listen, review life, identify meaning
Affirmation of relationship with higher being	Provide assistance in locating clergy, a religious community

To deal with all these questions, both PLWH and their loved ones have a need for spiritual care (see Table 7–6). Often that care comes from clergy and is known as pastoral care. However, health care workers can also provide spiritual care. Knowing the spiritual concerns of the PLWH is the first step. Approaching the PLWH with compassion, nurturance, and support is the second. Spiritual care for PLWH must respect their conscience and integrity, accept and affirm their lives and their relationships, and break through the perception that spirituality is the preserve of the religious. Spiritual care involves strengthening the person's sense of meaning, purpose, worth, dignity, and identity. A sense of meaning and hope is life-affirming and nourishing, whereas the collapse of a person's meaning system is a primary motivation for suicide.

In addition to meaning and hope, PLWH need love and acceptance. Filling this need is sometimes difficult for significant others and health care workers because sick or dying people may be irascible, demanding, hostile, and unreasonable. The assistance of clergy and the religious community with these needs can be invaluable. Not only can they provide PLWH with the love and acceptance needed, but they can also support health care providers and significant others in meeting these spiritual needs on a consistent basis.

A third step in providing spiritual care is being available to listen. Health care workers can be open to discussions about faith, belief, meaning in life, and mortality. They can help PLWH review their lives, identify what has given them meaning and hope in the past, and plan experiences that will provide purpose and identity in the present and future. Sometimes PLWH request help in reconnecting with traditional faith and organized religion. Some ask for the ritual and practices of a particular religion. These practices provide comfort and give the person a sense of continuity with his or her past. They can decrease feelings of anxiety, isolation, and alienation by offering an experience of community. The health care worker can find members of the clergy who are willing to work with PLWH and their families in approaching the spiritual dimension of the illness. Clergy can assist PLWH in reconciling with their families and their church. They can encourage PLWH, their families, and their congregations to forgive one another. Members of a congregation or religious community can provide an important support system, giving spiritual, emotional, physical, and financial assistance (Hart, 1993). Furthermore, acceptance by a religious congregation can help PLWH and their families and loved ones counter the feelings of guilt and sin that have been associated with the disease.

Spiritual well-being has been associated with hardiness and with long-term survival (Carson, 1993; Carson & Green, 1992; Pace & Stables, 1997; Rabkin & Remien, 1993). Therefore providing spiritual care may mean more than just spiritual and psychosocial comfort; it may involve physical strength and physiologic competence as well. An understanding and supportive response to the spiritual needs of the PLWH can benefit the person's overall health, well-being, and longevity. Responding to clients' spiritual needs will help them to live a life of meaning and purpose. It will also help them to die with dignity and a sense of completion. Health care workers can provide spiritual care or can facilitate the provision of spiritual care to their clients. In addition, health care workers must be aware of their own spiritual and psychosocial needs in caring for PLWH.

PSYCHOSOCIAL STRESSES ON FORMAL HEALTH CARE PROVIDERS

Caring for persons with HIV disease may put stresses on health care workers (HCWs) that go beyond caring for persons with other disease.

Health care workers may be subject to a wide range of emotional, social, and work-related stresses, some of which are experienced also by clients, lovers, spouses, families, children, and friends of the PLWH and some of which are unique to health care providers. In general, their reactions can be characterized as pertaining to disease and death, sexuality and intimacy, and the burdens and rewards of formal caregiving. (See Table 7–7.)

Health care workers may have anxiety and concerns about contagion and transmission (Lego, 1994; van Servellen & Leake, 1994). They may be in contact with the patient's body fluids, administer medications and intravenous fluids, change beds, bathe the patient, and provide toilet care. Their concerns include fears of personal exposure (e.g., needle sticks) and exposure of other staff members. In addition, they have concerns about appropriate infection-control procedures. The fear of transmission has had social consequences for health care workers, some of whose spouses or lovers have urged them to quit their jobs to avoid infection of themselves and their families. Others have experienced social stigma and avoidance by friends because they work with PLWH (Lego, 1994).

Stresses on health care workers also may result from the uncertain discomfort and prejudice they feel in relating to drug users, prostitutes, sexually promiscuous persons, homosexuals, and the lovers of gay PLWH (Lego, 1994; Tierney, 1995). Personal values, cultural background, and religious ideals are challenged by the different backgrounds of these clients.

Table 7–7 ▪ Psychosocial Stresses on Health Care Workers

Stresses	Interventions
Contagion and transmission	Education
Discomfort with homosexuality and drug use	Adequate staff and resources
Intensive complicated care	Psychosocial support groups
Facing own mortality	Crisis intervention and individual support
Repetitive grief	Clear institutional policies and treatment goals
Conflicts over goals of treatment	Personal stress reduction

The intense physical care and emotional needs of hospitalized PLWH can cause health care workers to become overtaxed, stressed, fatigued, and fearful of being overwhelmed by the burden of the intensive, complicated care (Lego, 1994; Tierney, 1995; van Servellen & Leake, 1994). Enormous demands are made on their energies by the frequent necessity to meet immediate needs and by serious time pressures and overwork. In addition, they feel distressed because inattention to other responsibilities and other patients is necessitated by the seemingly all-encompassing needs of the AIDS population. These stresses increase each day because of the mushrooming incidence of the disease and tax institutional resources to the limit.

Dealing with clients with AIDS has a special impact on health care workers because they and the patients are usually about the same age (Lego, 1994). Identification and a sense of personal vulnerability to disease and death are elicited when clients are young, hitherto healthy persons who may face rapid physical deterioration and death. Health care workers are forced to recognize the fact of their own death and dying and are faced with the need to reexamine the meaning and quality of their lives. These situations take their toll on health care workers in cumulative stress, depression, and psychic fatigue.

Health care workers may also become intensely involved with PLWH because of the time and closeness of the care demanded. To some degree they become the client's family. This relationship is highly stressful when the person dies, and often health care workers are beset with increased helplessness and hopelessness. Repetitive grief and demoralization occur because of the high mortality rate for AIDS (Lego, 1994).

The traditional goals of health care impose additional stresses on health care providers. In general, these goals are to cure, to prolong life, and to improve the quality of remaining life when its duration is beyond control (Voight, 1995; von Gunten et al., 1995). PLWH fall into the second and often the third categories. Prolonging life and improving quality of life become the prime focus of service. However, even these goals cannot be carried out without personal conflict and ambiguity (von Gunten et al., 1995). Many of the treatments of HIV disease produce debilitating and distressing side effects, so that prolonging life and im-proving quality of life can be at odds. Sometimes treatment fails. Health care workers become involved in questions about whether the treatment regimen is justified; they become pessimistic and wonder, "What's the use?" Their professional identity as persons who improve clients' lives is called into question, which results in a feeling of professional impotence (van Servellen & Leake, 1994). Some staff members may empathize with a PLWH's desire for suicide; they may even be supportive of medically assisted suicide on request. These conflicts can result in anxiety, depression, and anger among staff members (Voight, 1995).

The care of the PLWH presents a challenge to the health care worker's competence, professional and personal values, and ethical convictions. So that the psychosocial needs of health personnel caring for PLWH can be met, a multifaceted program of institutional support is required (von Gunten et al., 1995; Lego, 1994; Tierney, 1995; van Servellen & Leake, 1994):

1. All staff members should receive regularly scheduled educational and informational updates on HIV and its treatment. These educational programs must be repeated at intervals to reinforce and update information. Especially important is instruction on

   a. Transmission and contagion

   b. Sexual history taking and homosexuality

   c. Taking a drug history, drug use, drugs in use, and needle sharing

   d. Assessment of mental status and recognition of delirium

   e. Monitoring cognitive dysfunction and adjustment of expectations for the client's independent adherence to procedures and treatment

   f. Hospital and community resources to assist patients and families

2. Clear, consistent policies and procedures should be developed regarding infection control, the ethical and professional responsibility to care for PLWH, and HIV testing. Such policies, adhered to by all staff members, will decrease anxiety about transmission and ensure correct and appropriate behavior toward clients. Professionals most likely to experience occupational exposure (e.g., nurses and surgeons) should be involved in developing these policies.

3. Clear, consistent, and explicitly stated agreement among all agency staff members on the goals of treatment for PLWH will ensure a common approach and feelings of support for other staff members. This agreement on goals might address the issues of prolonging life through the use of available treatment; enhancing the quality of life for both client and family through excellence in symptom control and attention to psychologic, social, spiritual, legal, and financial needs; and providing supportive care until death.

4. Regular and as-needed small-group meetings to provide emotional support for staff members specifically related to the care of PLWH and their families will promote a sense of shared experience and social and professional group support to health care workers. Health care workers should be encouraged to discuss issues of grief and loss in this safe environment.

5. Easy access to mental health consultants who can provide emotional support for clients and staff members can be helpful in crisis situations. Referrals can be made for staff members who desire more long-term psychologic support.

6. Adequate institutional resources and support to provide the level of health and medical care needed will prevent staff members from becoming overwhelmed, fatigued, and overtaxed by the care of PLWH.

On a personal level, health care workers can implement several measures that may reduce their stress at work and away from work.

1. At work they can:
   a. Work regular (consistent) hours or shifts
   b. Take lunch and coffee breaks
   c. Take brief respite breaks (look out the window, wash hands and face, massage face, do isometric exercises)
   d. Acknowledge and reward work well done by one another
2. Away from work they can:
   a. Exercise, eat, and drink in moderation
   b. Create meaningful relationships and commit time to maintain them
   c. Develop an absorbing hobby or diversional activity
   d. Not bring work home
   e. Take regular vacations

Several psychosocial issues that usually arise separately are combined in the treatment of persons with AIDS, creating unusually difficult problems. These include fears of contagion, disease, and death in young persons; negative societal attitudes and personal prejudices; overworked, fatigued, and overwhelmed health care workers; and overtaxed institutional resources. Such difficult problems require that institutions provide a set of supportive guidelines for health care professionals in the care of persons with HIV disease.

PSYCHOSOCIAL TASKS OF HEALTH CARE WORKERS TREATING PERSONS WITH AIDS

In caring for persons with AIDS, health care workers engage in a variety of psychologic, social, and educational tasks to ensure that the persons' needs are met. Health models that emphasize care of the whole person provide guidelines for meeting the physiologic, psychosocial, and educational needs of the PLWH:

- Accept, value, and provide longitudinal psychosocial, physical health, and medical care to the PLWH.
- Support the person's capacity for hope, self-determination, independence, and control.
- Provide accurate medical information concerning treatment alternatives, benefits and risks, and the rationale for suggested interventions.
- Provide accurate information regarding health-enhancing behavioral options (e.g., diet, rest, exercise, and prevention of infection) in a sensitive, nonjudgmental manner.
- Understand common psychosocial issues surrounding AIDS and provide assistance or referral for problems.
- Familiarize oneself with community psychiatric, social, educational, political, and financial resources and appropriate referrals for PLWH, lovers, families, children, friends, and informal caregivers.
- Recognize and ensure treatment of neuropsychiatric syndromes common to AIDS.
- Control symptoms, reassure PLWH that this will be done, and provide supportive care or comfort measures.
- Carry out the person's wishes concerning life-sustaining treatment and reassure them that they will not be abandoned.

- Recognize the stress that coworkers experience in caring for persons with AIDS and work to minimize it.
- Assist survivors with bereavement support and grief counseling.

RESEARCH IN PSYCHOSOCIAL AND NEUROPSYCHIATRIC ASPECTS OF HIV DISEASE

Summary of Psychosocial Research

Studies focusing on psychosocial variables have examined HIV disease and its various stages (e.g., HIV testing, appearance of symptoms, mortality) from the perspective of a stressful life experience or event. Research has been conducted also on the role of coping and social support as reactions and mediators of HIV infection, psychologic reaction to HIV infection, and disease progression. The role of depression as a debilitating psychologic response to HIV disease and in disease progression has been investigated. Finally, certain personality variables and their role in HIV disease have been studied in relation to morbidity and mortality (Cole & Kemeny, 1997; McCain & Zeller, 1994). The stresses and supports of persons with HIV disease, their partners, families, children, and their informal caregivers and the stresses on health care providers themselves have been described. Those studies, which focus on generalized attitudes or coping styles, have not been shown to affect disease progression (Keet et al., 1994; Patterson et al., 1996). Studies of the effects of social support (positive social relationships) have provided mixed evidence, in some cases making a difference and in others making no difference in disease progression (Patterson et al., 1996; Theorell et al., 1995).

Psychosocial Research Needed

To advance knowledge for clinical practice, there is a need for studies of psychosocial variables and HIV disease that incorporate stringent methodologic criteria and measure clinical outcomes. Prospective longitudinal designs or randomized experimental designs should be employed, and potential confounders (age, gender, ethnicity, medications, drug use) should be controlled. It is necessary also to establish initial disease status, to include a large sample size, and to

follow up for at least 2 years for progression from HIV to AIDS and 6 months for progression of AIDS to death. Clinical outcomes (HIV morbidity, mortality) as well as immune paramaters should be examined.

Studies employing psychosocial variables that are needed include:

- Those that involve women, low-income groups, and ethnic people of color
- Those that identify psychosocial variables that affect HIV disease progression in different populations
- Those that examine the relationship of psychosocial variables to adaptation to HIV disease and to disease progression
- Those that examine differences in psychosocial needs among various populations and design interventions to meet those needs
- Those that test psychosocial interventions to promote immune response and slow disease progression

Neuropsychiatric Research

The psychiatric aspects of HIV disease have not been as well studied as the psychosocial aspects. Depression has probably been studied most often in an attempt to determine its effect on HIV disease progression. The relationship of depression to HIV disease progression has not been supported, although in some studies it has had an effect on immune parameters (Cole & Kemeny, 1997). Treatment of depression in persons with HIV disease has significantly improved the depressive symptoms but not immune function (Rabkin et al., 1994a; 1994b).

Depression in persons with HIV disease can occur as a reaction to the disease, but it can also occur as a discrete entity or as a comorbid condition. Any study of HIV and depression should consider chronic or recurrent depression, family history, and substance abuse. Depression should not be considered a natural outcome variable in studies of HIV disease; nor should it be considered a failure of coping or social support.

Other psychiatric illnesses commonly comorbid with HIV disease, such as anxiety/panic disorders, mania, psychosis, and delirium, have not been investigated as they relate to HIV disease progression or as stressors. As is true of depression, these comorbid conditions should not be studied as outcome variables of HIV disease. Psychopharmacologic treatment, together with stress-management training and cognitive-behavioral therapy, are interventions that should be tested in populations of PLWH who also have a psychiatric illness. Symptom control and quality of life may be appropriate client outcome variables in this type of research (Holzemer, 1997).

Substance abuse accompanies many psychiatric illnesses—depression, anxiety, psychosis, mania—and, in psychiatric terms, constitutes a dual diagnosis. Studies of any of the psychiatric illnesses comorbid with HIV should always consider the role of substance abuse in both the psychiatric illness and HIV disease. Substance abuse is the great confounding variable in any study of the role of psychiatric illness in HIV disease progression or immune functions. Studies that include this confounding variable are urgently needed. In all studies of psychiatric illnesses and HIV disease, it is necessary to isolate the effects of drug-induced, medication-induced, or HIV-induced neuropsychiatric disturbances from the relationship of the particular psychiatric illness (e.g., depression) and HIV progression.

There have been several recent studies of sexual and drug use risk behaviors among mentally ill persons. Beginning attempts to design psychoeducational interventions for this population are under way. This is an important and urgent area of research in a population in which behavior change is difficult.

Remediation of cognitive impairment in persons with HIV-1-related neurocognitive disorders should also be a focus of research. In conjunction with antiretroviral treatment and psychopharmacologic treatment, interventions should be designed to test the effects of cognitive-behavioral therapy and milieu management (e.g., reality orientation cues, memory compensation techniques, and so forth) on cognitive function and client autonomy. Informal caregivers in the home should also be a focus of study in the context of caregiving for both a PLWH with cognitive dysfunction and those with other debilitating symptoms. Reducing the burden and stress of caregivers and helping them adapt to loss and deal with their bereavement are outcomes that warrant testing.

In all studies of psychosocial and neuropsychiatric aspects of HIV disease, it is important to include critical populations within which the epidemic is now expanding rapidly. These populations are low-income persons, women, ethnic people of color, and all marginalized and stigmatized people who are most at risk of HIV disease and of psychosocial and neuropsychiatric complications.

Stress on formal health care providers also deserves study. However, to study the stress of AIDS caregiving on health care workers (HCWs), researchers must take a new direction and attempt a new set of studies from a theoretical and comparative perspective:

- Longitudinal studies using sequential measurement of HCW symptoms to assess cumulative effects and changes with time
- Controlled observations of the physical, psychologic, and social aspects of HIV-related work and stress in HCWs
- Investigations using standardized measures as well as psychodiagnostic interviews to (1) assess physical symptoms, anxiety, depression, and behavioral and cognitive symptoms and (2) determine whether HCWs are experiencing a stress-related disorder
- Comparative longitudinal studies that specify and quantify the stresses that HCWs experience in relation to the cumulative effects of care and to the type of care required for persons with HIV disease and for persons with other life-threatening disease
- Evaluations of intervention programs for HCWs with matched comparison groups of providers who are not receiving the particular intervention
- Hypothesis-testing studies that investigate the preexistence of undiagnosed occupational, physical, and psychiatric morbidity in health care workers involved in intensive caregiving to PLWH

SUMMARY

The diagnosis of AIDS presents psychologic and social dilemmas, conflicts, and stresses for everyone intimately involved with the PLWH, for less intimately involved acquaintances, and ultimately for society. An awareness of these stresses on the persons involved, of the psychosocial therapies and supports needed and available, and of new developments in the treatment of HIV disease and care of PLWH will help health professionals give optimal care. In addition, health care workers should become skilled in psychiatric and neuropsychiatric assessment and treatment and recognize the complicating role of substance abuse in psychiatric illness and HIV disease. Research in the psychosocial and neuropsychiatric aspects of HIV disease must focus on interventions to control symptoms and improve the quality of life for PLWH and their caregivers. Studies should include critical populations, including the poor, ethnic people of color, and women.

REFERENCES

Alonzo, A.A., Reynolds, N.R. (1995). Stigma, HIV and AIDS: An exploration and elaboration of a stigma trajectory. *Social Science and Medicine, 41*(3), 303–315.

Amaro, H. (1995). Love, sex and power. American Psychologist, 50(6), 437–447.

American Academy of Neurology AIDS Task Force. (1991). Nomenclature and research case definitions for neurologic manifestations of human immunodeficiency virus-type1 (HIV-1) infection. *Neurology, 41*, 778–785.

American Psychiatric Association. (1995). *Diagnostic and statistical manual of mantal disorders* (4th ed.). Primary care version. Washington, DC: Author.

Anastasio, C., McMahan, T., Daniles, A., et al. (1995). Self-care burden in women with human immunodeficiency virus. *Journal of the Association of Nurses in AIDS Care, 6*(3), 31–41.

Andrews, S., Williams, A.B., Neil, K. (1993). The mother-child relationship in the HIV-1 positive family. *IMAGE: Journal of Nursing Scholarship, 25*(3), 193–198.

Atkinson, J.H., Grant, I. (1994). Natural history of neuropsychiatric manifestations of HIV disease. *Psychiatric Clinics of North America, 17*(17), 33.

Aylward, E.H., Brettschneider, P.D., McArthur, J.C., et al. (1995). Magnetic resonance imaging measurement of gray matter volume reductions in HIV dementia. *American Journal of Psychiatry, 152*(7), 987–994.

Baumann, S.L. (1993). Problems in the mental health assessments of persons with HIV. *Journal of the Association of Nurses in AIDS Care, 4*(4), 36-44.

Bindels, P.J.E., Krol, A., van Ameijden, E., et al. (1996). Euthanasia and physician-assisted suicide in homosexual men with AIDS. *Lancet, 347*, 499–504.

Bornstein, R.A., Nasrallah, H.A., Para, M.F., et al. (1993). Neuropsychological performance in symptomatic and asymptomatic HIV infection. *AIDS, 7*, 519–524.

Boxall, B. (September 3, 1995). Young gays stray from safe sex: New data shows. *Los Angeles Times*, pp. 1, 18.

Boyle, J.S., Ferrell, J.A., Hodnicki, D.R., et al. (1997). Going home: African American caregiving for adult children with human immunodeficiency virus disease. *Holistic Nursing Practice, 11*(2), 27–35.

Brashers, D.E., Neidig, J.L., Reynolds, N.R., et al. (1998). Uncertainty in illness across the HIV/AIDS trajectory. *Journal of the Association of Nurses in AIDS Care, 9*(1), 66–77.

Breitbart, W., Rosenfeld, B.D., Passik, S.D. (1996). Interest in physician assisted suicide among ambulatory HIV-infected patients. *American Journal of Psychiatry, 153*, 238–242.

Broadley, R.C. (1993). Spiritual support at the end of life. *HIV Frontline, 13*, 16–17.

Bussing, R., Burket, R.C. (1993). Anxiety and intrafamilial stress in children with hemophilia after the HIV crisis. *Journal of American Academy of Children and Adolescent Psychiatry, 32*(3), 562–567.

Cabaj, R.P. (1996). Management of anxiety and depression in HIV-infected patients. *Journal of the International Association of Physicians in AIDS Care, 2*(6), 11–16.

Camacho, L.M., Brown, B.S., Simpson, D. (1996). Psychological dysfunction and HIV/AIDS risk behavior. *Journal of Acquired Immune Deficiency Syndromes and Human Retrovirology, 11*, 198–202.

Capaldini, L. (1997). HIV disease: Psychosocial issues and psychiatric complications. In M.S. Sande, P.A. Volberding (Eds.), *The medical management of AIDS* (pp. 217–238). Philadelphia: Saunders.

Carson, V.B. (1993). Prayer, meditation, exercise, and special diets: Behaviors of the hardy person with HIV/AIDS. *Journal of the Association of Nurses in AIDS Care, 4*(3), 18–28.

Carson, V.B., Green, H. (1992). Spiritual well-being: A predictor of hardiness in patients with acquired immunodeficiency syndrome. *Journal of the Professional Nurse, 8*(4), 209–220.

Centers for Disease Control and Prevention. (February 23, 1996). Continued sexual risk behavior among HIV-seropositive, drug-using men—Atlanta, Washington, D.C., and San Juan, Puerto Rico, 1993. *Morbidity and Mortality Weekly Report, 45*(7), 151–159.

Centers for Disease Control and Prevention. (September 27, 1996). Contraceptive method and condom use among women at risk for HIV infection and other sexually transmitted diseases. *Morbidity and Mortality Weekly Report, 45*(38), 820–831.

Centers for Disease Control and Prevention. (1997). HIV and AIDS trends: The changing landscape of the epidemic: A closer look. (On-line). Available at *www.cdcnac.org//hivtrend.html.*

Cherry, K., Smith, D.H. (1993). Sometimes I cry: The experience of loneliness for men with AIDS. *Health Communication, 5*(3), 181–208.

Choi, K., Catania, J.A. (1996). Changes in multiple sexual partnerships, HIV testing and condom use among U.S. heterosexuals 18–49 years of age, 1990–1992. *American Journal of Public Health, 86,* 554–556.

Choi, K.H., Catania, J.A., Docini, M.M. (1994). Extramarital sex and HIV risk behavior among U.S. adults: Results from the National AIDS behavioral survey. *American Journal of Public Health, 84*(12), 2003–2007.

Cleary, P., van Devanter, N., Rogers, T.F., et al. (1993). Depressive symptoms in blood donors notified of HIV infection. *American Journal of Public Health, 83*(4), 534–539.

Clipp, E.C., Adinolfi, A.J., Forrest, L., et al. (1995). Informal caregivers of persons with AIDS. *Journal of Palliative Care, 11*(2), 18.

Cole, S.W., Kemeny, M.E. (1997). Psychobiology of HIV Infection. *Critical Reviews in Neurobiology, 11*(4), 287–321.

Cole, S.W., Kemeny, M.E., Taylor, S.E., et al. (1996). Accelerated course of human immunodeficiency virus infection in gay men who conceal their homosexual identity. *Psychosomatic Medicine, 58*(3), 219–231.

Coverdale, J.H. (1996). HIV risk behavior in the chronically mentally ill. *International Review of Psychiatry, 8,* 149–156.

Crum, R.M., Anthony, J.M., Bassett, S.S., et al. (1993). Population-based norms for the mini-mental state examination by age and educational level. *Journal of the American Medical Association, 269*(18), 2386–2391.

Cummings, J. (1993). Mini-mental state examination: Norms, normals, and numbers. *Journal of the American Medical Association, 269*(18), 2391–2420.

Dal Pan, G.J., McArthur, J.C., Harrison, M.J.G. (1997). Neurological symptoms in human immunodeficiency virus infection. In J.R. Berger, R.M. Levy (Eds.), *AIDS and the nervous system* (2nd ed, pp. 141–172). New York: Lippinott-Raven.

Dannenberg, A.L., McNeil, J.G., Brundage, J.F., et al. (1996). Suicide and HIV infection: Mortality follow-up of 4147 HIV-seropositive military service applicants. *Journal of the American Medical Association, 276*(21), 1743–1746.

Depression Guideline Panel. (1993a). *Depression in primary care: Vol. 1. Detection and diagnosis. Clinical practice guidelines, no. 5.* Rockville, MD: U.S. Department of Health and Human Services, Agency for Health Care Policy and Research publication 93-0550.

Depression Guideline Panel. (1993b). *Depression in primary care: Vol. 2. Treatment of major depression. Clinical practice guidelines, no. 5.* Rockville, MD: U.S. Department of Health and Human Services, Agency for Health Care Policy and Research publication 93-0551.

Enger, C., Graham, N., Peng, Y., et al. (1996). Survival from early, intermediate, and late stages of HIV infection. *Journal of the American Medical Association, 275*(17), 1329–1334.

Erickson, J.R. (1997). Human immunodeficiency virus infection risk among female sex partners of intravenous drug users in Southern Arizona. *Holistic Nursing Practice, 11*(2), 9–17.

Flaskerud, J.H., Tabora, B. (1998). Health problems of low income female caregivers of adults with HIV/AIDS. *Health Care for Women International, 19,* 23–36.

Gorman, C. (June 23, 1997). If the condom breaks. *TIME,* p. 48.

Grimes, R.M., Grimes, D.E. (1995). Psychological states in HIV disease and the nursing response. *Journal of the Association of Nurses in AIDS Care, 6*(2), 25–32.

Grossman, A.H. (1994). Homophobia: A cofactor of HIV disease in gay and lesbian youth. *Journal of the Association of Nurses in AIDS Care, 5*(1), 39–43.

Grossman, A.H. (1995). At risk, infected, and invisible: Older gay men and HIV/AIDS. *Journal of the Association of Nurses in AIDS Care, 6*(6), 13–19.

Grossman, A.H. (1996). Families and children: The challenge of HIV/AIDS: NYU AIDS/SIDA Mental Hygiene Project. New York City Department of Mental Health, Mental Retardation and Alcoholism Services.

Hamburg, M.A.C. (1996). Public health and urban medicine. *Lancet, 348,* 1008–1010.

Hart, C.W. (1993). "Our minister died of AIDS": Pastoral care of a congregation in crisis. *Journal of Pastoral Care, 47*(2), 109–115.

Heaton, R.K., Velin, R.A., McCutchan, J.A., et al. (1994). Neuropsychological impairment in human immunodeficiency virus-infection: Implications for employment. HNRC Group. HIV Neurobehavioral Research Center. *Psychosomatic Medicine, 56,* 8–12.

Herman, R., Kaplan, M., Satriano, J., et al. (1994). HIV prevention with people with serious mental illness: Staff training and institutional attitudes. *Psychosocial Rehabilitation Journal, 17*(4), 97–103.

Hinkin, C.H., van Gorp, W.G., Mandelkern, M.A., et al. (1995). Cerebral metabolic change in patients with AIDS: Report of a six-moth follow-up using positron emission tomography. *Journal of Neuropsychiatry and Clinical Neuroscience, 7*(2), 180–187.

Holzemer, W.L. (1997). Commentary: Post-Vancouver: Implications for nursing practice and nursing research. *Journal of the Association of Nurses in AIDS Care, 8*(4), 62–65.

Irwin, K.L., Valdiserri, R.O., Holmberg, S.D. (1996). The acceptability of voluntary HIV antibody testing in the United States: A decade of lessons learned. *AIDS, 10,* 1707–1717.

Irving, G., Bor, R., Catalan, J. (1995). Psychological distress among gay men supporting a lover or partner with AIDS: A pilot study. *AIDS Care, 7*(5), 605–617.

Janssen, R.S. (1997). Epidemiology and neuroepidemiology of human immunodeficiency virus infection. In J.R. Berger, R.M. Levy (Eds.), *AIDS and the nervous system* (2nd ed., pp. 13–37). New York: Lippincott-Raven.

Kalichman, S.C., Sikkema, K.J., Kelly, J.A., et al. (1995). Use of a brief behavioral skills intervention to prevent HIV infection among chronic mentally ill adults. *Psychiatric Services, 46*(3), 275–280.

Kalichman, S.C., Center for AIDS Intervention Research, Medical College of Wisconsin, and Georgia State University. (1996). Human immunodeficiency virus (HIV) risk among the seriously mentally ill. *American Psychological Association, 3*(2), 130–143.

Katz, M.H., Gerberding, J.L. (1997). Postexposure treatment of people exposed to the human immunodeficiency virus through sexual contact or injection-drug use. *Sounding Board, 336*(15), 1097–1099.

Keet, I.P.M., Krol, A., Klein, M.R., et al. (1994). Characteristics of long-term asymptomatic infection with human immunodeficiency virus type 1 in men with normal and low CD4+ cell counts. *Journal of Infectious Disease, 169,* 1236.

Kemeny, M.E., Weiner, H., Taylor, S.E., et al. (1994). Repeated bereavement, depressed mood, and immune parameters in HIV seropositive and seronegative gay men. *Health Psychology, 13*(1), 14–24.

Kemeny, M.E., Dean, L. (1995). Effects of AIDS-related bereavement on HIV progression among New York City gay men. *AIDS Education and Prevention, 7*(Suppl. 5), 36–47.

Latkin, C., Mandell, W., Vlahov, D., et al. (1996). People and places: Behavioral settings and personal network characteristics as correlates of needle sharing. *Journal of Acquired Immune Deficiency Syndromes and Human Retrovirology, 13,* 273–280.

Lego, S. (1994). AIDS-related anxiety and coping methods in a support group for caregivers. *Archives of Psychiatric Nursing, 8*(3), 200–207.

Leiphart, J.M. (1997). Psychoneuroimmunology: A basis for HIV treatment. *Focus: A Guide to AIDS Research and Counseling, 12*(3), 1–4.

Levy, J.K., Fernandez, F. (1997). Neuropsychiatric aspects of human immuno-deficiency virus infection of the central nervous system. In S.C. Yudofsky, R.E. Hales (Eds.), *The American Psychiatric Press textbook of neuropsychiatry* (pp. 663–692). Washington, D.C.: American Psychiatry Press.

Lilleleht, E., Leiblum, S. (1993). Schizophrenia and sexuality: A critical review of the literature. *Annual Review of Sex Research, 4,* 247–276.

Lovejoy, N.C., Matteis, M. (1997). Cognitive-behavioral interventions to manage depression in patients with cancer: Research and theoretical initiatives. *Cancer Nursing, 20*(3), 155–167.

Lyketsos, C., Federman, E. (1995). Psychiatric disorders and HIV infection: Impact on one another. *Epidemiologic Review, 17,* 152–164.

Mascolini, M. (1996). HIV and the mind. *Journal of the International Association of Physicians in AIDS Care, 2*(6), 19–26.

McArthur, J.C., Hoover, D.R., Bacellar, H., et al. (1993). Dementia in AIDS patients: Incidence and risk factors. *Neurology, 43,* 2245–2252.

McCain, N.L., Zeller, H. (1994). Research priorities for psychosocial aspects of nursing care in HIV disease. *Journal of the Association of Nurses in AIDS Care, 5*(2), 21–26.

McEnany, G.W., Hughes, A.M., Lee, K.A. (1996). Depression and HIV. *Nursing Clinics of North America, 31*(1), 57–80.

McKeogh, M. (1995). Dementia in HIV disease: A challenge for palliative care? *Journal of Palliative Care, 11*(2), 30–33.

McKirnan, D.J., Ostrow, D.G., Hope, B. (1996). Sex, drugs and escape: A psychological model of HIV-risk sexual behaviours. *AIDS Care, 8*(6), 655–659.

Medical Letter. (1993). Drugs that cause psychiatric symptoms, *Medical Letter, 35,* 65–70.

Merson, M.H. (1996). Returning home: Reflections on the USA's response to the HIV/AIDS epidemic. *Lancet, 347,* 1673–1676.

Miller, E.N., Selnes, O.A., Satz, P. (1994a). Methods of controlling for demographic differences in neuropsychological studies of HIV infection. *AIDS, 8,* 280–281.

Miller, E.N., Satz, P., Selnes, O.A. (1994b). Problems with causal inference in cross-sectional studies of HIV infection *Journal of Neuropsychiatry and Clinical Neuroscience, 6,* 201–203.

Moore, L.H., van Gorp, W.G., Hinkin, C.H., et al. (1997). Subjective complaints versus actual cognitive deficits in predominantly symptomatic HIV-1 seropositive individuals. *Journal of Neuropsychiatry and Clinical Neuroscience, 9*(1), 37–44.

Neaigus, A., Friedman, S.R., Curtis, R., et al. (1994). The relevance of drug injectors' social and risk networks for understanding and preventing HIV infection. *Social Science Medicine, 38*(1), 67–78.

Neal, J.J., Fleming, P.L., Green, T.A., et al. (1997). Trends in heterosexually acquired AIDS in the U.S., 1988 through 1993. *Journal of Acquired Immune Deficiency Syndromes and Human Retrovirology, 14,* 465–474.

Norris, A.E., Ford, K., Shyr, Y., et al. (1996). Heterosexual experiences and partnerships of urban, low-income African and Hispanic youth. *Journal of Acquired Immune Deficiency Syndromes and Human Retrovirology, 11,* 288–300.

Pace, J.C., Stables, J.L. (1997). Correlates of spiritual well-being in terminally ill persons with AIDS and terminally ill persons with cancer. *Journal of the Association of Nurses in AIDS Care, 8*(6), 31–42.

Pace, J.C. (1996). Spirituality issues. In G.J. Moore (Ed.), *Women and cancer: A gynecologic oncology nursing perspective* (pp. 579–599). Sudbury, MA: Jones & Bartlett.

Pakenham, K.I., Dadds, M.R., Terry, D.J. (1995). Carers' burden and adjustment to HIV. *AIDS Care, 7,* 189–203.

Patterson, T.L., Shaw, W.S., Semple, S.J., et al. (1996). Relationship of psychosocial factors to HIV disease progression. *Annals of Behavioral Medicine, 18,* 30.

Perkins, D.O., Leserman, J., Stern, R.A., et al. (1995). Somatic symptoms and HIV infection: Relationship to depressive symptoms and indicators of HIV disease. *American Journal of Psychiatry, 152*(12), 1776–1781.

Perkins, D.O., Stern, R.A., Golden, R.N., et al. (1994). Mood disorders in HIV infection: Prevalence and risk factors in a nonepicenter of the AIDS epidemic. *American Journal of Psychiatry, 15*(2), 233–236.

Perrault, Y. (1995). AIDS grief: "Out of the closet and into the boardrooms": The bereaved caregivers. *Journal of Palliative Care, 11*(2), 34–37.

Peterson, J.L., Coates, T.J., Catania, J.A., et al. (1995). Help-seeking for AIDS high-risk sexual behavior among gay and bisexual African-American men. *AIDS Education and Prevention, 7*(1), 1–9.

Peterson, J.L., Coates, T.J., Catania, J., et al. (1996). Evaluation of an HIV risk reduction intervention among African-American homosexual and bisexual men. *AIDS, 10,* 319–325.

Phillips, K.D., Thomas, S.P. (1996). Extrapunitive and intrapunitive anger of HIV caregivers: Nursing implications. *Journal of the Association of Nurses in AIDS Care, 7*(2), 17–27.

Powell-Cope, G.M. (1996). HIV disease symptom management in the context of committed relationships. *Journal of the Association of Nurses in AIDS Care, 7*(3), 19–28.

Power, C., Selnes, O.A., Grim, J.A., et al. (1995). HIV Dementia Scale: A rapid screening test. *Journal of Acquired Immune Deficiency Syndromes, 8,* 273–278.

Rabkin, J.G., Johnson, J., Lin, S., et al. (1997). Psychopathology in male and female HIV-positive and negative injecting drug users: Longitudinal course over 3 years. *AIDS, 11,* 507–515.

Rabkin, J.G., Rabkin, R., Hanson, W., et al. (1994b). Effect of imipramine on mood and enumerative measures of immune status in depressed patients with HIV illness. *American Journal of Psychiatry, 151,* 516.

Rabkin, J.G., Remien, R. (1993). Resilience in adversity among long-term survivors of AIDS. *Hospital and Community Psychiatry, 44*(2), 162–167.

Rabkin, J.G., Wagner, G., Rabkin, R. (1994a). Effects of sertraline on mood and immune status in patients with major depression and HIV illness: An open trial. *Journal of Clinical Psychiatry, 55,* 433.

Regan-Kubinski, M.J., Sharts-Hopko, N. (1995). Illness cognition of HIV-infected mothers. *Issues in Mental Health Nursing, 16*(4), 327–344.

Rose, M.A., Clark-Alexander, B. (1996). Quality of life and coping styles of HIV-positive women with chil-dren. *Journal of the Association of Nurses in AIDS Care, 7*(2), 28–34.

Rose, M.A., Clark-Alexander, B. (1998). Caregivers of children with HIV/AIDS: Quality of life and coping styles. *Journal of the Association of Nurses in AIDS Care, 9*(1), 58–65.

Roy-Byrne, P.P., Fann, J.R. (1997). Psychopharmacologic treatments for patients with neuropsychiatric disorders. In S.C. Yudofsky, R.E. Hales (Eds.), *The American Psychiatric Press textbook of neuropsychiatry* (pp. 943–981). Washington, D.C.: American Psychiatry Press.

Saunders, J.M., Hughes, A. (1998). Nurses and assisted dying: Taking our roles to heart and mind. *Journal of the Association of Nurses in AIDS Care, 9*(2), 15–17.

Schiller, N.G. (1993). The invisible women: Caregiving and the construction of AIDS health services. *Culture, Medicine and Psychiatry, 17,* 487–512.

Selnes, O.A., Miller, E.N. (1993). Asymptomatic HIV-1 infection and aviation safety. *Aviation, Space, and Environmental Medicine, 64,* 172–173.

Sikkema, K.J., Heckman, T.G., Kelly, J., et al. (1996). HIV risk behaviors among women living in low income, inner city housing developments. *American Journal of Public Health, 86*(8), 1123–1128.

Sher, R. (1993). The role of women in the AIDS epidemic. *Medicine & Law, 12,* 467–469.

Singleton, J.A., Tabnak, F., Kuan, J., et al. (1996). Human immunodeficiency virus disease in California. *Western Journal of Medicine, 164,* 122–129.

Smith, M.Y., Rabkin, B.D. (1996). Social support and barriers to family involvement in caregiving for persons with AIDS: Implications for patient education. *Patient Education and Counseling, 27*(10), 85–94.

Snyder, C.M., Kaempfer, S.H., Ries, K. (1996). An interdisciplinary, interagency, primary care approach to case management of the dually diagnosed patient with HIV disease. *Journal of the Association of Nurses in AIDS Care, 7*(5), 72–82.

Solomon, L., Moore, J., Gleghorn, A., et al. (1996). HIV testing behaviors in a population of inner city women at high risk for HIV infection. *Journal of Immune Deficiency Syndromes and Human Retrovirology, 13,* 267–272.

Stall, R., Hoff, C., Coates, T.C., et al. (1996). Decisions to get HIV tested and to accept antiretroviral therapies among gay/bisexual men: Implications for secondary prevention efforts. *Journal of Acquired Immune Deficiency Syndromes and Human Retrovirology, 11,* 151–160.

Stewart, M.J., Hart, G., Mann, K.V. (1995). Living with hemophilia and HIV/AIDS: Support and coping. *Journal of Advanced Nursing, 22*(66), 1101–1111.

Sumner, C.H. (1998). Recognizing and responding to spiritual distress. *American Journal of Nursing, 98*(1), 26–30.

Susser, E., Miller, M., Valencia, E., et al. (1996). Injection drug use and risk of HIV transmission among homeless men with mental illness. *American Journal of Psychiatry, 153*(6), 794–798.

Swanson, B., Cronin-Stubbs, D., Zeller, J.M., et al. (1993a). Characterizing the neuropsychological functioning of persons with human immunodeficiency virus infection. Part 1. Acquired immunodeficiency syndrome dementia complex: A review. *Archives of Psychiatric Nursing, 7*(2), 74–81.

Swanson, B., Cronin-Stubbs, D., Zeller, J.M., et al. (1993b). Characterizing the neuropsychological functioning of persons with human immunodeficiency virus (HIV) infection. Part II. Neuropsychological functioning of persons at different stages of HIV infection. *Archives of Psychiatric Nursing, 7*(2), 82–90.

Sweeney, C., Agger, W. (1997). AIDS-related lymphomas with neurologic manifestations. *Western Journal of Medicine, 167*(1), 40–44.

Tabet, S.R., de Moya, A., Holmes, K.K., et al. (1996). Sexual behaviors and risk factors for HIV infection among men who have sex with men in the Dominican Republic. *AIDS, 10,* 201–206.

Theis, S.L., Cohen, F.L., Forrest, J., et al. (1997). Needs assessment of caregivers of people with HIV/AIDS. *Journal of the Association of Nurses in AIDS Care, 8*(3), 84.

Theorell, T., Blomkvist, V., Jonsson, H., et al. (1995). Social support and the development of immune function in human immunodeficiency virus infection. *Psychosomatic Medicine, 57,* 32.

Tierney, A.J. (1995). HIV/AIDS knowledge, attitudes and education of nurses: A review of the research. *Journal of Clinical Nursing, 4*(1), 13–21.

Torian, L.V., Weisfuse, I.B., Makki, H.A., et al. (1996). Trends in HIV seroprevalence in men who have sex with men: New York City Department of Health, Sexually Transmitted Disease, 1988–1993. *AIDS, 10,* 187–192.

Valente, S.M., Saunders, J.M. (1997). Diagnosis and treatment of major depression among people with cancer. *Cancer Nursing, 20*(3), 168–177.

van Haastrecht, H.J.A., Mientjes, G.H.C., van den Hoek, A.J., Coutinho, R.A. (1994). Death from suicide and overdose among drug injectors after disclosure of first HIV test results. *AIDS, 8,* 1721–1725.

Van Servellen, G., Leake, B. (1994). Emotional exhaustion and distress among nurses: How important are AIDS-care specific factors? *Journal of the Association of Nurses in AIDS Care, 5*(2), 11–19.

Voight, R.F. (1995). Euthanasia and HIV disease: How can physicians respond? *Journal of Palliative Care, 11*(2), 38–41.

Von Gunten, C.F., Martinez, J., Neely, K.J., et al. (1995). AIDS and palliative medicine: Medical treatment issues. *Journal of Palliative Care, 11*(2), 5–11.

Ward, D., Brown, M.A. (1994). Labor and cost in AIDS family caregiving. *Western Journal of Nursing Research, 16*(1), 10–22.

Wells, E.K. (1997a). New prognosis for HIV: A mental health perspective. *HIV Frontline, 26,* 4–6.

Wells, E.K. (1997b). When new treatments don't work: A mental health perspective. *HIV Frontline, 27,* 4–5.

Wells, E.K., Mayer, R.R. (1997). HIV-negative women in serodiscordant couples. *HIV Frontline, 29,* 4–5, 8.

Williams, A.B., Shahryarinejad, A., Andrews, S., et al. (1997). Social support for HIV-infected mothers: Relation to HIV care seeking. *Journal of the Association of Nurses in AIDS Care, 8*(1), 91–98.

Wood, A.J.J. (1996). Drug therapy. *New England Journal of Medicine, 334*(1), 34–40.

Zeifert, P., Leary, M., Boccellari, A. (1995). *AIDS and the impact of cognitive impairment.* San Francisco, CA: UCSF AIDS Health Project.

Zung, W.W., Broadhead, E., Roth, M.E. (1993). Prevalence of depressive symptoms in primary care. *Journal of Family Practice, 37*(4), 337–344.

8

The Needs of Special Populations

■ Men Who Have Sex with Men

ARNOLD H. GROSSMAN

In the United States, men who have sex with men (MSM) have constituted the largest category of people diagnosed with AIDS. Originally they were almost all white (non-Hispanic) men; however, they have increasingly become men of color (CDC, 1995, 1996). Although most health care providers believe that all HIV-positive men who have had sex with men are *gay* men, this is not the case. Sexual identity and sexual behavior are two distinct constructs, and one is not always predictive of the other (Irvine, 1995). Some men who identify themselves as heterosexual or bisexual have also become infected by having sex with men (de la Vega, 1995; Manalansan, 1996). Their same-sex fantasies, desires, and erotic experiences, as well as those of self-identified gay men, are labeled homosexual by society; and this label and the reactionary homophobia (i.e., antigay feelings and behaviors) that it generates continue to shape the needs of HIV-positive MSM (Altman, 1988; Powell, 1996; Shilts, 1987).

Although homophobia is a complex set of beliefs and activities, cultural patterns of certain groups have proved to be more fertile ground for the growth of antigay perspectives than others (Irvine, 1995). Therefore the impact of homophobia on the needs of HIV-positive MSM will be greater among certain groups of people.

Coping with a Double Stigma

Many HIV-positive MSM became infected during their adolescent years. Engaging in same-sex behaviors or identifying oneself as gay or bisexual means having to live with the stigma of ho-

mosexuality, and that stigma leads to the person's being assigned a "spoiled identity" (Goffman, 1963). For many, this stigma leads to hiding and passing; for others, it engenders the challenge to come out and claim an authentic identity, usually accompanied by verbal abuse and other types of sexual-orientation victimization. Both of these responses, along with internalizing of society's homophobia, place many gay and bisexual youth in situations in which they are at risk of depression, suicide, alcohol and other substance abuse, homelessness, prostitution, and HIV infection (Grossman, 1994, 1997).

The fear of being discovered or discredited because of their same-sex behaviors continues into adulthood; therefore, when they perceive themselves as being HIV-infected, many MSM need to learn how to cope with the repercussions of living with a *double stigma* (Grossman, 1991; Public Media Center, 1995). In addition, research has indicated that greater internalized homophobia among HIV-positive, asymptomatic gay men predicts higher levels of distress at a 2-year follow-up (Wagner et al., 1996).

Because this internalized homophobia is compounded by the shame of having a sexually transmitted infection, these men also need help in seeking HIV counseling and testing. If they receive an HIV-positive test result, they often need aid in confronting their fear, anger, and denial. Assistance in helping them to accept their diagnosis and seek early medical care meets a primary need. Often they need encouragement in disclosing their HIV-positive diagnosis to significant others (both male and female) whom they may have unknowingly exposed to HIV through sexual activity (Cohen, 1995). At the same time, they need emotional support, as they frequently do not have a social support network of friends and family to whom they have publicly acknowledged their same-sex sexual behaviors.

The social isolation of many HIV-positive MSM "is a psychological death experience that precedes the physical death" (Elia, 1997, p. 72). Consequently, they need opportunities to interact with other HIV-positive MSM (Barney & Duran, 1997), and they ultimately need assistance in establishing communication with family members and significant others before the disease interferes with their functioning (Powell, 1996). These underlying issues related to same-sex behaviors, along with the presence of such factors as poverty, substance abuse, limited education, low self-esteem, ethnicity, religion, homelessness, and mental illness, continue to have enormous effects on the ongoing needs of HIV-positive MSM throughout the course of the disease.

Getting Quality Health and Medical Care

The primary needs of HIV-infected MSM are access to and receipt of quality health and medical care that is provided in nondiscriminatory, confidential, and safe environments. Labels referring to behaviors as deviant, immoral, and sinful and judgments by health care providers about the mode of infection tend to bring back painful memories of name calling, jeers, abuse, hostility, and blame to MSM. Assumptions about people's sexual orientation and behaviors based on their looks are often inaccurate and tend to lead to behaviors of health care providers that are not beneficial to their clients (NYC Department of Health, 1996). MSM need health care providers who keep their personal prejudices out of their professional decision-making processes and who understand the negative impact of religious policies that are being made to subjugate gay people (Powell, 1996). When health care providers act on their personal moral and religious beliefs or stigmatize HIV-positive MSM, they compound the health problems of these men. On the other hand, when health care workers build into their health care plans experiences that lead to greater self-esteem and a healthy identity, MSM can make positive life changes, frequently leading them to make radical changes in their health and social behaviors (Barney & Duran, 1997).

Managing Stress and Coping with Losses

Living with HIV infection is a stressful experience. It requires adaptation and adjustments in activities of daily living and patterns of relationships, while its impact on the immune system often leads to unfamiliar and unpredictable opportunistic infections. Coping longer with the uncertainty of the disease and the lack of control it imparts to careers and finances does not guarantee survival, but it often brings personal losses and the difficulty of surviving the deaths of loved ones (Remien & Rabkin, 1995).

Not only does the person have to adapt to living with chronic sadness and loss, but he also develops a feeling of being stalked by grief and loss: Who will be next? When will it happen? How will it affect me? These are some of the questions that HIV-positive MSM continually ask of themselves, as dealing with massive loss and anticipated individual losses often goes unspoken (Elia, 1997). Fears of physical deterioration, loneliness, and living as a statistic are frequently compounded by feelings of hopelessness, alienation, and depression. These feelings point to needs with which health care providers can help HIV-positive MSM cope, such as not seeing themselves as victims, not giving in to the disease, learning to live in the present, rechanneling negative emotions (i.e., not giving the virus the power to kill), and being proactive with regard to their lifestyle and medical treatment.

Dealing with Failed Promises

For some HIV-positive men, the needs discussed above become major ones when they do not benefit from the new combination therapies. The HIV in their bodies is either resistant or unresponsive to the treatments, or intolerable side effects to the drug regimens may develop. For others, the treatments may succeed initially but then lose their effectiveness, or adherence to the medication regimen may become too difficult. These failed promises lead to psychosocial sequelae of despair and depression emanating from feelings of being left out, left behind, and condemned to die. In addition to exploring these feelings, MSM may also need help in examining feelings of guilt—for not perfectly adhering to an onerous drug schedule and for loss of control over their destinies—as there are no known therapies to stop the progression of HIV in their bodies and time is running out (Rabkin & Ferrando, 1997).

Meeting Uncertainty and a Shifting Horizon

For other HIV-positive men, 1996 will be recorded in their lives as the year the tide turned in their war against HIV/AIDS. Their positive reactions to the new antiretroviral treatments, which include the protease inhibitors, are leading these HIV-positive MSM to have viral loads that have become undetectable. Along with the hope that these medical successes are bringing come needs related to uncertainty and the challenges of coping with a shifting horizon. An undetectable viral load does not equal eradication of the virus from their bodies, and success now does not rule out failure, resistance, or intolerable side effects in the future. The long-term effects of combination therapies, including the protease inhibitors, are unknown. This uncertainty is accompanied by the challenges of learning to live instead of waiting to die.

Having anticipated the end of life when given a diagnosis of a number of opportunistic infections (OIs) associated with HIV disease, many HIV-positive MSM are now having to reevaluate their end-of-life decisions. Their lives now mirror those of long-term survivors of the 1980s, characterized by psychologic resilience and positive survival rather than preoccupation with impending decline (Remien & Rabkin, 1995). These men now have mental health dilemmas related to whether they should return to work, change careers, start a new relationship, or end an existing personal relationship, having previously settled for less or anticipated a diminished life expectancy (Rabkin & Ferrando, 1997). Compounding these decisions are others related to the consequences of terminating disability benefits in the face of the uncertainty of long-term treatment effects and to dealing with debts that may have accumulated (along with creditors who may come knocking on the door). Concomitantly, many may have to learn to build lives without shame as MSM who are not dying of HIV/AIDS. These men frequently need assistance in confronting issues related to their internalized homophobia and challenging discrimination based on sexual orientation. A parallel need relates to a new type of survivor guilt, i.e., the potential of living much longer with AIDS whereas many friends died before the introduction of protease inhibitors and others continue to die because they are unresponsive to new treatments.

Minimizing Risky HIV-Transmission Behaviors

If the new hope generated by the antiretroviral treatments is realized, the greatest number of HIV-positive MSM will be living for the longest periods of time since the advent of the HIV epidemic. Although this fact brings joy to many, it also creates an increasing cadre of men who have the potential of transmitting HIV, as "undetectable" HIV does not mean noninfectious HIV. ("Undetectable" means that the assay cannot detect viral copies, if they are present, below a specified threshold.) If some of these men are still hiding their sexual orientation for fear of discrimination or alienation, they are likely to place themselves in situations that are not conducive to safer sex practices (McNeill, 1993). In addition, they need to explore the triggers that precede or lead to risky behaviors (e.g., use of alcohol or drugs, loneliness, or cognitive biases that justify unsafe sexual practices) (Klotz, 1995). Furthermore, reduced viral loads, elevations in T-cell counts, reduced numbers of hospital stays, extended disease-free survival, and improved quality of life may lead many of these HIV-positive men to deny the fact that they remain capable of transmitting HIV. Therefore these HIV-positive MSM have needs related to secondary prevention (Parish, 1997). They need assistance in continuing to perceive themselves as infectious and in recognizing that lapses in safer sex practices and in clean-needle drug use can lead to their transmitting HIV. This need is further complicated by those who have come to believe that the powerful new drugs currently being used to treat established infections can be used as "morning-after" pills to forestall infection after risky sexual encounters (Zuger, 1997). Also, uninfected young gay men who want to experience the reported liberated sexual experiences of gay men in the 1970s may now be less concerned about having unprotected sex with HIV-positive men, as they erroneously believe that HIV/AIDS is curable.

Meeting Multiple Needs

Some HIV-positive MSM have multiple needs. Having declared that they are HIV-positive and that the mode of transmission was engaging in same-sex behaviors, these men may have been rejected in their homes, fired by their employers, barred from their places of worship, and discriminated against in their communities. They may have needs related to (1) being poor or homeless, (2) domestic violence or sexual abuse, (3) coping with stress through substance use and abuse, or (4) a psychiatric disorder. Therefore they need case management services to help them achieve a better quality of life, rehabilitation to engage them in harm-reduction activities or to move them toward a clean and sober lifestyle, and mental health interventions to help them become emotionally stable and cope with their internalized homophobia. Concurrently, they need assistance in dealing with dual or triple diagnoses of HIV, substance abuse, and mental illness. Interventions should be focused on helping them achieve a consistent and committed approach to their health and to succeeding on combination-therapy regimens. The role of the health care provider is to act as an advocate for these HIV-positive MSM with regard to meeting their coexisting needs and to provide interventions that are consistent and empowering.

REFERENCES

Altman, D. (1988). Legitimation through disaster: AIDS and the gay movement. In E. Fee, D.M. Fox, *AIDS: The burdens of history* (pp. 301–315). Berkeley: University of California Press.

Barney, D.D., Duran, E.S. (1997). Case management: Coordinator of service delivery for HIV-infected individuals. In M.G Winiarski (Ed.), *HIV mental health for the 21st century* (pp. 241–256). New York: New York University Press.

Centers for Disease Control and Prevention [CDC]. (December 31, 1995). *HIV/AIDS Surveillance Report, 7*(2), 11–16.

Centers for Disease Control and Prevention [CDC]. (December 31, 1996). *HIV/AIDS Surveillance Report, 8*(2), 11–16.

Cohen, E.D. (1995). Ethical standards in counseling sexually active clients with HIV. In W. Odets, M. Shernoff (Eds.), *The second decade of AIDS: A mental health practice handbook* (pp. 233–254). New York: Hatherleigh Press.

de la Vega, E. (1995). Considerations for presenting HIV/AIDS information to U.S. Latino populations. In W. Odets, M. Shernoff (Eds.), *The second decade of AIDS: A mental health practice handbook* (pp. 255–274). New York: Hatherleigh Press.

Elia, N. (1997). Grief and loss in HIV/AIDS work. In M.G. Winiarski (Ed.), *HIV mental health for the 21st century* (pp. 67–81). New York: New York University Press.

Goffman, E. (1963). *Stigma: Notes on the management of a spoiled identity.* Englewood Cliffs, NJ: Prentice Hall.

Grossman, A.H. (1991). Gay men and HIV/AIDS: Understanding the double stigma. *JANAC: Journal of the Association of Nurses in AIDS Care, 2*(4), 28–32.

Grossman, A.H. (1994). Homophobia: A cofactor of HIV disease in gay and lesbian youth. *JANAC: Journal of the Association of Nurses in AIDS Care, 5*(1), 39–43.

Grossman, A.H. (1997). Growing up with a "spoiled identity": Lesbian, gay and bisexual youth at risk. *Journal of Gay & Lesbian Social Services, 6*(3), 45–56.

Irvine, J.M. (1995). *Sexuality education across cultures: Working with differences.* San Francisco: Jossey-Bass.

Klotz, D.E. (1995). Safer sex maintenance and reinforcement for gay men. In W. Odets, M. Shernoff (Eds.), *The second decade of AIDS: A mental health practice handbook* (pp. 219–232). New York: Hatherleigh Press.

Manalansan, M.F., IV. (1996). Double minorities: Latino, black and Asian men who have sex with men. In R.C. Savin-Williams, K.M. Cohen, *The lives of lesbians, gays, and bisexuals: Children to adults* (pp. 393–415). Fort Worth, TX: Harcourt Brace.

McNeill, J.J. (1993). *The church and the homosexual* (4th ed.). Boston: Beacon Press.

New York City Department of Health/Bureau of HIV Program Services. (1996). *Giving the best care possible: Unlearning homophobia in the health and social service setting.* New York: Author.

Parish, K. (1997). Secondary prevention: Working with people with HIV to prevent transmission to others. In M.G. Winiarski (Ed.), *HIV mental health for the 21st century* (pp. 116–133). New York: New York University Press.

Powell, J. (1996). *AIDS and HIV-related diseases: An educational guide for professionals and the public.* New York: Plenum.

Public Media Center. (1995). *The impact of homophobia and other social biases on AIDS.* San Francisco: Author.

Rabkin, J.G., Ferrando, S. (1997). A "second life" agenda: Psychiatric research issues raised by protease inhibitor treatments for people with HIV/AIDS. *Archives of General Psychiatry, 54*(11), 1049–1053.

Remien, R., Rabkin, J. (1995). Long-term survival with AIDS and the role of community. In G.M. Herek, B. Greene, *AIDS, identity, and community: The HIV epidemic and lesbians and gay men* (pp. 169–186). Thousand Oaks, CA: Sage.

Shilts, R. (1987). *And the band played on: Politics, people and the AIDS epidemic.* New York: St. Martin's Press.

Wagner, G., Brondolo, E., Rabkin, J. (1996). Internalized homophobia in a sample of HIV+ gay men, and its relationship to psychological distress, coping and illness progression. *Journal of Homosexuality, 32*(2), 91–106.

Zuger, A. (1997, June 10). "Morning after" treatment for AIDS. *The New York Times,* pp. C1, C5.

▪ Older Adults

Arnold H. Grossman

HIV/AIDS in the United States is seen as primarily a disease of young adults. Whereas at one end of the spectrum infants born to HIV-infected mothers have received much attention, at the other end older adults with HIV remain invisible and underserved. Health care providers and others have failed to notice that older persons are becoming infected, getting sick, and dying (Anderson, 1994, p. 1). HIV-infected persons over the age of 50 years make up the most overlooked population, even though they have consistently accounted for 10% to 11% of persons in whom AIDS is diagnosed (Ungvarski, 1997). They account for 59,424 of the cumulative number of reported AIDS cases through December 31, 1996, with 87% being men and 13% being women (CDC, 1996). The modes of HIV transmission among these persons are as follows: 49.2% contact between MSM, 16.7% injecting drug use, 11.2% heterosexual contact, 6.4% receipt of transfusion, 2.5% MSM who are injecting drug users, 0.8% hemophilia or coagulation disorder, and 13% other or risk not reported. These routes of transmission among older HIV-infected adults provide a contextual framework for examining their needs, with special attention to the fact that 62.9% of them became infected by sexual transmission.

Learning About HIV Vulnerability

Older adults—men and women of all sexual orientations—need to learn that they are vulnerable to HIV infection. Professionals who provide health education and care must learn the same lesson. Physicians, nurses, and other health care providers must be prepared to take complete sexual histories and must learn about the drug-using behaviors of older persons, even if those persons are older than they are. Beliefs and myths that portray Grandma, Grandpa, Aunt Ethel, and Uncle Ernie as sexually inactive teetotalers must be confronted for what they are (Anderson, 1994, Grossman, 1997). Contrary to popular belief, studies have found that age does not inherently decrease sexual desire or activity, and in some cases sexual activity actually increases (Grossman,

1995). Recent studies indicate that 40% to 65% of those 60 to 71 years of age reported they had sexual intercourse (Whipple & Scura, 1996); and more than two thirds of gay and bisexual men aged 50 or over said they were sexually active (Kooperman & Hemenway, 1994).

Kooperman and Hemenway (1994) also found that almost two thirds of the 191 participants knew between 1 and 10 persons in whom AIDS had been diagnosed; therefore AIDS had a human face for them, which might have increased their own concern about HIV risk and led to their reporting moderate- to low-risk sexual activity.

The belief that older adults do not engage in risky behaviors that make them vulnerable to HIV infection often means that early signs and symptoms of HIV infection are overlooked or are inappropriately attributed to the physical changes associated with the aging process or to age-related diseases (Whipple & Scura, 1996). Meeting their educational needs to prevent HIV reinfection or another sexually transmitted disease (STD), as well as protecting their sexual partners, then becomes a lost option. Opportunities for meeting treatment needs through early antiretroviral and prophylaxis therapies and for monitoring viral loads are missed. These forfeited chances may be particularly troublesome for older adults, as HIV (like other infections), appears to have a faster disease progression in older persons than in younger ones, leading to a more rapid clinical deterioration (Emlet, 1993; Whipple & Scura, 1996). Once treatments have been started, however, older adults may need more frequent and more sensitive monitoring, as they are more prone than younger persons to adverse effects of individual drugs and to drug interactions in polypharmacy (Whipple & Scura, 1996).

Coping with a Triple Stigma

Approximately one half of the older adults with HIV disease are MSM. These men not only have to learn to confront the stigmas associated with homosexuality and HIV (see section on Men Who Have Sex with Men in this chapter) but also have to cope with beliefs and stereotypes associated with old age. Frequently labeled "ageist," these beliefs associate old age with being unattractive, asexual, out of date, valueless, over the hill, mentally incompetent, and physically incapable.

Many older gay men grew up before gay liberation and have been consistently confronted with the decision as to whether, to whom, and when to disclose their sexual orientation. Because they lived most of their lives in a sex-negative and extremely homophobic society, they frequently contributed to the conspiracy of silence that surrounded homosexuality. They have lived with an increasing amount of internalized homophobia and have faced invisibility and aging in a society in which gay and lesbian lives were acknowledged to only a limited extent (Grossman, 1997). These life experiences have placed older gay men at continual risk of HIV infection. Among their risk factors are anonymous sexual encounters (with prostitutes or in private clubs and gay theaters), denial of risk (they see AIDS as a young gay man's disease), and not responding to educational efforts of HIV/AIDS service organizations (Kooperman, 1993). Other risk factors include weariness with condom use, returning to a sexual intimacy without condoms, high rates of alcohol and other drug use, and participation in sexual activities while under the influence of these substances. Also, many of these men consider anal sex as central to their definition of male homosexuality (Dowsett, 1996), and returning to sexual intimacy without condoms is the symbolic center of their gay identity.

Older HIV-positive MSM and their health care providers need to learn that

1. Homosexuality is a normal variation of both sexual orientation and sexual behavior.
2. Understanding homosexuality does not require understanding its cause.
3. Homophobic attitudes (including internalized homophobia) create pain, stress, and inner conflicts.
4. Increased self-esteem, greater social support of peers, and more effective skills to cope with stress associated with HIV disease increase mental health and quality of life.

Learning to Negotiate Safer Sex and Use of Clean Needles

Increases in divorce and widowhood are leading many heterosexual people to reenter the dating scene after 20, 30, or even 50 years of marriage. The rise in visibility of gay liberation and the increase of services to older gay and lesbian persons are providing images and opportunities for some to acknowledge their same-sex attractions and to participate in homoerotic behaviors (Jacobson & Grossman, 1996). All of these older adults need help and practice in (Drost, 1996; Grossman, 1995)

1. Learning to talk about sexuality, including same-sex behaviors
2. Going to the pharmacy and purchasing condoms
3. Discussing HIV counseling and testing with current or prospective sexual partners
4. Negotiating safer sex practices
5. Identifying the "triggers" (e.g., alcohol use or loneliness) that lead to lapses in safer sex behaviors

Through these types of experiences, older HIV-positive adults will learn how to prevent reinfection and transmission of the virus to their sexual partners. These learning experiences, however, will not be effective unless health care providers establish environments that older adults perceive as safe and that recognize that to be human is to be sexual and that gay sex is part of the diversity of human sexuality (Grossman, 1995).

Although abstinence from drugs remains a priority, a narrow focus on it is regarded as unrealistic in containing HIV infections. The emphasis has shifted to harm reduction, i.e., minimizing the harm associated with particular drug use, usually injection. Older HIV-positive adults who inject drugs need to be educated (King, 1993)

1. Away from injection and towards oral drug use
2. About the benefits of needle-exchange programs
3. On the dangers of sharing syringes and needles with trusted friends or sexual partners
4. About techniques for cleaning drug paraphernalia

Meeting Emotional and Social Needs

An HIV diagnosis often leads to feelings of fear, anxiety, and humiliation, regardless of age. In older adults the HIV-positive test result is further compounded by chronic illnesses, loneliness, and the fears associated with growing old. Feelings of shame and fears of isolation and rejection, especially by friends and neighbors, become preoccupations. Disclosing HIV infection to family members, children, and grandchildren is often traumatic for older adults because of the grief it causes and the stigma attached to the disease. It is often difficult and humiliating to admit extramarital sex, gay sex, or drug use (Whipple & Scura, 1996). It is not surprising that feelings and fears lead many older adults to keep their HIV-positive status a secret, often leaving them feeling isolated, lacking a support network, and being at risk of depression (Emlet, 1993; Whipple & Scura, 1996). These feelings and fears are more acute for those older adults in whom AIDS dementia complex (HIV encephalopathy) has also been diagnosed.

Older adults with HIV infection need access to confidential counseling and to support groups that will enable them to discover, examine, and meet their emotional and social needs. Older adults, in general, are less likely to seek and use these services. Those with HIV infection also have feelings of remorse and guilt over using scarce resources that they believe should go to the young people who did not have much of a chance at life before receiving their HIV diagnoses. Additional access barriers for older adults are their limited experience with mental health services and their lack of experience in group settings. To overcome these barriers and to meet the psychosocial needs of older adults with HIV, health care providers have to design outreach strategies that invite older adults to mental health services that can be viewed as comfort zones and places of support. For those with AIDS-dementia complex, standard principles for dementia should also be applied.

Some older adults with HIV have additional emotional and social needs. They have become the caregivers for their children or grandchildren who may be infected with or affected by HIV. The stress caused by the awareness of their own vulnerability to HIV disease is compounded by the needs of their dependents. Learning not to neglect their own treatment needs and wants, to set limits for their caregiving activities, and to participate in a respite program becomes paramount among their needs. The role of the health care provider is to assist these adults in enrolling in case management programs and to advocate inclusion of emotional support services in their individualized care plans.

REFERENCES

Anderson, G. (1994, Summer). AIDS and older adults. *Outword, 1*(1), 1, 8.

Centers for Disease Control and Prevention [CDC]. (December 31, 1996). *HIV/AIDS Surveillance Report, 8*(2), 15–16.

Dowsett, G.W. (1996). *Practicing desire: Homosexual sex in the era of AIDS.* Palo Alto, CA: Stanford University Press.

Drost, M. (1996). Older adults' knowledge and attitudes about HIV/AIDS. *Outword, 2*(4), 6, 8.

Emlet, C.A. (1993). Service utilization among older people with AIDS: Implications for case management. *Journal of Case Management, 2*(4), 119–124.

Grossman, A.H. (1995). At risk, infected, and invisible: Older gay men and HIV/AIDS. *JANAC: Journal of the Association of Nurses in AIDS Care, 6*(6), 13–19.

Grossman, A. H. (1997). The virtual and actual identities of older lesbians and gay men. In M. Duberman (Ed.), *A queer world: The Center for Lesbian and Gay Studies reader* (pp. 615–626). New York: New York University Press.

Jacobson, S., Grossman, A.H. (1996). Older lesbians and gay men: Old myths, new images, and future directions. In R.C. Savin-Williams, K.M. Cohen (Eds.), *The lives of lesbians, gays, and bisexuals: Children to adults* (pp. 345–373). Fort Worth, TX: Harcourt Brace College Publishers.

King, M.B. (1993). *AIDS, HIV and mental health.* Cambridge, England: Cambridge University Press.

Kooperman, L. (Speaker). (1993). *AIDS and the elderly* (Cassette recording). San Francisco: American Society on Aging.

Kooperman, L., Hemenway, B. (1994). A research brief on the impact of the AIDS epidemic on sexual behavior in gay and bisexual men over 50. *Outword, 1*(2), 6.

Ungvarski, P.J. (1997). Update on HIV infection. *American Journal of Nursing, 97*(1), 44–52.

Whipple, B., Scura, K.W. (1996). The overlooked epidemic: HIV in older adults. *American Journal of Nursing, 96*(2), 22–28.

▪ Adolescents and Persons with Hemophilia

RICHARD FERRI

ADOLESCENTS

Adolescents are generally overlooked and underrepresented in the HIV/AIDS pandemic (Ferri, 1995). According to the Centers for Disease Control and Prevention (CDC), the number of reported adolescents with HIV infection is relatively small. However, one out of every five cases of AIDS is diagnosed in the 20- to 29-year age group. The World Health Organization (WHO) estimates that 50% of the approximately 14 million people infected with HIV worldwide were infected between the ages of 15 and 24 years (Hein et al., 1995) Given the long period preceding development of symptoms and the lack of adequate testing options for adolescents, it is clear that many young adults became infected as teenagers (Kaplan & Schonberg, 1994; Report to the President, 1996).

Often adolescents do not have the maturity and life experiences that are available to adults. Also, the adolescent is at a distinct social and political disadvantage, without the required clout to affect social change and self-advocacy.

The time of adolescence is viewed by adult society as a transition from childhood to adulthood. This view generally regards children as needing protection and believes that adults generally take care of themselves. It is the adolescent in the middle of the developmental spectrum who is frequently lost with respect to health and social issues.

Many adolescents are short-term thinkers who will act on the here and now and place themselves at risk. The primary care clinician needs to be aware of the special developmental and medical needs of adolescents. When health care workers fail to understand youth-specific needs, they fail to provide comprehensive quality care.

Epidemiology of HIV Infection in Adolescents

Although the CDC reported a 19% decrease in U.S. AIDS deaths in 1997, AIDS remains the leading cause of death of all persons 25 to 44 years of age (CDC, 1997). The death rate in women declined by only 7% between 1995 and 1996. AIDS is the third leading cause of death among American woman in the same age group, with a No. 1 ranking among African-American women. The rate of decline was 10% in the African-American community and 16% among Hispanics. Women and minorities are not showing the same demographic decline in the AIDS death rate that is seen in the their white male counterparts. Not surprisingly, these data suggest that female and minority adolescents are at greater risk than other groups.

Programs and interventions need to be developed that address the issues faced by the general adolescent community and its specific subgroups, such as runaway/throwaway youths, gay youths,

drug users, and adolescent sex workers. Clinicians must be certain that they are addressing HIV issues with their adolescent clients in a culturally inclusive manner. Adolescents in society carry virtually no political clout and are dependent largely on the adult society to champion their issues.

Adolescents have "fallen through the cracks" in the HIV pandemic. They have been considered either "large children" or "small adults." They are neither—they are adolescents, unique in their developmental needs. The current epidemiologic data do not accurately reflect demographics of the adolescent population.

Current CDC AIDS reporting data are grouped from the ages of 13 to 19 years. This age frame is too restrictive, since most adolescents do not develop AIDS by age 19, and therefore gives a false impression of a low incidence rate in teens. Also, this age frame overemphasizes the transfusion-related acquired infection of adolescent males affected by hemophilia.

The broader scope of adolescent HIV infection can be viewed by examining several other demographic factors instead of stagnant age-specific reporting methods. In 1990 youth entering the federal Jobs Corps program, which provides training for disadvantaged persons 16 to 21 years of age, reported that 3 out of every 1000 applicants tested positive for HIV (St. Louis et al., 1991). Back-calculation of HIV statistics indicates that between the years of 1989 and 1992 one out of every four persons newly infected with HIV in the United States was under the age of 22 (Rosenberg et al., 1992). Therefore it is important to view people in their twenties and thirties as having potentially become infected as teens.

Developmental Issues

Adolescents have developmental and age-specific issues that place them at increased risk of contracting HIV disease. Developmentally, adolescents live in the "here and now"; they are focused on the present without regard for future consequences (Moon, 1995). Teenage bravado, described as a sense of invulnerability, is another major developmental issue that increases the risk-taking behavior of teens (Cates, 1990). The adolescent does not perceive himself or herself at risk of harm or of acquiring a disease (Remafedi, 1990; Ferri, 1992).

Specific adolescent risk factors include hemophilia, gay/lesbian/bisexual identity formation ("coming out"), nonconsensual sexual activity, economically coerced sexual behaviors ("survival sex"), recreational sexual activity ("comfort sex"), and substance misuse (Savin-Williams & Rodriguez, 1993).

According to the CDC as of June 1997, there was a cumulative total of 22,070 reported cases of AIDS in persons under the age of 25 years. In addition, states with coincidental HIV infection–reporting mandates report that 12,673 persons under the age of 25 are seropositive for HIV (CDC, 1997). The office of the National AIDS Policy Advisor to the President of the United States is estimating that one in four new infections is occurring in a person below the age of 20 (Report to the President of the United States, March 1996).

Kral and colleagues (1997) examined the prevalence of HIV risk behaviors and substance use among homeless and runaway youth in three major epicenters of the epidemic. Of the 775 youth involved in the survey, 98% reported having had sexual intercourse. Forty-nine percent stated that they experienced coitus by the age of 13. Seventy-five percent reported having had sex while under the influence of alcohol or drugs.

In a national school survey Resnick and colleagues (1997) assessed eight areas of adolescent risk behaviors in 12,118 youth in grades 7 through 12. Seventeen percent of the seventh and eighth graders indicated that they had sexual intercourse. Among students in grades 9 to 12, 49.3% reported sexual activity. Among female adolescents aged 15 and older, 19.8% reported having been pregnant.

This increase in the sexual activity of adolescents is troubling, since the increase in the rate of sexual activity corresponds with the time frame of the AIDS pandemic. Pearlberg (1991) noted this relationship and identified "barrier" issues for the adolescent in the age of AIDS. The "barriers" identified were the adolescents' perception that they are impervious to harm; adolescents not seeing their peers die of AIDS because of the long time from infection to appearance of clinical symptoms of the virus; and the fact that AIDS-prevention curricula are often adult-centered.

The increase in the sexual activity of the adolescent coupled with the younger age at sexual debut can potentially increase the number of sexual partners and thus increase the opportunity for exposure to HIV infection. The adolescent years comprise many factors that increase the possibility of becoming infected.

Adolescents frequently experiment with alcohol and drug use. The use of marijuana and alcohol has been identified as contributing to high-risk sexual behaviors in adolescents (DiClemente et al., 1992); 17.9% of high school students reported drinking alcohol more than once a month, and 9.9% reported weekly alcohol consumption. One fourth (25.2%) of students have smoked marijuana (Resnick et al., 1997).

Cates (1990) examined the behavioral determinants of drug use and the increasing STD rates in adolescents. The overall percentage of cocaine use among high school students decreased, but the use of crack increased. This is significant, since the use of crack facilitates high-risk sexual behavior and stimulates the sex drive.

The use of alcohol, drugs, or both decreases compliance with condom use in the sexually active adolescent. Hingson and Strunin (1990) performed a statewide anonymous random digit dial telephone survey of 1773 adolescents (response rate 82%) in Massachusetts. The survey explored respondents' knowledge and beliefs about HIV transmission; alcohol, marijuana, and other illegal drug use; and behavioral changes related to the AIDS pandemic. Also, the study specifically asked the adolescent respondent about beliefs identified in the Health Belief Model. The Health Belief Model questions were developed to assess the adolescent's perceptions of susceptibility to HIV infection, the severity of the disease, the effectiveness of condom use, and any barriers to action. Standard demographic data were collected also. The results demonstrated that alcohol and drug use decreased condom use among the sexually active adolescents. Sixteen percent (73/465) were less likely to use condoms after drinking alcohol, and 25% (40/160) reported decreased condom use after taking drugs. One possible limitation of this study is that low-income households were the least likely to own a phone and may have represented a high risk of acquiring HIV. This could result in an underestimate of the actual prevalence of the risk behaviors of alcohol and drug use in the adolescent.

It should not be surprising that HIV infection is a growing phenomenon in adolescents, given the sexual activity of adolescents, their experimentation with sexual orientation, and substance use. It is also prudent to recognize the scope of STDs in the adolescent population.

STDs are transmitted through sexual contact and are epidemic in the United States (Kurth, 1993). This is the same mode of transmission of HIV infection. The epidemic is compounded in adolescents because of their feelings of being "immortal and invincible" to disease (Keating, 1990). These data on STDs in adolescents have limitations because of state-by-state differences in reporting mandates in and completeness of reports by public and private clinics. Therefore these data should be viewed as part of an interactive whole and not in isolation (Aral & Holmes, 1990).

Cates (1990) suggested that trends in gonorrhea reporting are the best indicators of STD patterns in adolescents because of the large numbers and reporting stability. Although the overall number of gonorrhea cases decreased, the rate of gonorrhea infection in adolescents has declined more slowly than in any other age group. In fact, the incidence of gonorrhea in males and females 15 to 19 years of age increased during the 1990s as compared with all other age groups.

Risk Behaviors Associated with Acquiring HIV Infection

There are developmental specific risk behaviors associated with acquiring HIV infection in the adolescent community. These behaviors are frequently influenced by physical and psychosocial developmental growth during adolescence.

SEXUAL ACTIVITY. Adolescents may be more biologically vulnerable to infection than their adult counterparts. The metamorphosis of the uterine cervix epithelium may determine the pathophysiology of some STDs. Columnar epithelium that extends from the endocervical canal into the vagina lacks the protection of cervical mucus. These sites and cells are targeted for infection with chlamydial and gonococcal agents in adolescents. As a public health issue, it may be important to delay sexual debut and to ensure that the sexually active adolescent uses appropriate contraception. However, not all contraceptive choices offer protection against STDs, and the adolescent needs counseling and access to condoms (Mann & Tartantola, 1996). The best method of how to or, indeed, even *if* to make condoms available is

the basis of dramatically polarized debate. What cannot be debated, however, is the alarming rate of adolescent sexual activity, STDs, and unintentional pregnancies. Education and prevention programs are needed for provision of adequate adolescent health care (DiClemente et al., 1992).

However, many prevention programs meet with adult disapproval. Many adults worry that when sex education materials and contraceptive devices are provided, the rate of sexual activity in the adolescent population will increase. To address these concerns, the World Health Organization (WHO) Global Programme on AIDS commissioned a review of the studies of the effects of sex education on adolescent beliefs and behaviors. Rates of teen pregnancy, abortion, birth, STDs, and self-reporting of sexual activity were measured. The review showed that sex education did not lead to or increase sexual activity of youth, even when contraceptive devices were offered in the program. Second, sex education programs may actually delay sexual debut, decrease sexual activity, and increase safer sex practices for the already sexually active adolescent (Fisher et al., 1992). These findings have been supported by other researchers (Ferri & Tannebring, 1993).

Education and prevention programs are critical for decreasing the number of STDs, including HIV infection, in the adolescent. Not all STDs are curable, and many go undetected in the adolescent because there are no symptoms. Adolescents who receive little or no health care are at increased risk. Innovative psychosocial and behavioral programs must be developed and delivered to all adolescents (Boyer, 1990).

Strategies in safer-sex education that are congruent with adolescent development and learning patterns need to be employed. Many STD-prevention education programs require the adolescent to process complex information. Skills and knowledge, not just the simple imparting of knowledge, should be incorporated into the curriculum. Brooks-Gunn and associates (1988) found that multimethod and multimedia programs increased effectiveness of education. Use of didactic education, skills-building, role-playing, vignettes, and transmission games assisted in modifying risk behaviors. Boyer (1990) found that prevention programs need to be developed for heterogeneity and within-group differences. Building on sociocultural values will enhance learning effectiveness. The specific factors that should be accounted for are language, culture, socioeconomic status, gender, sexual orientation, and age. Independent of curriculum development, the major obstacle in program management and implementation is the perceived notion by adults of associated increased sexual activity.

Kirby and colleagues (1991) evaluated the reproductive health care programs of six diverse school-based clinics and measured their impact on adolescent sexual behavior and the use of contraceptives. The six clinics that were evaluated were selected because of their geographic diversity and differences in political and cultural milieus. The sites included urban and rural areas: Gary, Indiana; San Francisco; Muskegon, Michigan; Jackson, Mississippi; Quincy, Florida; and Dallas. All of the clinics were based on school property and served large populations of minority students. The clinics had been operational for 3 to 14 years at the time of the study. The clinics were staffed by one part-time or full-time physician and one or more part-time or full-time clinical practitioners, plus support staff. The primary focus of the clinics was comprehensive primary adolescent health care and was not limited to reproductive and contraceptive issues. To evaluate the impact of the school-based clinics, a comparison set of schools that were geographically close and demographically similar to the clinic schools was recruited. A comprehensive survey that measured social and demographic characteristics, clinic use, use of medical services in general, risk-taking behavior, sexual activity, contraceptive use, and pregnancy was designed to be administered at all clinic and nonclinic schools.

The researchers believed that their data on sexual activity and contraception were valid because the survey data were consistent with previously published findings and with the clinics' data.

At three of the sites the data on sexual activity revealed no significant difference in sexual debut. At the Dallas site, males but not females were significantly ($P < .01$) less likely to have sex. At the San Francisco site, females but not males were more likely to have had sex since the clinic was opened ($P < .05$). The Muskegon site revealed the same significant results as the San Francisco site. These results were further examined to establish age at first intercourse. The mean age at first intercourse indicated that many of the students

were sexually experienced before entering high school and using the clinic services. The researchers thought it improbable that the school-based clinics affected adolescents' sexual activity before they entered high school and merged data to perform a regression analysis. This analysis revealed no significant differences between the clinic and nonclinic schools, at any site, related to sexual activity. This study is limited by the population that the clinics served, which were largely African-Americans. Therefore it is not representative of a larger, culturally inclusive community. Also, the San Francisco site had a well-established HIV-prevention program and community support that may have affected the data.

School-based sexuality education increased the adolescents' knowledge of sexuality but had no significant effect on sexual activity (Newman et al., 1993). The data on sexuality education and sexual debut are inconclusive because they mainly examine adolescents of high school age who are presumed to be heterosexual in orientation (Ferri & Tannebring, 1993).

Without a cure or vaccine for AIDS, the best hope for controlling the rate of infection, especially among adolescents, is through education and social marketing skills (Report to the President, 1996).

SEXUALLY TRANSMITTED DISEASE. A decrease in gonorrhea has been reported in the general adult population. However, although the overall number is down, the rate of gonorrhea infection in teens is on the rise. Both male and female adolescents have increased their rates of gonococcal infection compared with other age groups.

SUBSTANCE USE. Issues surrounding drug and alcohol use are not new to the teen community. However, today's consequences are very different and sometimes fatal. Some of the more alarming statistics include the finding that 1% of students reported using heroin and 6% had used cocaine in the National Survey of High School Seniors. This survey did not control for dropout students, and therefore the numbers are generally considered underrepresentative of the true picture.

Also, injection drug behavior is the sole reason for 10% of all cases of AIDS in adolescents in the United States, and it includes heroin, cocaine, amphetamines, and anabolic steroids. Adolescent athletes are being pressured to perform at very high standards and may become performance dependent on steroids. Needle-sharing for nonhallucinatory drugs is mistakenly considered "safe" because no one is getting "high."

Runaway and throwaway youths who are living on the streets are becoming addicted to crack cocaine in increasingly large numbers. In addition to standard concerns about using a hallucinogenic agent is the concern that crack cocaine, which is highly addictive, is associated with high-risk sexual behaviors. Crack acts a sexual stimulant and social disinhibitor. Also, many teens on the street do not have any marketable job skills and therefore turn to prostitution as a means of support. Heterosexual adolescent males are engaging in high-risk sex with men, who are usually older, to support their drug habits.

The use of alcohol continues to be a major adolescent health problem. Many college campuses are reporting high student absentee rates and an alcohol-related decrease in academic performance. However, it is important to examine not only the abusive drinker but also those who engage in "socially acceptable drinking." Alcohol as a social disinhibitor can dramatically affect youths who are not proficient with its influence.

PSYCHOSOCIAL FACTORS. Teenage "bravado" is a common developmental issue with adolescents. The adolescent does not perceive himself or herself as being vulnerable to disease and death. This phenomenon may influence the use of alcohol, drug experimentation, reckless driving, and unprotected sex.

The influence of adolescent peers is paramount. This influence can be positive or negative. The adolescent is developmentally engaged in the process of separating from family and identifying with peer groups. In early adolescence youths strive to remove themselves from the family group and to intensify their peer relationships, while in later adolescence there is a redirection of emotions, with the older teens identifying their own values with reintegration of family norms (Herdt, 1994).

For these reasons, one of the most effective methods of altering teen behaviors regarding such issues as tobacco use, alcohol use, and safer sex choices is peer education. Providing age-appropriate peer leaders with the correct information can help them promote health behaviors among other teens.

Adolescents are developmentally vulnerable to HIV infection, and primary care providers must address issues regarding peer pressure and sexual behaviors in all contacts with them.

Primary Prevention Issues

Primary prevention strategies must be multidimensional and targeted to the adolescent's developmental needs and issues. Some basic principles have been identified for behavioral change in adolescents (Kunins et al., 1993):

- Adolescents must believe that they are personally at risk.
- Multiple options for behavioral change need to be provided. Offering only one option for prevention will not be effective.
- Positive peer pressure is very effective. Peer norms have a major influence on adolescent behavior.
- Skills-building workshops are necessary to assist the adolescent with negotiation skills and the ability to resist negative peer pressure.
- Development of self-efficacy is essential. Adolescents who believe in their ability to carry out behavioral change will have lower levels of risk behavior.
- Behavior and beliefs that are adolescent-centered must be valued and respected.
- Cultural identity inclusion will assist in risk-reduction skills and behaviors.
- Heterosexuality should not be presumed to be the norm for the group. Homosexual and bisexual identities should be included in a comprehensive manner and not as separate items.

Prevention Strategies

Prevention strategies that are effective in the adolescent community are those that are adolescent-centered and targeted to a specific group. This goal is hampered by three major barriers to primary prevention education: the adolescents' perception that they are impervious to harm, adolescents not seeing their peers dying of AIDS, and AIDS-prevention curricula that are often adult-centered in their approach (Pearlberg, 1991). In addition, youths who are gay, lesbian, or bisexual are often dismissed as nonexistent (Friedman & Downey, 1994; Lynch & Ferri, 1997).

Behavioral change in sexual activity for the adolescent community needs to be personalized regardless of the prevention strategy that is advocated—abstinence, monogamy, or explicit safer-sex instructions (Rotheram-Borus & Koopman, 1991). The adolescent needs to view the possibility of becoming infected with HIV as a potential in the present.

Generally the adolescent community is divided into either school-based or street-based groups. For the school-based adolescent, a peer leadership model appears to be an effective model (Rickert et al., 1991). Ability of teens educated on the issues of HIV infection and its transmission to talk to their peers provides a mechanism that makes the information "real" to the teen. The adolescent will value and personalize the information provided by a peer more than that provided by an adult.

Many school systems have struggled with the issue of condom availability as a prevention strategy. The pros and cons have been greatly debated. There is a generalized fear that condom-availability programs will increase sexual activity of students and therefore lead to higher rates of infection. There is little evidence to support this assumption (Rotheram-Borus & Koopman, 1991).

The issues and problems encountered by runaway, homeless, and "throwaway" adolescents are numerous and complicated. Implementation of primary prevention programs in this environment can be daunting. Moon (1995) reviewed four exceptional programs for street youth. Each program examined the needs and lifestyles of street adolescents in their community and developed specific interventions. Generally, development of life skills and improvement of self-esteem are core issues that affect disenfranchised youth living on the street or in homeless shelters.

HIV Antibody Counseling and Testing Issues

Like their adult counterparts, adolescents need appropriate support and counseling in making the decision to learn their HIV antibody status. When an adolescent inquires about "getting tested," it is appropriate and important for the provider to help the teen clarify why he or she feels at risk of becoming infected with HIV. This is an opportune time to help clarify misinformation and to assess risk behaviors.

The major challenge is to interact with the adolescents on their developmental level. Cognitive development of adolescents may differ from that of adults in the following ways:

1. Concrete thinkers (very "black and white with no shades of gray")
2. Magical thinkers (wishing away any "bad situations")
3. Denial ("it can't happen to me because . . .")
4. Feeling immortal (teenage bravado)
5. Peer pressure sensitivity
6. Difficulty in weighing options

HIV antibody-testing opportunities need to be scheduled to complement, not compete with, school schedules (Report to the President, 1996). Ideally, HIV antibody testing should occur within a system where the adolescent could receive primary care. If this is not the case, then a relationship should be established between the testing site or individual and a primary care source.

Primary Care

The adolescent with HIV infection is one of the biggest missing pieces in the clinical care puzzle. There appears to be a gap between HIV infection found in children and that found in adults. This lack of information on primary care of adolescents with HIV is going to grow as children with HIV begin to age with advanced medical therapies and the adolescent cohort begins to grow (Riddel & Moon, 1996). Development of adolescent-specific protocols and interventions needs to be a clinical priority.

One should approach the adolescent with HIV infection as someone with a chronic, manageable disease that mandates the collection of a significant data base. These data will have to be refined over time.

1. Health history
   a. All past health problems
   b. The usual diseases of childhood
   c. Status of immunizations
   d. Seroconversion illness syndrome
   e. Recurrent yeast infections
   f. Any history of STDs
   g. Any history of pregnancy, miscarriage, termination
   h. Any surgical history

2. Social history
   a. Current living situation
   b. School status (Is grade appropriate to age?)
   c. Work status
   d. Social supports
   e. Persons who know of his or her HIV infection
3. Psychologic history
   a. Past or present depression, anxiety, suicidal thoughts
   b. Past inpatient or outpatient treatments
4. Sexual history. Sexual history is important in helping to formulate a risk-reduction plan for the adolescent and to establish a therapeutic relationship in which sexual concerns can be addressed in a nonthreatening manner. It is important to use nonjudgmental terms. Also, it is important to use whatever language is acceptable to the adolescent. Chapter 2 contains a sexual history–taking assessment tool.
5. Substance history
   a. Assess for use of both licit and illicit substance use
   b. Assess for any "works" sharing
   c. Assess whether sex has ever been exchanged for drugs or money
6. Review of HIV-specific systems/physical assessment
   a. General. Fever, night sweats, weight loss, skin lesions, rashes. Stable weight patterns are not signs of good health in the adolescent since he or she is still developing physically. Stable weight patterns or continued weight loss during Tanner Stages II to IV may be indicators of HIV disease. HIV-infected children who progress into adolescence may signal advance of their condition by growth failure. This may be an indicator *prior to any drop in the CD4 cell counts.*
   b. Update of immunizations:
      (1) Pneumococcal vaccine
      (2) Influenza (yearly)
      (3) Tetanus (Td)
      (4) Mumps, measles, and rubella (MMR) (Assess all females for immunity to rubella; immunize those without prior immunity.)
      (5) Hepatitis B vaccine if no prior immunity
7. Laboratory data and medication management. There does not *appear* to be any significant need for additional blood and other laboratory

specimens. Once again, however, the true data on the age-specific needs of adolescents have not yet been fully studied.
8. Medication management. If the child is in Tanner Stage I, use pediatric dosage guidelines; if in Tanner Stage V, use adult dosage guidelines; appropriate dosing for children in Tanner Stages II to IV has not been established.

Special Populations: Gay, Lesbian, Bisexual, and Questioning Youths

The lack of understanding and acknowledgment of gay and bisexual adolescents contributes to increasing stressors and places adolescents at high risk of physical and psychosocial dysfunction (Friedman & Downey, 1994). Studies of youths who are struggling with their sexual identities have found that gay and bisexual adolescents were two to three times more likely to attempt suicide than other youths are (Rotheram-Borus et al., 1992). The dysfunction of the gay and bisexual adolescent may manifest in sexual acting out and even suicide (Remafedi et al., 1991).

Gay, lesbian, bisexual, and questioning youths do not find the popular public heath messages, such as abstinence until marriage, relevant. These heterosexist messages further isolate the adolescents, and do not address their need for meaningful primary prevention messages (Remafedi, 1990; Ferri, 1992). Gay adolescents are often isolated from positive adult and peer role models. Internalized and societal homophobia often limits their access to information and opportunities contributing to a sense of worthlessness.

The gay, lesbian, or bisexual youth has numerous and difficult challenges to master:

1. The "invisibility" of gay, lesbian, and bisexual youths may be compounded with sexual activity and risk taking (Remafedi, 1990).
2. The gay or bisexual adolescent male's first sexual partner is typically 7 years older than he is, which may increase potential exposure to HIV infection.
3. Gay, lesbian, and bisexual teens may be in the process of "coming out" (see Box, p. 306) to themselves and to society and may engage in heterosexual activity to "prove themselves straight."
4. Gay, lesbian, and bisexual teens who are not enculturated into the gay community may be-

---

■ **COMING OUT STAGES** ■

Although "coming out" is not a static experience four stages have been identified with the homosexual adolescent.

Stage 1: Occurs up to age 11. The child feels "different" from other children—not explicitly connected with sexual feelings.

Stage 2: Ages 11 to 14. First experiences related to sexual differences. The youth is very confused about his or her sexual feelings and realizes that he or she is drawn to same-sex partners. The youth is also aware (socialized homophobia) of the social stigma attached to such feelings and may deny or avoid them.

Stage 3: Age 15 and up. Identity assumption takes place. The adolescent self-identifies as a gay person and develops coping mechanisms for dealing with a heterosexist society.

Stage 4: Age 20 and up. Commitment. A solidification of one's identity as a gay person.

---

lieve that safer-sex messages are not directed toward them and that therefore they are exempt from having to practice safer sex.

PERSONS WITH HEMOPHILIA

Any discussion of HIV infection in the adolescent community must review the special issues and needs of the person living with the dual diagnoses of hemophilia and HIV infection. By definition, hemophilia is a sex-linked genetic disorder characterized by a deficiency or absence of a plasma-clotting protein.

There are two major classifications of hemophilia:

1. Classic hemophilia (hemophilia A), which is characterized by a lack of clotting factor VIII
2. Christmas disease (hemophilia B), which is characterized by a lack of clotting factor IX

Hemophilia A is four times more prevalent than hemophilia B and occurs in 1 of 7500 live male births in the United States.

The rate of HIV infection in persons with hemophilia is approximately 70% for any person who received clotting factor VIII between the years of 1978 and 1985 (Augustyniak, 1990). HIV-positive persons with hemophilia can transmit the virus to their sexual partners in the same manner as other people living with HIV.

The natural history of HIV disease in people with hemophilia is similar to that of others with HIV. Karposi's sarcoma is a rare AIDS-defining illness in people with hemophilia, whereas immune thrombocytopenia purpura is more likely to occur after an episode of bleeding. The general course of HIV infection may be complicated by the person's clotting disorder.

Adolescents with Hemophilia and HIV Infection

Since hemophilia is an X-linked genetic disorder, with the majority of factor VIII recipients being HIV-positive if they received blood products before 1985, special needs of the adolescent and young adult should be examined by clinicians. In addition, although the blood supply in the United States is generally considered the safest in the world, persons with hemophilia who are not infected with HIV must deal with the psychologic stressor of fear of infection at virtually every infusion they receive. This increased stress may potentiate inappropriate coping behaviors.

Obviously, there are going to be the unique issues related to living with a genetic disorder that is often debilitating and disfiguring. Coupling this with the multiple issues of being a person with HIV infection complicates matters more fully.

Drotar and colleagues (1997) studied psychologic distress of HIV-positive adolescents with hemophilia and their mothers in comparison with HIV-negative hemophiliacs and their mothers. There was a significant interaction between the HIV-positive status and the frequency of stressful life events. Therefore the family unit was affected in the overall coping methods and levels of psychologic distress. Brown and colleagues (1995) examined the coping strategies of HIV-positive adolescents with hemophilia. Daily reminders of their HIV status created increased stress and ineffective coping strategies. Anger was the most commonly reported emotion.

Clinicians need to develop a comprehensive treatment plan that addresses these psychologic factors and to make the appropriate mental health referrals as needed. Generally, however, the provider needs to help persons living with hemophilia and HIV understand certain issues and incorporate them into their lives.

1. Sexual partners of HIV antibody–positive persons with hemophilia are at increased risk of HIV infection. Issues surrounding discordant couples need to be considered.
2. Education and reinforcement of the need for universal precautions in the home setting and safe handling of blood products to prevent spread among family members are needed.
3. All treatments should be carefully reviewed on a regular basis to assess for any interaction that may increase bleeding. HIV therapies that may increase the likelihood of thrombocytopenia may be contraindicated.

REFERENCES

Aral, S., Holmes, K. (1990). Epidemiology of sexual behavior and sexually transmitted diseases. In K. Holmes et al. (Eds.), *Sexually transmitted diseases* (2nd ed., pp. 19–36). New York: McGraw-Hill.

Augustyniak, L. (1990). *Regional seropositivity rates for HIV infection in patients with hemophilia (abstract)*. Presented at the Sixth International Conference on AIDS, San Francisco.

Boyer, C. (1990). Psycho-social, behavioral and educational factors in preventing sexually transmitted diseases. *Adolescent Medicine, 1*(30), 597–615.

Brooks-Gunn, J., Boyer, C.B., Hein, K. (1988). Preventing HIV infection and AIDS in children and adolescents: Behavior research and intervention strategies. *American Psychologist, 43,* 958.

Brown, L., Schultz, J., Gragg, R. (1995). HIV-infected adolescents with hemophilia: Adaptation and coping; the Hemophilia Behavioral Intervention Evaluation Project. *Pediatrics, 3,* 459–463.

Cates, W. (1990). The epidemiology and control of sexually transmitted disease in adolescents. *Adolescent Medicine, 1*(3), 409–427.

Centers for Disease Control and Prevention. (June 30, 1997). *HIV/AIDS Surveillance Report, 9*(1), 1–39.

DiClemente, R.J., Durbin, M., Siegel, D., Kranovsky, F., Lazarus, N., Comacho, T. (1992). Determinants of condom use among junior high school students in a minority, inner-city school district. *Pediatrics, 89,* 197–202.

Drotar, D., Agle, D., Eckl, C., Thompson, P. (1997). Correlates of psychological distress among mothers of children and adolescents with hemophilia with HIV infection. *Journal of Pediatric Psychology, 22,* 1–14.

Ferri, R. (1992). Adolescents and HIV infection. *Journal of the Association of Nurses in AIDS Care, 3*(3), 49–50.

Ferri, R. (1995). HIV and adolescents: A primary care perspective. *Advance for Nurse Practitioners, 3*(7), 36–52.

Ferri, R., Tannebring, E. (1993). *Safer sex education and adolescent sexual behavior.* Unpublished manuscript.

Fisher, J.D., Misovich, S.J., Fisher, W.A. (1992). Impact on perceived social norms on adolescents' AIDS-risk behavior and prevention. In R.J. DiClemente (Ed.), *Adolescents and AIDS.* Newbury Park, CA: Sage Publications.

Friedman, R., Downey, J. (1994). Homosexuality. The New England Journal of Medicine, 331(14), 923–930.

Gibson, P. (1989). *Gay male and lesbian youth suicide. Report of the Secretary's Task Force on Youth Suicide. Volume 3: Prevention and intervention in youth suicide.* Washington, DC: U.S. Department of Health and Human Services.

Greenberg, J., Magder, L., Aral, S. (1992). Age at first coitus: A marker for risky sexual behavior in women. *Sexually Transmitted Diseases, 19,* 331–334.

Hein, K., Dell, R., Futterman, D., Rotheram-Borus, M.J., Shaffer, N. (1995). Comparisons of HIV+ and HIV– adolescents: Risk factors and psychosocial determinants. *Pediatrics, 95,* 96–104.

Herdt, G. (1994). *Third sex, third gender.* New York: Zone.

Hingson, R., Strunin, L. (1990). Beliefs about AIDS, use of alcohol and drugs, and unprotected sex among Massachusetts adolescents. *Journal of Adolescent Health Care, 80*(3), 295–299.

Horton, M. (1993, June). *Homosexually active men and the evolving global epidemic of HIV.* Presented at IX International Conference on AIDS, Berlin, Germany (abstract PS-08-2).

Kaplan, M.E., Schonberg, S.K. (1994). HIV in adolescents. *Clinical Perinatology, 21,* 75–84.

Keating, D.P. (1990). Adolescent thinking. In S. Feldman, G. Elliott (Eds.), *At the threshold* (pp. 54–90). Cambridge, MA: Harvard University Press.

Kirby, D., Waszak, C., Ziegler, J. (1991). Six school-based clinics: Their reproductive health services and impact on sexual behavior. *Family Planning Perspective, 23*(1), 6–16.

Kral, A.H., Molnar, B.E., Booth, R.E., Watters, J.K. (1997). Prevalence of sexual risk behavior and substance use among runaway and homeless adolescents in San Francisco, Denver, and New York City. *International Journal of STD AIDS, 8*(2), 109–117.

Kunins, B.A., Hein, K., Futterman, D., Tapley, E., Elliot, A. (1993). Group education and support for adolescents. *Journal of Adolescent Health, 14*(5), 100–106.

Kurth, A. (1993). *Until the cure.* New Haven, CT: Yale University Press.

Lynch, M., Ferri, R. (1997). Health care needs of lesbian women and gay men. *Clinician Review, 7*(1), 85–118.

Mann, H., Tartantola, D. (1996). Youth and HIV/AIDS. In H. Mann, D. Tartantola (Eds.), *AIDS in the world II* (pp. 236–251). New York: Oxford University Press.

Moon, M. (1995). Nursing care of the adolescent. In J.H. Flaskerud, P. Ungvarski (Eds.), *HIV/AIDS: A guide to nursing care* (3rd ed., pp. 220–242). Philadelphia: Saunders.

Newman, C., DuRant, C., Ashworth, C., Gaillard, G. (1993). Evaluation of a school based AIDS/HIV education program for young adolescents. *AIDS Education and Prevention, 5,* 327–339.

Pearlberg, G. (1991). *Women, AIDS and communities.* Metuchen, NJ: Women's Action Alliance.

Remafedi, G. (1987). Homosexual youth: A challenge to the contemporary society. *Journal of the American Medical Association, 258,* 222–225.

Remafedi, G. (1990). Sexually transmitted diseases in homosexual youth. *Adolescent Medicine: State of the Art Reviews, 1*(3), 565–581.

Remafedi, G., Farrow, J., Deisher, R. (1991). Risk factors for attempted suicide in gay and bisexual youth. *Pediatrics, 87,* 869–875.

Report to the President of the United States. (1996, March). *Youth & HIV/AIDS: An American Agenda.*

Resnick, M., Bearman, P., Blum, R., Bauman, K., Harris, K., Jones, J., Tabor, J., Beuhring, T., Sieving, R., Shew, M., Ireland, M., Bearinger, L., Udry, J. (1997). Protecting adolescents from harm. *Journal of the American Medical Association, 278*(10), 823–832.

Rickert, V.I., Jay, M.S., Gottlieb, A. (1991). Effects of a peer-counseled AIDS education program on knowledge, attitudes, and satisfaction of adolescents. *Journal of Adolescent Health, 12,* 38–43.

Riddel, J., Moon, M. (1996). Children with HIV becoming adolescents: Caring for long term survivors. *Pediatric Nursing, 22,* 220–223, 227, 255.

Rosenberg, P.S., Gail, M.H., Carroll, R.J. (1992). Estimating HIV prevalence and projecting AIDS incidence in the United States: A model that accounts for therapy and changes in the surveillance definition of AIDS. *Statistics in Medicine, 11*(13), 1633–1655.

Rotheram-Borus, M.J., Koopman, C. (1991). HIV and adolescents. *Journal of Primary Prevention, 12*(1), 65–82.

Rotheram-Borus, M.J., Meyer-Bahlburg, H.F.L., Rosario, M. (1992). Lifetime sexual behaviors among predominantly minority male runaway and gay/bisexual adolescents in New York City. *AIDS Education and Prevention (special edition),* 34–42.

Savin-Williams, R.C., Rodriguez, R.G. (1993). A developmental, clinical perspective on lesbian, gay male, and bisexual youths. In T.P. Gullotta, G.R. Adams, R. Montemayor (Eds.), *Adolescent sexuality* (pp. 141–160). Newbury Park, CA: Sage.

St. Louis, M.E., Conway, G.A., Hayman, C.R. (1991). HIV infection in disadvantaged adolescents: Findings from the U.S. Job Corps. *Journal of the American Medical Association, 266,* 2387–2391.

▪ Women, Pregnant Women, Lesbians, and Transgender/ Transsexual Persons*

ANN KURTH

HIV disease in the United States has followed certain trends but is best described overall as a series of subepidemics, presenting unique concerns and configurations of need in a variety of affected populations. This section will discuss the clinical and psychosocial needs of women in general, then will do so for women who are pregnant or considering pregnancy, for women who have sex with women, and for persons who are transgendered. Providers who work with these populations play a role by discussing reduction of HIV risk and integrating the latest clinical advances to help those identified as HIV-positive live longer with their HIV disease.

Women and HIV

EPIDEMIOLOGY. Women with AIDS were first identified in 1981, with cases retrospectively identified in the United States to the late 1970s. Of the 612,078 cases of adult/adolescent AIDS reported to the Centers for Disease Control and Prevention (CDC) in the United States through mid-1997, the 92,242 cases of AIDS in women represented 15% of the cumulative total; however, women and girls represented 20% of the new adult/adolescent cases of AIDS reported during 1996. Women also comprise an increasing proportion of HIV cases (30% in 1996) reported to the CDC (CDC, 1996a; CDC, 1997a).

The rate of HIV infection is growing fastest among women, particularly young women. While the estimated increase in AIDS incidence for men slowed to 5% in 1994, the rate of increase in women rose to 10% that year (CDC, 1996b). Of cases of AIDS among adolescents nationally, female incidence tripled from 14% in 1987 to 47% of the cases by December 1996

---

*Adapted in part from "AMA Treatment Guidelines for Women with HIV," a manuscript written for the American Medical Association by Ann Kurth.

(CDC, 1996a). An analysis of 37,000 cases of AIDS diagnosed in New York City between 1984 and 1993 found that most of the persons under age 30 were female, came from communities of color, and had heterosexual contact as their source of transmission (Shevitz et al., 1996).

Thirty-three percent of women with AIDS reported between June 1996 and June 1997 acquired HIV from their own injecting drug use (IDU), and 40% did so from heterosexual contact; nearly one in three of these reported having sex with an injecting drug user. The majority of women (63%) who acquired HIV from heterosexual contact could not identify a specific risk factor to account for the HIV infection in their sexual partners (CDC, 1997a). While heterosexual contact is growing as a risk for women, continued attention to the risks related to substance abuse is critical.

The impact of HIV/AIDS in communities of color has been disproportionate, with more than three fourths of all reported cases of AIDS occurring in African-American (55%), Latina (20%), Asian, and Native American populations (1% through December 1996). Race and ethnicity have long stood not as risk factors per se for communicable and chronic disease but as indicators of underlying lower socioeconomic status and the reduced access to preventive and other health care that attends poverty (National Commission on AIDS, 1992). These factors illuminate why the AIDS case rate for black females is approximately 15 times the rate for white females.

AIDS is the third leading cause of death for all women 25 to 44 years of age, and it is the leading cause of death for African-American women in the same age category. Advances in treatment led to declining AIDS death rates for the first time ever in 1996. However, these advances were not shared equally across gender and race; while deaths among men declined by 15% in the first 6 months of 1996, they *increased* among women by 3%. Declines in AIDS deaths were greater among whites (21%) than among blacks (2%) and Hispanics (10%) (CDC, 1997a), raising questions about access to health care options. HIV disease is the leading cause of death in women of reproductive age in a number of U.S. cities, but it is by no means limited to certain urban epicenters. Case increases have been seen in small cities, rural areas (particularly in the South), and in "bridge" cities that are connected to emigration pathways between the United States, Puerto Rico, and some Caribbean islands.

MANIFESTATIONS OF HIV DISEASE. Large cohort studies to track the natural history of HIV disease in women, such as the Women's Interagency HIV Study (WIHS) and the HIV Epidemiological Research Study (HERS), began in the 1990s. Earlier small cohort studies of women with HIV disease demonstrate that universalities are seen with HIV disease in women and men as regards OIs and HIV disease progression, and there are some distinct differences, largely gynecologically related (Clark, 1997). *Pneumocystis carinii* pneumonia (PCP) generally is the most common cause of death in HIV-infected women and men, although it may not be the first AIDS-defining illness in women. Kaposi's sarcoma, commonly seen in MSM and now known to have a viral origin, occurs more rarely in women (approximately 2% of cases)—usually in situations in which the male partner was bisexual. Early manifestations of HIV in women may be non-AIDS defining and may occur in the reproductive tract.

MANAGEMENT. In the 1980s distinct differences in survival rates were seen between men and women with HIV, although by the early 1990s studies began to show that when men and women had *equal access* to treatment, there appeared to be no difference in survival rates due to gender alone. However, assuring access to care and achievement of equivalent treatment regimens is still an issue. Several studies document that women enter care at later stages of disease and may receive fewer services than men (Hellinger, 1993), including lower rates of antiretroviral and prophylactic therapies than are recommended at certain CD4+ cell count levels. In one national study HIV-positive women had a higher risk of death than HIV-positive men, even with no higher risk of progressing to AIDS (Melnick et al., 1994). Delays in receiving an HIV/AIDS diagnosis or treatment (Melnick et al., 1994) and differences in access to health care, treatment regimens, and support services may account for the population differences seen.

Poverty, chemical dependence, and responsibilities for child care already have sapped the health of many women by the time their HIV disease is diagnosed. Many HIV-positive women are necessarily crisis-oriented in their approach to health care, since concerns for food, shelter, and safety take precedence. Suspicion of institutions and agencies that have been experienced as hostile or judgmental; lack of health insurance; a dearth of child care, transportation, and other supportive services; self-identification as a caretaker and not a care receiver; and clinician or client belief that HIV infection is primarily a disease of white gay men or injecting drug users may lead many women to ignore symptoms of HIV disease until they are very ill.

Provision of family-centered, culturally competent services by an interdisciplinary team should be arranged so that primary care, HIV specialty care, contraceptive, obstetrical, and gynecologic care (including colposcopy and neoplasia management), pediatric services, subspecialties such as neuropsychiatry, and addiction treatment are all linked to facilitate care for women with HIV disease and their families. A case-management approach can enhance continuity in the provision of clinical and psychosocial services by tracking each client's needs and addressing impediments to accessing care (e.g., lack of child care or difficult public transit routes). Especially in lower HIV-seroprevalence areas, woman-specific HIV services may not be readily available and staff members may have to spend time advocating needed services. Community outreach may be accomplished by using "inreach" methods, where clients themselves are used as peer educators in the clinic setting (Sunderland & Holman, 1993).

CLINICAL CARE NEEDS. Provision of preventive care is critical in this immunocompromised population. Teaching avoidance of coinfections (including other STDs), stress-management techniques, and other supportive advice should be part of the clinical encounter. It is important not to neglect nutritional status; many HIV-positive women have borderline malnutrition related to poor dietary patterns, concurrent drug use, or HIV disease itself. Women's caloric intake, weight, and, ideally, lean body mass should be tracked, with recommendations for nutritional intake and exercise made in consultation with nurses, dietitians, and other members of the health care team (Hanna, 1994).

The impact that protease inhibitor combination therapies may have on the course of HIV disease (i.e., fewer hospitalizations, longer time frame of illness) likely will necessitate chronic management for HIV-positive women over many years and result in a lifetime context of sexual, reproductive, and health care concerns.

GYNECOLOGIC CARE. Clinicians often see a high prevalence (more than 70%) of treatable gynecologic conditions in HIV-positive women (Burdge & Money, 1996). Reproductive care, including gynecologic screening and management, must be an integrated part of the service continuum for women with HIV disease.

Little is known about the impact of HIV on the local immune system of the female genital tract, although there is evidence that the reduction in immunocompetence of vaginal Langerhans' and plasma cells, as well as local CD4+ and CD8+ T-cells, may be related to sexual and perinatal transmission as well as to chronic viral and fungal infections of the genital tract (Olaitan et al., 1996).

Cervical intraepithelial neoplasia (CIN) is found in HIV-positive women at a rate 4 to 10 times higher than in HIV-negative women, with the prevalence of cervical dysplasia often related to the client's degree of immunosuppression (Olaitan & Johnson, 1997). There is strong evidence of an association between coinfection with human papillomavirus (HPV) infection and HIV infection, immune deterioration, and the development of cervical dysplasias or neoplasms. In one cohort of women with HPV infection, for example, those who were infected with HIV-1 and HIV-2 were 23.3 and 9.3 times more likely, respectively, to have a cytologic diagnosis of dysplasia than those women who were HIV-seronegative (Seck et al., 1994).

All women with HIV disease should receive a thorough gynecologic examination with Papanicolaou (Pap) smear or cervical cytology, cultures, and anal examination at least once a year. Although there has been some concern about the sensitivity of Pap smears in detecting cervical abnormalities, small comparison studies have found that Pap smears are an adequate screening tool (Norton et al., 1994), and a federal panel convened to develop HIV guidelines concluded that annual Pap smears are sufficient for HIV-infected women with no history of abnormal Pap smears (El-Sadr et al., 1994). However, many clinicians and those providing care to HIV-positive women believe that Pap smears should be obtained at least twice a year, particularly in those women with CD4+ cell counts below 200/mm³, and support the liberal use of colposcopy when Pap smears in HIV-positive women are uninterpretable or yield abnormal results, including only inflammation (Hankins et al., 1994). For HIV-positive women with a history of genital warts, prior abnormal Pap smears, or other evidence of HPV infection, colposcopic examination is recommended at least twice a year, and some recommend anal screening or anoscopic examination as well for women with extensive and aggressive HPV infection (Williams et al., 1994). Cross-sectional cohort studies have shown that HIV infection is an independent risk factor for both anal HPV infection and anal cytologic abnormalities, with a stronger association in women with lower CD4+ T-lymphocyte counts (Hillemanns et al., 1996).

Given the risk of more rapid disease progression, any HIV-positive woman with atypical squamous cells of undetermined significance (ASCUS) or low-grade squamous intraepithelial lesion (LSIL) is advised to have a colposcopic examination, endocervical curettage, and directed biopsy of abnormal areas of the ectocervix (Williams, 1995). Aggressive management with specialty consultation is required, especially for SIL or squamous carcinoma. In these women, cryotherapy may not be as effective, and choice of ablative or excisive treatment should be determined by client choice and clinical/immune status. (Chemosurgery with 5-flourouracil may be preferable to loop electrocautery excision [LEEP] and other surgical procedures in a severely immunocompromised client, for example.) Recurrence of CIN in HIV-infected women is common, and the prognosis for those with cervical cancer is poor, highlighting the need for aggressive screening and more innovative therapies (El-Sadr et al., 1994).

Genital ulcer disease (GUD) caused by herpes, chancroid, and syphilis may be more fulminant, take longer to treat, and require more intensive therapy in HIV-positive women (Tannenbaum, 1992). Idiopathic GUD has been noted with HIV infection, and genital ulcers can result from the use of foscarnet in cytomegalovirus (CMV)

treatment and, sometimes, from irritation caused by use of nonoxynol-9. Herpes simplex virus (HSV) may be more systemic and more severe, with acyclovir-resistant strains seen.

Pelvic inflammatory disease (PID), if diagnosed early, can be managed with standard therapy. However, symptoms may be masked in an immunocompromised woman with fewer white blood cells, thus leading to rapid progression that requires intravenous inpatient treatment. Clinicians should be vigilant about symptoms that suggest PID and should treat quickly according to current standards, hospitalizing HIV-positive women as necessary (Barbosa et al., 1997).

Vulvovaginal manifestations of candidiasis can occur months before oral thrush is noted or throughout the course of HIV infection. Although vaginal candidiasis is a problem common to all women, a study that matched seronegative controls with seropositive subjects found a nearly twofold risk of vulvovaginal candidiasis in HIV-positive women (Spinillo et al., 1994a). Not every HIV-infected woman will have florid vaginal yeast infections, but for those who do such episodes can be refractory and have an adverse impact on quality of life. HIV-infected women whose CD4+ cell counts are less than 300/mm³ have high rates of mucosal candidiasis; prior episodes of oropharyngeal and vaginal candidiasis appear to be the main risk factors or predictors of recurrence (El-Sadr et al., 1997).

Assessment of vaginal discharge should be done under the microscope to differentiate *Candida, Trichomonas,* and bacterial vaginosis (BV). For treatment, it is best to avoid short-course therapy, using antifungal creams or suppositories such as clotrimazole or nystatin and oral/systemic regimens for treatment failures. Prophylaxis for oral and vaginal candidiasis has been shown to be effective; a 1996 clinical trial demonstrated that 200 mg of fluconazole once a week reduced the risk of oral candidiasis by 50% and of vaginal candidiasis by 38%; there were too few cases to assess the effect of fluconazole on prevention of oropharyngeal and invasive fungal disease (NIAID, 1996). Antifungal resistance has been seen with HIV-associated candidiasis, including fluconazole-resistant strains. As usual, women should be advised that the use of antibiotics can lead to development or exacerbation of vaginal candidiasis and should be managed accordingly.

Because there is an association between STDs and the risk of acquiring or exacerbating HIV disease, prevention, diagnosis, and treatment of STDs are paramount. There is some evidence that women with HIV disease are at high risk of asymptomatic genitourinary *Chlamydia* colonization (Spinillo et al., 1994b). Screening every 6 months, or more routinely as indicated, is recommended. Gonorrhea is usually asymptomatic, involving more complications; a gonococcus culture always should be obtained if another STD is diagnosed. Syphilis screening should be done by means of a nontreponemal test (RPR, VDRL). Syphilis treatment will be the same for women as for men except during pregnancy, when inpatient, aggressive treatment is warranted to prevent disease progression and congenital spread.

Amenorrhea, oligomenorrhea, and infertility may occur with higher frequency in women with HIV disease although it is not clear whether this is due to drug use, to weight loss or wasting, to OIs, or to HIV disease itself. Studies assessing the effect of HIV disease on menstrual function and symptoms have been conflicting. For example, one prospective cohort trial that controlled for confounders did find higher rates of amenorrhea, longer intervals between menstrual cycles, and lower rates of dysmenorrhea among HIV-positive women with no or mild symptoms than among HIV-negative women, although it did not attribute these differences directly to secondary complications of HIV disease (Chirgwin et al., 1996). Another study matching 55 HIV-negative and HIV-positive women found no significant differences in the prevalence of oligomenorrhea, amenorrhea, menorrahgia, dysmenorrhea, or dyspareunia between the two groups or between the symptomatic and asymptomatic HIV-infected women (Shah et al., 1994). Amenorrhea, dysmenorrhea, premature menopause, and premenstrual syndrome should all be managed with the same standard of care as in HIV-negative women.

Because there has not been much research into the interactions between HIV and the reproductive endocrine and immune systems, not enough is known about the use of exogenous hormones, such as with oral contraceptives (OCPs), hormone replacement, or hormone maintenance for transsexual persons. Until more is known, use of exogenous hormones by HIV-positive women is neither recommended nor contraindicated (Denenberg, 1993).

PSYCHOSOCIAL NEEDS, INCLUDING ADDICTION TREATMENT. Many women with HIV infection have enormous burdens. Often they are primary caretakers of partners, children, and other loved ones, but they may not always get timely care themselves. They may face social isolation as well as economic and social powerlessness. These multiple stressors require support and the availability of a variety of resources.

Women with HIV infection often have high rates of past or current abuse in their lives, including rape and other sexual trauma. Preexisting depression, as well as sometimes repeated exposure to domestic and community violence, requires ready access to competent psychologic and psychiatric assistance and social service consultation where appropriate.

Just as adjustment to living with an HIV diagnosis can take various forms and can change over time, so too will the type of support needed by each woman. Services should be culturally relevant and suited to what the woman requires at her stage of psychologic and clinical adaptation to her HIV disease. Community-based resources can be very helpful. Peer-based and psychotherapeutic support (Chung & Magraw, 1992) provides evidence to the client that she is not alone in facing problems common to other women living with HIV infection, such as child care and reproductive concerns, whether or how to disclose the child's or the woman's HIV status, treatment decision making, and relationship concerns.

Psychiatric morbidity associated with HIV disease includes organic causes (OI) as well as nonorganic causes, such as grief reactions, adjustment disorders, anxiety disorders, major depression, and exacerbation of underlying personality or substance-abuse disorders. Little has been published regarding the neuropsychiatric considerations unique to women with HIV disease. However, the cognitive, behavioral, and motor dysfunction generally seen with HIV-related encephalopathy should be assessed. A neuropsychiatric workup for HIV-infected women should include evaluation by a psychiatrist and a neurologist of laboratory data (electroencephalogram, thyroid function, syphilis serology, sedimentation rate, complete blood cell count, and

CD4+ T-lymphocyte subsets), lumbar puncture, neuropsychologic testing, and magnetic resonance and SPECT brain imaging (Sanders, 1993).

Substance-abusing women may avoid the health care system out of fear that they will be imprisoned or that their children will be taken from them. Ideally, gender-appropriate addiction treatment will be available, both to reduce harm to the woman's own health and to prevent transmission of HIV. However, the availability of addiction-treatment centers, which are limited in many parts of the country, is almost nonexistent for women with children or women who are pregnant. Providers not only should be aware of where to refer women for pertinent addiction treatment (crack detoxification, treatment for alcohol or polysubstance use) but should know which facilities are most successful in addressing women's particular needs through the provision of child care and use of a supportive peer-based approach, which has been found to be more successful in treating chemically dependent women.

Family law issues are of great concern to many women with HIV. These needs include arranging custody, temporary child care when the client is physically unable to care for her children, and establishing who will care for the children (HIV-negative or HIV-positive) when she dies. Child care in many communities is based on kinship, where the grandmother, an aunt, or some other member of an extended family assumes responsibility for the children. However, these kinship providers may not receive the same amount of financial support from entitlement programs as do persons who legally adopt. Financial and other support has to be arranged for them and for the children. A National Institute of Mental Health (NIMH) study of 360 mothers with AIDS found that most of the parents' plans failed to address important contingency issues such as housing, financial support, and connection with the extended family for their children and guardians (Rotheram-Borus & Draimin, 1992). Some states have now adopted laws that allow naming of a "standby guardian" when the mother is in crisis, thus allowing the mother to retain parental rights.

Women also need life planning for themselves, including execution of wills (property and living will or other advanced medical directives) and designation of a decision-making proxy if they become incapacitated.

PREVENTION OF HIV IN WOMEN. As with other diseases that are sexually transmitted, rates of HIV acquisition around the world may be highest during adolescence and young adulthood. Young women are at risk biologically because of thinner vaginal mucosa and cervical ectopy (where endocervical transition zone cells that are more susceptible to HIV infection are everted). They also are at social risk because of patterns of sex with older men (who may have more likelihood of being infected with HIV), the practice of anal sex to preserve virginity in some groups, and the lack of sexual negotiation power as well as risk-taking behaviors around substance use.

Trends of HIV disease among older women also are of concern, however, as women represent nearly one in five (17%) of all cases of HIV disease in persons over the age of 50 reported to the CDC (CDC, 1996a). These older women, who may be at increased transmission risk because of postmenopausal atrophic vaginal mucosa, may be the least likely to practice safer sex or to consider the need for HIV testing. Similarly, clinicians might not consider HIV disease as a differential diagnosis in an older female client with symptoms of fatigue, muscle weakness, rashes, or cognitive and neurologic deficits (Editor, 1994).

It is important to recognize that potentially harmful behaviors, such as unprotected sex and substance abuse, occur heterogeneously and that defining stereotypical categories of "persons at risk" based on race, age, or clinician assumption is likely to result in missed opportunities for identifying actual risk and interventions. Every clinical provider should take a thorough sexual and substance-use history with each new client, asking at least "What are you doing to protect yourself from AIDS?" (Hatcher et al., 1994).

Although much policy focus has been on preventing perinatal transmission, it is imperative that energy and resources focus on preventing transmission of HIV *to* women (Goedert & Cote, 1994), including the targeting of men for HIV prevention. Programs that have been successful in getting women to reduce their sexual or substance-use risks tend to be those that engage peers or "target" group members in designing the intervention, emphasize relevant risk-reduction strategies, and use enhancement of self-esteem and self-empowerment as vehicles for behavioral change (Maldanado, 1996). Health workers can assist by discussing risks and reduction strategies with every client.

Many of the recommendations commonly made to women to reduce sexual transmission of HIV (e.g., limit the number of sexual partners or use condoms) require social and economic empowerment for implementation. Women tend to be socialized to associate trust with love, but sexual partners do not always know or tell the truth about their risk history. An increasing number of HIV-infected women cannot identify their risk factor for HIV beyond heterosexual contact with men they presumably thought to be HIV-negative.

Safer-sex precautions include both the use of technologies (such as barrier methods) and communication. Sexual negotiation is a learned skill but often one that is dictated by circumstances beyond an individual woman's control, such as whether she will face physical violence or economic and emotional abandonment if she suggests that her partner use a condom. Assertiveness training, including the use of role playing and other skills development, can provide some reinforcement, but, wherever feasible and appropriate, women's sex or substance-sharing partner(s) also should receive counseling about prevention and health promotion. The CDC encourages the use of latex male condoms with or without spermicide, or the use of female condoms if it is not possible to use male condoms, and does not recommend the use of spermicide alone until safe and effective vaginal microbicides are developed (NIAID, 1997).

Women desperately need protective methods that are under their control and that do not require the approval of the sexual partner. Ideally, these methods would include safe, nonirritating, inexpensive, and invisible agents that will kill HIV/STD organisms but not sperm. Vaginal microbicide trials are under way, although it may be some time before these products are widely available. The other, limited methods available include the polyurethane female condom (which has a lower pregnancy-prevention rate than the male condom but which does have the advantage of covering the vaginal vault as well as the perineum); the cervical cap and diaphragm (which protect the cervical cells most vulnerable to HIV

infection but which do not cover the vaginal epithelium and thus leave exposure to HIV possible); and vaginally applied spermicides. It always should be emphasized to women that hormonal contraceptives (oral, injectables, and implants) and sterilization provide a high degree of protection from pregnancy but *none* from HIV and STDs. Providers are not adequately meeting their responsibility to convey the need for *dual protection;* one national study of women at risk of HIV found that many women who were potentially well protected against pregnancy were underprotected against STDs (CDC, 1996c). Concern about the use of progesterone-containing contraceptives (such as Norplant and Depo-Provera) was highlighted by a 1996 study in which it was found that rhesus monkeys that received subcutaneous progesterone implants were 7.7 times more likely to become infected with simian immunodeficiency virus (SIV). An NIH meeting convened in mid-1996 concluded that women should not be discouraged from taking progestin-based contraceptives but should be counseled to always use a latex condom with intercourse (Maldonado, 1996).

Contributing causes of risk-taking behaviors, such as underlying depression (which may make adoption of healthier behavior difficult to attain [Orr et al., 1994] or may impede adoption by the effects of "psychiatric self-medication" through street drugs and alcohol), should not be overlooked. It takes time and repetition to change health behaviors. Health providers can support such change by reinforcing the benefit to a client of reducing harmful behaviors in her life while acknowledging that there may be difficulties. This approach recognizes that, as with other chronic illnesses, periods of exacerbation and remission may occur in addictive behaviors. By expressing nonjudgmental concern, setting clear, consistent limits, and listening to the client's cues, the clinician may be able to prevent or minimize the impact of relapses (Williams & O'Conner, 1995).

HIV and Pregnancy

PERINATAL TRANSMISSION TRENDS AND FACTORS. Eighty-four percent of all adult and adolescent American women and girls with AIDS are between the ages of 13 and 44 (CDC, 1996a), the peak years of reproductive potential. The impact of HIV disease as an intergenerational family illness results in HIV-infected and HIV-negative orphans. The CDC estimates that by the year 2000 American women will represent more than half of the cases of adult HIV disease, and another study estimates that between 72,000 and 125,000 U.S. children (30,000 of them in New York City alone) will be motherless because of AIDS (Michaels & Levine, 1994). Approximately 95% of the 7629 pediatric cases of AIDS identified through December 1996 were due to perinatal HIV transmission (CDC, 1996a). Whereas the number of women living with HIV infection continues to grow, the number of babies born with HIV infection peaked in 1991 and declined by 43% from 1992 to 1996.

Rates of transmission of HIV-1 from mother to infant (vertical or perinatal transmission) seen in cohort studies range from 16% to 60% (Heymann & Brubaker, 1997), with rates of 13% to 32% seen in industrialized and 25% to 48% in developing nations (Peckham, 1993). It is thought that the majority of transmissions occur in late pregnancy or during the intrapartum period (labor and delivery), although transmission can occur in utero and in the postpartum period through breast-feeding, which adds a risk of around 15%.

In 1994 the ACTG 076 clinical trial provided evidence that administration of zidovudine (AZT) to the mother during pregnancy after the first trimester and during labor and delivery and postpartally to the infant can reduce the risk of transmission by around two thirds (from 22.6% to 7.6%). Although this reduction is dramatic, the relative impact of the period of AZT administration or of the woman's disease state is not clear. Other small studies have shown a similar transmission reduction impact in women with lower CD4+ cell counts than the 076 cohort (Boyer et al., 1994). Two recent studies also showed that use of AZT can lead to vaginal and other tumors in laboratory rats, although generalization from this animal model to predict a human impact may not be applicable.

In 1995 the U.S. Public Health Service recommended that health care providers ensure that all women are routinely counseled about HIV and encouraged to be tested for HIV infection "to allow women to know their infection status both for their own health and to reduce the risk for perinatal HIV transmission" (CDC, 1995a). It

was estimated that one third of all American women of reproductive age that year had been tested for HIV. The fact that the number of infants born with HIV infection has declined significantly is attributed to more widespread discussion of the benefits of testing and of antiretroviral therapy during the perinatal period. Nonetheless, there are renewed calls for mandatory testing of newborns (which became law in New York State) and of women of reproductive age. Testing for HIV is only one step, however. Women need to be partners in their care and in choosing and adhering to options for reducing the risk of transmitting HIV to their fetuses and infants.

A number of factors have been found to be associated with higher rates of vertical HIV transmission, including maternal factors (disease state, CD4+ cell count, HIV viral load and type, neutralizing antibody); placental status (chorioamnionitis); fetal and infant considerations (delivery before 34 weeks, immune response); and intrapartal events (mode of delivery, duration of labor, use of invasive procedures), especially premature (by more than 4 hours) rupture of membranes (Kuhn et al., 1994). The exact role of maternal viral load in perinatal transmission remains undefined. Some studies have suggested a "threshold" level at which transmission appears more likely, while others have shown that HIV can be transmitted at all maternal RNA levels (Gilden, 1996). Also, viral load in the genital tract may differ from that in plasma. An understanding of when transmission is most likely to occur is critical for developing management strategies to reduce risk.

PERINATAL MANAGEMENT OF HIV DISEASE. Pregnancy has not been found to hasten women's HIV disease unless severe immunocompromise is already present. If the client has advanced HIV disease, aggressive monitoring to diagnose and manage the opportunistic infections, neoplasias, or neurologic events that can occur with AIDS is required. CD4+ cell counts should be assessed every trimester, especially in women whose T-helper cell counts are below $300/mm^3$. HIV has not been found definitively to adversely affect obstetric or fetal outcome (European Collaborative Group, 1994a).

The antenatal period provides an opportunity to establish a relationship with the woman, to discuss her coping strategies, available support, need for treatment of addiction and other health concerns, and to review her sexual, reproductive, and life-planning goals. Clinical care in pregnancy involves establishing baseline history, physical examination data, and laboratory work that will include immunologic monitoring. All the usual components of prenatal care should be provided, with the addition of CD4+ cell counts and HIV viral load monitoring, baseline cytomegalovirus and toxoplasmosis titers, purified protein derivative (PPD) anergy panel, and heightened vigilance on the part of the health provider to distinguish between complaints that are pregnancy-related from those that are HIV-related.

Opportunistic infections should be treated on a case-by-case basis to prevent harm to the mother and thus fetal compromise. The fact that *Pneumocystis carinii* pneumonia (PCP) is the most common cause of pregnancy-associated deaths in HIV-positive women highlights the importance of prevention and treatment of OIs in pregnancy for the mother and for the infant. Although the use of certain medications in pregnancy should be avoided altogether (Watts, 1997), others may be used (preferably after the first trimester) when the risk of not treating poses a known compromise to mother or fetus. CD4+ cell counts of $200/mm^3$ warrant PCP prophylaxis (aerosol pentamidine has the advantage of localized delivery, with trimethoprim-sulfamethoxazole the oral drug of choice). Syphilis should be screened regularly and treated aggressively.

The use of antiretroviral agents for the health of the mother, as well as for a possible role in reducing transmission to the fetus, needs to be considered carefully. With an enhanced understanding of HIV pathogenesis and the need for combination drug therapy to combat viral replication, the use of antiretroviral monotherapy is no longer considered a standard of care. In fact, many HIV specialists believe that monotherapy can be harmful in terms of viral resistance. The standard is moving toward three- and four-drug combinations, none of which by 1997 had clinical trial data in terms of perinatal transmission impact and impact on the health of the fetus or infant or on the mother's long-term antiretroviral treatment strategy. Federal guidelines for HIV treatment recognize this dilemma and, while recommending that all women be offered the ACTG 076 regimen, state that "[w]hile zidovudine monotherapy has been shown to significantly reduce the risk of perinatal HIV transmission, appropriate combinations of antiretroviral drugs should be administered if indicated on the basis of the mother's health....In general, pregnancy should not compromise optimal HIV therapy for the mother" (USPHS, 1998). HIV-positive women who are pregnant or considering pregnancy will need to discuss the risks and benefits of antiretroviral regimens on an individualized basis until there are more clinical data available regarding the safety and efficacy of various combination therapies for the health of the woman and the infant and for their impact on perinatal transmission. Treatment decisions are the woman's to make, and a long-term treatment plan should be discussed by the woman and her provider (USPHS, 1998).

Research is under way to determine whether intervention strategies such as passive (immune globulin, monoclonal antibodies) and active (HIV vaccines) immunoprophylaxis to the mother, the baby, or both, vitamin A administration, chemoprophylaxis with combination antiretroviral therapies, or mechanical innovations to reduce the amount of fluid to which an infant may be exposed during birth can be efficacious in reducing perinatal transmission. This latter method, called vaginal lavage, was shown in one study using chlorhexidine not to have a statistically significant impact on perinatal transmission rates (Biggar et al., 1996).

In individual studies mode of delivery itself has not been found to be predictive of HIV transmission. Although some see a possible protective effect from cesarean delivery (European Collaborative Group, 1994b), HIV-infected infants have been born by cesarean delivery. Meta-analysis supports a protective effect of cesarean over vaginal delivery (Villari et al., 1993). However, this advantage may not pertain to all women, and there are risks of surgical sequelae in immunocompromised clients. Until such time as randomized controlled trials that evaluate mode of delivery are conducted, delivery determination should be based on individual clinical indicators.

Breast milk–associated transmission can occur, and for this reason it is recommended that HIV-positive women who have access to safe alternatives for infant nutrition not breast-feed. (This recommendation is controversial in developing nations, where the additional risk of HIV transmission may be outweighed by the risk of infant malnutrition and diarrheal illness). Women should receive support and information about universal precautions in the home setting and the importance of self-care and infant care after discharge.

HIV and Lesbians

Women who have sex with women (WSW) have been involved in the HIV epidemic since the beginning, as providers, caregivers, activists—and as persons living with HIV infection.

EPIDEMIOLOGY. The CDC's HIV/AIDS surveillance report has never included a single category of WSW, instead showing other risk factors for WSW such as injecting drug use. The assumption has been that women who have sex with women are at low risk of acquiring HIV. However, this assumption—what some have labeled the "myth of lesbian immunity"—is dangerous for two reasons. First, a handful of cases of HIV transmission between two women who have no other risk factors (female-to-female or FTF transmission) has been reported (Chu et al., 1994), although, according to a study of HIV-discordant lesbian couples, such transmission appears to be rare (Raiteri et al., 1996). Second, and perhaps most important to bear in mind, is that a person's sexual behavior and preferred sexual identity are not synonymous and may be fluid over time. Many WSW, whether or not they identify themselves as lesbians, also have unprotected sex with men (often gay and bisexual men). Other behavioral factors that put lesbians at risk of HIV include substance abuse or injecting drug use and alternative insemination, often with unscreened donor semen (Kennedy et al., 1995).

Studies bear out the fact that people's behaviors and labels do not correlate and that rigid classification into set "categories" may well ignore a person's risks. In the WIHS natural history study of HIV-positive women, for instance, 14% of self-identified heterosexual women reported having sex with a woman in the last 6 months (Barkan et al., 1996). Among groups of women who report same-sex contact, the rates of sex with men range from 22% (San Francisco Department of Public Health, 1995) to 93%. WSW may be at

risk because of their own injecting drug use, sex with an injecting drug user (IDU), or sex with men who engage in high-risk behaviors. One study of the HIV risk patterns of lesbian and bisexual women who frequented gay bars in 16 small or medium-sized cities across the United States found that 39% of bisexual women had sex with a gay man and 20% with an IDU; the majority of respondents who reported sex with a man did not consistently use condoms (Norman et al., 1996). Among female IDUs, WSW have been reported to inject more often, share works or inject with used works more often, use shooting galleries, and have higher rates of HIV seroconversion than do women who have sex with men only (CDC, 1995b). Perhaps because of higher rates of unsafe sex and injecting drug use, women reporting same-sex contacts have shown higher rates of HIV infection than women reporting sex only with men: 17% vs. 11% in one New York City sample (Bevier et al., 1995), 1.12% vs. 0.55% in a Los Angeles sample (Smith, 1997), and 1.2% among lesbian and bisexual women living in the San Francisco Bay Area, a prevalence three times higher than that estimated for other adolescent and adult women in the area (Lemp et al., 1995). In a study of HIV seroprevalence data for women at four of New York State's counseling and testing programs from 1993 to 1994, rates of HIV infection were highest in bisexual women (4.8%), followed by women who were sexually active exclusively with women (3.0%), and then by women who had sex exclusively with men (2.9%); injecting drug use was by far the predominant risk factor for seropositive WSW (Shotsky, 1996).

An underlying factor putting lesbians at risk is societal and interpersonal homophobia. This may be particularly true for lesbian, gay, bisexual, or questioning youths, who experience cognitive, emotional, and social isolation, feelings of alienation and despair, leading to higher rates of suicidal ideation, alcohol and polysubstance use, and sexual encounters that are often unsafe (Grossman, 1994).

MANAGEMENT. WSW need access to the same woman-specific primary and preventive care as other women, including screening and management of STDs, since some lesbians may be exposed through sex with men. Furthermore, various STDs and vaginal infections, such as human papillomavirus, HSV disease, syphilis, hepatitis B and C, and *Chlamydia* infections, trichomoniasis, and bacterial vaginosis, can be spread between women. Providers should not make assumptions about the sexual practices of their lesbian clients; instead, they should discuss together the actual behaviors, with screening for STDs based on individual assessment (Lynch & Ferri, 1997).

Psychologic or psychiatric support and assessment and treatment for addictions are important components of comprehensive care for lesbians. One national study of rates of depressive distress and suicidal thoughts among 829 gay men and 603 lesbian African-Americans found that the female subjects were as distressed as HIV-infected gay black men (Cochran & Mays, 1994). Issues of access to care for lesbians who do not feel comfortable "coming out" to their health care providers are only exacerbated by coexisting conditions of poverty, exposure to violence, and racism.

History taking by primary care and other women's health providers working with lesbians and women who are sexually active with women should use principles of communication that are not heterosexist-biased, that describe behaviors in language that the client understands, and that facilitate open communication. Such assessment will include reviewing the risk of STDs and HIV infection, and methods to reduce that risk, including appropriate safer-sex techniques for contact with both women and men (White, 1997), cancer risk and screening (including Pap smear screening intervals that, on the basis of the woman's sexual history and risk factors, may be similar to those that are advised for heterosexual women) (O'Hanlan & Crum, 1996), parenting issues, depression, alcohol and other substance use, and violence (White & Levinson, 1995).

PREVENTION. Lesbian and bisexual women need information about those behaviors that enhance their risk of HIV acquisition. They may be having unprotected sex with men (and these men may be more likely to be bisexual and have a higher likelihood of being infected with HIV). They may be injecting or abusing drugs and need to be aware of harm-reduction techniques. Like other populations, particularly those that are socially and economically disenfranchised, WSM

face a number of barriers to prevention. More immediate survival needs, such as housing, sex work for survival, and active addiction, can take precedence over future concerns of HIV infection (DeCarlo & Gomez, 1996). Small studies have indicated that, while high-risk behavior occurs with some frequency among WSW, many of those surveyed do not use safer-sex practices (Einhorn & Polgar, 1994).

Safer-sex practice information should be tailored to the actual behaviors of the person, based on whether she is having sex with women, with men, or with both or is engaging in substance-abuse patterns that put her at risk of HIV infection. All persons who inject drugs should be counseled regarding the importance of not sharing needles and of receiving information on the availability of clean needles, needle cleaning with bleach (though this is not 100% effective in killing HIV), and the availability of harm-reduction and drug-treatment programs. Although there is a dearth of research on the risks of HIV transmission during cunnilingus (Young, 1994), this activity is not without risk and can be practiced more safely with the use of vulvar barriers (such as latex squares from a cut-up condom, dental dams, or household food wraps such as Saran wrap). However, it should be emphasized that cunnilingus is less risky than is having unprotected vaginal or anal sex with a male partner and that condoms and lubricant should be used consistently for sex with a man (Gorna, 1996). Sex toys should not be shared, and blood-to-blood contact should be avoided. Bisexual women or women who indicate that they have sex with men should receive information and support regarding choice of a partner (i.e., higher HIV seroprevalence among gay and bisexual men), negotiation skills, and use of latex condoms during vaginal and anal sex.

Women who are considering becoming pregnant through self-insemination or alternative insemination should receive information about how to reduce the risks from donor sperm through screening for HIV and should be given help to overcome barriers (such as cost, concern about gynecologic examinations, or discriminatory practices) to the use of medical insemination from sperm banks and fertility clinics (Macauley et al., 1995), where such screening procedures already are in place.

HIV and Persons Who Are Transgender or Transsexual

Transsexualism, a form of gender-identity discordance,* involves incongruity between a person's anatomic/natal sex and personal sense of gender identity (Cole et al., 1994; Money, 1994). Just as there is no definitively identified single cause of sexual orientation, the reason for this feeling of "having been born the wrong sex" is unknown; perhaps it is due to an interaction between the developing brain and sex hormones (Zhou et al., 1995). The incidence of transsexualism, based on studies outside the United States, appears to be about 1 per 20,000 to 50,000, with the ratio favoring male-to-female transsexualism about 2.3 to 2.5:1 (Weitze & Osburg, 1996; Bakker et al., 1993), although in Sweden transsexualism is found equally in men and women (Landeb et al., 1996).

Standards of care for treating transsexualism, including psychologic assessment, hormone therapy for desired secondary sex characteristics, and sex-reassignment surgery, were developed relatively recently (around 1979). A transsexual person's HIV status should not be seen as an impediment to hormonal treatment or surgical sex-reassignment therapy.

Persons experiencing gender identity discordance or gender dysphoria, of which transsexualism can be said to be the most extreme form, are at risk of HIV infection through unsafe sexual behavior and injecting drug use (Pang et al., 1994), including potential factors such as sharing of needles when injecting exogenous hormones. Transgender and transsexual persons are socially and often economically vulnerable to engaging in risk behavior as well, since they are an unaddressed minority that may not be fully accepted in either the gay or the straight culture and for whom few specific prevention programs have been developed. Recognizing this fact, Australia conducted a national needs assessment on transsexuals and HIV/AIDS, outlining specific needs for planning and service provision and discussing the human and civil rights abuses experienced by transsexuals

---

*People who are "transgendered" exhibit full-time cross-gender behavior but have not made any major alteration to their bodies; persons who are "transsexual" wish to *be* the other gender and undertake hormonal and surgical alteration to achieve this.

that have allowed HIV infection to have such a severe impact on this minority (Alan et al., 1992).

In small studies, the incidence of HIV seropositivity in transsexuals has ranged from 4% in a population of California state prison inmates (Valenta et al., 1992), to 21% in an Australian study (Alan et al., 1989), to 50% in a small sample of street-involved transsexuals from Canada. Noting the high-risk behaviors in this latter group, the authors point out the need for counseling, social support, medical care, access to gender dysphoria care, and sex-change surgery where desired, as well as opportunities for education and involvement in training and for more sensitivity on the part of caregivers (Rekart et al., 1993).

Although transsexualism is not in itself a psychopathologic disorder (Cole et al., 1997), higher levels of depression, anxiety, and associated symptoms have been reported as being more common in HIV-positive men who are gender dysphoric (Weinrich et al., 1995). There are almost no reported studies on the psychologic needs of female-to-male (FTM) transsexuals.

Model programs have been developed to provide transgender and transsexual populations with access to appropriate prevention education and early intervention services. One such project in New York City combined the transgender-specific services of five community-based providers to develop specific educational tools, initiate street and club outreach, develop protocols, and engage a corps of transgender peer educators. The success of the program was attributed to the fact that peers and professionals worked together to deliver relevant, credible materials and services (Warren et al., 1996).

REFERENCES

Alan, D., Alexander, R., Monroe, J. (1992, July). *Transsexuals—don't think about them and they go away and die.* Presented at VIII International Conference on AIDS, Florence, Italy.

Alan, D.L., Guinan, J.J., McCallum, L. (1989, June). *HIV seroprevalence and its implications for a transsexual population.* Presented at V International Conference on AIDS, San Francisco.

Bakker, A., van Kesteren, P.J., Gooren, L.J., Bezemer, P.D. (1993). The prevalence of transsexualism in the Netherlands. *Acta Psychiatry Scandinavia, 87,* 237–238.

Barbosa, C., Macasaet, M., Brockmann, S., et al. (1997). Pelvic inflammatory disease and human immunodeficiency virus infection. *Obstetrics & Gynecology, 89,* 65–70.

Barkan, S., Deamont, C., Young, M., et al. (1996, July). *Sexual identity and behavior among women with female sexual partners: The Women's Interagency HIV Study WIHS.* Presented at XI International Conference on AIDS, Vancouver, British Columbia.

Bevier, P.J., Chiasson, M.A., Hefferman, R.T., Castro, K.G. (1995). Women at a sexually transmitted disease clinic who reported same-sex contact: Their HIV seroprevalence and risk behaviors. *American Journal of Public Health, 85,* 1366–1371.

Biggar, R.J., Miotti, P.G., Taha, T.E., et al. (1996). Perinatal intervention trial in Africa: Effect of a birth canal cleansing intervention to prevent HIV transmission. *Lancet, 347,* 1647–1650.

Boyer, P.J., Dillon, M., Navaie, A., et al. (1994) Factors predictive of maternal-fetal transmission of HIV-1. *Journal of the American Medical Association, 271*(24), 1925–1930.

Burdge, D.R., Money, D.M. (1996). Bridging the gender gap in HIV diagnosis and care. *Medscape Women's Health, 1*(10), 4.

Centers for Disease Control and Prevention (CDC). (1995a). U.S. Public Health Service recommendations for human immunodeficiency virus counseling and voluntary testing for pregnant women. *Morbidity and Mortality Weekly Report, 44*(RR-7), 9.

Centers for Disease Control and Prevention (CDC). (1995b, April). *Report on lesbian HIV issues meeting.* Atlanta: CDC/National Center for HIV, STD, and TB Prevention, Division of HIV/AIDS Prevention.

Centers for Disease Control and Prevention (CDC). (1996a). *HIV/AIDS Surveillance Report Year End Edition, 8*(2), 10, 12, 14, 16, 31.

Centers for Disease Control and Prevention. (1996b). *HIV & AIDS trends.* Atlanta: Author, p. 3.

Centers for Disease Control and Prevention. (1996c). Contraceptive method and condom use among women at risk for HIV infection and other STDs—selected US sites, 1993–1994. *Morbidity and Mortality Weekly Report, 45*(38), 820–823.

Centers for Disease Control and Prevention. (1997a). *HIV/AIDS Surveillance Report, 9*(1), 3–33.

Centers for Disease Control and Prevention. (1997b). *1996 HIV/AIDS trends provide evidence of success in HIV prevention and treatment.* Atlanta: Author, p. 2.

Chirgwin, K., Feldman, J., Muneyyirci-Delale, O., et al. (1996). Menstrual function in HIV-infected women with acquired immunodeficiency syndrome. *Journal of AIDS and and Human Retrovirology, 12,* 489–494.

Chu, S.Y., Conti, L., Schable, B.A., Diaz, T. (1994). Female-to-female sexual contact and HIV transmission [Letter]. *Journal of the American Medical Association, 272,* 433.

Chung, J., Magraw, M. (1992). A group approach to psy-chosocial issues faced by HIV-positive women. *Hospital & Community Psychiatry, 43*(9), 891–894.

Clark, R. (1997). Clinical manifestations and the natural history of human immunodeficiency virus infection in women. In D. Cotton, D.H. Watts (Eds.), *The medical management of AIDS in women* (p. 115). New York: Wiley-Liss.

Cochran, S.D., Mays, V.M. (1994). Depressive distress among homosexually active African-American men and women. *American Journal of Psychiatry, 151,* 524–529.

Cole, C.M., Emory, L.E., Huang, T., Meyer, W.J., 3rd. (1994). Treatment of gender dysphoria. *Texas Medicine, 90,* 68–72.

Cole, C.M., O'Boyle, M., Emory, L.E., Meyer, W.J., 3rd. (1997). A comorbidity of gender dysphoria and other major psychiatric diagnoses. *Archives of Sexual Behavior, 26,* 13–26.

DeCarlo, P., Gomez, C. (1996, January). *What are women who have sex with women's HIV prevention needs?* San Francisco: Center for AIDS Prevention Studies, UCSF.

Denenberg, R. (1993). Female sex hormones and HIV. *AIDS Clinical Care, 5*(9), 69–71, 76.

Editor. (1994). The impact of HIV/AIDS upon women. *HIV Hotline, 4*(8), 7–8.

Einhorn, L., Polgar, M. (1994). HIV-risk behavior among lesbians and bisexual women. *AIDS Education and Prevention, 6,* 514–523.

El-Sadr, W., Oleske, J.M., Agins, B.D., et al. (1994, January). *Evaluation and management of early HIV infection. Clinical Practice Guideline No. 7.* Washington, D.C.: AHCPR.

El-Sadr, W., Schuman, P., Peng, G., et al. (1997, May). *Predictors of mucosal candidiasis among HIV-infected women.* Presented at National Conference on HIV & Women, Washington, D.C.

European Collaborative Group. (1994a). Perinatal findings in children born to HIV-infected mothers. *British Journal of Obstetrics & Gynecology, 101,* 136–141.

European Collaborative Group. (1994b). Cesarean section and risk of vertical transmission of HIV-1. *Lancet, 343,* 1464–1467.

Gilden, D. (1996). The (viral) burden of motherhood. *GMHC Treatment Issues, 10*(4), 3.

Goedert, J.J., Coté, T.R. (1994). Editorial: Public health interventions to reduce pediatric AIDS. *American Journal of Public Health, 84*(7), 1065–1066.

Gorna, R. (1996, July). *Lesbian safer sex: Alarmist or inadequate?* Presented at XI International AIDS Conference, Vancouver, British Columbia.

Grossman, A.H. (1994). Homophobia: A cofactor of HIV disease in gay and lesbian youth. *Journal of the Association of Nurses in AIDS Care, 5,* 39–43.

Hankins, C., Lamont, J., Handley, M. (1994). Cervico-vaginal screening in women with HIV infection: Need for increased vigilance? *Canadian Medical Association Journal, 150*(5), 684.

Hanna, L. (1994). Nutritional considerations for women with HIV. *BETA,* December.

Hatcher, R., Trussell, J., Stewart, F., et al. (1994). *Contraceptive technology* (16th ed., p. 30). New York: Irvington Publishers, Inc.

Hellinger, F. (1993). The use of health services by women with HIV infection. *Health Services Research, 28*(5), 543–561.

Heymann, J., Brubaker, J. (1997). Breastfeeding and HIV infection. In D. Cotton, D.H. Watts (Eds.), *The medical management of AIDS in women* (p. 61). New York: Wiley-Liss.

Hillemanns, P., Ellerbrock, T., McPhillips, S., et al. (1996). Prevalence of human papillomavirus infection and anal cytologic abnormalities in HIV-seropositive women. *AIDS, 10,* 1641–1647.

Kennedy, M.B., Scarlett, M.I., Duerr, A.C., Chu, S.Y. (1995). Assessing HIV risk among women who have sex with women: Scientific and communication issues. *Journal of the American Medical Women's Association, 50,* 3–4.

Kuhn, L., Stein, Z.A., Thomas, P.A., et al. (1994). Maternal-infant HIV transmission and circumstances of delivery. *American Journal of Public Health, 84*(7), 1110–1115.

Landeb, M., Walinder, J., Lustrom, B. (1996). Incidence and sex ratio of transsexualism in Sweden. *Acta Psychiatry Scandinavia, 93,* 261–263.

Lemp, G.F., Jones, M., Kellogg, T.A., et al. (1995). HIV seroprevalence and risk behaviors among lesbians and bisexual women in San Francisco and Berkeley, California. *American Journal of Public Health, 85,* 1549–1552.

Lynch, M., Ferri, R. (1997). Health needs of lesbian women and gay men. *Clinician Reviews, 7*(1), 98–102.

Macauley, L., Kitzinger, J., Green, G., Wight, D. (1995). Unconventional conceptions and HIV. *AIDS Care, 7,* 261–276.

Maldonado, M. (1996). *The challenges of HIV/AIDS for women of color and their families.* Washington, DC: National Minority AIDS Council, 8, 9, 11.

Melnick, S., Sherer, R., Louis, T.A., et al. (1994). Survival and disease progression according to gender of clients with HIV infection. *Journal of the American Medical Association, 272*(24), 1915.

Michaels, D., Levine, C. (1994). Estimates of the number of motherless youth orphaned by AIDS in the United States. *Journal of the American Medical Association, 268*(24), 3457–3461.

Money, J. (1994). The concept of gender identity disorder in childhood and adolescence after 39 years. *Journal of Sexuality and Marital Therapy, 20,* 163–177.

National Commission on AIDS. (1992, December). *The challenge of HIV/AIDS in communities of color.* Washington, DC: Author.

National Institute of Allergy and Infectious Diseases (NIAID). (1996, July). *Fluconazole prevents yeast infections in women with HIV.* Washington, DC: Author.

National Institute of Allergy and Infectious Diseases (NIAID). (April 2, 1997). *NIAID evaluates N-9 film as microbicide.* Washington, DC: Author.

Norman, A.D., Perry, M.J., Stevenson, L.Y., et al. (1996). Lesbian and bisexual women in small cities—at risk for HIV? *Public Health Reports, 111*(4), 347.

Norton, D., Brosgart, C., Barkin, M., et al. (1994). *Papanicolaou smears versus colposcopy as screening tests for cervical intraepithelial neosplasia (CIN) in HIV seropositive women.* Presented at X International Conference on AIDS, Yokohama, Japan.

O'Hanlan, K.A., Crum, C.P. (1996). Human papillomavirus-associated cervical intraepithelial neoplasia following lesbian sex. *Obstetrics and Gynecology, 88,* 702–703.

Olaitan, A., Johnson, M. (1997, May). Cervical intraepithelial neoplasia in women with HIV. *Journal of the International Association of Physicians in AIDS Care, 3*(5), 15–17.

Olaitan, A., Johnson, M., MacLean, A., Poulter, L. (1996). The distribution of immunocompetent cells in the genital tract of HIV-positive women. *AIDS, 10,* 759–764.

Orr, S.T., Celentano, J., Santelli, D.D., et al. (1994). Depressive symptoms and risk factors for HIV acquisition among black women attending urban health centers in Baltimore. *AIDS Education and Prevention, 6*(3), 230–236.

Pang, H., Pugh, K., Catalan, J. (1994). Gender identity disorder and HIV disease. *International Journal of STDs and AIDS, 2,* 130–132.

Peckham, C. (1993, June). *Mother-to-child transmission of HIV: Risk factors and timing.* Presented at IX International Conference on AIDS, Berlin, Germany.

Raiteri, R., Fora, R., Russo, R., Sinnicco, A. (1996, July). *HIV transmission in HIV-discordant lesbian couples.* Presented at XI International Conference on AIDS, Vancouver, British Columbia.

Rekart, M.L., Manzon, L.M., Tucker, P. (1993, June). *Transsexuals and AIDS.* Presented at IX International Conference on AIDS, Berlin, Germany.

Rotheram-Borus, M.J., Draimin, B. (1992). Interventions for adolescents whose parents live with AIDS. NIMH Grant MH49958-03.

Sanders, K.M. (1993). Neuropsychiatric aspects of infection. In A. Kurth (Ed.), *Until the cure: Caring for women with HIV* (pp. 81–93). New Haven, CT: Yale University Press.

San Francisco Department of Public Health AIDS Prevention Services Branch/Surveillance Branch. (1995). Health behaviors among lesbian and bisexual women: Research report. San Francisco: Author, p. 15.

Seck, A.C., Faye, M.A., Critchlow, A.D., et al. (1994). Cervical intraepithelial neoplasia and human papillomavirus infection among Senegalese women seropositive for HIV-1 or HIV-2 or seronegative for HIV. *International Journal of STDs and AIDS, 5*(3), 189–193.

Shah, P., Smith, J., Wells, C., et al. (1994). Menstrual symptoms in women infected with the human immunodeficiency virus. *Obstetrics and Gynecology, 83,* 397–400.

Shevitz, A., Pagano, M., Chiasson, M.A., et al. (1996). The association between youth, women, and acquired immunodeficiency syndrome. *Journal of Acquired Immune Deficiency Syndromes and Human Retrovirology, 13*(5), 427–433.

Shotsky, W.J. (1996). Women who have sex with other women: HIV seroprevalence in New York State counseling and testing programs. *Women's Health, 24,* 1–15.

Smith, L. (1997, May). *Characteristics of and HIV seroprevalence among medically underserved women utilizing a mobile testing and outreach van in LA County.* Presented at National Conference on Women and HIV, Washington, D.C.

Spinillo, A., Gorini, G., Regazzetti, F., et al. (1994b). Asymptomatic genitourinary *Chlamydia trachomatis* infection in women seropositive for human immunodeficiency virus infection. *Obstetrics and Gynecology, 83*(6), 1005–1010.

Spinillo, A., Michelone, C., Cananna, L., et al. (1994a). Clinical and microbiological characteristics of symptomatic vulvovaginal candidiasis in HIV seropositive women. *Genitourinary Medicine, 7*(4), 268–272.

Sunderland, A., Holman, S. (1993). Optimizing the delivery of services. In A. Kurth (Ed.), *Until the cure: Caring for women with HIV* (pp. 212–227). New Haven, CT: Yale University Press.

Tannenbaum, I. (1992, June/July). The impact of HIV on women: Gynecology, pregnancy, and family planning considerations. *SIECUS Report, 20*(4), 1, 4.

U.S. Public Health Service. (1998). Public Health Service task force recommendations for the use of antiretroviral drugs in pregnant women infected with HIV-1 for maternal health and for reducing perinatal HIV-1 transmission in the U.S. *MMWR Morbidity and Mortality Weekly Report, 47*(RR-2), 1–30.

Valenta, L.J., Elias, A.N., Domurat, E.S. (1992). Hormone pattern in pharmacologically feminized male transsexuals in the California state prison system. *Journal of the National Medical Association, 3,* 241–250.

Villari, P., Spino, C., Chalmers T., et al. (1993). Cesarean section to reduce perinatal transmission of human immunodeficiency virus. *Online Journal of Current Clinical Trials* (Doc. No. 74).

Warren, B.E., Capozuca, J., Pols, B., Otto, B. (1996, July). *AIDS prevention for transgender and transsexual persons: A collaborative community-based program.* Presented at XI International Conference on AIDS, Vancouver, British Columbia.

Watts, H. (1997). Care of the HIV-positive pregnant woman. In D. Cotton, D.H. Watts (Eds.), *The medical management of AIDS in women* (pp. 195–198). New York: Wiley-Liss.

Weinrich, J.D., Atkinson, J.H., Jr, McCutchan, J.A., Grant, I. (1995). Is gender dysphoria dysphoric? Elevated depression and anxiety in gender dysphoric and nondysphoric homosexual and bisexual men in a HIV sample. *Archives of Sexual Behavior, 1,* 55–72.

Weitze, C., Osburg, S. (1996). Transsexualism in Germany: Empirical data on epidemiology and application of the German Transsexuals' Act during its first ten years. *Archives of Sexual Behavior, 25*(4), 409–425.

White, J.C. (1997). HIV risk assessment and prevention in lesbians and women who have sex with women: Practical information for clinicians. *Health Care of Women International, 18,* 127–138.

White, J.C., Levinson, W. (1995). Lesbian health care. What a primary care physician needs to know. *Western Journal of Medicine, 162,* 463–466.

Williams, A. (1995). Clinical management of HIV infection in women. In N. Clumeck, G. Friedland (Eds.), *Handbook of supportive care in AIDS.* New York: Marcel Dekker.

Williams, A., Darragh, T.M., Vranizan, K., et al. (1994). Anal and cervical human papillomavirus infection and risk of anal and cervical epithelial abnormalities in HIV-infected women. *Obstetrics and Gynecology, 84,* 591–597.

Williams, A., O'Conner, P.G. (1995). Substance abuse issues. In P. Kelly, S. Holman, R. Rothenberg, S. Holzemer (Eds.), *Primary care of women and children with HIV infection.* Boston: Jones & Bartlett.

Young, R.M. (1994). The scarcity of data on cunnilingus in the risk of HIV transmission from oral-genital intercourse. *Infections in Urology, 7*(6), 170–183.

Zhou, J.N., Hofman, M.A., Gooren, L.J., Swaab, D.F. (1995). A sex difference in the human brain and its relation to transsexuality. *Nature, 6552,* 68–70.

▪ Injecting Drug Users, Incarcerated Persons, and Commercial Sex Workers

Mary McCarthy

Some of the most pressing issues of the current HIV pandemic concern the delivery of quality and compassionate services to infected injecting drug users (IDUs), incarcerated persons, and commercial sex workers. Medical and social needs in these groups are often unique and frequently go unmet; thus they merit attention apart from others infected with HIV. The measures required to reduce high-risk behavior and to prevent viral transmission in these groups are controversial and politically sensitive. Developing and implementing effective outreach and treatment modalities for them will undoubtedly offer caregivers challenges well into the next century.

Injecting Drug Users

In 1993 the CDC redefined AIDS to include bacterial pneumonia and tuberculosis, diseases common among IDUs (CDC, 1993). This resulted in a significant increase in the percentage of cases attributable to injecting drug use. As of December 1996, injecting drug use accounted for approximately 36% of the 573,000 reported cases of AIDS (CDC, December 31, 1996). Most AIDS cases among women of childbearing age are associated with injecting drug use, as a direct result of either sharing contaminated paraphernalia (e.g., needles, syringes, sterilizing equipment, and cotton swabs) or engaging in unprotected sexual relations with an HIV-infected IDU. A study by MaWhinney et al. of various risk groups (1996) revealed that IDUs account for the majority of new cases of HIV infection in New York City, and it is expected that other parts of the country will soon mirror this finding. Nationwide, IDUs are second only to heterosexual women in the number of new cases of AIDS (CDC, December 31, 1996).

RISK REDUCTION. The injecting drug user typically acquires HIV infection by engaging in the high-risk behavior of sharing injection paraphernalia, especially needles and syringes. To verify placement of a needle in a vein, IDUs draw blood into their syringes before injection. The aspirated blood and the drug are then injected directly into the user's bloodstream. Some amount of blood will unavoidably remain in the needle and syringe, which, if reused without proper cleansing, will efficiently transfer any bloodborne pathogens in the residual blood into the bloodstream of the next user. If this blood is infected with HIV, users of the contaminated equipment are essentially injecting themselves with the virus.

Injecting drug use is also associated with other high-risk behaviors, most notably unprotected sex with multiple partners, often in exchange for more drugs. Rhodes et al. (1996) examined the existing research on risk behaviors in IDUs and found that the majority are sexually active with both drug injectors and noninjectors, rarely use condoms, and show only scant indications of sexual behavior changes necessary to prevent HIV transmission. Neaigus and colleagues (1996) suggest that sharing needles or syringes and having high-risk personal networks (those with whom IDUs share drugs or sex) significantly increase the risk of HIV transmission. In addition, the disinhibiting effects of certain drugs have been implicated with sexual activity that is highly risky (Finelli, et al., 1993).

The statistics indicate that reducing the risk of HIV transmission in IDUs is imperative to slow the spread of AIDS. Providing IDUs with easy access to clean needles and syringes has been shown to reduce disease transmission and to engage users in treatment. A model needle-exchange program in Tacoma, Washington, showed a sixfold decrease in the number of cases of hepatitis B and a sevenfold decrease in hepatitis C infections among participants. It may be inferred that this type of program can also be successful in reducing the transmission of HIV (Hagan et al., 1995). The National Academy of Sciences has endorsed syringe-exchange programs (SEPs) as an effective strategy to combat the spread of HIV and other infectious diseases in the IDU community (Normand et al., 1995).

The Beth Israel Medical Center in New York City and the North American Syringe Exchange Network conducted a survey of 101 SEPs. The 87 responding SEPs were operating in 71 cities in 28 states and one territory. In follow-up telephone interviews, 46 of the programs reported that they were legal, 20 were illegal but tolerated, and 21 operated underground (CDC, September 22, 1995). SEPs remain highly controversial and inaccessible to many IDUs. Opponents of SEPs believe that providing clean needles for IDUs will foster the further abuse of injection drugs, whereas advocates of this approach stress the overlooked services they offer, such as condom and bleach distribution, testing for HIV and tuberculosis, screening for STDs, counseling, and referral for treatment. Legalizing the purchase of syringes in pharmacies may also encourage IDUs to use clean needles when injecting (Schoenbaum et al., 1996).

An encouraging study by Iguchi et al. (1996) showed that the majority of the IDUs interviewed reported a decline in injection-related risks. Other studies have reported similar trends (Des Jarlais, 1991; Guydish et al., 1990). Reducing rates of sexual risk behaviors in IDUs, however, have shown promising but smaller declines in comparison with risks of injecting drug use. The importance of continuing to provide education to IDUs is evident. Psychoeducational programs such as Training in Interpersonal Skills (TIPS) are an important component of successful treatment. Developed by Platt and colleagues (1995), TIPS helps participants learn to build the skills required to effect behavioral changes.

PRIMARY CARE. Along with a current knowledge of the treatment issues involved in providing competent health care to those with HIV infection, all primary health care providers in today's society must have a working knowledge of "street" drugs and the culture of addiction. Past or current histories of mental illness, physical or sexual abuses, and discrimination make the establishment of rapport and trust with an IDU a long-term process. HIV-infected IDUs respond well to caregivers who avoid the traditional, more inflexible approaches to care ("disease models") and who acknowledge that the priorities of the client and of the provider may not be the same. The harm-reduction model of care (Springer, 1991) recognizes and accepts the IDU's substance use and potential for relapses. Also understood is the fact that not every IDU will be able to comply with prescribed therapies.

Occasionally, written contractual agreements between client and provider may be used to foster safer behaviors or appropriate use of certain medications, such as those prescribed for pain and anxiety, and the complicated regimens required by current antiretroviral treatment. Any care plans developed for HIV-positive IDUs are structured to individual needs, which may be many and complex. A multidisciplinary health care team comprising providers, social/outreach workers, and case managers works collaboratively and respects the autonomy of the client, who is included in all decision making regarding care. Since the chaotic lifestyles caused by substance abuse make it difficult for the client to keep appointments, health systems guided by this model offer urgent care and drop-in times, providing simpler access

to helpful personnel in the event of emergencies. Because homelessness is a common problem among IDUs, more street-based operations should be established to deliver outreach and referral to drug treatment, health care, and social services in the places where IDUs congregate.

ADDICTION TREATMENT. HIV-infected IDUs will be unable to successfully pursue treatment of addiction without a commitment to lifestyle changes. When the decision is made to seek treatment, gaining access to therapy may not be possible, as obstacles often interfere with the process. The existence of waiting lists at methadone detoxification centers and other programs offering treatment to IDUs underscores the need to establish more drug-treatment services in general and for the HIV-infected user in particular. Some drug programs themselves may have barriers to HIV-infected IDUs seeking treatment. Lacking trained personnel to provide physical care in the event of serious illness, a therapeutic community, for example, may bar the admission of someone with advanced disease.

Most treatment programs require abstinence as a condition of inclusion, but Schoenbaum and colleagues (1996) noted that continued injecting drug use was common in methadone-treated IDUs. They suggested that access to clean needles and syringes be included in the strategies designed for IDUs who inject even occasionally. Some HIV-positive IDUs may require permission to continue to use drugs in moderation as a way to cope with physical symptoms (e.g., the use of marijuana for nausea and for appetite enhancement). Concepts such as these are likely to stimulate lively debate and encounter resistance before they can be implemented. The severity of addiction, medical status, social support, psychiatric and drug-treatment histories, as well as program availability, must all be considered before any treatment is offered. Although social workers, community workers, and primary caregivers are able to direct most IDUs for appropriate treatment, referral to a substance-abuse treatment professional may be necessary (Selwyn & O'Connor, 1992).

SOCIAL NEEDS. Most IDUs distrust the institutions established to provide them with assistance, viewing them as confusing, filled with barriers to access, and possibly leading to their arrest. Like health care workers, employees of social service organizations must be educated about the disease of addiction and must acquire negotiating skills to work competently with these clients and provide them with needed services without discrimination, regardless of ethnicity, gender, or sexual orientation. More service organizations need to develop drop-in times if they hope to provide accessible benefits for their clients. Situating various agencies that provide financial, health, nutrition, and housing support in one location, preferably one that is near public transportation, provides an ideal situation but is seldom a reality.

SUMMARY. Working successfully with HIV-infected IDUs is a complex undertaking, which will likely challenge our society for years to come. IDUs must be committed to making significant lifestyle changes. This goal is attainable but requires support from personal social networks and a multidisciplinary health care team using interventions based on harm reduction. Progress may be slow, and relapses will likely occur. Health, social service, and community agencies must recognize and remove barriers to those seeking care before successful outcomes can be expected in this difficult-to-reach group. Education for caregivers and service providers, as well as for HIV-infected IDUs, must be culturally sensitive and directed toward behavioral change. As injecting drug use increases, so too will the incidence of HIV infection unless agressive public health programs to prevent HIV transmission are implemented.

The Incarcerated

The effects of HIV infection are having a serious impact on the nation's correctional facilities, which are unquestionably loci of HIV concentration. HIV infection rates among inmates are reportedly four to six times those of the general population (Gaynes, 1996; CDC, 1993). Considering the many persons detained or confined for drug-related crimes, a significant percentage of whom are HIV-infected IDUs, such statistics are not surprising. In a cross-sectional study of incarcerated persons done in Quebec (Dufour et al., 1996), 9% of the male IDU participants included were infected with HIV.

RISK REDUCTION. Injecting drug use and sexual activity take place behind bars, whether or not a facility provides the means for these activities to occur in a safe manner (Mahon, 1996). Most U.S. correctional facilities expressly forbid risk-reducing measures, such as the provision of clean needles or bleach for IDUs and condoms for sexually active inmates. Attempts to reduce HIV transmission are perceived as encouraging inmates to engage in the prohibited behaviors of sexual relations and injecting drug use and are, therefore, nonexistent in the vast majority of jails and prisons (Ward, 1996). Consequently, noninfected inmates can easily acquire HIV infection during their imprisonment.

Outreach services, such as New York State's AIDS/HIV hotline for prisoners, have been quite successful in assisting incarcerated HIV-positive persons. Unlike most AIDS hotlines, this bilingual service responds to collect calls and is staffed by volunteers, many of whom are ex-offenders living with HIV infection or AIDS. In addition to general HIV treatment and prevention information, the hotline provides prerelease planning services (Nesselroth & Lopez, 1996).

Other prisoner outreach programs have been described. Although the methods used may vary from program to program, their goals remain similar: to increase trust between inmates and prison staff; to educate inmates about high-risk behaviors and ways to prevent HIV transmission; to create a support network for those who are infected with HIV; and to help inmates plan for their release from prison.

TREATMENT. Arrest is frequently the first point of contact with a health provision system for an HIV-infected IDU. Inmates therefore need access to HIV testing and counseling, support groups, competent medical care, and current therapies. Unfortunately, most correctional facilities are unable to meet these requirements because of financial constraints. Ray and associates (1996) reported that it costs nearly 13 times as much to provide medical care for an HIV-infected IDU ($51.40 a day) as it does to care for a noninfected, drug-free inmate ($4.10 a day). Correctional facilities that are experiencing financial problems in providing care to HIV-infected prisoners today will note increased expenses as the disease progresses in those who are already infected and spreads to those who are not.

SUMMARY. All inmates, HIV-infected or not, need the ability to freely discuss their concerns, find constructive ways to deal with them, and overcome the feelings of powerlessness and apathy related to their personal histories and exposure to the criminal justice system. Peer counselors, especially those who are living with HIV or AIDS, appear to improve the chances for successful outcomes in this population (Nesselroth & Lopez, 1996; Schoenfisch & Walsh, 1996). Any outreach programs aimed at reducing risk behaviors and slowing the spread of HIV infection, among both inmates and those in postrelease populations, must be accessible to every inmate and parolee. The importance of providing multilingual HIV education and prevention programs in a culturally sensitive manner cannot be understated.

As of the spring of 1996, the 1991 recommendations made by the National Commission on AIDS, which included programs for distribution of condoms and bleach kits, assurance of bilingual intervention and prevention programs, and aggressive treatment of patients with AIDS, had not been implemented as standards in any U.S. prison (CDC, 1995; Vasquez, 1996).

Commercial Sex Workers

The sex industry employs men, women, and transgendered persons who provide sexual activity in exchange for money or drugs. Services offered, such as brothels, performance, and pornography, are not always illegal. Multiple sexual partners and the high rate of injecting drug use among prostitutes place this subgroup of sex workers at highest risk of HIV infection. Female prostitutes represented 39% of street IDUs in Bern, Switzerland, according to a 1995 study (Burki et al., 1996). In many non-Western countries, the sex industry has been the primary source of HIV transmission to heterosexuals. Serosurveillance studies from India (Pais, 1996) reveal an alarming fact: between 1986 and 1994, the HIV-prevalence rate among sex industry workers rose from 1.6% to 40%, mainly through heterosexual intercourse.

In a study conducted among prostitutes working in legal brothels in Victoria, Australia, sexual activities with clients were found to entail low risk of transmission of HIV, although many prostitutes were at risk of HIV through injecting drug use and unprotected sex with nonpaying private partners (Pyett et al., 1996).

Commercial sex workers may represent one of the most sensitive and difficult-to-reach high-risk populations among those discussed here. They are often wary of outreach programs, whether governmental or privately sponsored, especially when they are also IDUs. Female prostitutes have also been found to be the least likely, among all IDU subgroups, to seek services from rehabilitation clinics or needle-exchange centers (Schoenbaum et al., 1996). Peer outreach, often accomplished within a penal system, has been shown to be a successful method of intervention in these disenfranchised members of society.

SUMMARY. As the incidence of HIV/AIDS infection has declined in homosexual and bisexual men, new high-risk populations have emerged, the most significant being IDUs, who now account for the majority of new AIDS cases in the United States. Injecting drug use is related to other high-risk factors for HIV transmission, particularly unprotected sexual relations with multiple partners. Drug-related offenses and the policies that mandate imprisonment for these crimes are largely responsible for the number of people in U.S. jails and prisons, where HIV infection rates far exceed those seen in the general population. Injecting drug use is also common in commercial sex workers, particularly among prostitutes.

Although each of these special populations has needs that are distinct to them as a group, their basic requirements are commonly shared: recognition as human beings with the potential for change; HIV-prevention education, which focuses on behavioral change, preferably presented by their peers; and obstacle-free access to health and social services provided by people who are knowledgeable and compassionate.

HIV disease has reached epidemic proportions among the most marginalized members of our society, but controversy, paternalism, and political sensitivity have hindered the implementation of strategies that have proved effective in protecting them from a preventable disease. Collaboration between health and social service professionals as well as policy makers, community activists, and members of these special populations must continue until the alarming trends toward increased incidence of AIDS in these populations can be reversed.

REFERENCES

Burki, C., Egger, M., Haemmig, R., et al. (1996). HIV-risk behaviour among street IVDUs attending a shooting room in Bern, Switzerland, 1990 and 1995 (abstract NP/WeC3549). *International Conference on AIDS, 11*(2), 152.

Centers for Disease Control and Prevention. (December 18, 1992). 1993 revised classification system for HIV infection and expanded surveillance case definition for AIDS among adolescents and adults. *Morbidity and Mortality Weekly Report, 41*(RR-17), 1–19.

Centers for Disease Control and Prevention. (June 30, 1993). *HIV/AIDS Surveillance Report, 5*(1).

Centers for Disease Control and Prevention. (June 30, 1995). *HIV/AIDS Surveillance Report, 7*(1).

Centers for Disease Control and Prevention. (1995). AIDS education and prevention programs for adults in prisons and jails and juveniles in correctional facilities, United States, 1994. *Morbidity and Mortality Weekly Report, 45*(13), 268.

Centers for Disease Control and Prevention. (September 22, 1995). Syringe exchange programs—United States, 1994–95. *Morbidity and Mortality Weekly Report, 44*(37), 684–692.

Centers for Disease Control and Prevention. (December 31, 1996). *HIV/AIDS Surveillance Report, 8*(2), 1–39.

Des Jarlais, D.C., Abdul-Quader, A., Tross, S. (1991). Immune deficiency syndrome education project: The impact of indigenous outreach workers as change agents for injecting drug users. *International Journal of Addictions, 26*(12), 1279–1292.

Dufour, A., Alary, M., Poulin, C., et al. (1996). Prevalence and risk behaviours for HIV infection among inmates of a provincial prison in Quebec City. *AIDS, 10*(9), 1009–1015.

Finelli, L., Budd, J., Spitalny, K.C., et al. (1993). Early syphilis: Relationship to sex, drugs, and changes in high-risk behaviors from 1987–1990. *Sexually Transmitted Diseases, 20*(2), 23–28.

Gaynes, E.A. (1996). Prison changes everything: A criminal justice agency serving prisoners living with AIDS/HIV. *International Conference on AIDS, 11*(2), 171.

Guydish, J.R., Abramowitz, A., Woods, W., et al. (1990). Changes in needle sharing behavior among intravenous drug users: San Francisco, 1986–1988. *American Journal of Public Health, 80*(8), 995–997.

Hagan, H., Des Jarlais, D.C., Friedman, S.R., et al. (1995). Reduced risk of hepatitis B and hepatitis C among injecting drug users participating in the Tacoma syringe exchange program. *American Journal of Public Health, 85*(11), 1531–1537.

Iguchi, M.Y., Bux, D.A., Lidz, V., et al. (1996). Changes in HIV risk behavior among injecting drug users: The impact of 21 versus 90 days of methadone detoxification. *AIDS, 10*(14), 1719–1728.

Mahon, N. (1996). New York inmates' HIV risk behaviors: The implications for prevention policy and programs. *American Journal of Public Health, 86*(9), 1211–1215.

MaWhinney, S., Gieseker, K.E., Chiasson, M.A., et al. (1996). Incidence trends by risk group accounting for CDC 1993 definition change (abstract no. MoC 1561). *International Conference on AIDS, 11*(1), 152.

Neaigus, A., Friedman, S.R., Jose, B., et al. (1996). High-risk personal networks and syringe sharing as risk factors for HIV infection among new drug users. *Journal of Acquired Immune Deficiency Syndromes and Human Retrovirology, 11,* 499–509.

Nesselroth, S.L., Lopez, W. (1996). AIDS/HIV hotline for prisoners: Education, counseling and services to an underserved population (abstract no. WeD 3668). *International Conference on AIDS, 11*(2), 172.

Normand, J., Vlahov, D., Moses, L.E. (Eds.). (1995). *Preventing HIV transmission: The role of sterile needles and bleach.* Washington, D.C.: National Academy Press.

Pais, P. (1996). HIV and India: Looking into the abyss. *Tropical Medicine and International Health, 1*(3), 295–304.

Platt, J.J., Husband, D.S.D., Steer, R.A., et al. (1995). Problem-solving skills training: Addressing high-risk behaviors in Newark and Jersey City. In B.S. Brown, G.M. Beschner (Eds.), *Handbook on risk of AIDS* (pp. 483–498). Westport, CT: Greenwood Press.

Pyett, P.M., Haste, B.R., Snow, J. (1996). Risk practices for HIV infection and other STDs amongst female prostitutes working in legalized brothels. *AIDS Care, 8*(1), 85–94.

Ray, R., Stafford, K., Hewett, M., et al. (1996). Medical care costs associated with jail incarceration of people with HIV/AIDS (abstract no. WeD 3667). *International Conference on AIDS, 11*(2), 72.

Rhodes, T., Stimson, G.V., Quirk, A. (1996). Sex, drugs, intervention, and research: From the individual to the social. *Substance Use and Misuse, 31*(3), 375–407.

Schoenbaum, E., Hartel, D., Gourevitch, M. (1996). Needle exchange use among a cohort of injecting drug users. *AIDS, 10*(14), 1729–1734.

Schoenfisch, S., Walsh, M.A. (1996). Meeting the HIV/AIDS prevention needs of high-risk incarcerated populations across Florida's correctional continuum. *International Conference on AIDS, 11*(1), 379.

Selwyn, P., O'Connor, P. (1992). Diagnosis and treatment of substance users with HIV infection. *Primary Care, 19*(1), 119–148.

Springer, E. (1991). Effective AIDS prevention with active drug use: The harm reduction model. In M. Shernoff (Ed.), *Counseling chemically dependent people with HIV illness* (pp. 141–157). New York: Haworth Press.

Vasquez, E. (1996). Prison within a prison. *Positively Aware, 7*(3), 12–14.

Ward, K. (1996). AIDS/HIV in prison: The importance of prevention. *Nursing Standards, 11*(4), 51–52.

9

Culture and Ethnicity

Jacquelyn Haak Flaskerud

Culture and ethnicity have become important concepts in understanding the transmission and prevention of HIV/AIDS because of the disproportionate occurrence of the disease in ethnic communities of color and because AIDS affects so many aspects of life that have cultural meaning: reproduction, birth, death, the roles of women, sexuality, and so forth. The Public Health Service has become aware that standard prevention messages about condom use, multiple sexual partners, anal-receptive intercourse, and sharing of needles have met cultural roadblocks that increase the complexity of the AIDS education campaign. The nature of HIV/AIDS lends itself to different cultural interpretations and explanations (Nicoll et al., 1993; O'Connor, 1996). It is a sexually transmitted disease (STD); it appeared relatively recently without a demonstrable reason; it has a long incubation period, separating infection from death by many years; it is usually lethal and is spreading worldwide; and scientific knowledge of HIV is growing constantly but frequently changing (Nicoll et al., 1993; O'Connor, 1996). Therefore AIDS is important, mysterious, and subject to legitimate speculation. It is a strong candidate for alternative lay beliefs and explanations. Frequently these are rooted in existing, workable lay explanations of the cause, transmission, prevention, and treatment of disease. Beliefs and practices acquired through the family and cultural explanations about other illnesses will also be applied to AIDS. Values and practices related to sexuality, the role of women, the importance of children, and so forth will not be changed simply because of the threat of a new and dangerous disease. This is especially so when

the lay public perceives the health professional and scientific communities as limited in their knowledge of the disease, frequently changing their explanations and proscriptions, and, in some cases, not to be trusted. The force of a cultural worldview is much more persuasive and pervasive than a scientific explanation based on Western biomedicine, not only in ethnic communities of color but in all sociocultural groups (Hufford, 1995).

Health care workers will have to become culturally competent if they are to work credibly and effectively with their various client groups in preventing and treating HIV disease (AAN Expert Panel Report, 1992; Holtgrave et al., 1995). Cultural competence involves a set of congruent behaviors, attitudes, and policies between a health care system, health care professionals, and their clients (Grossman, D. 1994; Misener et al., 1997; Office for Substance Abuse Prevention [OSAP], 1992). Cultural competence facilitates effective assessments and interventions in cross-cultural situations. A culturally competent system of care (health care agency) acknowledges and incorporates at all structural and management levels the importance of culture; an assessment of cross-cultural relations between workers, workers and clients, and communities; and vigilance in policies, procedures, and methods toward the dynamics resulting from cultural differences (AAN Expert Panel Report, 1992; Grossman, D., 1994; OSAP, 1992). Culturally competent caregivers acknowledge and actively pursue expansion of cultural knowledge specific to their clients and the communities they serve and adapt their services to meet culturally unique needs (Misener et al., 1997; O'Connor, 1996). This adaptation might include a change in focus, method, timing, and emphasis, as well as concrete services and treatments that will be accepted. Before cultural competence can be achieved, a basic understanding of the constructs of culture and ethnicity is needed.

CULTURE AND ETHNICITY

There are as many definitions of culture as there are cultural theorists and conceptual models of culture. The definition of culture given here was chosen because of its universality and its goodness-of-fit with the current situation of HIV disease, particularly as it affects ethnic communities of color and gay communities in the United States. Theories of cultural ecology or cultural adaptation (Anderson, 1973; Edgerton, 1971) provide a conceptualization of culture and environment that includes the major variables identified by the relevant social, behavioral, and medical scientists in the field (see Amaro, 1995; Belgrave & Randolph, 1993; CDC, May 10, 1996; Cochran & Mays, 1993; Holtgrave et al., 1995; Jenkins et al., 1993; Doll & Beeker, 1996; Marin & Gomez, 1994; McKirnan et al., 1996).

Culture is passed on by the family of origin through child-rearing practices from infancy onward; it is learned, shared, and transmitted in patterned ways. Theories of cultural ecology or cultural adaptation propose that the culture of a social group arises in response to the environmental resources available to that particular group (Fig. 9–1). The environment includes natural and physical habitat, resources available, and other human groups competing for these same resources. It includes also constraints imposed by the environment, such as racism, discrimination, segregation, and limited access to health care (Northridge & Shepard, 1997).

Culture embodies and consists of economic structures, social structures, ideology, and art and artifacts. Economic structures include economic opportunities and power differentials, sources of income, and available occupations provided by the particular environment into which one is born. Social structures arise to support the economic structures. Type and function of social structures are influenced by the economic structures and income opportunities. Social structures

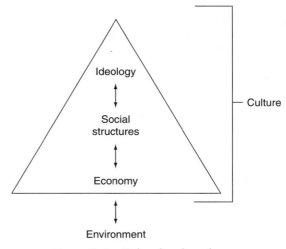

Figure 9–1 ■ Cultural ecology theory.

include family, kin, fictive kin and friend networks, gender roles and dynamics, social status, political organizations, social and religious organizations, and so forth. Finally, there arises an ideology that endorses, validates, and legitimates the social structures and economy. Ideology consists of values, beliefs, attitudes, behaviors, morals, ideals, ethics, and so forth. Art and artifacts are expressions of ideology, social structures, and economic structures.

Members of a particular social group who share a culture learn and transmit it in patterned ways, often without being cognitively aware that their worldview differs from that of persons with other cultural backgrounds (O'Connor, 1996; Wenger, 1993). In the United States the worldview of ethnic people of color is influenced by their native cultures (e.g., West African, Mexican, Chinese, and so forth), by Anglo-American orientation and values, and by minority experiences of discrimination, prejudice, and segregation (Airhihenbuwa et al., 1992; Jagers, 1996).

Beyond their familial cultures of origin and rearing, people are influenced by group cultures in which they have membership (O'Connor, 1996). In that sense, the term *culture* has been applied to gay culture, teen culture, rock culture, drug culture, and so on. From this perspective, culture may also be taught through the social group rather than the family (Misener et al., 1997; O'Connor, 1996). It is acquired in adolescence or young adulthood, and not from infancy on. It embodies the beliefs and practices of social groups other than the family. Finally, it functions to integrate a person into his or her social group. In some groups (for instance, white gay men) the culture may be well developed, strong, supportive, and sustaining. It may include shared social and community structures and resources; shared political structures; a political agenda; shared discrimination, stigma, and isolation; and shared values, lifestyle, and practices (Grossman, 1994, 1995). In other cases (for example, teen culture) it may mark only a passing phase in one's life.

Ethnicity differs from the formal definition of culture given here. Ethnicity is based on a shared sense of peoplehood related to national or regional origin and sometimes on shared language, religion, and customs. However, despite this difference, several investigators have presented an argument for ethnic culture (CDC, June 25, 1993; Hu et al., 1995; Wyatt, 1991). Ethnic culture includes a body of shared cultural meanings that influence beliefs, practices, and relationships with other members of the ethnic group and with the larger society. The term *ethnicity* is chosen here as opposed to *race* or *racial groups* because of its better fit with HIV disease. Use of the term *race* would imply a biologic or genetic risk factor for HIV disease in members of a particular racial group; in the case of HIV, this risk factor is not known to exist (CDC, June 25, 1993; Hu et al., 1995; Kaufman & Cooper, 1995; Wyatt, 1991). Ethnicity, on the other hand, may reflect cultural or learned values, behavioral patterns, social class and other psychosocial factors, and demographic and regional variations (CDC, June 25, 1993; Wyatt, 1991). Ethnicity is here considered a risk marker rather than a risk factor for HIV disease (CDC, June 25, 1993; Hu, et al., 1995).

It should be established at the outset that levels of ethnic association or identification differ within ethnic groups and with individual members of a particular ethnic group (O'Connor, 1996). Levels of ethnic identification are usually measured and observed in frequency and exclusivity of personal and social contacts, language used and preferred, preferred media, values endorsed and practiced, and preference for foods, dress, and other customs (Daroszewski, 1995; Keefe & Padilla, 1987; Marin et al., 1987; Marin & Marin, 1990; Suinn et al., 1987; Wyatt, 1991). For persons with low levels of ethnic identification or association, ethnicity might be recognized only at holidays or in awareness of surnames.

ETHNICITY AND EPIDEMIOLOGY OF HIV DISEASE

HIV surveillance data are collected for four broad ethnic communities of color in the United States and for an equally broad community of white persons. These groups are categorized here as African-Americans, Latinos/Hispanics, Asian-Americans and Pacific Islanders, American Indians and Alaskan Natives, and European-Americans. These broad divisions do not account separately for other groups, such as those from the Middle East and Near East or from Australia and New Zealand.

African-Americans make up the largest ethnic community of color in the United States, comprising 12% of the population (Bureau of the Census, 1997). African-Americans include those whose ancestors were brought here as slaves in the seventeenth century, as well as recent immigrants from the Caribbean, Africa, and Europe (National Commission on Acquired Immune Deficiency Syndrome [NCA], 1992). Latinos/Hispanics make up 11% of the U.S. population and include Spanish-speaking and Spanish-surnamed persons from Central and South America, the Caribbean, and Spain (Bureau of the Census, 1997). The largest group are Mexican-Americans (64%), followed by other Central and South Americans (14%), Puerto Ricans (11%), and Cubans (5%) (NCA, 1992). Asian-Americans and Pacific Islanders are the third largest community of color in the United States (3.6%) and the fastest growing. They speak more than 100 different languages and are grouped together because of similar regional origins. Asian-Americans include Japanese, Chinese, Koreans, Pilipinos, and Southeast Asians. Pacific Islanders include Native Hawaiians and immigrants from Guam, Samoa, and other small island nations having a close relationship with the United States (NCA, 1992). American Indians and Alaskan Natives make up less than 1% of the U.S. population and include 557 tribes and villages with government-to-government relationships with the United States (Bureau of Indian Affairs, 1998). Each has its own language, customs, and history (Kutenai, 1996; Bureau of the Census, 1997). About half live in urban areas of the United States, one fourth on reserved lands, and one fourth in rural areas (NCA, 1992). For HIV surveillance purposes, European-Americans (whites) compose the remainder of the U.S. population (75%), presumably including Australians and New Zealanders and encompassing people from the Middle East (Arab countries) and Near East (e.g., India, Pakistan). As may be seen from each of these broad categorizations, a wide range of ethnic groups, cultures, languages, value systems, beliefs, and practices are included within each category.

The African-American community has been affected the most severely by the HIV epidemic. African-Americans make up 35% of all persons with AIDS (CDC, June 30, 1997). Among-African American men, those who risk exposure to HIV are men who have sex with men (MSM) (38%), injecting drug users (IDUs) (36%), and MSM who are also IDUs (8%). From January 1989 to June 1994, the largest proportionate increase of HIV (79%) among MSM occurred among black men (CDC, June 2, 1995). For African-American MSM in the youngest age group (13 to 24 years), rates increased by 31%. Together with Latino young MSM, African-American young MSM now account for the majority of young MSM with AIDS (Denning et al., 1996). Other investigators have reported a 65% increase in AIDS incidence through heterosexual contact among youthful (13 to 25 years) African-Americans (Denning & Fleming, 1997). These data represent a spread of HIV disease to youthful populations, especially young women. African-American women make up 55.7% of all adult women in the United States with AIDS (CDC, June 30, 1997). Injecting drug use is the most common means of exposure (46%), followed by heterosexual contact with an IDU or with an HIV-infected person who is not an IDU (36%). In one study, exposure to AIDS among black women as a result of sex with bisexual men was higher than among white women because black bisexual men were more likely to have sex with women than were white men (McKirnan et al., 1995). Although the highest seroprevalence rates of HIV are concentrated in urban areas, primarily along the East Coast, several studies have documented the spread of HIV to nonurban African-American women, principally those living in the U.S. South and East (Neal et al., 1997; Solomon et al., 1996; Sowell et al., 1996, 1997). In these studies, women were unaware that they were at risk of acquiring infection that was occurring principally through heterosexual exposure. African-American children account for 58% of all pediatric AIDS cases in the United States. Of these, 95% acquired HIV infection perinatally from infected mothers and 3% from transfusion with blood products. Contrasting rates of AIDS by ethnic group are provided for men, women, and children in Tables 9–1 to 9–3.

Latinos/Hispanics make up 18% of reported AIDS cases and, together with African-Americans, account for 53% of all cases. Among Latino

Table 9–1 ▪ Percent of Total AIDS Cases in Men by Ethnicity and by Exposure Category, June 30, 1997

Total (n = 511,934*) 100% Exposure Category	European-American (n = 256,353) 50%	African-American (n = 160,984) 31.4%	Hispanic/Latino (n = 88,756) 17.3%	Asian/Pacific Islander (n = 3850) <1%	American Indian/ Alaskan Native (n = 1390) <1%
Male-male sexual contact (MSM)	76	38	44	75	59
Injecting drug use (IDU)	9	36	37	5	15
MSM/IDU	8	8	7	3	17
Receipt of blood products†	2	1	1	5	3
Heterosexual contact	2	7	5	3	2
Unidentified risk	3	11	7	9	5

*Includes 601 men whose ethnicity is unknown.
†Includes factor VIII concentrate (hemophilia).
Total United States: 612,078
Total Adults: 604,176
Total Children: 7,902

men, 44% were exposed to HIV through male-male sexual contact, 37% through injecting drug use, and 7% through male-male sexual contact and injection drug use. Among Latino MSM, rates of AIDS increased 61% from June 1989 to June 1994 (CDC, June 2, 1995). Among young Latino MSM (13 to 24 years), rates increased 39% and the proportion of young MSM who were Latino increased from 15% to 21% (Denning et al., 1996). Of the total persons with AIDS among U.S. adolescents (13 to 19 years of age), 20% are Latino/Hispanic (Denning & Fleming, 1997). Latino women account for 20.2% of the total AIDS cases among women. For women, exposure is principally through injecting drug use (43%) and heterosexual contact with IDUs or bisexual men (46%) (CDC, June 30, 1997; Martinez & Diaz, 1997). Pediatric cases of AIDS among Latinos make up 23% of all U.S. pediatric cases. Perinatal transmission accounts for 92% of cases.

Exposure to HIV varies among Latinos according to ethnicity (Martinez & Diaz, 1997). Among men born in Central and South America, Cuba, and Mexico, about 53%, 58%, and 60%, respectively, of reported cases were associated with male-male sexual contact and fewer than 10% with injection drug use. In contrast, among men born in Puerto Rico, 61% were exposed through injection drug use and 22% through male-male sexual contact. A similar pattern was seen in women. Women born in Central and South America, Cuba, and Mexico were exposed through heterosexual contact with HIV-infected men. According to Ramirez and colleagues (1994), a study in Mexico showed that about 59% of these men were infected through sex with other men (35% homosexual and 23.7% bisexual). In contrast, women born in Puerto Rico or in the United States but of Puerto Rican ancestry are more likely to be infected through injecting drug use or sex with IDUs (Martinez & Diaz, 1997; Murphy et al., 1996).

Currently, Asian-Americans and Pacific Islanders account for fewer than 1% of AIDS cases in the United States, whereas these groups make up 3% of the total population of the United States. For a variety of reasons, there may be underreporting in this group (Choy, 1995). The distribution of AIDS in these groups resembles the epidemiology of HIV disease in the early years of the epidemic for other ethnic groups. Among men, 75% have been exposed through male-male sexual contact, 5% through injecting drug use, and 3% through male-male sexual contact combined with injection drug use. Among Asian/Pacific Islander MSM, rates of AIDS have increased 55% from June 1989 to June 1994 (CDC, June 2, 1995). Women have been exposed to HIV through heterosexual contact (46%), receipt of blood products (19%), and injecting drug use (17%). Asian-American and Pacific Islander children have been exposed through perinatal transmission (66%) and receipt of blood or blood products (31%). The Asian-American–Pacific Islander community is considered to be in

Table 9–2 ▪ Percent of Total AIDS Cases in Women by Ethnicity and by Exposure Category, June 30, 1997

Total (n = 92,242*) 100% Exposure Category	European-American (n = 21,319) 23%	African-American (n = 51,410) 55.7%	Hispanic/Latino (n = 18,663) 20.2%	Asian/Pacific Islander (n = 479) <1%	American Indian/ Alaskan Native (n = 26) <1%
IDU	43	46	43	17	48
Sexual contact IDU MSM Other	39	36	46	46	36
Receipt of blood products[†]	8	2	3	19	5
Unidentified risk	9	16	8	19	11

*Includes 110 women whose ethnicity is unknown.
[†]Includes factor VIII concentrate (hemophilia).

Table 9–3 ▪ Percent of Total AIDS Cases in Children by Ethnicity and by Exposure Category, June 30, 1997

Total (n = 7902*) 100% Exposure Category	European-American (n = 1400) 17%	African-American (n = 4586) 58%	Hispanic/Latino (n = 1833) 23.2%	Asian/Pacific Islander (n = 41) <1%	American Indian/ Alaskan Native (n = 26) <1%
Perinatal	74	95	92	66	96
Receipt of blood products	13	2	5	24	—
Hemophilia	11	1	2	7	4
Risk not identified	2	2	1	2	—

*Includes 16 children whose ethnicity is unknown.

the early stages of a growing HIV epidemic in this group in the United States (Choi et al., 1996). Because of the relative insularity of the ethnic groups composing these communities, once an infectious disease takes hold, it spreads rapidly. If prevention efforts are not instituted, the epidemic in the United States in these groups is expected to resemble that in the African-American and Latino communities. Meanwhile, a changing epidemiology is projected worldwide by the year 2000, with the largest proportion of HIV infections occurring in Asian and Pacific Rim countries (Mann & Tarantola, 1996, pp. 5–40; Weniger & Brown, 1996).

Currently, fewer than 1% of AIDS cases in the United States have occurred among American Indians and Alaskan Natives. However, there is evidence that AIDS may be undercounted in these groups and misrepresented as occurring in white or Latino groups (Barney, 1996; CDC, March 6, 1998). AIDS surveillance data show that, among Native American men, 58% were exposed through male-male sexual contact, 16% through injecting drug use, and 17% through a combination of these exposure routes (CDC, March 6, 1998). The rates of AIDS in American Indian/Alaskan Native MSM increased 77% from June 1989 to June 1994 (CDC, June 2, 1995). Among women, 44% were exposed through injecting drug use, 36% through heterosexual contact, and 5% through receipt of blood products. Of pediatric cases, 96% occurred through perinatal transmission. Seroprevalence studies of HIV infection in Native Americans have demonstrated that rates may be much higher than those reflected in AIDS surveillance data

(Barney, 1996; CDC, March 6, 1998). AIDS cases have been reported in every age group for Native Americans and in every Indian Health Service Area (NCA, 1992). From 1993 to 1996, AIDS cases in Native Americans more than doubled, which is higher than the rate of increase in Latinos and African-Americans (CDC, March 6, 1998).

Americans of European origin (whites) account for the remainder of AIDS cases (45%) (CDC, June 30, 1997). European-Americans comprise 72.7% of the total population of the United States. White men account for 50% of AIDS cases among men. White men were exposed through male-male sexual contact (76%) and through injecting drug use (9%); 8% were exposed through these two categories combined (CDC, June 30, 1997). Among white MSM, rates of AIDS increased 14% from June 1989 to June 1994 (CDC, June 2, 1995). In young white MSM (13 to 24 years), the rates decreased 31% during this same time period (Denning et al., 1996). White women account for about 23% of total AIDS cases among women. White women have been exposed to HIV through injecting drug use (43%), heterosexual contact (39%), and receipt of blood products (8%). Of children with AIDS, fewer than 18% are European-Americans. White children with AIDS were exposed principally through perinatal transmission (74%) and through the receipt of blood products, including factor VIII concentrate (24%).

The epidemiology of AIDS makes it clear that the disease is affecting ethnic communities of color disproportionately in the United States (AIDS Alert, 1997; Denning & Fleming, 1997;

Denning et al., 1996). Of all ethnic groups, the rate of reported AIDS cases per 100,000 people in 1995 was highest among African-Americans (92.6 per 100,000). The rate among Latinos was 46.2 per 100,000; the rate among whites was 15.4 per 100,000; the rate among American Indian/Alaska Natives was 12.3 per 100,000; and the rate among Asian/Pacific Islanders was 6.2 per 100,000. In 1995, for the first time, African-Americans and Latinos combined represented the majority of cases in the United States (CDC, 1997).

ENVIRONMENTAL AND HEALTH SYSTEM CONSTRAINTS

As noted in the discussion of the conceptualization of culture, a group's economic and social structures, and values, beliefs, and practices do not arise in isolation. Instead, they are a response to the environmental resources available and to environmental and health system constraints imposed on the group. So, too, AIDS is not only the result of individual behavior but occurs in an environmental and societal context. For ethnic communities of color, this environmental context includes poverty, crime, gang violence, poor schools, deteriorating housing, segregation, economic and social racism and discrimination, and often an absence of social, political, and economic structures and of health and human services (Airhihenbuwa et al., 1992; Blank, 1995; Cochran & Mays, 1993; Seals, 1996).

Ethnic communities of color are affected adversely by differentials in income and employment. On average, people of color have lower income and higher unemployment than whites. The poverty rate in 1996 was 28.4% for African-Americans, 29.4% for Latinos, 14.5% for Asian-Americans and Pacific Islanders, 31.6% for American Indians/Alaskan Natives, and 11.2% for whites (Bureau of the Census, 1996). The unemployment rate was 14.8% for American Indians/Alaskan Natives, 13.7% for African-Americans, 11.9% for Latinos, and 6.7% for whites in 1997 (Department of Labor, 1997). Poverty and ill health are often correlated, probably because of decreased access to resources, health education, and health care (Carlisle et al., 1996; Guralnik & Leveille, 1997; Link & Phelan, 1996). The relationship of poverty and ill health plays a large part

in any explanation of the proportionately high prevalence of HIV disease among people of African descent in both the United States and Africa. Poverty is only one indicator of social inequalities that create vulnerability to increased morbidity and mortality from HIV disease (Evans et al., 1994; Flaskerud, 1998; Link & Phelan, 1996). Other resource inequalities occur in knowledge, power, prestige and social connections.

Since World War II, African-Americans have become an increasingly urbanized population, moving from rural areas in the South to Northern urban centers that are experiencing inner-city decay (abandonment by commerce, by social, political, and economic structures, and by health and human services). The same kind of migration from rural to urban areas has occurred in several of the Latino ethnic groups and in Native Americans. The inner-city areas to which people have migrated are characterized by open drug markets, oppressive environmental and social conditions, and few economic opportunities (Seals, 1996). High rates of addiction to injection drugs have been disproportionately associated with inner-city urban life, especially in the Northeast (Montoya & Atkinson, 1996; Pivnick et al., 1994). Among Native Americans, however, high rates of drug use are found also in those residing on reservations (CDC, March 6, 1998). Significantly, injecting drug use has played a major role in spreading HIV not only through the use of shared needles but also through sexual contact and perinatal transmission among IDUs.

Racism and discrimination have resulted in differentials in the reporting of cases of HIV, in health education, and in health care (CDC, December 27, 1996; Crystal et al., 1995; Hu et al., 1995). AIDS cases in blacks and Hispanics are counted more stringently than in whites, and blacks and Hispanics are undercounted in the census (Hu et al., 1995). This results in underreporting of cases in whites rather than overreporting in other groups. Health education is limited in communities of color from several perspectives. There are fewer resources and programs in black and Hispanic middle and secondary schools; a higher dropout rate in these schools results in less education; ethnic people of color entering the health professions are underrepresented; and much of prevention education focuses on a white gay lifestyle (Dalton, 1993; Hu et al., 1995; McClary, 1996). Conversely, in the Asian community, HIV infection may be underreported because of stigma and the masking of illness as cancer or leukemia for fear of deportation (Choy, 1995). Underreporting also leads to differentials in health education and health care.

Health care is limited in impoverished urban communities (Guralnik & Leveille, 1997) and in rural areas, including reservations (CDC, March 6, 1998). The preexisting health of populations in these communities is poor, increasing the risk of transmission. Concurrent sexually transmitted diseases, pregnancy, and drug use may all undermine immunity and thereby facilitate transmission. The quality of health care may also be lower in poor urban areas and on reservations because there are fewer health professionals and other resources (CDC, December 27, 1996, March 6, 1998). Significantly, clinical trials of drugs for the treatment of HIV disease have failed to adequately enroll people of color (CDC, February 28, 1997; Simon et al., 1996). This failure may be related to the high numbers of IDUs in these communities and the stigma of drug abuse and to issues related to poverty and gender (CDC, February 28, 1997; Crystal et al., 1995; Lester et al., 1995). As a result, however, ethnic people of color have not had early access to experimental treatments available through clinical trials (CDC, February 28, 1997; Battle et al., 1996; Diaz et al., 1995; Lauver et al., 1995). Crystal and colleagues (1995) reported ethnic differences in survival time of patients treated with zidovudine. African-Americans had decreased survival time because their disease was more advanced when zidovudine therapy was started and because use of prophylaxis therapy for *Pneumocystis carinii* pneumonia was less frequent.

The social, political, and economic resources that the gay white community has been able to mobilize in the fight against HIV are not available in poor communities or in gay communities of color (Croteau et al., 1993; Roman, 1993; McKirnan et al., 1995; Ramirez et al., 1994). The absence of health and human services has resulted in notable disparities in health status between the general U.S. population and ethnic communities of color. Average life expectancy is lower and the infant and maternal mortality rates are higher in African-Americans, Latinos, and Native Ameri-

cans than in the general population (CDC, March 1, 1996; Singh & Yu, 1996). Particular diseases affect each community disproportionately. High rates of other STDs, substance abuse, diabetes, tuberculosis, and death from cardiovascular disease, stroke, and homicide affect the African-American community (Carlisle et al., 1996; CDC, August, 1993; Guralnik & Leveille, 1997; Morris, 1996). Among Latinos, the rates of tuberculosis, gonorrhea, hypertension, heart disease, arthritis, and diabetes are disproportionately high (Artemis, 1996; Campos-Outcalt & Ryan, 1995; Carter et al., 1996; Guralnik & Leveille, 1997). Health problems are exacerbated in this population by alarmingly low levels of health insurance coverage (CDC, December 27, 1996). The health status of Native Americans is affected by high rates of STDs, tuberculosis, diabetes, heart disease, drug use, and alcoholism (Campos-Outcalt et al., 1995; Carter et al., 1996; CDC, March 6, 1998). Among other health problems, Asian-Americans and Pacific Islanders are affected by two infectious diseases—hepatitis B and tuberculosis—at much higher rates than the general population (NCA, 1992; Pickwell, 1996). Poor health status and the various diseases described contribute to the AIDS epidemic by compromising immunity and facilitating transmission of the virus or expression of disease (Royce et al., 1997). It is possible also that competing health and social concerns of ethnic communities of color (cancer, heart disease, poverty, violence) dominate people's attention and thereby indirectly contribute to the AIDS epidemic (Stevenson & Davis, 1994). Lack of access to health care means that the opportunistic infections and neoplasms associated with AIDS go untreated and the death rate from AIDS is higher than in those persons with adequate health care and treatment (CDC, June 27, 1997; Crystal et al., 1995). With this background in environmental and health system constraints and societal inequalities, the knowledge, attitudes, and practices of the various ethnic groups are discussed. These are placed in the context of the social structures and ideology associated with various cultures. However, it is important to remember that the cultures of ethnic people of color in the United States reflect a combination of their native culture (e.g., West African, Mexican, Korean, and so forth), Anglo-American orientation and values, and minority experience (e.g., discrimination, prejudice, and so forth) (Airhi-henbuwa et al., 1992; Jagers, 1996).

KNOWLEDGE AND BELIEFS

Since 1987 the National Health Interview Survey has included questions about AIDS (see Barrios et al., 1993; Choi et al., 1994; Grinstead et al., 1997; Schoenborn et al., 1994). From this survey, it is possible to compare by gender, ethnicity, and age the knowledge, attitudes, beliefs, and behaviors of African-Americans, Latinos, and whites. Asians and Native Americans have not been included in this national survey to date. More regional surveys of AIDS knowledge, attitudes, and behaviors have been conducted in all these groups (see, for instance, Chang & Hill, 1996; Choi et al., 1996; Flaskerud et al., 1996, 1997; Kalichman et al., 1996; Peterson et al., 1996; Marin & Gomez, 1994; Norris et al., 1996; Tabet et al., 1996). In these studies, general knowledge of the virus and the three primary modes of HIV transmission was uniformly high. Greater levels of knowledge were correlated with higher education and level of acculturation; however, the large majority of all respondents were aware of the major exposure categories (Chang & Hill, 1996; Erickson, 1997; Flaskerud & Uman, 1993; Flaskerud et al., 1997; Marin & Gomez, 1994).

Despite knowledge of transmission and willingness to learn, perception of personal risk often is not related to knowledge or, in other cases, to actual practices (Battle et al., 1996; Lauver et al., 1995; Ramirez et al., 1994; Flaskerud & Nyamathi, 1996; Flaskerud et al., 1996, 1997). As of this writing, 55% of cases of AIDS now occur in ethnic people of color, with African-Americans (35%) and Latinos (18%) making up the bulk of that number. Regardless, the belief persists that AIDS is a white person's disease, specifically a gay white man's disease. For example, African-American adolescents are not aware of their own particular risk. African-American and Latino women do not recognize their risk; and Asians believe that they are not at risk (Choi et al., 1996; Stevenson & Davis, 1994; Wells & Mayer, 1997). It is possible that women may be unaware of their risk, even though they are aware of the major transmission routes, because bisexual behavior is often not acknowledged in ethnic communities

of color (Doll & Beeker, 1996; McKirnan et al., 1995; Ramirez et al., 1994). In addition, perception of risk (multiple sexual partners) did not affect risk behaviors of a sample of women attending a family-planning clinic because of a perception of invulnerability to HIV (Eversley et al., 1993). In other cases, perception of risk among women did not affect risk behaviors because of power differentials in the male-female relationship (Amaro, 1995; Bayer, 1994; Jenkins et al., 1993).

There is less knowledge of the availability of HIV testing than there is of modes of transmission (Grinstead et al., 1997). In addition, in several studies fewer respondents were aware of the availability of medications to extend life (Graham et al., 1994; Fahs et al., 1994; Simon et al., 1996). The majority of respondents were aware of the efficacy of condoms but, again, fewer than were aware of the modes of transmission (Flaskerud & Uman, 1993; Grinstead et al., 1997; Simon et al., 1996). There are also inaccurate beliefs that the use of other forms of contraception (e.g., diaphragms, spermicidal foams, vasectomy) will prevent AIDS (Flaskerud et al., 1996).

Although correct knowledge of HIV transmission is high, many inaccurate beliefs about casual transmission have continued. Chief among these are beliefs about transmission by mosquitos, airborne transmission through coughing and sneezing, and transmission through eating food or from dishes handled by someone with HIV (Choy, 1995; Flaskerud et al., 1997; Flaskerud & Uman, 1993; Herek & Capitanio, 1994). Beliefs also persist about transmission through other body fluids (sweat, tears, saliva) or through contact with germs, dirty toilet seats or furniture, or water in swimming pools and spas. In addition, there are beliefs that AIDS is the result of evil forces, "bad" spirits, offense of ancestors, or a punishment from God for individual or collective sins characterized by sexual excess and drug use (Flaskerud & colleagues, 1989, 1991a, 1991b; Kerr, 1993; Martin et al., 1995; Nicoll et al., 1993; Suarez, et al., 1996). Many of these beliefs persist because of their congruence and intuitive fit with general conceptualizations of the cause of disease (Flaskerud & colleagues, 1989, 1991a, 1991b; Kerr, 1993; Martin et al., 1995; Nicoll et al., 1993; O'Connor, 1996; Suarez et al., 1996). Beliefs about casual transmission, although they are not dangerous, should be corrected because they lead to unnecessary fear, stigmatization, and isolation of persons who are infected.

More dangerous beliefs are those concerned with how AIDS may be prevented or avoided (Erickson, 1997; Flaskerud et al., 1996). Among these are beliefs that AIDS can be prevented by washing after sex or by ejaculating outside the partner and then drinking a lot of water to induce copious urination. Other dangerous beliefs are that one can use antibiotics prophylactically, that antibiotics (especially penicillin), if taken immediately after intercourse, can prevent or cure AIDS, and that there is a vaccine available to cure AIDS.

Recently, a series of dangerous beliefs have evolved surrounding the use of protease inhibitors and the consequent reduction in viral load, sometimes to undetectable levels (Gorman, 1997; Randolph, 1997; Shernoff & Ball, 1997). A religious interpretation of this occurrence is that the virus has disappeared from the infected person's blood because of a miracle, God's direct intervention in healing the person. This belief is based on a deep and profound spiritual faith that is common among some religious groups (Gregonis, 1997; Martin et al., 1995; Randolph, 1997). The danger in this belief is that infected persons will believe they are no longer infected and pass on the virus through risky sexual or other transmission routes. There is also a danger that people will no longer avoid infection because they believe there is a religious cure. Community-based AIDS researchers and physicians have warned against the dangers of this interpretation in the African-American community (Wyatt et al., 1997).

Another belief that has surfaced is that the protease inhibitors can be used as "morning-after pills" (CDC, July 1997). In this belief, the risk of transmission is minimized and AIDS seems more benign because people think that if they take the medications after sexual intercourse or other exposure they can prevent infection with HIV (Shernoff & Ball, 1997; Katz & Gerberding, 1997). These beliefs are furthered by physicians at some U.S. clinics who are willing to prescribe a cocktail of drugs that include protease inhibitors as morning-after AIDS treatment (Gorman, 1997) and by public knowledge of the availability of these agents to health care workers as postexposure prophylaxis for occupational exposure to HIV (CDC, July 1997). Related dangerous beliefs are that people can have unprotected sex because their viral load is low as a result of the use of protease inhibitors (Shernoff & Ball, 1997). In all of these beliefs the risk of HIV transmission is minimized, as are the serious and debilitating side effects of the anti-HIV drug cocktail and its huge cost (McDuffie, 1997). Furthermore, it is possible that overuse of the antiviral cocktail could unleash a new strain of drug-resistant HIV viruses (Katz & Gerberding, 1997).

There also are inaccurate beliefs about vulnerability. For example, some believe that people who are thin or look sick are more vulnerable to infection or are already infected. Others believe that people who are fat or well nourished are protected from AIDS and are therefore safer as sexual partners (CDC, August 1993; Flaskerud & colleagues, 1989, 1991a, 1991b; Martin et al., 1995; Nicoll et al., 1993). Unlike beliefs about casual transmission of HIV, these beliefs represent an increased risk of infection if they are used to justify unsafe behavior.

Finally, there is a distrust of the medical and scientific communities and government, as well as fear and anger born of past and current medical and government practices in the gay community and ethnic communities of color that may discourage people from following public health service proscriptions for the prevention of HIV transmission (Bayer, 1994; Herek & Capitanio, 1994; Ostrow, 1993). There are several beliefs related to genocide. In the gay community there was a belief that HIV was introduced by the government in the hepatitis B vaccine trials in gay men (Ostrow, 1993). In the Asian community there is the belief that AIDS is a form of genocide brought to them by white men (Choy, 1995). In African-American communities, one powerful source of the fear of genocide has a basis in past experience with public health professionals and the government—the Tuskegee syphilis study (Guinan, 1993; Richardson, 1997; Thomas & Quinn, 1991). The Tuskegee study by the U.S. Public Health Service of untreated syphilis in black men extended from 1932 to 1972, long beyond the advent of effective treatment. The legacy of that study in the AIDS epidemic has led to legitimate mistrust by African-Americans of the Public Health Service and to the belief that AIDS is a form of genocide (Thomas & Quinn, 1991).

Current fears of genocide include the belief that HIV was deliberately introduced into the African-American community by scientists who were studying the virus (Cochran & Mays, 1993; Richardson, 1997). An alternative belief is that U.S. scientists accidentally introduced the virus but are allowing its spread among African-Americans because of racist motives to control population (Guinan, 1993; Nicoll et al., 1993).

Fueling these beliefs are reports from South Africa that the AIDS-prevention campaign in the black townships has been abandoned. The suspicion is that the intention of this move is to allow the majority black population to be devastated by AIDS within the next 10 years, so that it will pose no political threat (Ryan, 1997, pp. 268–284). In addition, in both Africa and the United States the emphasis on the use of condoms to prevent AIDS is viewed as an attempt to reduce pregnancies and births among African-Americans and thus control the size of the black population on both continents (Bayer, 1994; Cochran & Mays, 1993; Nicoll et al., 1993; Ostrow, 1993; Stevenson & Davis, 1994). Finally, needle-exchange programs are viewed by some as an attempt to increase the use of injection drugs in the African-American community (Bradley-Springer, 1997; Ostrow, 1993; Schilling et al., 1991).

Among Latinos and other immigrant populations, there is a distrust of government related to HIV testing programs. These programs are seen as a means of locating undocumented immigrants and deporting them. Alternatively, HIV testing is seen as a means of uncovering infection in documented immigrants and then deporting them because persons with HIV are not eligible to immigrate (Artemis, 1996; Pickwell, 1996). In a study offering free HIV testing and counseling to low-income Latino women in Los Angeles, these barriers to testing had to be overcome before participants would enroll (Flaskerud, personal observation, 1994; Flaskerud et al., 1997). The same fears of deportation may affect HIV testing and prevention programs in Asian-American communities. Compounding this situation is the fact that persons who have HIV disease may not seek treatment because they fear that they will be reported to the Immigration and Naturalization Service.

Several other lay beliefs about prevention and treatment practices may have positive influences on the prevention of HIV transmission and on the expression of disease. These are addressed in depth later in this chapter, in the section on Behaviors and Practices.

ATTITUDES AND VALUES

In addition to knowledge and beliefs, attitudes, moral ideals, and values also influence behaviors and practices. Homophobia and the stigmatization of gay men is a major problem in ethnic communities of color as well as in society at large (Alonzo & Reynolds, 1995; Grossman, 1994, 1995; Herek & Capitanio, 1994). Homophobia results in social and emotional isolation from family and friends, disapproval, prejudice, judgments of shame and immorality, and even violence against persons identified as gay (Alonzo & Reynolds, 1995; Armendariz et al., 1997; Grossman, 1994, 1995; Herek & Capitanio, 1994). Homophobia and the stigmatization of gay men has been reported to be especially intense in ethnic communities of color, causing both the community and gay persons to practice denial and concealment (Armendariz et al., 1997; Chang & Hill, 1996; Choi et al., 1996; Choy, 1995; Martin et al., 1995; Peterson et al., 1995). These attitudes have been reported for African-Americans, Latinos, Asian-Americans and Pacific Islanders, and Native Americans. In these communities, homosexuality is generally denied, AIDS is often seen as a gay white disease, and bisexuality may be practiced to conceal male-male sexual contact (Doll & Beeker, 1996; Chang & Hill, l996; Choy, 1995; Jenkins et al., 1993; McKirnan et al., 1995; Ramirez et al., 1994). In contrast, in some Native American communities, homosexuality has a traditional social role for men but not for women (CNA, 1993).

Negative attitudes of families toward homosexuality may be one reason for concealment and denial (Choy, 1995; Croteau et al., 1993; Grossman, 1994, 1995; Peterson et al., 1995; Ramirez et al., 1994). The absence of a viable gay subculture to support and sustain gay men may be another reason for concealment (Croteau et al., 1993; Doll & Beeker, 1996; McKirnan et al., 1995). Gay subcultures may not develop in communities of color because of severe stigma, hatred, and even violence, and also for economic reasons. Living separately from one's family may be a choice available only in affluent communities. Choices of living situations may be limited in ethnic communities of color for both economic and social-attitudinal reasons. Another reason for concealment of homosexuality may be related to the primacy of social group identification (Croteau et al., 1993; Grossman, 1996). If a man who has sex with men considers his ethnic identity to be primary, he may conceal his sexual identity out of deference to community morals and attitudes. If, on the other hand, his sexual orientation is considered primary, he may join a gay community rather than remain part of an ethnic community (Doll & Beeker, 1996). If economic and material resources are not available, he may have no choice but to remain with his family and ethnic community.

Within mainstream society, people of color who are homosexual or bisexual experience prejudice and discrimination based on their ethnic identity and their sexual orientation (Choi et al., 1996; Peterson et al., 1995). AIDS creates an additional stigma (Grossman, 1994, 1995, 1996). First, it may reveal or expose persons as those who have engaged in a stigmatizing lifestyle (for instance, male-male sexual contact or injecting drug use). Second, the disease itself creates a stigma because of its infectious, or "dirty," nature and its association with death and dying. Both of these circumstances make people want to distance themselves from persons with HIV disease. According to several investigators, AIDS was not considered a problem in ethnic communities of color until 1986 and that belief still exists (Chang & Hill, 1996; Erickson, 1997; MRC Collaborative Study Group, 1996). Denial of AIDS by leaders in the Asian community and promulgation of this information by the Asian-language media have resulted in a common belief that Asians are immune to AIDS (Chang & Hill, 1996; Choy, 1995). Reasons for denying the existence of AIDS in communities of color are related to the stigma associated with the disease, with homosexuality, and with drug use. Person(s) living with HIV disease (PLWH) may face tremendous alienation within their own ethnic and cultural communities. The stigma is compounded by the revelation of homosexuality or injection drug use.

Several investigators have discussed differences in mental distress and social support among African-American, Latino, and white persons with HIV disease as a result of this multiple stigma.

Linn and colleagues (1996) reported that African-American women with HIV were more depressed and had poorer perceptions of their health than men and that men and women with small support networks were more depressed. Peterson and colleagues (1995) found that African-American gay men with HIV sought support from peers and professionals as opposed to family and clergy. This situation was due to the family's difficulty in accepting their gay lifestyle and to their limited involvement with the family to avoid disclosure or discussion of their homosexuality. Several investigators have found a sense of shame and disempowerment among gay and bisexual Latino men because of machismo, homophobia, and racism in their own communities (Diaz, 1994; Zimmerman et al., 1997). Among bisexual men, there is a tendency to be covert about homosexual behavior because of high levels of stigmatization, especially in communities of color (Doll & Beeker, 1996; McKirnan et al., 1995). Bisexual men have been reported to use drugs to ease their shame. Asian gay men also have been reported to use drugs because of the pain of being gay and unaccepted in the community (Choy, 1995).

Attitudes of the family toward homosexuality and AIDS play a large role in determining both who will care for PLWH and the stresses on the caregiver (Flaskerud & Tabora, 1998). In most ethnic communities of color, the value of the family overrides that of the individual (Martinez & Diaz, 1996; Choy, 1995; Cochran & Mays, 1993). PLWH, to protect their family from the disgrace of public exposure, may choose not to seek support from the family (Peterson et al., 1995). However, support agencies and services for PLWH in ethnic communities are limited, and the health of the PLWH is therefore affected (Croteau et al., 1993; McKirnan et al., 1995; Ramirez et al., 1994). When families do provide care for the PLWH, they may be overly protective and overly involved in an effort to keep the disease a secret (Flaskerud et al., 1996; Flaskerud & Tabora, 1998; Rose & Clark-Alexander, 1996). By not using or not having available support agencies and services, families may become severely distressed and overwhelmed by the care of the PLWH. In communities of color, the caregivers often are female family members (mothers, sisters) (Flaskerud & Tabora, 1998; Schiller, 1993; Sher, 1993).

Attitudes of various ethnic communities toward homosexuality, drug use, and AIDS may be influenced by organized religion, conceptualizations of male-male sexual contact, and the value placed on civil liberties (Doll & Beeker, 1996; Herek & Capitanio, 1994; Peterson et al., 1995). Herek and Capitanio (1994) found that African-Americans expressed greater support than whites for policies separating persons with AIDS from others (quarantine, publishing their names) and a stronger desire to avoid these persons along with a tendency to overestimate their own risk of acquiring HIV from casual contact. In contrast, whites expressed more negative feelings toward PLWH and a greater willingness to blame them for their illness. African-Americans may also be less tolerant of homosexuality because of the strong disapproval expressed by black churches with fundamentalist origins (Icard et al., 1992; Peterson et al., 1995), although there is disagreement on this characterization (Crawford et al., 1992). Latinos may have a narrower conceptualization of homosexuality, considering only the receptive partner to be homosexual (Flaskerud et al., 1996). This view may result socially in less moral judgment; however, personal and family shame and pain contribute to the stigma attached to homosexuality and efforts to conceal a family member who is homosexual (Doll & Beeker, 1996; Flaskerud et al., 1996). On the other hand, African-Americans and Latinos may be more tolerant of departures from mainstream norms in many areas of sexuality, such as teen pregnancy and single motherhood (Linares et al., 1992; Smith & Weinman, 1995).

Attitudes toward male and female sexuality in general also influence the transmission of HIV. Several sexual values of lower-class and working-class African-Americans are barriers to AIDS prevention (Choi et al., 1994). One is the myth of black male sexual superiority that has carried over into the nation's conventional folklore but is believed also by some African-Americans. Placing a value on sexual superiority carries with it a need to demonstrate and affirm this superiority through sexual contacts (Caetano & Hines, 1995; Icard et al., 1992; Wright, 1993). According to Jenkins and colleagues (1993), these "machismo behaviors" play a part in the increasing heterosexual transmission of HIV among African-Americans. Similar values have been described in Latino and Asian cultures (Choi et al., 1996; Diaz, 1994; Norris et al., 1996; Weniger & Brown, 1996). Mexican men may measure themselves against other men through an emphasis on multiple uncommitted sexual contacts that begin in adolescence (Doll & Beeker, 1996). High rates of sexual activity have been found among Hispanic men outside their primary relationships. Investigators have related this activity to traditional values that emphasize the need for men to express themselves sexually (Norris et al., 1996). Such values may encourage the transmission of HIV. These values and practices have been validated by other investigators as well (Flaskerud et al., 1996).

A second sexual value that may be a barrier to AIDS prevention is the importance of children in affirming masculinity or femininity, claiming status as an adult, and perpetuating the family and its name (Choi et al., 1996; Flaskerud et al., 1996). Failing to father children may be considered socially deviant at least and a contribution to genocide at most (Choi et al., 1996; Icard et al., 1992). Fathering children becomes an obligation to the ethnic group and a mark of manhood, and there are also strong social incentives for women to have children (Amaro, 1995). The value placed on having children is one of the reasons for the reluctance to use condoms; this, in turn, may contribute to the spread of HIV. Another negative attitude toward condoms is their association with prostitution and extramarital relationships in some cultures (Choi et al., 1994; Doll & Beeker, 1996; McKirnan et al., 1995; Norris et al., 1996).

Finally, attitudes toward the role of women in society and in sexual relationships cannot be minimized in their effect on the transmission of HIV. The unequal status of women in U.S. society extends to many aspects of HIV disease and may be more pronounced in ethnic communities of color, where power differentials are more apparent (Amaro, 1995; Bayer, 1994; Chavkin, 1997; Schopper & Vercautern, 1996). Cultural attitudes toward the role of women that appear to have a direct association with the spread of HIV often involve sexual relationships. Dual standards for men and women extend to cultural attitudes toward virginity, monogamy, expression of sexuality, talking about sexuality, condom use, who may initiate sexual intercourse, and reproduction (Amaro, 1995; Chang & Hill, 1996; Choy, 1995; Martinez & Diaz, 1996; Norris, et al., 1996;

Weniger & Brown, 1996). Women are expected to be virgins until married, to be monogamous during marriage, to bear children, and not to initiate sexual activities. They are not expected to negotiate condom use or to question their partners' sexual activities. As a consequence, women frequently may be unaware of a partner's risk behaviors, such as multiple sexual partners or male-male sexual contact, or injection drug use (Chang & Hill, 1996; Flaskerud et al., 1996; McKirnan et al., 1995; Neal et al., 1997; Wells & Mayer, 1997; Weniger & Brown, 1996). Bisexual men of color are more likely to be infected with HIV, more likely to have sex with women, less likely to disclose their homosexual behavior, and less likely to introduce condoms into their heterosexual relationships than are white bisexual men (Doll & Beeker, 1996; McKirnan et al., 1995). In addition, according to investigators studying IDUs, women are expected to share their needles with their partners, a behavior tied to gender role socialization (Latkin et al., 1996; Neaigus et al., 1994; Wayment et al., 1993). Furthermore, addicted women may be more stigmatized than their male counterparts because of society's expectations of nurturant role obligations (Amaro, 1995; Bayer, 1994). Attitudes toward the role of women in gender and sexual relationships places them at increased risk of exposure to HIV. Attitudes that lead to exposure of women to HIV also lead to perinatal transmission.

BEHAVIORS AND PRACTICES

Knowledge, beliefs, cultural attitudes, and values are all related to the behaviors and practices that put people at risk of exposure to HIV. Sexual behaviors and drug use behaviors are either directly or indirectly related to the majority of exposures to HIV for all ethnic groups. Sexual behaviors in association with condom use, reproductive practices, and drug use account for the majority of all adult and pediatric exposures.

Sexual Behaviors

It is important to note that there is a difference between sexual identity and sexual behaviors. A man who has sex with men may label himself as heterosexual, bisexual, or homosexual (CDC, January 15, 1993; Doll & Beeker, 1996; Flaskerud et al., 1996; McKirnan et al., 1995; Magana

& Carrier, 1991). These labels are probably influenced by middle socioeconomic class and white ethnocentric distinctions but may have different interpretations among the various ethnic groups. Cultural values, moral ideals, and attitudes influence sexual practices and how sexual behavior is labeled. Jenkins and colleagues (1993) reported that African-Americans are taught that homosexuality is not indigenous to the black community; men who are homosexual are pressured also to maintain heterosexual relationships. Men who are bisexual are expected to conceal homosexual contacts (McKirnan et al., 1995). Similar values and consequent practices are ascribed to Asian-Americans (Choi et al., 1996). In the traditional Latino community, a narrower conceptualization of homosexuality has been described by several investigators (Doll & Beeker, 1996; Flaskerud et al., 1996). Only men who practice anal-receptive intercourse ("feminine" men) are labeled as homosexual. "Masculine" men, who play the anal-insertive role, are not stigmatized as homosexual. In this role, their masculine self-image is not threatened by sexual contact with other men as long as they also have sex with women. The same practices have been reported in the black community (Doll & Beeker, 1996; Wright, 1993).

As a result of these cultural values, norms, and labels, African-American and Latino MSM may not identify themselves as homosexual (Doll & Beeker, 1996; McKirnan et al., 1995). In some MSM a discordance has been noted between sexual identity and sexual behavior. Some MSM may identify themselves as heterosexual, some as homosexual, and some as bisexual. In several studies more white MSM identified themselves as homosexual than did MSM of color. MSM who identified themselves as bisexual or heterosexual were more likely to be African-American or Latino (Doll & Beeker, 1996; McKirnan et al., 1995). There was a trend among men whose behavior and sexual identity were discordant, especially men of color, to report multiple HIV risk, to have risky sex with men and women, and not to disclose their homosexual activities to female partners. Because of such findings, researchers have begun to use categories based on sexual behaviors rather than on sexual self-identification (Doll & Beeker, 1996; McKirnan et al., 1995).

Several studies suggest that bisexuality might be more common among ethnic men of color than among white men (Doll & Beeker, 1996; McKirnan et al., 1995). Bisexual behavior may be influenced by socioeconomic and cultural contexts, such as sexual norms that facilitate bisexual behavior, homosexual stigma, unavailability of female partners, and exchanging sex for money or drugs. Bisexuality carries with it several risks for HIV infection. The first risk comes from failure to recognize risk because of failure to perceive oneself in a risk group and practice risk-reduction behaviors (McKirnan et al., 1995; Neal et al., 1997). Nationally, although AIDS incidence has stabilized among MSM, it has increased dramatically among African-American and Latino MSM, especially young MSM (CDC, 1997; Denning et al., 1996; Peterson et al., 1995, 1996). A second risk comes from higher rates of injection drug use in the bisexual group than in other sexual groups (Doll & Beeker, 1996; McKirnan et al., 1995). It has been proposed that men who practice bisexual behavior because of cultural proscriptions against homosexuality may abuse drugs because of the stress of concealment and denial (Choy, 1995). Supporting this assumption, Doll and Beeker (1996) reported that bisexual men were more often IDUs than were heterosexual men. Bisexuality carries with it also the risk of HIV transmission to women and, by extension, to children through perinatal exposure (Choi et al., 1996; Flaskerud et al., 1996; McKirnan et al., 1995). Latin-American bisexual men are more likely to be married than are other ethnic bisexual men (Diaz et al., 1993b). It has been suggested that bisexuality may be even higher than reported in ethnic people of color but may not be acknowledged as a risk factor because of stigma or, in the case of women, because of lack of awareness of a partner's bisexuality (Doll & Beeker, 1996; MRC Study Group, 1996). The relatively high numbers of cases that fall in the "unidentified risk" category in these communities is thought to be related to a failure to report bisexual behavior (Jenkins et al., 1993; Neal et al., 1997) (see Tables 9–1 and 9–2).

Sexual behavior may differ in relation to the level of acculturation, ethnic identification, and social class (Chang & Hill, 1996; Diaz et al., 1993b; Martinez & Diaz, 1997; Norris et al., 1996). Several investigators reported that married Latino men were more likely to have additional sex partners than were non-Latinos. However, highly acculturated Latino men were less likely to have multiple partners than were less acculturated men. The opposite was true of Latino women (Martinez & Diaz, 1997; Norris et al., 1996). Choi and colleagues (1994) described differences in extramarital sexual behavior related to social class among white, African-American and Hispanic men and women. Other investigators support their findings (Caetano & Hines, 1995). Men in all ethnic groups engaged in more extramarital sex than did women. African-American and Hispanic respondents endorsed more monogamy beliefs than whites. Among men, however, African-Americans and Hispanics engaged in extramarital sex twice as often as white men (Choi et al., 1994; Caetano & Hines, 1995). This finding was interpreted as reflecting traditional sex role expectations in the African-American community and Hispanic cultures. Respondents with less education and income were involved in more extramarital sex (Choi et al., 1994). Level of acculturation and sexual socialization were found to be the most important determinants of whether adult men of Mexican origin who have sex with men were influenced by Mexican or Anglo homosexuality (Ramirez et al., 1994). Unacculturated and less acculturated MSM in California preferred a single sexual role (i.e., either anal-insertive or anal-receptive but not both) and a focus on anal intercourse, whereas more acculturated men played both roles and engaged in a variety of behaviors, fellatio being most common. In addition, oral and anal intercourse with women has been found to be more prevalent among Latino heterosexual men than among others (Norris et al., 1996). Anal-receptive sex carries with it the same risks of HIV transmission among women as it does among men.

Condom use is a practice related to sexual behavior and is promoted by the Public Health Service as a method of reducing the risk of HIV transmission. According to some reports, Latinos and African-Americans may not use condoms because of cultural proscriptions against their use except with prostitutes and in extramarital affairs, because of suspicion that condoms are being promoted out of motivation to control the population, and because of feelings of invulnerability to HIV or, conversely, fatalistic beliefs about the outcome of diseases such as HIV infection and cancer (Amaro, 1995; Bayer, 1994; Doll &

Beeker, 1996; McKirnan et al., 1995; Martinez & Diaz, 1996; Ramirez et al., 1994). Reports about condom use among Asians reveal that condoms are used infrequently among heterosexual or homosexual partners (Chang & Hill, 1996; Choi et al., 1996; Weniger & Brown, 1996). Early in the HIV epidemic, it was assumed by some Asian leaders and health professionals that AIDS might not occur in the Asian community (Choy, 1995; Weniger & Brown, 1996). This assumption may have provided a false sense of security, in addition to any cultural proscriptions against the use of condoms as a risk-reduction practice. Furthermore, the lack of gay and bisexual subcultures in communities of color and the lack of funding for prevention programs for these same populations allow risk behaviors to continue unchecked (Croteau et al., 1993; Grossman, 1996; Jenkins et al., 1993; McKirnan et al., 1995). The CDC (January 15, 1993) reported that condom use among MSM is significantly higher among those who identified themselves as homosexual or bisexual them for those who identified themselves as straight. As noted earlier, there is less willingness among MSM to self identify as homosexual in ethnic communities of color.

Among women, other reasons for not using condoms are the personal desire and the cultural mandate to bear children (Amaro, 1995; Chang & Hill, 1996; Weniger & Brown, 1996). Women may choose to have a child because it makes them feel good about themselves—special, worthwhile, mature, and responsible (Linares et al., 1992; Smith & Weinman, 1995). They may bear children also because fertility is highly valued in their sociocultural group or because they have no choice but to take on a maternal role (CDC, May 28, 1993; Flaskerud et al., 1996; Linares et al., 1992). Negotiating safer sexual practices with a partner may encounter male resistance anchored in class and culture and may jeopardize a woman's economic survival (Amaro, 1995; Erickson, 1997; Mays & Cochran, 1993; Nyamathi et al., 1995). These same reasons may extend to women with HIV disease. In addition, for a woman with HIV disease, having a child ensures that she will leave a legacy of herself after death (Rose & Clark-Alexander, 1996).

Finally, both women and men may not use condoms because they do not perceive a risk of acquiring HIV disease. MSM who do not identify themselves as homosexual or bisexual may not perceive themselves at risk when prevention messages are couched in these terms (McKirnan et al., 1995; Neal et al., 1997). Likewise, women who are unaware of a partner's bisexuality, extramarital activity (or activity outside the primary partnership), or drug use may not perceive themselves at risk (Wells & Mayer, 1997). One finding that appears to be consistent across studies is that persons with multiple partners and casual partners are least likely to use condoms (Norris et al., 1996). Finally, for poor people the perceived risk of HIV infection may be low on a list of priorities of more serious life problems, such as employment, child care, and single parenting (Croteau et al., 1993; Stevenson & Davis, 1994).

Drug Use Behaviors

Injecting drug use or being the sexual partner of an IDU is the leading route of exposure to HIV for women of color (CDC, June 30, 1997). The great majority of perinatal exposures of children of color is linked to injection drug use (CDC, June 30, 1997). For men of color, injecting drug use is the second most frequent exposure category after male-male sexual contact. Native American men, however, are more than twice as likely to be categorized as MSM/IDU as all other men with AIDS in the United States (CDC, March 6, 1998). Behaviors associated with the use of injection drugs that increase the risk of exposure to HIV are unprotected sexual practices and sharing of injecting equipment. In addition to the reasons cited for unprotected sexual behavior, the use of crack cocaine and amphetamines has been associated with high-risk sexual practices. High-risk sexual behaviors are related to both crack injection and crack smoking (Turner & Solomon, 1996; Montoya & Atkinson, 1996). Cocaine and amphetamine injectors report a greater interest in sex and a greater frequency of intercourse. They also report exchanging sex for drugs, money, or a place to sleep and the use of drugs before or during sex (Doll & Beeker, 1996; Erickson, 1997; Montoya & Atkinson, 1996). The use of opioids and alcohol has recently been differentiated from the use of cocaine and amphetamines in their effects on sexual practices. Some investigators have suggested that the use of alcohol and opioids may not increase sexual risk practices (Montoya & Atkinson, 1996). Others continue to report an association between high-risk sexual practices and alcohol and opioid use, sometimes in relation to the degree of addiction and the necessity of exchanging sex for drugs (Caetano & Hines, 1995; Turner & Solomon, 1996). African-American, Hispanic, and white women in Arizona who were sexual partners of IDUs were reported to use alcohol, marijuana, cocaine, and crack frequently (Erickson, 1997). In a study of predominantly African-American female drug users enrolled in a methadone program in New York City, 72% were currently using illicit drugs, chiefly crack; 40% reported being HIV-positive and 50% were living with a sexual partner (Pivnick et al., 1994). Despite knowledge of sexual risk behaviors and perception of their own risk, IDUs were reported often to continue high-risk sexual behaviors (Erickson, 1997; Lester et al., 1995; Turner & Solomon, 1996).

Behaviors related to cleaning of injecting equipment, sharing equipment, using needle-exchange programs, and using "shooting galleries" to inject have been related to the type of drug used, the degree of dependence on the drug, and the gender, ethnicity, and social relationship of the users (Latkin et al., 1996; Neaigus et al., 1994; Nyamathi et al., 1995). Cocaine injection has been associated more strongly with HIV seropositivity than has heroin injection. Cocaine users inject more frequently, up to four or five times an hour during bingeing. Cocaine binges create anxiety for the drug, resulting in less ability to follow guidelines for bleach decontamination and reduced willingness to delay injection long enough to use bleach (CDC, June 24, 1994). Heroin injectors are typically more able to follow guidelines for using bleach. However, severely dependent heroin injectors are more likely than less dependent users to share equipment. More dependent users share with dealers because of the urgency of their need for drugs during withdrawal.

Women (more than men) have been found repeatedly to share injecting equipment (Neaigus et al., 1994; Wayment et al., 1993). Women most commonly share equipment with drug-injecting partners (Caetano & Hines, 1995; Neaigus et al., 1994). This behavior has been related to gender role socialization; the woman's most significant social relationship may be with her injecting partner, who also may be her sexual partner. The sub-ordinate status and role of the woman in the relationship require that she be giving and attentive to the needs of a male partner in this situation, just as she is in all other aspects of the female-male relationship (Bayer, 1994; Erickson, 1997; Wayment et al., 1993).

Sharing injecting equipment is also a means of expressing mutual friendship and kinship between persons in the drug-using community (Latkin et al., 1996; Neaigus et al., 1994). Sharing is a behavior that tends to integrate the individual into a family and social group and makes him or her part of the subculture.

Drug use practices have been related to ethnicity. Drug injectors' social and risk networks exhibit ethnic homogeneity. Sharing equipment often occurs for economic as well as social reasons. It has been reported that African-Americans have reduced their injecting risk behaviors (sharing, not cleaning equipment), but they have not reduced sexual risk behaviors that may accompany drug use. Other investigators have reported that Latinos continue to share unclean equipment and use "shooting galleries" to inject. The majority of Mexican-American men and women (81.6%) in a Los Angeles study ($n = 100$) who injected drugs shared uncleaned needles (Parra et al., 1993). In another study, Mexican-American women who used drugs were more likely than other women to have drug-using partners and to use drugs daily (Turner & Solomon, 1996). The use of "shooting galleries" and shooting up in semipublic places have been reported to be more frequent among IDUs in the Northeast (Montoya & Atkinson, 1996). It has been speculated that Latinos may be less likely to reduce their risks because of language barriers, sociocultural differences derived from specific histories of a particular ethnic group, or traditional cultural differences (Diaz et al., 1993a). Current place of residence in the United States and a traditional lack of experience with organizational behavior and power have been cited as examples (Diaz et al., 1993b; Montoya & Atkinson, 1996). Drug use as a means of exposure to HIV continues to be highest in the Northeast and Southeast and lower in the West than sexual activity as an exposure factor among African-Americans, Latinos, and Asians. In any case, the social dynamics of ethnicity seem to have an important impact on HIV risk associated with IDU.

The use of and support for needle-exchange programs as a means of reducing HIV risk have met with skepticism and criticism in some parts of the African-American community (Bayer, 1994; Ostrow, 1993; Bradley-Springer, 1997). These programs have been viewed by some in the community as encouraging drug use and as part of a racist conspiracy to commit genocide against the African-American population. It has been argued persuasively that ethnic communities of color need drug-rehabilitation programs instead. Other African-American leaders have encouraged risk-reduction programs that provide needle exchange, bleach to clean equipment, and information on not sharing equipment, in conjunction with more drug rehabilitation programs being made available to African-Americans and Latinos.

A frequent practice among Latinos in the Southwest and West may also be a risk of HIV transmission through the sharing of needles and syringes. The home use and reuse of needles for injection of medications may be common in some social groups and may pose a risk of HIV transmission (Martinez & Diaz, 1997). Flaskerud and Nyamathi (1996) found, in a sample of 216 low-income women in California, that the use of injectable medications (penicillin, vitamins, birth control agents) purchased in Mexico was fairly common (43.5%). Reuse of disposable needles and syringes among injectors (48%) and sharing of equipment (36%) were also common. Methods of cleaning needles and syringes were inadequate by CDC-recommended guidelines (CDC, June 24, 1994).

Several other behaviors and practices are related to HIV risk reduction or disease progression. Involvement in HIV testing and in clinical trials are two such practices. The others are health promotion behaviors and practices. All may be related to ethnicity and traditional cultural practices.

HIV Antibody Testing

Several investigators have noted that ethnic communities of color do not participate in voluntary HIV testing programs at the same rate as whites (Battle et al., 1996; CDC, October 15, 1993; Grinstead et al., 1997; Lauver et al., 1995; Lester et al., 1995; Schwarcz et al., 1993). These rates may be influenced by the high rates of gay white men who participate in voluntary testing and parturient women who participate knowingly

or unknowingly through the testing of umbilical cord blood and placental tissue. In addition, Latinos and other immigrants are tested involuntarily as part of an immigration requirement. Various reasons have been given for failure to participate in HIV testing. One is skepticism among people of color about medical research and medical professionals. The stigma associated with AIDS or the behaviors that put persons at risk of HIV may be another reason (Grinstead et al., 1997; Lester et al., 1995). An additional reason may be that mandatory testing has been widely viewed as punitive; voluntary testing may engender a similar attitude. For women in one study, HIV testing and seropositive status were related to discrimination in health care delivery (Lester et al., 1995). Health care facilities became a site of public exposure and personal stress.

Other reasons are related to perception of risk. Many persons are unaware of their risks because of failure to identify culturally with the risk behaviors as they are currently labeled. In the case of women, lack of perception of risk may be related to lack of awareness of a partner's drug use or sexual activity (CDC, October 15, 1993; Grinstead et al., 1997; Wells & Mayer, 1997). Finally, some persons may not be tested because of a fatalistic attitude toward HIV disease (If I am positive, there's nothing to be done about it anyway. Why make myself worried?). Many of these reasons should carry less weight because HIV testing is thought of differently today than in the past. Today, early testing can result in enrollment in clinical trials, prophylactic treatment, better treatment outcomes, and increased longevity (Diaz et al., 1995; Lester et al., 1995). Several recent studies have documented that women and people of color are less likely to be enrolled in clinical trials programs (CDC, February 28, 1997; Crystal et al., 1995; Diaz et al, 1995; Lester et al., 1995). Consequently, they are not receiving the new HIV treatments. Efforts to increase voluntary testing among people of color are warranted for these reasons.

Health Promotion Practices and Behavior

Despite attributions of fatalism to some social and cultural groups, studies of low-income Latino, African-American, and white women in Los Angeles revealed that all groups were involved in lay disease-prevention and treatment practices that were being applied to HIV/AIDS (Flaskerud, 1994; Flaskerud & Calvillo, 1991a; Flaskerud et al., 1997; Flaskerud & Rush, 1989; Flaskerud & Thompson, 1991b). In these studies and others, AIDS was conceptualized generally as an attack from external forces on the immunity or resistance of the person (Martinez & Diaz, 1996). The same type of conceptualization has been reported for Haitian women (Martin et al., 1995; Walker, 1996). This conceptualization is congruent with beliefs in an external locus of control, often attributed to persons of color and lower social class (Jenkins et al., 1993; Marin & Gomez, 1994) and to the military metaphors used to describe the epidemic in the United States (Sontag, 1990; Wenger, 1993).

Regardless, the women in these studies had well-developed prevention and treatment practices that were being used to ward off illness in general and also were being applied to AIDS. These practices involved the use of foods, vitamins, and herbs to keep the body healthy and as remedies for illness. Preventing chills, avoiding extremes in temperature, and keeping the body warm during illness were other common practices. An emphasis on cleanliness to decrease germs in the body, the home, and the environment was practiced by all groups for both prevention and treatment. Moderate lifestyle behaviors, or a balance in rest and exercise, work and play, and food and fluids, together with a limited use of alcohol and tobacco, were endorsed by all to promote health and to treat illness. All groups also noted the importance of spirituality, friends, and family in maintaining health and in combating illness (Suarez et al., 1996). These behaviors and practices were recommended for all illnesses and for AIDS as well. The usefulness and applicability of these practices to AIDS are apparent in their relation to both HIV prevention and progression to disease in PLWH. The use of traditional healing practices, many of which are preventive in nature, has been reported also among Native Americans to treat and prevent AIDS (Barney, 1996; Kutenai, 1996).

These practices and behaviors and the beliefs and values they are founded on have been reported by other investigators who have studied other groups (Martinez & Diaz, 1996; Suarez et al., 1996). Similar practices and beliefs have been described for Haitians, Asians, Middle Easterners, and East Indians (Martin et al., 1995; Pliskin, 1992; Ramakrishna & Weiss, 1992; Reid, 1994; Walker, 1996). These beliefs and practices should be viewed as a rich foundation for integrating and implementing HIV-prevention and intervention programs. Education, prevention, and treatment within the context of existing ethnocultural beliefs and practices (rather than in the context of biomedical beliefs) are more likely to succeed because they represent the worldview of the community served.

HIV PREVENTION AND TREATMENT

Designing Programs

Numerous investigators, clinicians, and community-based organizations have made similar recommendations for designing and delivering HIV-prevention and treatment services in communities of color (Bayer, 1994; CDC, May 10, 1996; Fishbein, 1996; Flaskerud et al., 1996, 1997; Halloran et al., 1996; Holtgrave et al., 1995; Kalichman et al., 1996; Kegeles et al., 1996; Kerr, 1993; Marin & Gomez, 1994; Nicoll et al., 1993; Rogers et al., 1996; Zimmerman et al., 1997). Many suggestions have come from people of color and from community-based organizations that can be relied on to provide the best direction and guidance for prevention and treatment services (Casimir, 1996). These recommendations are summarized here.

Communities of color have benefited most from programs that have been funded directly to minority organizations and to community-based organizations. However, better targeting of these programs is needed: programs specifically designed for men of color who have sex with other men (almost 50% of AIDS cases among men of color occur in this group), for IDUs (more than 75% of cases are in adults of color), and for women (about 76% of cases are in women of color) (Casimir, 1996; CDC, June 30, 1997; Jenkins et al., 1993). The unwillingness and inadequacy of traditional leadership organizations and efforts such as churches, tribal councils, and beneficent societies to confront AIDS suggest that funding should go to new organizations and leaders who are more fully involved in HIV/AIDS efforts (Choi et al., 1996; Croteau et al., 1993). Traditional organizations may provide inadequate leadership because of long-standing cultural and moral proscriptions against homosexuality, drug use, and abortion; the perceived need to remain focused on long-standing social, political, and health problems in the community; and the fear that AIDS will tarnish their image (Jenkins et al., 1993).

A second recommendation is that programs be part and parcel of the target community, that they emerge from the community and be delivered by persons of that same community. These persons include not only professionals, policy makers, and customary leaders but also lay persons indigenous to the community representing homosexuals and bisexuals, IDUs, women, poor persons, and persons of varying levels of education and acculturation. Persons delivering HIV-prevention and treatment services should speak the language(s) of the community and share the cultural values and practices. In some cases they also should share the gender of the group served. Both staff and agencies should be culturally competent. Even staff members who share gender, language, and ethnicity with their clients and are indigenous to the community need workshops on homophobia, sexuality, and drug use. Agencies must formulate clear, explicit, and enforceable policies, and agency leaders and managers must enforce these policies. Education and prevention programs should be communicated by common, familiar, and accepted methods (for example, by the use of oral traditions, storytelling, popular novellas, small discussion groups, role playing, and role models) (Croteau et al., 1993; Flaskerud et al., 1996, 1997; Holtgrave et al., 1995; Kalichman et al., 1996; Marin & Gomez, 1994; Peterson et al., 1996; Zimmerman et al., 1995).

LOCATION OF PROGRAMS. In ethnic communities of color, AIDS occurs within the context of ongoing, serious health problems as well as social and political problems, including drug abuse, unemployment, violence, teen pregnancies, and STDs. Many community leaders, health professionals, and minority national organizations have recommended that AIDS prevention should be integrated into broad, comprehensive goals of community change and service. This integrated approach is believed to carry with it a greater efficacy in reducing HIV infection than an isolated HIV-prevention approach (CDC, March 6,

1998; Hu et al., 1995; Jenkins et al., 1993; Kalichman et al., 1996). In Chapter 2 a case was made for integrating AIDS-prevention programs and treatment services into existing community programs and institutions such as the U.S. Public Health Service Nutrition Program for Women, Infants, and Children (WIC), STD clinics, family-planning clinics, drug-rehabilitation programs, and the school system. It was argued that these agencies have a history, expertise, and experience and are currently accepted and used by the members of the community. An alternative argument is given here. These existing programs and institutions may reflect the current negative attitudes toward homosexuality, drug use, and AIDS; they may be perceived by the community as external rather than internal sources of help; and they may be viewed as tired and ineffective in meeting the health and social problems of the community. In such an argument, established programs and institutions would be ineffective in meeting and defeating AIDS at a community level. It could be argued persuasively that new institutions are needed to provide a broad, comprehensive approach to health care, including AIDS treatment. These new institutions would enhance ethnic group identity, solidarity, and political advocacy and activism. They would enlist community members in the development of effective responses to the conditions that contribute to AIDS, drug abuse, teen pregnancies, STDs, tuberculosis, cancer, heart disease, and so forth. These agencies would develop, implement, and enforce social policy strategies that enhance sensitivity to the groups most affected by HIV, eradicate discrimination and prejudice within the community, and build a sense of unity and support throughout the community. Additional benefits of such activities are the therapeutic effect on participants and the community when purpose, direction, and self-determination are fostered and the degree of power and control over participants' lives that they provide (Bayer, 1994; Croteau et al., 1993; Holtgrave et al., 1995; Kalichman et al., 1996; Singer, 1991; Zimmerman et al., 1997).

SUCCESS OF PROGRAMS. On the basis of cultural proscriptions, several specialized interventions have attempted to change AIDS knowledge, beliefs, attitudes, and practices among Latino, African-American, Asian, and white (European-

American) program participants. Other studies have made recommendations for culturally competent interventions based on study findings (Bayer, 1994; Choi et al., 1996; Doll & Beeker, 1996; Flaskerud & Nyamathi, 1996; Flaskerud et al., 1996, 1997; Halloran et al., 1996; Kegeles et al., 1996; Kalichman et al., 1996; Marin & Gomez, 1994; McKirnan et al., 1996; Peterson et al 1996; Ramirez et al., 1994; Zimmerman et al., 1997). These studies employed risk-reduction interventions and measured changes in knowledge, beliefs, attitudes, and practices. All studies reported significant changes, and some of the interventions were related to sustained change over time. To measure changes in behavior, almost all studies employed self-report measures. A few measured actual behavior changes: HIV antibody testing, requests for condoms, maintenance of seronegativity. Some innovative approaches used the extended family in the intervention, life-enhancement counseling, videotapes, games, counseling, role playing, demonstration–return demonstration, problem solving, coping, oral traditions and storytelling, novellas, photo novellas, comic books, and grounding of the intervention in a personal (ethnic and gender match) and cultural (values related to family and community) context. Some programs targeted to persons with little formal education used messages that were concrete and rooted in temporal reality (rather than general premises), that is, messages related to current environment and life circumstances (Doll & Beeker, 1996; Hu et al., 1995; Zimmerman et al., 1997). Acknowledging the environmental constraints on subjects, many studies reimbursed participants with cash, subway tokens, and video-game tokens; some provided child care and food. Although all these studies offered specialized AIDS interventions, some of the interventions were offered in such existing community agencies and services as WIC programs, the school system, homeless shelters, STD clinics, and drug rehabilitation programs. Some also used an existing social network (the family) in the intervention. Less traditional locations, such as gay bars, migrant labor camps, pornographic bookstores, street corners, county jails, and alternative test sites, were also used.

GOALS AND STRATEGIES OF PROGRAMS. Recommendations drawn from the literature on community-based programs and specialized AIDS interventions pertinent to ethnic communities of color emphasized cultural values, customs and traditions, and social networks. On the basis of these studies and building on existing beliefs and practices, HIV prevention and treatment programs can be based on five goals:

1. Consciously mobilize and enhance cultural beliefs, values, and roles as core elements of the intervention process.
2. Use traditional gender roles and the role of the family in health education and care as a starting point.
3. Enhance beneficial beliefs and practices that may be related to HIV disease.
4. Clarify misperceptions that may create fear and stigma.
5. Modify detrimental beliefs or negative attitudes and practices within the context of positive ethnocultural and community values.

To reach these goals, prevention programs will benefit from the strategies used and tested in other successful programs (CDC, May 10, 1996; Croteau et al., 1993; Dearing et al., 1996; Flaskerud et al., 1997; Halloran et al., 1996; Kegeles et al., 1996; Nyamathi & Bennett, 1997; Nyamathi et al., 1993, 1995; Peterson et al., 1996; Rogers et al., 1996; Zimmerman et al., 1997). Based on a number of successful community programs, three strategies are recommended. These occurred consistently in the field study programs cited.

First and foremost, all successful community-based prevention programs used members of the targeted group (homophiles) to convey the message. Targeted groups were defined very *narrowly* by specific HIV risk factors, age, ethnicity, gender, language, and other situational or behavioral characteristics (e.g., homelessness, runaways, prostitution, and so forth). Members of the targeted group were full partners in the development and maintenance of the program, as well as in delivering the message and serving as advocates for prevention. Peer leaders were a source of advice that would be accepted by the target audience because they were persons who had "walked in the shoes" of the targeted group. The emphasis was not as much on message content as on establishing a trusting relationship with members of the target audience so that they would be receptive to an HIV-prevention message.

Second, successful programs collaborated with other community programs to share resources and information. This strategy requires a thorough knowledge of the community and its resources: formal and informal, mainstream, and counterculture. The goal is to identify both barriers and facilitators of community intervention and to create an integrated communitywide network of services. This may include HIV education of some community service providers. In the process of involving the community, norms and values will become apparent, effective and credible settings for program delivery will be identified, and the necessary content and language of programs will become clear. Communication acceptable to the target community in form and language will become apparent (i.e., use of the vernacular or street talk, use of role model stories or theater skits, awareness of reading level). The intervention will develop a social and cultural focus relevant to the target group. A successful intervention operates at several levels: small group, one-on-one, use of media, inclusion of public health efforts, and so forth.

Finally, successful programs foster group pride and empower the community to respond constructively to the epidemic. Esteem-building cultural activities as well as leadership positions in the prevention effort are part of this approach (Diaz, 1994; Zimmerman et al., 1997).

CHANGING CULTURAL NORMS AND BEHAVIORS. There is one important warning for community education and prevention programs that cannot be minimized (Bayer, 1994). HIV-prevention programs are aimed at *changing behavior.* As noted in this chapter, behaviors are based on deep-seated cultural norms. HIV-prevention programs, by their nature, must challenge the cultural norms that inform and structure sexual and drug-using behavior. The subordination of women to men in their sexual relationships requires a rupture in current cultural norms in this society and in some ethnic groups in particular. The culture of promiscuity in gay men must be challenged as a norm that encourages deadly behavior in the case of HIV. The cultural norms of some fundamentalist religions and conservative communities deny education to high school students for whom sexual activity poses a risk of HIV transmission. There has been cultural resis-

tance to programs for needle exchange and condom use by some ethnic groups and gay groups who fear genocide. In all these instances, cultural norms that inform behavior are being challenged.

Public health efforts to control the HIV epidemic demand radical behavior change. By advocating culturally sensitive and competent programs, are efforts at behavior change being thwarted? Allowing cultural beliefs and norms to stand as barriers to behavioral change is *incompatible* with HIV prevention. Clearly, to the extent that AIDS-prevention messages are sensitive to target group language, style, and format, public health efforts are not being thwarted. Furthermore, acknowledgment of cultural conflict and the ineffectiveness and counter-productiveness of solutions imposed by powerful social groups on ethnic and social minorities does not hinder public health efforts. Seeking an understanding of the cultural context of behavior in order to redefine cultural values and facilitate behavior change does not thwart public health efforts. However, as Bayer (1994) so forthrightly states, cultural sensitivity is ultimately incompatible with the goals of AIDS prevention if it is not acknowledged that AIDS prevention requires radical behavioral and normative change. AIDS-prevention efforts at the community level must acknowledge and facilitate cultural change and cultural competence.

RESEARCH IN CULTURE, ETHNICITY, AND AIDS

Summary of Research

Much of the content of this chapter has been based on studies investigating the relationship of culture, ethnicity, and HIV. Several studies have included ethnicity as a variable and some have focused on cultural values, beliefs, attitudes, and practices; social structures, roles, status, and social networks; economic structures and power differentials; and environmental constraints. These aspects of culture are involved with behavior and provide a framework for culturally competent interventions. More and more investigators are designing field studies to test the effects of culture-compatible interventions on changes in AIDS-risk behavior. Since the last edition of this text, more researchers are focusing their efforts on Asian populations, groups that were ignored in earlier studies. Studies of prevention efforts focusing on American Indians and Alaskan Natives are still needed. Two other areas of study become dramatically clear and urgent when the progress of HIV-prevention research with ethnic people of color is reviewed. In the United States the majority of AIDS cases (55%) now occur in ethnic people of color and not in gay white men. African-American men, women, and children make up more than one third of all persons with AIDS (35%). HIV incidence has leveled off in the white gay community but continues to rise among women and ethnic people of color, including young MSM (CDC, February 28, 1997; Denning & Fleming, 1997; Neal et al., 1997). Clearly, there is an urgent need for effective AIDS-prevention interventions in the African-American and Latino communities. Field studies of interventions that demonstrate behavior change are of high priority. Secondly, there is cultural resistance to acknowledging that certain risk behaviors occur in some communities (e.g., gay sexual behavior) and to changing certain values and norms (e.g., status and roles of women). Studies are needed that can demonstrate success in reducing cultural resistance and changing cultural norms and behaviors.

Issues in Research

Studies of culture and HIV disease are susceptible to a plethora of methodologic pitfalls that result essentially from taking "shortcuts." Some of these pitfalls are summarized here. Chief among them is the use of Anglocentric measures based on an Anglocentric worldview or conceptualization of the values, attitudes, and behaviors related to HIV disease. An obvious example is the use of the Anglocentric labels "homosexual" or "bisexual" in questioning persons about their sexual preferences and activity. As several investigators (Doll & Beeker, 1996; McKirnan et al., 1995; Ramirez et al., 1994) have pointed out, some MSM identify themselves as homosexual, others as bisexual, and still others as heterosexual. These labels appear to be related to ethnic culture and community and to societal homophobia and stigma. The difficulties that arise from the bias inherent in these labels result in inaccurate data about how AIDS is being transmitted, uninformed intervention protocols, and a waste of resources on community prevention programs that are addressing the wrong set of behaviors.

One devastating result is a total lack of community services for members of some ethnocultural groups with HIV disease who, as a consequence, are physically sicker and die earlier, psychologically and spiritually bereft. Compounding this situation is the Anglocentric value placed on these labels, which asserts that MSM should be calling themselves homosexuals and would do so if they were just a little better educated or more assimilated.

Another construct that has been applied frequently to research with ethnic people of color is locus of control (Jenkins et al., 1993; Martinez & Diaz, 1996; Suarez et al., 1996). The importance of control is apparent in most Western biomedical and psychologic writing about health and illness. Internal control is valued by European-Americans and is considered necessary to a health-promoting and disease-preventing lifestyle. According to the locus-of-control conceptualization, when disease does occur, internally controlled persons are more likely to believe that they have some control over its course and to marshall their personal, social, and spiritual resources to fight it. Most frequently, ethnic people of color, lower-class persons, and older persons are found to have an external locus of control. Theoretically, external control is associated with fatalism; in practice, it is greeted with frustration and labels such as "hard-to-reach" and "noncompliant" by health professionals and academicians. Persons with an external locus of control believe that illness is the result of external forces and that they have little control over their environment. When they become ill, they are more likely to accept their fate gracefully and not embarrass, shame, or dishonor themselves or their families by anger, complaining, challenging, or resistant behavior.

Some of the difficulties with using this construct in research occur because of the Anglocentric positive value placed on internal control, the negative attitudes toward external control, and consequent interventions designed to change a person's locus of control if it is external. Furthermore, an uninformed and incorrect assumption that accompanies the findings of an external locus of control is that persons with this orientation are believed not to possess or engage in health-promotion, disease-prevention, and treatment behaviors. As noted in the earlier section on behaviors and practices, many health-promotion, disease-prevention, and treatment behaviors are practiced by persons who believe that illness is caused by external forces. Given the different worlds and environments in which people live, it is difficult to say whether an internal or an external orientation is better, more realistic, or more comforting when a person is confronted with a life-threatening disease.

There are many other concepts that are equally problematic when they are defined and developed in one ethnocultural group and then applied to other groups. Depression is one such concept that has been investigated and clarified cross-culturally, with the result that it is now known that there are different idioms for dysphoria in some groups and no idiom for dysphoria in others. The question that researchers must consider seriously is whether the instruments that they are using are measuring the same attribute from one culture to another. In other words, are the instruments valid?

As noted at the beginning of this chapter, in the section on culture and ethnicity, some theoreticians and investigators have questioned whether commonly used attitude-behavior social science models and theories are applicable to research involving people of color, women, and people other than heterosexuals (Amaro, 1995; Cochran & Mays, 1993; Doll & Beeker, 1996; McKirnan et al., 1996). These same investigators have noted that the health-belief model, the theory of reasoned action, and the self-efficacy theory were developed without a view to cultural, ethnic, gender, sexual, and socioeconomic class differences. These theories are based on individualistic as opposed to collectivistic values; they do not account for significant concepts and variables such as environmental constraints, economic and social resources, and identity/behavior discordance; and they assume mainstream-defined motivations, decision-making processes, and personal control. These theories also do not address the realities of women in society or the HIV epidemic (Amaro, 1995). Women's social status is a central feature in women's risk and must be addressed in research and prevention programs. Traditional theories of development do not address a central aspect of women's identity: relationship to others. This orientation increases risk of HIV through sexual relationships with men but is ignored in most research and prevention programs.

Finally, any model of HIV sexual risk reduction in women must address women's fear of or the experience of abuse (Amaro, 1995). All of these factors may play a greater or lesser role, depending on ethnicity, culture, and socioeconomic status. The challenge to HIV health research is to capture the worldview and life experiences of a specific ethnocultural or gender group and then to design interventions congruent with these situations and instruments that measure these conceptualization variables.

A variety of other methodologic problems exist in cross-cultural research. Several problems involve translation of English-language instruments into other languages. One problem is the assumption that labels or concepts from one language can be directly and literally translated into another language. Compounding this problem is the use in many languages of circumlocutions rather than direct and explicit terms for sexual activity and drug use-activity (Flaskerud & Nyamathi, 1988). Another problem involves the idiomatic differences within the same language from one ethnic or regional group to another (Hendricson et al., 1989; Gomez et al., 1995). It is clear that establishing semantic equivalence is necessary but not sufficient for understanding or for valid and reliable responses. Rather, idiomatic equivalence is needed and should be based on ethnicity, social class, age, geographic region, and so forth.

Response formats may create additional problems. The use of Likert scale formats may be culturally biased (Flaskerud, 1988). The use of a true/false or dichotomous response format, although it decreases sensitivity and variability, may be preferable because of its universal practicality and familiarity (Flaskerud, 1988; Kelly et al., 1989). Response sets also may be influenced by cultural traits that encourage or minimize extremes or that encourage acquiescence on verbal measures. Acquiescence or extremes may be the result of cultural politeness, social desirability, the reimbursement offered to the participants in a study, or the shock value of the response on the interviewer (Bowser, 1992; Mays & Jackson, 1991). In addition, Kauth and colleagues (1991) questioned the reliability of retrospective assessments of behavior. They studied biweekly, 3-month, and 12-month self-reports of sexual behavior and found that the consistency and reliability of the data decreased as the recall period lengthened. Flaskerud & colleagues (1996, 1997) found that low-income women were highly likely to report no sexual activity in the preceding 12 months unless they were reminded of certain markers, such as a holiday, their birthday or anniversary, the birth of a child, or an abortion. Part of this failure to report may have been related to difficulty in recall, but part was also attributed to cultural modesty about sexual behavior, even with a husband or monogamous partner.

Other issues in measurement involve the use of validated and standardized measures of HIV knowledge, risk, and practices (Kelly et al., 1989). To plan, implement, evaluate, and refine interventions and risk-reduction programs, one must make a systematic outcome assessment. Many instruments are currently in use, but they often do not have preexisting established validity or reliability and their psychometric properties are not established in the study in which their use is reported. Consequently, data resulting from their use are not comparable. The National Health Interview Survey has included a survey of AIDS knowledge, behavior, and risk since 1988. This questionnaire is available in English and Spanish. The results of the survey are published by the National Center for Health Statistics every 2 years for a national sample of African-American, Latino, and white respondents. Data are published in a form that allows comparison of local samples with the national sample (see, for instance, Flaskerud & Uman, 1993) and that allows analysis of the effects of gender, age, and education on responses. Although the instrument is lengthy, if more investigators were to use it either totally or partially, comparisons and measurement of regional differences and changes over time would be facilitated. Arguments against its use are that it was constructed to measure a universal, vast middle of the U.S. population and not persons who have limited literacy, use idiomatic vocabulary, or come from nonacculturated groups.

Measurement of change is another issue in research on culture and HIV disease. The reliability of self-reported change has been questioned frequently (Choi & Catania, 1996; Rietmeijer et al., 1996; Ramirez et al., 1994). The extent to which reported behaviors and attitudes correspond with actual skills and behaviors is a limitation cited by most of the investigators whose research provided a basis for this chapter. In addition, the correspondence between intended behavior and actual behavior in the case of HIV disease has been challenged, especially as it applies to ethnic people of color (Cochran & Mays, 1993). The influences of poverty, racism, economic and social opportunity, and availability of resources separate the intention to change and the successful prediction of actual behavior. All these influences have an arbitrary and unpredictable nature.

Another measurement issue related to change is how it is conceptualized. Prochaska and colleagues (1994) conceptualized change in lifestyle and behaviors as a process that occurs in stages. If this conceptualization is applied to change in HIV risk behaviors, then an assessment must first be made of a person's current stage of change. Next, interventions are developed to move him or her to the next stage—from A to B. This approach is considered to have a greater chance of success than attempting to move persons from A to F with one intervention. It also provides the investigator with more information and validation of change than the more usual measures of community intervention, which often fail to achieve a significant effect. The CDC (May 10, 1996) has recommended the use of this model for community-level programs with high-risk populations. The cardinal rule is that the outcome variable selected must be consistent with and sensitive to the purpose of the intervention; the outcome measure must validly assess the outcome variable. Behavior-change interventions are designed to change behaviors, and the most appropriate outcome measure for evaluating a behavior-change intervention is a measure of the behavior per se (Fishbein, 1996). An attitude or normative change is measured by a change in attitude but does not reflect or predict a change in behavior. Changing behaviors (or norms) in stages has been shown to be related to more permanent change.

Research Needed

As may be noted from the preceding discussion, much of the research that needs to be done in the area of culture, ethnicity, and HIV involves discovery of the cultural basis of behavior, followed by development of culturally valid constructs, concepts, and theoretical models and then by development of instruments to measure these variables. Another research need is for culturally competent interventions that are designed and implemented by the target group, related to the stage of change of a particular group or community, and scientifically validated. Finally, research that measures actual change in behavior as opposed to reported change or intended change is needed. Some examples of the research base needed in the area of culture and HIV are provided; however, a much wider range of studies is needed than can be summarized here.

1. Research that discovers and describes
   a. Models for predicting health-related behavior change that include key constructs to ethnic communities of color, including gay and bisexual communities of color and to women: values, norms, social roles and structures, social status, power differentials, economic resources, environmental constraints, abuse, racism, and so forth
   b. Models for explaining and addressing cultural resistance
   c. Cultural models of health promotion, disease prevention, and treatment
   d. Cultural models of sexuality that include roles, gender, expression, interpersonal relationships, and power differentials
2. Methodologic research that develops and tests culturally valid instruments to measure concepts and variables related to values, attitudes, normative change, behaviors, behavior change, and so forth
3. Research that tests the effects of culturally competent interventions:
   a. Community-based studies that are designed, implemented, and evaluated by ethnic people of color who are most affected by HIV, such as MSM, IDUs, and women
   b. Community-based behavior change interventions that are longitudinal and attempt to move persons across the stages of change (for example, from fear induction to risk sensitization, to risk contemplation, and finally to risk reduction) with the introduction of the necessary skills and resources at each stage to facilitate change to the next stage
   c. Behavior change studies that measure actual behavior change on either a personal or a community level as the result of a culturally competent intervention; for example, number of condoms requested, participation in HIV testing and returning for test results, maintaining a seronegative HIV status, a decrease in community STDs, a decrease in teen pregnancies, a decrease in the number of new AIDS cases, and an increase in enrollment in drug-rehabilitation programs.
   d. Studies that employ large enough numbers of participants to detect effects with a high probability
   e. Hypothesis-testing interventional studies in community settings that employ experimental field conditions and comparison groups

SUMMARY

Culture and ethnicity are important constructs in understanding HIV disease because they are apparent in values, attitudes, and behaviors associated with reproduction, sexuality, intimacy, family relationships, death and dying, drug use, stigma, and so forth. The disproportionate effect of HIV on ethnic communities of color is related to ethnocultural differences in values and behaviors but also to poverty, racism, discrimination, and lack of opportunity and resources. An understanding of ethnocultural differences in AIDS knowledge and beliefs, attitudes and values, and practices and behaviors is necessary for effective and culturally competent health care. The goal of this chapter is to increase an awareness of culture and the consequent competence of health care practice and research at individual, agency, and community levels. Health care practice and research should be based on an understanding of the cultural foundations of behavior; ethnocultural models of health, illness, prevention, and treatment; and culturally valid models of behavior change. Health care providers should involve their clients in the assessment of symptoms and behaviors, in the interpretation of illness, and in the planning and implementation of health care and interventions. Researchers and clinicians can continue the tradition they have begun in transcultural studies to discover cultural beliefs and practices. However, they also must go beyond discovery to implementation of cultural mandates for health promotion and care as these relate to HIV disease. The progression of HIV disease in ethnic communities of color makes these activities urgently important.

REFERENCES

AAN Expert Panel Report. (1992). Culturally competent health care. *Nursing Outlook, 40*(6), 277–283.

AIDS Alert. (1997, May). Minorities miss out on AIDS survival increase. *AIDS Alert, 12*(5), 55–57.

Airhihenbuwa, C.O., Diclemente, R.J., Wingood, G.M., et al. (1992). HIV/AIDS education and prevention among African-Americans: A focus on culture. *AIDS Education and Prevention, 4*(3), 267–276.

Alonzo, A.A., Reynolds, N.R. (1995). Stigma, HIV and AIDS: An exploration and elaboration of a stigma trajectory. *Social Science and Medicine, 41*(3), 303–315.

Amaro, H. (1995). Love, sex and power. *American Psychologist, 50*(6), 437–447.

Anderson, J.N. (1973). Ecological anthropology and anthropological ecology. In J. Honigman (Ed.), *Handbook of social and cultural anthropology* (pp. 179–246). Chicago: Rand McNally College Publishing Company.

Armendariz, A., Saunders, J.M., Poston, S.L., et al. (1997). Exploring a life history of HIV disease and self-caring: Alfredo's story. *Journal of the Association of Nurses in AIDS Care, 8*(2), 72–82.

Artemis, L. (1996). Migrant health care: Creativity in primary care. *Advanced Practice Nursing Quarterly, 2*(2), 45–49.

Barney, D. (1996). The National Database for HIV-infected American Indians, Alaskan Natives, and Native Hawaiians is up and running. *Innovations,* (Summer), 4–5.

Barrios, D.C., Hearst, N., Coates, T.J., et al. (1993). HIV antibody testing among those at risk for infection: The National AIDS Behavior Surveys. *Journal of the American Medical Association, 270*(13), 1576–1580.

Battle, R.S., Cummings, G.L., Yamada, K.A., et al. (1996). HIV testing among low-income African-American mothers. *AIDS Education and Prevention, 8*(2), 165–175.

Bayer, R. (1994). AIDS prevention and cultural sensitivity: Are they compatible? *American Journal of Public Health, 84,* 895–898.

Belgrave, F.Z., Randolph, S.M. (1993). Introduction: Psychosocial aspects of AIDS prevention among African Americans. *Journal of Black Psychology, 19,* 103–107.

Blank, R.M. (1995). Poverty and public policy in the 1990s. In Demko, G.J., Jackson, M.C. (Eds.), *Populations at risk in America* (pp. 60–76). Boulder, CO: Westview Press.

Bowser, B.P. (1992). Cross-cultural medicine a decade later: African-American culture and AIDS prevention from barrier to ally. *Western Journal of Medicine, 157*(3), 286–289.

Bradley-Springer, L. (1997). Needle and syringe exchange: Pride and prejudice. *Journal of the Association of Nurses in AIDS Care, 8*(5), 18–20.

Bureau of the Census, U.S. Department of Commerce. (1996). Poverty in the United States: 1996. *Current population reports,* pp. 60–194. Washington, DC: Author.

Bureau of the Census, U.S. Department of Commerce. (1997). *Resident population of the United States by race and Hispanic origin: September, 1997.* Washington, DC: Author.

Bureau of Indian Affairs. (1998, March). Indian entities recognized and eligible to receive services from the U.S. Bureau of Indian Affairs. Washington, DC: U.S. Department of the Interior.

Caetano, R., Hines, A.M. (1995). Alcohol, sexual practices, and risk of AIDS among blacks, Hispanics, and whites. *Journal of Acquired Immune Deficiency Syndromes and Human Retrovirology, 10*(5), 554–561.

California Nurses' Association (CNA). (1993). *Cultural issues. Women at risk: AIDS/HIV training for care providers* (pp. III-1 to III-58). San Francisco, CA: The Association.

Campos-Outcalt, D., Ellis, J., Aickin, M., et al. (1995). Prevalence of cardiovascular disease risk factors in a southwestern Native American tribe. *Public Health Reports, 110*(6), 742–748.

Campos-Outcalt, D., Ryan, K. (1995). Prevalence of sexually transmitted diseases in Mexican-American pregnant women by country of birth and length of time in the United States. *Sexually Transmitted Disease, 22*(2), 78–82.

Carlisle, D.M., Leake, B.D., Brook, R.H., et al. (1996). The effect of race and ethnicity on the rise of selected health care procedures: A comparison of South Central Los Angeles and the remainder of Los Angeles County. *Journal of Health Care for the Poor and Underserved, 7*(4), 308–322.

Carswell, W. (1993). HIV in South Africa. *Lancet, 342*(8864), 132.

Carter, J.S., Pugh, J.A., Monterrosa, A. (1996). Non-insulin-dependent diabetes mellitus in minorities in the United States. *Annals of Internal Medicine, 125*(3), 221–232.

Casimir, B.T. (1996). Why is it necessary to have agencies targeted and run by people of color? *Innovations: Issues in HIV Service Delivery,* (Summer), 2–3.

Centers for Disease Control and Prevention. (January 15, 1993). Condom use and sexual identity among men who have sex with men—Dallas, 1991. *Morbidity and Mortality Weekly Report, 42*(1), 7–14.

Centers for Disease Control and Prevention. (May 28, 1993). Sexual behavior and condom use—District of Columbia January–February 1992. *Morbidity and Mortality Weekly Report, 42*(20), 390–397.

Centers for Disease Control and Prevention. (June 25, 1993). Use of race and ethnicity in public health surveillance. *Morbidity and Mortality Weekly Report, 42*(RR-10), 11–12.

Centers for Disease Control and Prevention. (1993, August). Study of behavior in non-identifying gay men. *HIV/AIDS Prevention, 4*(2), 6–7.

Centers for Disease Control and Prevention. (October 15, 1993). Self-reported HIV-antibody testing behaviors: Southern Los Angeles County, 1991–1992. *Morbidity and Mortality Weekly Report, 42*(40), 786–789.

Centers for Disease Control and Prevention. (June 24, 1994). Knowledge and practices among injecting-drug users of bleach use for equipment disinfection—New York City. *Morbidity and Mortality Weekly Report, 43,* 439–446.

Centers for Disease Control and Prevention. (June 2, 1995). Update: Trends in AIDS among men who have sex with men—United States, 1989–1994. *Morbidity and Mortality Weekly Report, 44*(21), 401–404.

Centers for Disease Control and Prevention. (March 1, 1996). Mortality patterns, U.S. 1993. *Morbidity and Mortality Weekly Report, 45*(8), 161–163.

Centers for Disease Control and Prevention. (May 10, 1996). Community-level prevention of human immunodeficiency virus infection among high-risk populations. The AIDS community demonstration projects. *Morbidity and Mortality Weekly Report, 45*(no. RR-6).

Centers for Disease Control and Prevention. (December 27, 1996). State and sex specific prevalence of selected characteristics—behavioral risk factor surveillance system, 1992 and 1993. *Morbidity and Mortality Weekly Report, 45*(no. SS-6).

Centers for Disease Control and Prevention Report. (1997). HIV & AIDS trends: The changing landscape of the epidemic: A closer look. *Centers for Disease Control and Prevention. (www.cdcnac.org/hivtrend.html).*

Centers for Disease Control and Prevention. (February 28, 1997). Update: Trends in AIDS incidence, deaths, and prevalence—United States, 1996. *Morbidity and Mortality Weekly Report, 46,* 165–173.

Centers for Disease Control and Prevention. (May 2, 1997). Contraceptive practices among women—Selected U.S. sites, 1993–1995. *Morbidity and Mortality Weekly Report, 46*(17), 373–377.

Centers for Disease Control and Prevention. (June 27, 1997). Opportunistic infections in persons infected with human immunodeficiency virus. *Morbidity and Mortality Weekly Report, 46*(RR-12), 1–43.

Centers for Disease Control and Prevention. (June 30, 1997). *HIV/AIDS Surveillance Report, 9*(1), 1–39.

Centers for Disease Control and Prevention. (1997, July). HIV postexposure prophylaxis registry for HCWs is established to study side effects and effectiveness. *HIV/AIDS Prevention,* p. 12.

Centers for Disease Control and Prevention. (March 6, 1998). HIV/AIDS among American Indians and Alaskan Natives—United States, 1981–1997. *Morbidity and Mortality Weekly Report, 47*(8), 154–160.

Chang, S.B., Hill, M.N. (1996). HIV/AIDS related knowledge, attitudes, and preventive behavior of pregnant Korean women. *IMAGE: Journal of Nursing Scholarship, 28*(4), 321–324.

Chavkin, W. (1997). Topics for our times: Affirmative action and women's health. *American Journal of Public Health, 87*(5), 732–734.

Choi, K., Catania, J.A. (1996). Changes in multiple sexual partnerships, HIV testing, and condom use among U.S. heterosexuals 18 to 49 years of age, 1990–1992. *American Journal of Public Health, 86,* 554–556.

Choi, K., Catania, J.A., Dolcini, M.M. (1994). Extramarital sex and HIV risk behavior among US adults: Results from the National AIDS Behavioral Survey. *American Journal of Public Health, 84,* 2003–2007.

Choi, K., Lew, S., Vittinghoff, E., et al. (1996). The efficacy of brief group counseling in HIV risk reduction among homosexual Asian and Pacific Islander men. *AIDS, 10,* 81–87.

Choy, C. (1995). *Out in silence, AIDS in the Asian Pacific American Community.* Videotape produced by Fear of Disclosure Project, Christine Choy, Director, Filmmakers Library, New York, NY.

Cochran, S.D., Mays, V.M. (1993). Applying social psychological models to predicting HIV-related sexual risk behaviors among African Americans. *Journal of Black Psychology, 19*(2), 142–154.

Crawford, I., Allison, K.W., Robinson, W.L., et al. (1992). Attitudes of African-American Baptist ministers towards AIDS. *Journal of Community Psychology, 20,* 304–308.

Croteau, J.M., Nero, C.I., Prosser, D.J. (1993). Social and cultural sensitivity in group-specific HIV and AIDS programming. *Journal of Counseling & Development, 71,* 290–296.

Crystal, S., Sambamoorthi, U., Merzel, C. (1995). The diffusion of innovation in AIDS treatment: Zidovudine use in two New Jersey cohorts. *Health Services Research, 30*(4), 593–614.

Dalton, H.L. (1993). AIDS in blackface. In E.S. Nelson (Ed.), *Critical essays: Gay and lesbian writers of color* (pp. 205–225). Binghamton, NY: The Haworth Press.

Daroszewski, E. (1995). African American Ethnocultural Association Scale. In *Dietary risk, readiness to change and dietary choices of African American women.* Unpublished dissertation. UCLA School of Nursing, Los Angeles.

Dearing, J.W., Rogers, E.M., Meyer, G., et al. (1996). Social marketing and diffusion-based strategies for communicating with unique populations: HIV prevention in San Francisco. *Journal of Health Communication, 1,* 343–363.

Denning, P., Fleming, P. (1997). *Estimating recent patterns of HIV infection among adolescents and young adults* (abstract 375). Presented at 4th Conference on

Retroviruses and Opportunistic Infections, Washington, DC.

Denning, P., Ward, J., Chu, S., et al. (1996). *Current trends in AIDS incidence among young men who have sex with men, United States* (abstract Tu.C. 2405). Presented at XI International Conference on AIDS, Vancouver, British Columbia.

Department of Labor. (1997, August). News: The employment situation. Publication No. USDLA 97-309.

Diaz, R.M. (1994). *Latino gay men and the psychocultural barriers to AIDS prevention.* Unpublished manuscript, Stanford University Center for AIDS Prevention Studies, UCSF, San Francisco.

Diaz, T., Buehler, J.W., Castro, K.G., et al. (1993a). AIDS trends among Hispanics in the United States. *American Journal of Public Health, 83*(4), 504–509.

Diaz, T., Chu, S.Y., Frederick, P., et al. (1993b). Sociodemographics and HIV risk behaviors of bisexual men with AIDS: Results from a multistate interview project. *AIDS, 7*(9), 1227–1232.

Diaz, T., Chu, S.Y., Sorvillo, F., et al. (1995). Differences in participation in experimental drug trials among persons with AIDS. *Journal of Acquired Immune Deficiency Syndromes and Human Retrovirology, 10*(5), 562–568.

Doll, L.S., Beeker, C. (1996). Male bisexual behavior and HIV risk in the United States: Synthesis of research with implications for behavioral interventions. *AIDS Education and Prevention, 8*(3), 205–225.

Edgerton, R.B. (1971). *The individual in cultural adaptation* (pp. 1–22). Los Angeles: University of California Press.

Erickson, R.E. (1997). Human immunodeficiency virus infection risk among female sex partners of intravenous drug users in Southern Arizona. *Holistic Nursing Practice, 11*(2), 9–17.

Evans, R.G., Barer, M., Marmor, T.R., et al. (1994). Review: Why are some people healthy and others not? The determinants of health of populations. *American Journal of Public Health, 86*(4), 598–599.

Eversley, R.B., Newstetter, A., Avins, A., et al. (1993). Sexual risk and perception of risk for HIV infection among multiethnic family-planning clients. *American Journal of Preventive Medicine, 9*(2), 92–95.

Fahs, M.C., Waite, D., Sesholtz, M., et al. (1994). Results of the ACSUS for pediatric AIDS patients: Utilization of services, functional status, and social severity. *Health Services Research, 29*(5), 549–568.

Fishbein, M. (1996). Editorial: Great expectations, or do we ask too much from community-level interventions? *American Journal of Public Health, 86*(8), 1075–1076.

Flaskerud, J.H. (1988). Is the Likert scale format culturally biased? *Nursing Research, 37*(3), 185–186.

Flaskerud, J.H. (1994). AIDS and traditional food therapies. In R. Watson (Ed.), *Nutrition and AIDS* (pp. 235–247). Boca Raton, FL: CRC Press.

Flaskerud, J.H. (1998). Vulnerable populations. In J. Fitzpatrick (Ed.), *Encyclopedia of nursing research.* New York: Springer Publishing Company.

Flaskerud, J.H., Calvillo, E.R. (1991a). Beliefs about AIDS, health, and illness among low-income Latino women. *Research in Nursing and Health, 14*(6), 431–438.

Flaskerud, J.H., Nyamathi, A.M. (1988). An AIDS education program for Vietnamese women. *New York State Journal of Medicine, 88*(12), 6327.

Flaskerud, J.H., Nyamathi, A.M. (1996). Home medication injection among Latino women in Los Angeles: Implications for health education and prevention. *AIDS Care, 8*(1), 95–102.

Flaskerud, J.H., Nyamathi, A.M., Uman, G.C. (1997). Longitudinal effects of an HIV testing and counseling program for low income Latino women. *Ethnicity and Health, 2*(1/2), 89–103.

Flaskerud, J.H., Rush, C.E. (1989). AIDS and traditional health beliefs and practices of black women. *Nursing Research, 38*(4), 210–215.

Flaskerud, J.H., Tabora, B. (1998). Health problems of low income female caregivers of adults with HIV/AIDS. *Health Care for Women International, 19,* 23–36.

Flaskerud, J.H., Thompson, J. (1991b). Beliefs about AIDS, health, and illness in low-income white women. *Nursing Research, 40*(5), 266–271.

Flaskerud, J.H., Uman, G. (1993). Directions for AIDS education for Hispanic women based on analyses of survey findings. *Public Health Reports, 108*(3), 298–304.

Flaskerud, J.H., Uman, G., Lara, R., et al. (1996). Sexual practices, attitudes, and knowledge related to HIV transmission among low income Los Angeles Hispanic women. *Journal of Sex Research, 33*(6), 1–11.

Gomez, V.M., Stewart, A., Ritter, P.L., et al. (1995). Translation and validation of arthritis outcome measures into Spanish. *Arthritis & Rheumatism, 38*(10), 1429–1446.

Gorman, C. (June 23, 1997). If the condom breaks. *Time Magazine,* 48.

Graham, N.M.H., Jacobson, L.P., Kuo, V., et al. (1994). Prevention of HIV/AIDS and other blood-borne diseases among injection drug users. *Journal of the American Medical Association, 277*(1), 53–62.

Gregonis, S.W. (1997). Magic Johnson and Lazarus: The new syndromes. *Journal of the Association of Nurses in AIDS Care, 8*(5), 75–76.

Grinstead, O.A., Peterson, J.L., Faigeles, B., et al. (1997). Antibody testing and condom use among heterosexual African Americans at risk for HIV infection: The National AIDS Behavioral Surveys. *American Journal of Public Health, 87*(5), 857–859.

Grossman, A.H. (1994). Homophobia: A cofactor of HIV disease in gay and lesbian youth. *Journal of the Association of Nurses in AIDS Care, 5*(1), 39–43.

Grossman, A.H. (1995). At risk, infected, and invisible: Older gay men and HIV/AIDS. *Journal of the Association of Nurses in AIDS Care, 6*(6), 13–19.

Grossman, A.H. (1996). *Families and children: The challenge of HIV/AIDS* (2nd ed.). New York: Department of Mental Health, Mental Retardation and Alcoholism Services.

Grossman, D. (1994). Enhancing your cultural competence. *American Journal of Nursing, 94,* 58, 60, 62.

Guinan, M.E. (1993). Black communities' belief in "AIDS as genocide": A barrier to overcome for HIV prevention. *Annals of Epidemiology, 3*(2), 193–195.

Guralnik, J.M., Leveille, S.G. (1997). Annotation: Race, ethnicity, and health outcomes. Unraveling and mediating role of socioeconomic status. *American Journal of Public Health, 87*(5), 728–729.

Halloran, J.P., Ross, M.W., Huffman, L. (1996). Training persons with HIV disease for involvement in community planning process: Project LEAP. *Journal of the Association of Nurses in AIDS Care, 7*(6), 39–56.

Hendricson, W.D., Russell, I.J., Prihoda, T.J., et al. (1989). An approach to developing a valid Spanish language translation of a health-status questionnaire. *Medical Care, 27*(10), 959–966.

Herek, G.M., Capitanio, J.P. (1994). Conspiracies, contagion, and compassion: Trust and public reactions to AIDS. *AIDS Education and Prevention, 6,* 365–375.

Holtgrave, D.R., Qualls, N.L., Curran, J.W., et al. (1995). An overview of the effectiveness and efficiency of HIV prevention programs. *Public Health Reports, 110*(2), 134–146.

Hu, D.J., Fleming, P.L., Castro, K.G., et al. (1995). How important is race/ethnicity as an indicator of risk for specific AIDS-defining conditions? *Journal of Acquired Immune Deficiency Syndromes and Human Retrovirology, 10*(3), 374–380.

Hufford, D. (1995). Cultural and social perspectives on alternative medicine: Background and assumptions. *Alternative Therapies, 1*(1), 53–61.

Icard, L., Schilling, R.F., El-Bassel, N., et al. (1992). Preventing AIDS among Black gay men and Black gay and heterosexual male intravenous drug users. *Social Work, 37*(5), 440–445.

Jagers, R.J. (1996). Culture and problem behaviors among inner-city African-American youth: Further explorations. *Journal of Adolescence, 19,* 371–381.

Jenkins, B., Lamar, V.L., Thompson-Crumble, J. (1993). AIDS among African Americans: A social epidemic. *Journal of Black Psychology, 19*(2), 108–122.

Kalichman, S.C., Carey, M.P., Johnson, B.T. (1996). Prevention of sexually transmitted HIV infection: A meta-analytic review of the behavioral outcome literature. *Annals of Behavioral Medicine, 18*(1), 6–15.

Katz, M.H., Gerberding, J.L. (1997). Postexposure treatment of people exposed to the human immunodeficiency virus through sexual contact or injection-drug use. *New England Journal of Medicine, 336*(15), 1097–1110.

Kaufman, J.S., Cooper, R.S. (1995). In search of the hypothesis. *Public Health Reports, 110,* 662–666.

Kauth, M.R., St. Lawrence, J., Kelly, J.A. (1991). Reliability of retrospective assessments of sexual HIV risk behavior: A comparison of biweekly, three-month, and twelve-month self-reports. *AIDS Education and Prevention, 3*(3), 207–214.

Keefe, S., Padilla, A.M. (1987). *Chicano ethnicity.* Albuquerque, NM: University of New Mexico Press.

Kegeles, S.M., Hays, R.B., Coates, T.J. (1996). The Mpowerment project: A community-level HIV prevention intervention for young gay men. *American Journal of Public Health, 86*(8), 1129–1136.

Kelly, J.A., St. Lawrence, J., Hood, H.V., et al. (1989). An objective test of AIDS risk behavior knowledge: Scale development, validation, and norms. *Journal of Behavioral Therapy and Experimental Psychiatry, 20*(3), 227–234.

Kerr, H.D. (1993). White liver: A cultural disorder resembling AIDS. *Social Science Medicine, 36*(5), 609–614.

Kutenai, K. (1996). A Native-American nurse's view. Advanced Practice. *Nursing Quarterly, 2*(2), 59–61.

Latkin, C., Mandell, W., Vlahov, D., et al. (1996). People and places: Behavioral settings and personal network characteristics as correlates of needle sharing. *Journal of Acquired Immune Deficiency Syndromes and Human Retrovirology, 13,* 273–280.

Lauver, D., Armstrong, K., Marks, S., et al. (1995). HIV risk status and preventive behaviors among 17,619 women. *Journal of Obstetric, Gynecologic, and Neonatal Nursing, 24*(1), 33–39.

Lester, P., Partridge, J.C., Chesney, M.A., et al. (1995). The consequences of a positive prenatal HIV antibody test for women. *Journal of Acquired Immune Deficiency Syndromes and Human Retrovirology, 10,* 341–349.

Linares, L.O., Leadbetter, B.J., Jaffe, L. (1992). Predictors of repeat pregnancy outcome among Black and Puerto Rican adolescent mothers. *Journal of Developmental and Behavioral Pediatrics, 13*(2), 89–94.

Link, B.G., Phelan, J.C. (1996). Editorial: Understanding sociodemographic differences in health—The role of fundamental social causes. *American Journal of Public Health, 86*(4), 471–475.

Linn, J.G., Anema, M.G., Hodess, S., et al. (1996). Perceived health, HIV illness, and mental distress in African-American clients of AIDS counseling centers. *Journal of the Association of Nurses in AIDS Care, 7*(2), 43–51.

Magana, J.R., Carrier, J.M. (1991). Mexican and Mexican American male sexual behavior and spread of AIDS in California. *Journal of Sex Research, 28*(3), 425–441.

Mann, J.A., Tarantola, D. (Eds.). (1996). *AIDS in the*

world II: Global dimensions, social roots, and responses. New York: Oxford University Press.

Marin, B.V., Gomez, C. (1994). Hispanic culture: Latinos, HIV disease and culture: Strategies for AIDS prevention. In P.T. Cohen, M.A. Sande, P.A. Volberding (Eds.), *The AIDS knowledge base* (2nd ed., pp. 10.81–10.813). Boston: Little, Brown.

Marin, B.V., Marin, G. (1990). Effects of acculturation on knowledge of AIDS and HIV among Hispanics. *Journal of Behavioral Sciences, 12*(2), 110–121.

Marin, G., Sabogal, F., Marin, B., et al. (1987). Development of a short acculturation scale for Hispanics. *Hispanic Journal of Behavioral Sciences, 9*(2), 183–205.

Martin, M.A., Rissmiller, P., Beal, J.A. (1995). Health-illness beliefs and practices of Haitians with HIV disease living in Boston. *Journal of the Association of Nurses in AIDS Care, 6*(6), 45–56.

Martinez, L.I., Diaz, J.A. (1996, Spring/Summer). Reach out to the Hispanic community. *¡ADELANTE!* American Red Cross, pp. 1–2.

Martinez, L., Diaz, J. (1997, Summer). HIV and AIDS among Hispanics: Statistical update for better outreach. *¡ADELANTE!* American Red Cross, pp. 1–2.

Mays, V.M., Cochran, S.D. (1993). Ethnic and gender differences in beliefs about sex partner questioning to reduce HIV risk. *Journal of Adolescent Research, 8*(1), 77–88.

Mays, V.M., Jackson, J.S. (1991). AIDS survey methodology with black Americans. *Social Science and Medicine, 33*(1), 47–54.

McClary, R. (1996). The fortune society: Reaching out to Latino ex-offenders. *Innovations: Issues in HIV service delivery,* Summer, 10–15.

McDuffie, J.F. (1997, June). Letters to the editor. *Ebony,* p. 10.

McKirnan, D.J., Ostrow, D.G., Hope, B. (1996). Sex, drugs and escape: A psychological model of HIV-risk sexual behaviours. *AIDS Care, 8*(8), 665–669.

McKirnan, D.J., Stokes, J.P., Doll, L., et al. (1995). Bisexually active men: Social characteristics and sexual behavior. *Journal of Sex Research, 32*(1), 56–76.

Misener, T., Sowell, R.L., Phillips, K.D., et al. (1997). Sexual orientation: A cultural diversity issue for nursing. *Nursing Outlook, 45*(4), 178–181.

Montoya, I.D., Atkinson, J.S. (1996). Determinants of HIV seroprevalence rates among sites participating in a community-based study of drug users. *Journal of Acquired Immune Deficiency Syndromes and Human Retrovirology, 13*(2), 169–176.

Morris, R.I. (1996). Bridging cultural boundaries: The African American and transcultural caring. *Advanced Practice Nursing Quarterly, 2*(2), 31–38.

MRC Collaborative Study Group. (1996). Ethnic differences in women with HIV infection in Britain and Ireland. *AIDS, 10,* 89–93.

Murphy, J., Mueller, G., Whitman, S. (1996). Epidemiology of AIDS among Hispanics in Chicago. *Journal of Acquired Immune Deficiency Syndromes and Human Retrovirology, 11*(1), 83–87.

National Commission on Acquired Immune Deficiency Syndrome (NCA). (1992, December). *The challenge of HIV/AIDS in communities of color.* Washington, DC: The Commission.

Neaigus, A., Friedman, S.R., Curtis, R., et al. (1994). The relevance of drug injectors' social and risk networks for understanding and preventing HIV infection. *Social Science and Medicine, 38*(1), 67–78.

Neal, J.J., Fleming, P.L., Green, T.A., et al. (1997). Trends in heterosexually acquired AIDS in the United States, 1988 through 1995. *Journal of Acquired Immune Deficiency Syndromes and Human Retrovirology, 14,* 465–474.

Nicoll, A., Laukamm-Josten, U., Mwizarubi, B., et al. (1993). Lay health beliefs concerning HIV and AIDS: A barrier for control programs. *AIDS Care, 5*(2), 231–241.

Norris, A.E., Ford, K., Shyr, Y., et al. (1996). Heterosexual experiences and partnerships of urban, low-income African-American and Hispanic youth. *Journal of Acquired Immune Deficiency Syndromes and Human Retrovirology, 11,* 288–300.

Northridge, M.E., Shepard, P.M. (1997). Comment: Environmental racism and public health. *American Journal of Public Health, 87*(5), 730–731.

Nyamathi, A., Bennett, C. (1997). Visual coping scenarios: An innovative strategy to facilitate discussion of coping responses with impoverished women at risk for AIDS. *Journal of Psychosocial Nursing and Mental Health Services, 35*(8), 17–23.

Nyamathi, A., Bennett, C., Leake, B., et al. (1993). AIDS-related knowledge, perceptions, and behaviors among impoverished minority women. *American Journal of Public Health, 83,* 65–71.

Nyamathi, A., Lewis, C., Leake, B., et al. (1995). Barriers to condom use and needle cleaning among impoverished minority female injection drug users and partners of injection drug users. *Public Health Reports, 110,* 166–172.

O'Connor, B.B. (1996). Promoting cultural competence in HIV/AIDS care. *Journal of the Association of Nurses in AIDS Care, 7*(Suppl. 1), 48–52.

Office for Substance Abuse Prevention (OSAP). (1992). *Cultural competence for evaluators.* Rockville, MD: United States Public Health Service.

Ostrow, D. (1993). AIDS conspiracy theories: Minireview. *AIDS Targeted Information, 7*(3), 1.

Parra, E.O., Shapiro, M.F., Moreno, C.A., et al. (1993). AIDS-related risk behavior, knowledge, and beliefs among women and their Mexican-American sexual partners who used intravenous drugs. *Archives of Family Medicine, 2*(6), 603–610.

Peterson, J.L., Coates, T.J., Catania, J.A., et al. (1995). Help-seeking for AIDS high-risk sexual behavior among gay and bisexual African-American men. *AIDS Education and Prevention, 7*(1), 1–9.

Peterson, J.L., Coates, T.J., Catania, J., et al. (1996). Evaluation of an HIV risk reduction intervention among African-American homosexual and bisexual men. *AIDS, 10,* 319–325.

Pickwell, S.M. (1996). Providing health care to refugees. *Advanced Practice Nursing Quarterly, 2*(2), 39–44.

Pivnick, A., Jacobson, A., Eric, K., et al. (1994). AIDS, HIV infection, and illicit drug use within inner-city families and social networks. *American Journal of Public Health, 84*(2), 271–274.

Pliskin, K.L. (1992). Dysphoria and somatization in Iranian culture. *Western Journal of Medicine, 157*(3), 295–300.

Prochaska, J., Redding, C., Harlow, J., et al. (1994). The transtheoretical model of change and HIV prevention: A review. *Health Education Quarterly, 21*(4), 471–486.

Ramakrishna, J., Weiss, M.G. (1992). Health, illness, and immigration: East Indians in the United States. *Western Journal of Medicine, 157*(3), 265–275.

Ramirez, J., Suarez, E., de la Rosa, G., et al. (1994). AIDS knowledge and sexual behavior among Mexican gay and bisexual men. *AIDS Education and Prevention, 6*(2), 163–174.

Randolph, L.B. (1997, April). The Magic "miracle": The Lord has healed Earvin. *Ebony,* pp. 73–76.

Reid, D. (1994). *The complete book of Chinese health and healing.* Boston: Shambhola Press.

Richardson, L. (April 21, 1997). Experiment leaves legacy of distrust of new AIDS drugs. *New York Times,* p. A1.

Rietmeijer, C.A., Kane, M.S., Simons, P.Z., et al. (1996). Increasing the use of bleach and condoms among injecting drug users in Denver: Outcomes of a targeted, community-level HIV prevention program. *AIDS, 10,* 291–298.

Rogers, E.M., Dearing, N.R., et al. (1996). San Francisco's response to the AIDS epidemic triggered a dramatically altered sense of community. *Communication Research, 22*(6), 664–678.

Roman, D. (1993). Fierce love and fierce response: Intervening in the cultural politics of race, sexuality, and AIDS. In E.S. Nelson (Ed.), *Critical essays: Gay and lesbian writers of color* (pp. 195–219). Binghamton, NY: The Haworth Press.

Rose, M.A., Clark-Alexander, B. (1996). Quality of life and coping styles of HIV-positive women with children. *Journal of the Association of Nurses in AIDS Care, 7*(2), 28–34.

Royce, R.A., Sena, A., Cates, W., et al. (1997). Sexual transmission of HIV. *New England Journal of Medicine, 336*(15), 1072–1078.

Ryan, F. (1997). *Virus X: Tracking the new killer plagues* (pp. 268–284). Boston: Little, Brown.

Schiller, N.G. (1993). The invisible women: Caregiving and the construction of AIDS health services. *Culture, Medicine & Psychiatry, 17,* 487–512.

Schilling, R.F., El-Bassel, N., Schinke, S.P., et al. (1991). Sexual behavior, attitudes toward safer sex and gender among a cohort of 244 recovering IV drug users. *International Journal of Addiction, 26*(8), 859–877.

Schoenborn, C.A., Marsh, S.L., Haroy, A.M. (1994). AIDS knowledge and attitudes for 1992. Data from the National Health Interview Survey. *Advanced Data, 23*(243), 1–16.

Schopper, D., Vercauteren, G. (1996). Testing for HIV at home: What are the issues? *AIDS, 10*(13), 1455–1465.

Schwarcz, S.K., Bolan, G.A., Kellogg, T.A., et al. (1993). Comparison of voluntary and blinded human immunodeficiency virus type 1 (HIV-1) seroprevalence surveys in a high prevalence sexually transmitted disease clinical population. *American Journal of Epidemiology, 137*(6), 600–608.

Seals, B.F. (1996). Viewpoint: The overlapping epidemics of violence and HIV. *Journal of the Association of Nurses in AIDS Care, 7*(5), 91–93.

Shernoff, M., Ball, S. (1997, April). Sex, secrets and lies. *OUT,* 105–147.

Sher, R. (1993). The role of women in the AIDS epidemic. *Medicine & Law, 12*(6-8), 467–469.

Simon, P.A., Weber, M., Ford, W.L., et al. (1996). Reasons for HIV antibody test refusal in a heterosexual sexually transmitted disease clinic population. *AIDS, 10,* 1549–1553.

Singer, M. (1991). Confronting the AIDS epidemic among IV drug users: Does ethnic culture matter? *AIDS Education and Prevention, 3*(3), 258–283.

Singh, G.K., Yu, S.M. (1996). U.S. childhood mortality, 1950 through 1993: Trends and socioeconomic differentials. *American Journal of Public Health, 86*(4), 505–512.

Smith, P., Weinman, M.L. (1995). Cultural implications for public health policy for pregnant Hispanic adolescents. *Health Values, 19*(1), 3–9.

Solomon, L., Moore, J., Gleghorn, A., et al. (1996). HIV testing behaviors in a population of inner-city women at high risk for HIV infection. *Journal of Acquired Immune Deficiency Syndromes and Human Retrovirology, 13,* 267–272.

Sontag, S. (1990). *AIDS and its metaphors.* New York: Anchor Books.

Sowell, R.L., Moneyham, L., Guillory, J., et al. (1997). Self-care activities of women infected with human immunodeficiency virus. *Holistic Nursing Practice, 11*(2), 18–26.

Sowell, R.L., Seals, B.F., Phillips, K.D. (1996). Knowledge of risk behaviors of people seeking HIV antibody testing at a community site. *Journal of the Association of Nurses in AIDS Care, 7*(3), 33–42.

Stevenson, H.C., Davis, G. (1994). Impact of culturally sensitive AIDS video education on the AIDS risk knowledge of African-American adolescents. *AIDS Education and Prevention, 6*(1), 40–52.

Suarez, M., Raffacelli, M., O'Leary, A. (1996). Use of folk healing practices by HIV-infected Hispanics living in the United States. *AIDS Care, 8*(6), 683–690.

Suinn, R.M., Rickard-Figueroa, K., Lew, S., et al. (1987). The Suinn-Lew Asian self-identity acculturation scale: An initial report. *Educational and Psychological Measurement, 47,* 401–407.

Tabet, S.R., Antonio de Moya, E., Holmes, K.K., et al. (1996). Sexual behaviors and risk factors for HIV infection among men who have sex with men in the Dominican Republic. *AIDS, 10,* 201–206.

Thomas, S.B., Quinn, S.C. (1991). The Tuskegee syphilis study, 1932–1972: Implications for HIV education and AIDS risk education programs in the Black community. *American Journal of Public Health, 81*(11), 1498–1505.

Turner, N.H., Solomon, D.J. (1996). HIV risks and risk reduction readiness in hard-to-reach, drug-using African American and Mexican American women: An exploratory study. *AIDS Education and Prevention, 8*(3), 236–246.

Walker, J. (1996). Targeting Haitians. *Innovations,* Summer, 8–9.

Wayment, H.A., Newcomb, M.D., Hannemann, V.L. (1993). Female and male intravenous drug users not-in-treatment: Are they at differential risk for AIDS? *Sex Roles, 28*(1/2), 111–125.

Wells, E.K., Mayer, R.R. (1997). HIV-negative women in serodiscordant couples. *HIVFrontline, 29,* 4–5.

Wenger, A.F.Z. (1993). Cultural meaning of symptoms. *Holistic Nursing Practice, 7*(2), 22–35.

Weniger, B.G., Brown, T. (1996). The march of AIDS through Asia. *New England Journal of Medicine, 335*(5), 343–344.

Wright, J.W. (1993). African-American male sexual behavior and the risk for HIV infection. *Human Organizations, 52,* 421–431.

Wyatt, G.E. (1991). Examining ethnicity versus race in AIDS related sex research. *Social Science and Medicine, 33*(1), 37–45.

Wyatt, G.E., Chen, I.S.Y., Tucson, R.V., et al. (1997, June). Letters to the editor: The magic miracle. *Ebony,* p. 10.

Zimmerman, M.A., Ramirez-Valles, J., Suarez, E., et al. (1997). An HIV/AIDS prevention project for Mexican homosexual men: An empowerment approach. *Health Education and Behavior, 24*(2), 177–190.

10

Community-Based and Long-Term Care

JOAN SCHMIDT ■ MICHELE CRESPO-FIERRO

For the first time since the beginning of the epidemic, the number of AIDS-related deaths declined in 1996 (CDC, 1997a). The mortality among persons with advanced HIV infection decreased from 29.4 per 100 person-years in 1995 to 8.8 per 100 person years in the second quarter of 1997 (Palella et al., 1998). With deaths decreasing, the number of persons living with AIDS continued to rise. The CDC estimated that 235,470 persons were living with AIDS as of 1996. Increased life expectancy results in an increased demand for health care services, especially in the community.

When planning for the health care and social services of persons living with HIV disease (PLWHIV), health care providers (HCPs) must look at the full range of services that may be required throughout the course of illness. In June 1988 the members of the Presidential Commission on the HIV Epidemic noted, in their final report, that a continued focus on AIDS, rather than on the entire spectrum of the HIV epidemic, has left the United States unable to deal effectively with the epidemic. Most important, the report looked at health care delivery "through the lens of the HIV epidemic and found gaping holes, huge problems" (Gebbie, 1989, p. 869). In essence, the HIV epidemic has vividly exposed the many weaknesses inherent in health care in the United States.

Gebbie (1989) noted that the HIV epidemic has revealed major deficits, such as (1) failure to offer each child born a comprehensive health and health education program that would provide a basis for a healthy adult life; (2) failure to construct a coherent system of delivering care services for ill persons and a method of paying for such services; and (3) failure to understand the dangers of creating a permanent under class, a drug-linked culture that does not participate in the ordinary obligations and benefits of our social service system. In fact, the HIV epidemic has shown that there is no such thing as a "health care system" in the United States (Ungvarski, 1989). The definition of the word *system* implies an interdependence and interrelationship between elements, which forms a collective entity. In the United States we have the antithesis to this definition: a fragmented array of health care services provided by federal, state, local, nonprofit, voluntary, and proprietary agencies. Brook (1996) summed up the current situation when he noted, "The American health care nonsystem of the 1990s might best be described by the words cost and chaos" (p. 1005).

In many respects, the phrase *health care system* is a misnomer. What is actually provided in the United States is a system of acute care, not health care. Essentially, a person who becomes seriously ill is provided a bed in a hospital. The emphasis is on hospitals, with limited focus on both long-term care and primary care or prevention. The latter is available to those who can afford it and who seek it out.

The consequence for Americans without health insurance is an increase in morbidity and mortality rates. Burstin and associates (1992), in a study of 51 hospitals in New York State, found that uninsured patients were at greater risk of suffering medical injury as a result of substandard medical care. Franks and colleagues (1993) studied 4694 Americans prospectively and concluded that lack of health insurance is associated with an increased risk of death. Both these studies underscore the inequities that currently exist in delivery of health care service and the urgent need for reform in the United States.

In 1996 the Clinton administration announced an AIDS strategy that included six goals:

1. Developing a cure and a vaccine
2. Reducing and eventually eliminating new infections
3. Guaranteeing care and services for those carrying HIV
4. Fighting AIDS-related discrimination
5. Translating scientific advances quickly into improved care and prevention
6. Providing strong, continuing support for international efforts to deal with AIDS (Associated Press, 1996)

However, the strategy did not include lifting the federal ban on funding for needle-exchange programs, a move that experts believe is essential to stem the tide of HIV infection among injecting drug users (Normand et al., 1995). Although funding for HIV/AIDS increased under the Clinton administration, the announcement of the AIDS strategy did not include a specific legislative agenda to meet the proposed goals.

AIDS AS A CHRONIC DISEASE

In 1989 the concept that AIDS should be viewed as a chronic disease was introduced (Fee & Fox, 1992). This approach was based on the premise that antiretroviral agents plus preventive and suppressive therapies for opportunistic infections (OIs) would significantly prolong life, even if the underlying HIV infection could not be cured. However, Fee and Krieger (1993) argued that the chronic disease model alone is inadequate to describe the complexities of HIV disease because, unlike other chronic diseases such as diabetes and heart disease, HIV is infectious. They proposed that health professionals characterize HIV as a chronic infectious disease, thus reflecting the need to be concerned about the prevention of new infections as well as the health care needs of those who are already infected.

If HIV is to be treated as a chronic infectious disease in the 1990s, the focus must shift from the acute care, inpatient setting to ambulatory care (Imperato, 1990). However, in a nationwide survey of 401 nurse executives to determine the availability of health care services for persons with AIDS, Sowell et al. (1990) found that acute care services were still the most widely available. Only half of the urban hospitals and one third of the rural hospitals offered comprehensive, chronic ambulatory care services, and such services were neither available nor proposed by 60% of the hospitals. Home care services were more prevalent: 91% of the nurse executives indicated that their communities offered home health care and hospice care and 59.9% provided case management services. Only 47.9% of those surveyed stated that their communities had long-term care services for persons with AIDS, and 52.1% said that long-term care was neither available nor planned. When Piette et al. (1993) conducted a cross-sectional nationwide study to determine the perceived needs and unmet needs for PLWHIV, the respondents reported a need for mental health services (57%), housing (39%), entitlements (34%), transportation (34%), and home care (28%).

COMMUNITY NURSING CENTERS

The 1980s saw the growth of community nursing centers as a source of primary health care, including services for persons with HIV/AIDS. A study conducted by the National League for Nursing (NLN) used the following characteristics to define a nursing center:

1. A nurse must occupy the chief management position in the center
2. Accountability and responsibility for client care and professional practice remain with the nurse
3. Nurses are the primary providers seen by clients visiting the center [NLN, 1992, p. 1]

The NLN estimates there are approximately 250 nursing centers in the country; of the 98 centers that responded to the NLN survey, 2% specialize in the care of PLWHIV/AIDS.

Nursing centers offer health care services to populations that historically have been underserved. In the NLN survey, 52% of the nursing centers' clients were white, 31% were black, 13%

were Latino, and 2% were Asian; thus 46% of the clients served were from communities of color. The centers are also providing health care to uninsured persons. When the NLN reported how services were compensated, 27% were paid by the client and 13% were uncompensated. Insurance coverage was as follows: Medicare, 11%; Medicaid, 13%; private insurance, 19%; and others, 17%.

One example of a nursing center that specialized in HIV/AIDS was the Denver Nursing Project in Human Caring. This project opened in 1988 to provide comprehensive services to PLWHIV and their significant others. Nurses used Jean Watson's *Philosophy and Science of Human Caring* as the basis for practice (Lyne & Waller, 1990). Watson believes that nursing educators and clinical staff need to work together "to transform the system from a sick care system to a human care-healing model" (Darbyshire, 1992, p. 44). For clients to have a consistently available nurse to guide them through the health care maze and the unpredictable course of HIV/AIDS, the Denver Caring Center used nursing care partnerships (Schroeder & Maeve, 1992). A descriptive study of clients' perceptions of the Center found high levels of client satisfaction with care (Leenerts et al., 1996). Seventy-three percent of the respondents indicated that nurses taught them self-care skills that increased their independence at home so that they were less dependent on more costly care settings. By preventing hospitalizations and reducing the length of institutional stay, the Center was estimated to have saved more than $700,000 in 1991 and $1 million in hospital charges in 1992 (Schroeder, 1993).

Unfortunately, after the Caring Center set the standard for holistic HIV care in Denver, it found itself a casualty of competing funding sources. Hospitals that had previously referred clients to the Center obtained funding to expand their outpatient services to include those offered by the Caring Center. Having lost significant hospital referral support, the Center could no longer remain financially viable, and it closed in July 1996 (R. Neil, personal communication, June 26, 1997).

Realizing and acknowledging these issues, HCPs can appreciate that planning care for an HIV-infected person from the time of diagnosis through the course of illness can be not only difficult but also frustrating. What is needed in the early stages of HIV infection is clinical monitoring through primary care and psychosocial services, whereas in the later stages acute care, home care, long-term residential care, and hospice care are required. Many persons have limited access to primary care and support services; they may be refused access to long-term residential care because they are infected with HIV. Unfortunately, lack of entitlement and the inability to pay are barriers to care that are shared by many HIV-infected persons.

FUNDING FOR HIV-RELATED CARE

In 1990 Congress recognized that there were gaps in funding and services for PLWHIV, and these issues were addressed with the passage of the Ryan White Comprehensive AIDS Emergency (CARE) Act and the establishment of the AIDS Drug Assistance Programs (ADAP). The former provides funding for outpatient and ambulatory medical and support services for persons living with HIV/AIDS; the latter pays for medications and health care for the uninsured or for those with limited insurance coverage.

Title I of the Ryan White CARE Act was targeted to those urban areas with the greatest numbers of reported AIDS cases. Bowen et al. (1992) indicated that the following services received the bulk of the funding: primary care, 34.6%; case management, 13.4%; medications, 12.5%; support services (including transportation, food, peer support, and volunteer services), 9.6%; housing-related services, 7.4%; and mental health services, 7.3% (p. 495). The remainder of the monies were allocated to home health care, substance abuse services, and long-term care, including adult day care, hospice, and institutional care.

With the advent of combination drug therapies for HIV infection, state ADAP programs have been struggling to meet the demand. Even though federal funds for the ADAP programs were increased by $115 million nationwide in late 1996 (Cooper, 1996), each state decides how to administer the programs and whether or not to contribute funds. Although some states have increased their own contributions to cover the cost of protease inhibitors, other states have adopted various strategies to address the needs, such as (1) limiting enrollments and establishing waiting lists; (2) capping individual expenditures per patient; and (3) limiting access to protease inhibitors by adding only one or two drugs to their formularies (Kolata, 1996). As a result of the ADAP restrictions, primary care providers often find that their choice of drug therapies is limited. Four states—Arkansas, Nevada, Oregon, and South Dakota—do not cover protease inhibitors under ADAP (Bayer & Stryker, 1997). Although the drug companies offer patient-assistance programs, the programs have strict eligibility criteria and require extensive paperwork.

It is important that HIV-infected persons receive health care that is delivered by knowledgeable, competent health care providers. Stone and associates (1992) examined more than 800 persons with AIDS in 40 hospitals in Massachusetts and found that the relative risk of death was more than twice as high in hospitals with lower AIDS familiarity than in hospitals that were more experienced in AIDS care. The need to disseminate HIV/AIDS care information continues even as we progress through the second decade of this disease. This chapter not only discusses the various aspects of planning care in a nonacute setting but also attempts to describe the realities related to access and delivery of services.

CASE MANAGEMENT

Because the United States has no system of health care, and because the average consumer has great difficulty in understanding and negotiating the complexities of entitlements, such as private insurance policies, Medicaid, and Medicare, case management has become a necessity. Case management is not new. At the turn of the century, public health programs provided community service coordination that was the forerunner of case management (American Nurses' Association [ANA], 1988). Coordination of services has always been the focus of public health nursing (ANA, 1988).

After World War II, the term *case management* was used to describe the community services necessary for the care of discharged psychiatric patients (Grau, 1984). The term first appeared in social welfare literature in the early 1970s, followed closely by mentions in the nursing literature (ANA, 1988). In more recent years, the U.S. government policy on health care has moved to-

ward programs that offer a comprehensive, coordinated continuum of care at the community level. In 1981 the Omnibus Budget Reconciliation Act and the Medicare prospective reimbursement program encouraged case management to provide community-based alternatives to institutional placement. The Ryan White CARE Act authorized funds for case management services, thereby recognizing their importance for persons with HIV/AIDS.

In the clinical practice guidelines for the evaluation and management of early HIV infection (1994), the Agency for Health Care Policy and Research (AHCPR) defined case management as a "system under which the patient's health care and social services are coordinated by one or more individuals familiar with both the patient's needs and community resources" (p. 141). According to AHCPR, most case management systems have the following objectives (pp. 95–96):

1. Assist patients, family, and significant others in achieving a coordinated set of services with client advocacy as an emphasis
2. Provide counseling on diagnosis and its implications, education about prevention and treatment, and necessary health care
3. Complete psychosocial assessments and integrate these with medical and nursing assessments
4. Develop achievable care plans, integrating psychosocial and health care goals
5. Link patient to one or more needed services
6. Support the patient with follow-through and continuation of services
7. Monitor and track patients to determine use, availability, and appropriateness of services
8. Reassess, together with the patient, family, and significant other, the plan and goals if the original plan is not working or cannot be achieved
9. Maintain records of unmet needs to be used in planning and advocacy efforts
10. Maintain records on each patient for evaluation of case management services.

Ideally, case management should not only optimize the client's self-care capability through the efficient use of resources but also stimulate the creation of new services. The goals of case management are to provide high-quality care, minimize fragmentation of care across many settings, enhance the quality of the client's life, and contain cost (ANA, 1988; Morrison, 1990).

It is best to have a single designated case manager. However, because of the complex needs of clients with HIV disease and the numerous players involved with care, what actually takes place is multiagency case management (see Box below). To achieve the client's goals, the various health care professionals managing the case should be aware of each other's capabilities and limitations and should develop a milieu of cooperation. Communication between providers is esssential for succesful case management.

Synonymous terms for case management include *case coordination, service management, care management,* and *managed care.* Case management can provide facilitating functions, gatekeeping functions, or a combination of both. Facilitating functions include helping the client and significant other obtain the needed services in a maze of complex rules and regulations. The gatekeeping role of case management ensures that the client and significant others receive appropriate and cost-effective health care. However, it is important that case management address the full spectrum of health and social needs, rather than limiting the focus to cost containment or medical services (Sowell, 1995).

■ TEAM MEMBERS INVOLVED IN CASE MANAGEMENT OF A PERSON WITH HIV INFECTION ■

1. Client and significant other(s)
2. Primary physician
3. Consulting physicians (e.g., ophthalmologist managing cytomegalovirus retinitis)
4. Hospital-based staff, including resident physicians, nurses, nutritionists, pharmacists, and discharge planners
5. Home care staff, including visiting nurse, homemakers, home attendants, home health aides, continuous nurses in the home, and special teams providing home infusion therapy
6. Case workers and managers from AIDS organizations, Medicaid programs, child welfare agencies, drug-treatment programs, and health clinics
7. Mental health professionals
8. Clergy

As employee health plans and government funding sources shift from a fee-for-service approach to capitated managed care programs, payers must address ways to deal with expensive, complex diseases such as HIV/AIDS. For a typical Medicaid managed care plan, the reimbursement averages $100 per month per patient (Soloway & Hecht, 1997). New York, California, and Maryland have adopted a "carve-out" approach for HIV, creating separate HIV Medicaid managed care programs with a different capitation rate and a requirement that plans offer specialized HIV services with knowledgeable providers. Case managers need to be adept at communicating client needs to managed care companies that require preauthorization for services.

Because there are no clearly delineated job requirements for the position of case manager, the position has emerged as a subspecialty in nursing and social work. In the United States there are 125,000 to 150,000 case managers, of whom approximately 17,000 are certified in case management (Wolfe, 1997, p. 25).

Case management includes intake/assessment of client needs, development of a care plan, implementation of the plan, and monitoring and evaluation (AHCPR, 1994). Regardless of the professional discipline of persons hired to perform case management, they should be provided with the necessary education, reference tools, and resource persons to understand the complex biobehavioral and psychobehavioral responses that persons experience during the course of HIV disease. They should be good listeners and not make quick value judgments without a total picture of the situation. As part of their role preparation, they should be taught the etiquette and value of telephone case management; they should be told that the telephone is an invaluable asset and should not be viewed as an interruption. Above all, case managers should keep in mind that they are not the client's only advocates. Advocacy based on a collaborative process, with mutual respect, will do more to obtain the needed services than will an adversarial approach.

Intake/Assessment

The collection of baseline data provides the framework on which the case manager structures the plan of care. Assessment is an interaction with the client, significant others, family members, and service providers. This is a time to introduce the role of the case manager and to establish a relationship between the case manager and the other parties. It is wise to remember that first impressions are lasting.

Comprehensive evaluation includes, but is not limited to, collection of data that describe

1. Demographic and personal characteristics
2. Support persons
3. Functional status of the client
4. Clinical needs of the client
5. Family information
6. Legal issues
7. Social data
8. Financial data
9. Summary of service providers, both individuals and agencies, that are involved in the case

(See Box, pp. 367–369, for a detailed assessment outline.) The primary purposes of the assessment are to identify the client's care needs and problems, to evaluate what needs are being met, and to determine what should be improved.

Ideally, the initial interview with the client and significant others should take place in the client's home. The presence of a significant other is especially important when there is a potential for discrete or undiagnosed cognitive impairment of the client. For the initial interview, the home setting provides the case manager with an opportunity to assess the home environment and community resources. Although at the initial assessment the client may be relatively healthy and independent, this information will provide a basis for future evaluation of the feasibility of in-home service, should the need arise. If the initial assessment is performed at the hospital or in an office, the case manager should arrange an in-home visit at a later date for assessment purposes.

Development of a Care Plan

The cardinal rule for the development of a service plan is that the client and significant others actively participate in developing the plan, which must include mutual goals. Involvement of the client in setting goals is probably the rule that health care professionals most frequently ignore. Unilateral setting of goals by the case manager will eventually lead to the client's being labeled as noncompliant. In this case the true statement would be, "This client was noncompliant with the case manager's wishes"! For example, if the case manager decides that home attendant services are indicated, even though the client views them as intrusive and can still manage on his or her own, much time and effort will have been wasted when the home attendant arrives and the client refuses service. It is important to keep in mind that the plan of care belongs to the client, not to the case manager.

The plan of care should also include measurable objectives, types of services required, responsible party (provider, agency, client, family, or case manager), and a time frame (AHCPR, 1994, p. 99). Documentation throughout the process is important, and constraints on achieving goals or meeting time frames should be recorded. The case manager should realize that problems with the care plan are inevitable and should not view these problems as personal failures. Internalization of problems can lead to frustration and anger and can impede the process.

The final requirement of the planning process is selection of the services needed. In the case of the HIV-infected person, this may be limited because access to institutional long-term care has been limited throughout the HIV/AIDS epidemic. In many areas nursing homes and psychiatric facilities that will accept an HIV-infected person are scarce. Gaining access to addiction-treatment services may be even more difficult. Day care is also limited. Home care and hospice care, although available in most areas, may not be adequate or safe for the client's needs. From time to time, the case manager may reach a dead end when other service providers reject the referral.

Implementation

In the implementation phase of the care plan, access to services is accomplished by completion of applications and contact with providers. Advocacy for entitlements will require providing all necessary information and educating the client and significant others to prevent future denial of services or financing.

The case manager should anticipate problems and conflicts during the process of implementation; for example, checks may not arrive on time, transportation may be delayed, home care workers may fail to arrive, and clients may miss appointments. A backup plan is needed for such situations: petty cash for food until checks can be

■ CASE MANAGEMENT: INITIAL DATABASE FOR CLIENT ASSESSMENT ■

I. Demographics
   A. Personal data: name, age, date of birth, sex, race, ethnicity, marital status
   B. Address, telephone number(s)
   C. Social Security number
   D. Level of education
   E. Occupation/profession
   F. Country of origin
   G. Immigration status if not a citizen
   H. Language(s) spoken (note primary/preferred language)
   I. Risk behavior/factor for acquiring HIV infection
II. Support Person(s)
   A. Person(s) living with client (note relationship[s])
   B. Person designated by the client to act on the client's behalf in an emergency (telephone number[s])
   C. Person who is willing to participate in the plan of care and to provide care when necessary
      1. Is the person available 24 hours a day, 7 days a week?
      2. If not, who can be designated as an alternative care partner?
   D. Family members
      1. Who are the persons aware of the client's diagnosis?
      2. Where do they live (nearby or in another city, state, or country)?
      3. Are they in agreement with the client's chosen care partner or significant other?
   E. Community-based AIDS services
      1. Is the client, at present, receiving services from AIDS organizations?
      2. Types of services
III. Functional Status
   A. Physical impairments
      1. Sensory—speech, sight, hearing, or areas of anesthesia or paresthesias
      2. Motor—dominant arm and hand dysfunction; hemiparesis, paraparesis, or tetraparesis; hemiplegia, paraplegia, quadraplegia
      3. Functional—limitations caused by neurologic, cardiovascular, or respiratory disease
      4. Bladder and bowel control—continent, occasionally incontinent, or always incontinent
   B. Mental impairments
      1. Cognitive impairment—disoriented, short-term memory impairment, impaired judgment, calculation problems
      2. Communication—can the client make needs known, and can the client direct others?
      3. Emotional status—anxious, agitated, angry, abusive, depressed, or danger to others
      4. Does the client wander when left unattended?
      5. Any sleep disorders?
      6. Does the client need safety monitoring (e.g., because of smoking)?
   C. Activities of daily living
      1. Personal care—bathing, grooming, dressing, toileting, ambulation, feeding (independent or needs assistance)
      2. Chore services—cleaning, laundry, shopping, meal preparation, reheating prepared meals (independent or needs assistance)
IV. Clinical Needs of the Client
   A. Medical diagnosis—include all, noting whether chronic or resolved
   B. Medications
      1. Allergies—allergy and type of reaction
      2. Current drug therapy—names, dosages, routes, and frequency
      3. Client's ability to self-medicate—needs reminding, help with preparation, needs supervision, or requires preparation and administration by another person
      4. Can the client be taught to self-medicate?
      5. What arrangements need to be made for medication administration?

Box continued on following page

■ CASE MANAGEMENT: INITIAL DATABASE FOR CLIENT ASSESSMENT *Continued* ■

IV. Clinical Needs of the Client *Continued*
  C. Clinical trials
    1. Type
    2. Location of trial
    3. Frequency of visits
    4. Special information on trial
  D. Nutrition
    1. Method—oral, enteral, or parenteral
    2. Is the client independent or in need of assistance?
  E. Rehabilitation therapy
    1. Does the client require occupational, physical, or speech therapy?
    2. What are the goals—functional, restoration, or maintenance?
    3. What is the frequency of therapy sessions?
  F. Treatments
    1. Does the client require special treatments, including decubitus care; turning, positioning, and exercising because of confinement to bed; incontinence care; ostomy care (type); catheter care (type); tube irrigation; oxygen therapy; inhalation therapy (including pentamidine aerosol); suctioning; infusion therapy?
    2. Has frequency of special treatments been noted?
    3. Who is available to perform treatments? And has this person been taught how to perform the procedures?
  G. Equipment neeeded for care
    1. Assist devices—cane, crutches, walker, wheelchair, hospital bed with trapeze bar, side rails, commode, bedpan, urinal, bath bar, bath seat, handheld shower, Hoyer lift, etc.
    2. Disposasble supplies—incontinence pads, diapers, dressing supplies, etc.
    3. Infusion or tube-feeding supplies
    4. Respiratory equipment
  H. Medical follow-up
    1. Frequency of physician visits required
    2. Laboratory abnormailites that should be monitored—actual or potential—and frequency
  I. Addiction treatment
    1. Does the client wish:
      a. To seek addictions treatment?
      b. Needle-exchange programs (if available)?
      c. To continue to use drugs (specify type and route)?
    2. Is the client, if necessary, enrolled in an addiction-treament program?
    3. Specify type of treatment program and frequency of contact visits
V. Family Data
  A. Has the client's sexual partner been tested for HIV? What were the test results?
  B. Is the sexual partner in need of health care?
  C. If the client is pregnant:
    1. How many months?
    2. Is she receiving prenatal care? Where?
    3. Does she want abortion information?
  D. If the client is a parent:
    1. Is the client living with sexual partner, or is he or she a single parent?
    2. What are the children's names, ages, and HIV status?
    3. What are the health problems of the children?

▪ CASE MANAGEMENT: INITIAL DATABASE FOR CLIENT ASSESSMENT *Continued* ▪

VI. Legal Data
  A. Has the client legally:
    1. Provided for durable power of attorney?
    2. Appointed a health care proxy?
    3. Drawn up:
      a. A living will?
      b. A will for the estate?
    4. Provided for guardianship of children?
VII. Social Data
  A. Living arrangements
    1. Housing
      a. Owns own home
      b. Rents an apartment in the home of another
      c. Rents a room (shares facilities) in the home of another
      d. Rents home
      e. Rents apartment
      f. Rents hotel room
      g. Lives in shelter for homeless persons
      h. Lives in special housing—supportive housing for persons with HIV/AIDS
      i. Lives in senior citizen housing
    2. Facilities
      a. Wheelchair accessible, both inside and outside
      b. Utilities—heat, hot water, electricity, air conditioner, sink, tub, shower, telephone
      c. Toilet—own or shared
      d. Cooking facilities—stove, hot plate, toaster oven, microwave, refrigerator
      e. Elevator or walk-up—can or cannot be managed by client
      f. Laundry—appliances in the home, in the building, or nearby
  B. Community assessment
    1. Safety—neighborhood where in-home service can be provided if needed
    2. Available services—grocery, shopping, pharmacy, etc.
    3. Transportation
      a. Does the client own a car, and is he or she able to drive?
      b. Is public transportation available near client's home, and can client negotiate public transportation?
  C. Spiritual needs
    1. What are the client's spiritual (religious) preferences?
    2. Does the client participate in religious services? With what frequency?
    3. How important is religion to the client?
VIII. Financial Picture
  A. Is the client able to continue employment?
    1. How many hours per week?
    2. Benefits?
  B. Monthly income versus monthly expenditures
  C. Savings and financial assets
  D. Health care payments—including insurance and payments for service care or drugs not covered
  E. Eligibility for entitlements:
    1. Medicaid
    2. Medicare
    3. Special programs for financial aid to persons with AIDS
IX. Current Services Received by Client
  A. List all agencies and individuals providing services to the client
  B. Identify contact persons and telephone numbers to facilitate case planning and management

traced, alternative transportation or appointment rescheduling, and someone to stay with the client until a replacement home care worker is available. The more service providers involved with a case, the greater is the likelihood that problems will arise, often because of communication breakdowns or conflicting agendas.

The case manager should watch for and avoid duplications in service. As the number of AIDS service organizations increases, so does the number of duplicative services provided. For example, if a client moves into supportive housing for PLWHIV that provides health care monitoring and psychosocial support services as well as food and shelter, there is little need to provide for medical appointments, counseling, friendly visitors, or volunteer "buddies" as previously required.

Monitoring/Evaluation

Monitoring and evaluation should be ongoing and planned and should not be left to chance or until a crisis develops. Planned visits to the client at specified intervals, or at least telephone audits to verify services and to identify problems, can be invaluable tools in preventing a major crisis. Educating the client and significant others about the importance of self-care is essential in providing

services and containing costs. Documentation of positive outcomes is important to assure future funding of case management services (Sowell, 1995).

Unnecessary services should not be continued for the sake of convenience or because a provider has difficulty saying, "No." Likewise, the case manager should not provide services as "gifts" in an attempt to win the client's confidence. Providers must consistently enforce predetermined contracts, especially when dealing with HIV-infected clients who also have alcohol/drug problems, mental health disorders, or both (Snyder et al., 1996). Overservicing a client and significant others is antithetical to achieving and maintaining independence.

Family members or significant others providing care may experience role fatigue. Plans of care that specify intervals of respite to prevent psychologic or physical fatigue are usually successful. Periods of respite care vary from a few hours a week to a long weekend once every few months.

Redefining goals and modifying the care plan will be based on the ongoing assessment of the needs of the client and significant others, as well as on clinical advances and changes in available services. Advances in antiretroviral therapies have

---

▓ CONSTRAINTS ON CASE MANAGEMENT ▓

1. Case management usually is limited to the provision of services to persons with AIDS, thus excluding persons with HIV who are in the earlier stages of disease.
2. Health care facilities and organizations may not have funding for case management.
3. Communication channels between case managers and other service providers are not always well established.
4. Power struggles can emerge between case managers from different agencies.
5. There is a lack of specialized training and resource materials that prepare case managers to interpret and understand the complex clinical problems of their clients, such as clinical needs related to opportunistic infections, research protocols, medication regimens, and alternative/complementary therapies.
6. Many case managers do not adequately involve the client in the plan of care.
7. Many case managers are unprepared to deal with an HIV-seropositive person who continues to engage in unsafe sexual activity or drug use or who wishes to become pregnant and have a baby.
8. Undiagnosed HIV-related cognitive impairment can complicate the decision-making process.
9. Confidentiality laws may leave case managers reluctant to provide adequate information to other service providers involved in the case.
10. Hospital-based providers may lack experience with outpatient case management and may be unfamiliar with solutions to problems that face persons with HIV/AIDS when they are at home in the community.
11. Emphasis on cost saving may result in conflict over supplies and services ordered by case managers and denied by third-party payers.

significantly improved the functional abilities of many HIV-infected persons, resulting in a need to "reconstruct" case management to include persons who are redefining their options and wish to return to work (Sowell, 1997). See Box on page 370 for constraints on case management.

HOME CARE

In 1981 the only option for care of PLWHIV was acute care hospitalization. Nursing responded to the need, however, and by 1984 the first program of home care services for PLWHIV was organized and implemented at the Visiting Nurse Association and Hospice of San Francisco. This was followed 1 year later by the development of a formalized program of home care services at the Visiting Nurse Service of New York (VNSNY). Today VNSNY operates the largest home care program for PLWHIV of its kind in the world, with an average daily census of more than 1700 clients.

Home care providers have responded to the growing health care needs of PLWHIV by designing special programs and adapting current ones to meet their needs. When developing a care model for persons with HIV/AIDS, home care agencies need to analyze local epidemiologic and demographic patterns of HIV infection as well as the prevailing social and political attitudes (Ungvarski, 1996). Depending on the situation, agencies may then decide to cultivate either specialized HIV/AIDS providers or a "case-mix approach" that educates all providers to work with PLWHIV. The San Francisco model exemplifies the use of specialized HIV/AIDS providers (Morrison, 1993); the case-mix approach involves a commitment to extensive, comprehensive staff education and has been successfully implemented from urban to rural areas (Sowell & Opava, 1995; Ungvarski, 1996).

Home care is especially appropriate and effective for PLWHIV. It enables them to remain in familiar surroundings, thus providing maximum emotional support for them and their significant others. It provides maximum independence and control over decision making in the least restrictive setting. Home care can significantly improve the quality of life and can give PLWHIV the greatest use of their remaining time (Ungvarski, 1988). It promotes the participation of significant others

in the plan of care. Finally, it provides an opportunity for case finding and health teaching in the community (Ungvarski, 1987). Health teaching is especially important in preventing transmission of not only HIV but also tuberculosis, which has become a major HIV-related illness.

One misconception about home care is that it consistently costs substantially less than institutional care. The cost of service in the home (excluding supplies such as medications, dressings, and intravenous infusion equipment) can range from about $140 to $1000 per day (New York City Department of Health, 1989). In addition, estimates comparing home care costs with institutional care rarely include total costs of care and may fail to include the average daily cost of rent, food, utilities, etc.

Hurley and colleagues (1996) studied home care costs for a cohort of patients serviced by VNSNY. The average monthly cost per case was $2056, with a range of $107 to $17,999 (p. 7). The authors found that several factors increased costs: the number of activities of daily living (ADL) requiring assistance and living alone, the number of daily prescribed medications, and gender (higher costs for services for women).

Master and colleagues (1993) reported the costs of hospital alternative care for Medicaid recipients with AIDS enrolled in a health maintenance organization (HMO) in Boston. They reported the average costs as $90 per patient per month for case management, $328 per patient per month for home intravenous therapy, and $405 per patient per month for home nursing and support services. However, it is important to note that in an HMO with capitated monthly expenditures, the costs of services are usually distributed among all patients enrolled, whether or not they actually use the services that are available. In addition, in a capitated program of case management, costs cited may not reflect the actual needs of the client but may be limited to what is allowed by the dollar amount allocated to each client per month.

Another misconception is that home care is intended to take over or take the care and responsibility for the PLWHIV away from the significant others. Nothing could be farther from the truth. Home care is specifically designed to support the client and significant others in self-care activities and not to take over custody of the client. In this

Table 10–1 ▪ Formal Caregivers Providing Home Care Services

Category of Staff	Functions
Professional staff	
Physician	Provides for medical care (usually through periodic office or clinic visits and telephone contact with the visiting nurse)
Visiting nurse (usually the case manager)	Provides for nursing care and coordinates all professional and paraprofessional services needed; promotes and teaches self-care to client and significant others
Medical social worker	Provides for necessary concrete social services as well as counseling
Therapists	Provide maintenance or restorative therapies and teach self-care to client and significant other
Specialists	Provide specific services (e.g., respiratory therapists for aerosolized pentamidine or clinical nurse specialists for problems in case management)
Paraprofessional staff	
Housekeeper	Provides chore services such as shopping, cleaning, laundry, meal preparation (no personal care)
Personal care assistants (also referred to as home attendants or personal care attendants)	Provide, in addition to chore services, assistance with bathing, dressing, toileting, ambulation, and traveling to and from appointments
Home health aides	In addition to the above, assist with many nursing tasks such as taking temperatures, providing special exercises, taking care of and providing safety with oxygen therapy
Homemakers	Usually provide chore services and child care services; may provide child care in the presence of an ill parent or may also act as a surrogate parent, staying in the home 24 hours when the parent is hospitalized

respect, home care may be inappropriate for persons who require continuous care in an institutional setting and may not be feasible with an insurance plan that has capitated monthly costs.

Many health care professionals throughout the United States place undue pressure on home care agencies to accept all PLWHIV who are referred, because there are virtually no other options for long-term care outside the hospital. Therefore it is important for all health care professionals to understand the purposes of home care, as well as its limits and constraints, which are predominantly governed by reimbursement issues. In a nationwide survey of 68 home care agencies in areas of high AIDS prevalence, Allen and Fleishman (1992) found lack of adequate insurance reimbursement to be a major problem in providing services to PLWHIV.

As previously stated, home care is a supportive system of care for the client and significant others. Therefore, in addition to educating the client in self-care, the significant other, often referred to as the informal caregiver, must be educated as the most important provider of care. Education and counseling can help to mitigate barriers to family involvement. Smith and Rapkin (1996) surveyed 224 persons living with AIDS (PLWA) in New York City and found that the patients identified these barriers to family involvement:

1. Interpersonal costs (emotional, financial and physical)
2. Lack of access (because of geographic distance or estrangement)
3. Lack of acceptance (of AIDS diagnosis or sexual orientation)
4. Lack of intimacy
5. Negative interactions/family conflicts
6. Avoidance of disclosure (either AIDS diagnosis or homosexuality)

Formal caregivers include professional and paraprofessional health care workers who participate in the plan of care (Table 10–1). The informal and formal caregivers should work together to develop a plan of care that is mutually agreeable, is designed to meet the needs of the client and significant others, and is realistic about the care that can be safely provided by the home care agency.

Case Management Issues and Home Care

Schmidt (1992) reviewed 100 consultations that took place at the VNSNY and found that the case management problems for PLWHIV receiving home services fell into four general categories: client and significant others, housing and community, support services, and nurses' needs. At that time, nurses identified psychiatric and other mental health issues as their No. 1 case management problem in the home.

Cognitive impairment resulting from the neurotropic effects of HIV disease or an opportunistic central nervous system infection is a grossly underdiagnosed problem in the HIV-ill population. Once the client is at home, the visiting nurse or paraprofessional home care worker is often the first person to detect cognitive or motor impairment. In a study of 244 clients who were admitted to VNSNY, Hurley and Ungvarski (1994) found that the medical diagnosis of HIV encephalopathy was made in only 15% of the sample, whereas the nurses noted memory deficit in 34% of the clients and impaired judgment in 18%. In the case of clients who live alone, forgetting to take medications or miscalculation of doses can lead to disastrous problems such as under- or overmedication or the worsening or recurrence of an OI because of inability to comply with a suppressive therapy regimen. In addition, home care is not the best milieu for the cognitive stimulation therapy necessary to keep the client at an optimal level of functioning. Home care in conjunction with a program of day care is the most desirable.

Because there are few long-term care options for HIV-ill persons with psychiatric disorders, acute care facilities may withhold psychiatric diagnoses when making home care referrals. Once the client is at home, paraprofessional home care workers, as well as families and significant others, are often reluctant or unable to cope with combative, assaultive, or self-destructive behaviors. In some instances this behavior can pose a real threat to the safety and welfare of the home care staff.

Home care agencies have begun to recognize that PLWHIV need specialized mental health services (Pessin et al., 1993). The VNSNY and the Visiting Nurse Associations of Boston and Los Angeles all use psychiatric clinical nurse specialists to provide counseling and support to clients and significant others in the home. Psychiatric nurses also work with the home care staff to develop a safe plan of care. However, it is important to realize that there are clients who cannot be maintained safely in the community because they pose a danger to themselves or others, need 24-hour supervision, and have no significant others who can provide backup for the home care staff. When Allen and Fleishman (1992) asked home care agencies to identify problems in providing services to PLWA, 77% of the respondents indicated that care was compromised by the absence of caregivers. Long-term care facilities would be the most appropriate setting for such clients, but if local long-term care facilities are unwilling or unable to accept such persons, then the only safe plan of care would be to return the client to the hospital.

From 1994 to 1997, the HIV/AIDS clinical nurse specialists at VNSNY provided a total of 1612 case consultations to the nursing staff. Table 10–2 shows the percentage breakdown of consultations according to case management issues. Although psychiatric/mental health issues remain among the top five reasons for a consultation, the most prevalent reasons were questions regarding the medical/nursing management of specific AIDS-indicator diseases.

Clients referred for home care often present with a litany of AIDS-indicator diseases and comorbidities that challenge health care providers' abilities to control symptoms. In their study of 244 clients who were referred to VNSNY, Hurley and Ungvarski (1994) found the following signs and symptoms to be the most frequent: dyspnea, weakness, fatigue/lethargy, pain, ataxia, cough, skin lesions, oral lesions (including thrush), weight loss, and memory deficit. It is essential for HCPs to be knowledgeable about effective symptom management so that they can offer appropriate interventions to clients and caregivers (see Chapter 5).

Family cases referred for home care services provide a unique challenge. Among the possible situations are

1. Infection of husband and wife
2. Infection of both parents and children
3. The presence of uninfected children in the same household with infected parents and siblings
4. Infection of multiple generations of persons in the same household
5. Infection of a gay couple, with both partners being severely ill

In the case of households with children present, home care nurses need to assess whether parent(s)' functional limitations prevent them from caring for their children. Extended family members may be able to assist with child care; if not, referrals for homemaker services (where available) will be necessary.

Legal assistance is often required for preparing wills and planning guardianship. Referrals will be necessary to assist survivors (e.g., grandparents, aunts, uncles) in caring for both HIV-infected and affected children whose parents have died or are otherwise absent. In the absence of planned guardianship or relatives willing to provide child care, referrals to foster care agencies will be necessary. By the end of this decade, it is projected that an estimated 80,000 children in the United States will be left orphaned by HIV/AIDS (Michaels & Levine, 1992).

Management of Substance Use

Evidence suggests a failure to diagnose alcohol and drug dependencies when clients are referred for home care services (Hurley & Ungvarski, 1994). With the initiation of services, the prob-

lem becomes evident and directly affects the client's ability to comply with prescribed medical and nursing regimens, as well as the willingness of paraprofessional workers to go into the home to provide services. Even when the HIV-infected person is free of alcohol or drugs, the significant other(s) may be overtly using substances, which again leads to reluctance of paraprofessionals to enter the home or may result in abusive behavior toward home care workers. When the problem of drug or alcohol use is diagnosed by professional home care staff, treatment options for referral are limited. Alcohol- and drug-treatment programs that meet the needs of homebound clients are almost nonexistent. There is also a limited array of services for persons who are primary family caregivers for dependent children. In the absence of a treatment plan for the chemical dependency, home care may not be feasible.

Home care agencies are able to provide services to active substance abusers if clients are willing to cooperate with a plan of care (Schmidt, 1992). Such a plan should include the stipulation that clients and significant others do not engage in substance use or drug trafficking while home care

Table 10–2 ▪ Summary of Clinical Nurse Specialist Consults VNSNY 1994–1997 (N = 1612)

Care Management Issues Discussed in Consultation*	Percent of Consults†
1. Medical or nursing management of AIDS-indicator diseases	34.5
2. Mental health issues	29
3. Emotional support for nurse	28
4. Accessing community-based services	25
5. Level or amount of in-home sevvice	20
6. Referral process to Medicaid home care/ADAP	13.5
7. Nonadhererence to the plan of care	13.25
8. Medication information	13.25
9. Parenting	12.5
10. Nutrition	11
11. Client safety related to impaired cognition	8.5
12. Substance use problems	7.5
13. Staff abuse by patient or significant other	7.25
14. Housing or community problems	7
15. Client not at home for service	5.5
16. Financial concerns	5
17. Lack of a care partner	4.25
18. Safer-sex education	4
19. Alternative/complimentary therapies	2.75
20. Clinical care related to tuberculosis	2.5

*Other topics discussed in less than 2% of the consults included terminal care, the pathogenesis of HIV, pain management, pet care problems, spiritual counseling, HIV testing, treatment of needle-stick injury, and managed care.
†Percents cited exceed 100% when totaled because several consults involved multiple problems.

workers are present. Clients also need to be told that home care workers cannot be involved in the procurement of drugs or alcohol.

Clients or family members may disrupt the plan of care by selling medications (Ungvarski, 1996). Although narcotics and sedatives have always had "street value," the publicity regarding the effectiveness of antiretroviral "drug cocktails" has resulted in a lucrative street business in urban areas such as New York City. HCPs in the community should have a high index of suspicion when clients repeatedly report "missing or lost" prescriptions. Clients or family members need to be educated that taking a suboptimal dose of HIV medications and selling the rest will result in the development of drug resistance. When providers realize that clients have been obtaining medication refills from different pharmacies, they may need to "lock" the Medicaid into one pharmacy so that refills are controlled (Snyder et al., 1996).

Staff members need to be educated about how to set limits on manipulative behaviors, such as repeated requests for money. If clients have no money for food, they can be referred to food pantries or AIDS organizations that provide food or meals. Another issue that staff members may find disturbing is the clients' use of profanity. If clients use profanity to express themselves, it is unrealistic to expect them to alter their vocabularies, especially in their own homes. The staff should acknowledge legitimate expressions of anger and frustration. However, they should set limits on verbal abuse that is directed toward them or another person. Any threats of violence directed toward home care workers should be reported to a supervisor immediately.

Case conferences are an effective way for home care agencies to set up a contract with the client and significant others. During the case conference, the agency explains what services it can provide and what is expected of the client and the significant others. It is important for the home care staff to outline what behaviors are acceptable and unacceptable and what behaviors (such as threats of violence) may lead to termination of home care services.

The home care staff will have to rely on the assistance of other community agencies when they encounter child neglect or abuse, incest, or truancy. A parent who repeatedly succumbs to the need to spend all available money on drugs and is unable to provide food for the children may require intervention from agencies that provide protective services for children. Such services are usually more readily available than are treatment resources for the parent's drug addiction. Situations of abuse are not restricted to those involving substance use. Client abuse by family members or lovers also occurs and may necessitate referral to community-based agencies that provide protective services for adults.

Housing and Community Problems

Home care cannot be provided in inadequate or unsuitable housing. Examples of HIV-ill persons with unsuitable housing include

1. Persons with diarrhea who are housed in single-room-occupancy hotels (SROs), often referred to as welfare hotels, have no bathroom or sink in the room, and are required to use distant, shared bathroom facilities
2. Those with significant weight loss who live in places without facilities for cooking and food storage and are too weak to go out for meals
3. Those who require intravenous therapy but have neither a telephone to use in case of a medical emergency nor a refrigerator where solutions and drugs can be stored
4. Clients who can no longer walk and who live in buildings with broken elevators or no elevator service

The provision of home care services may require that the client be relocated to more suitable housing or that home care be delayed until necessary services are provided.

Home care cannot be provided in unsafe housing. Examples of unsafe housing include

1. Buildings in which previous home care staff members have been accosted or mugged
2. Buildings in which entrances and hallways are used as "shooting galleries" for injection drug users or in which crack and cocaine are sold
3. Buildings designated by local police departments as high-crime areas
4. Homes in which overt drug use and trafficking takes place in the presence of the home care staff

Although most home care agencies in large urban areas provide an escort service for visiting nurses, this service is expensive, is not directly reimbursable, and therefore is extremely limited. Escort service is not usually provided for paraprofessionals, so they may refuse to provide service to clients in unsafe environments. This should not be misconstrued as refusal to care for a PLWHIV, a commonly encountered misinterpretation. In some cases, home care workers can arrange to be met by the family or significant others and escorted to and from the home. If the staff is unable to provide care because the environment is judged unsafe, clients will need a referral to community housing organizations to help find safe, affordable housing.

Support Services

In the absence of previous experience, it is not uncommon, while the client is in the hospital, for the significant others to agree to participate in the home-based plan of care. However, once faced with the harsh realities of the intense levels of physical care and emotional support needed in the home, the significant others or family members may withdraw from active participation. Some family members or significant others will insist that a client be returned home with home care services but may themselves be unable to participate in care because they live far away. The participation of family and significant others is the foundation of safe home care. Reimbursement for services varies with the payer source (for example, private insurance, Medicaid, or Medicare) and from state to state in the case of Medicaid. Capitations on the amount of service often require that significant others participate. If they do not, modification of the original plan and referral to an institution for long-term care may be necessary.

Many community-based AIDS organizations (CBOs) provide buddy services. Buddies are usually volunteers who visit clients once or twice a week. The buddy can run errands, maybe cook a meal and eat with the client or, if the client is strong enough to go out, take the client for a walk or a ride or out to the movies. The use of buddies is a good way to increase socialization for clients who have little support; buddies can also provide respite for significant others.

When Baigis-Smith and colleagues (1995) surveyed 386 PLWHIV to identify their health care needs, 51% reported that their most "pressing problem" was a lack of financial resources to cover living and health care expenses. It is essential for clients to receive assistance in applying for entitlements. Because PLWHIV may lack the strength and endurance to negotiate the entitlement bureaucracy, many CBOs offer step-by-step guidance and entitlement advocacy (Katoff, 1992).

Home-delivered meal programs not only supply nutritious foods, but they also ensure that clients will not neglect nutrition when finances are scarce. According to Balsam et al. (1996), home-delivered meal programs have been developed in San Francisco, Los Angeles, San Diego, Santa Fe, Seattle, Minneapolis/St. Paul, St. Louis, Chicago, Atlanta, New Orleans, Denver, Philadelphia, Washington, D.C., Baltimore, New York, New Haven, and Boston. These programs try to consider cultural preferences in designing menus, and they recognize the need to feed the children of PLWA as well as other household members if necessary.

Problems of Medical Follow-up

When home care service is provided to persons covered by Medicaid, their hospital-based medical care is often provided by house staff (residents in training). At the time of home care referral, the resident providing the initial medical orders is usually not assuming the role of primary care physician. Once the client is at home, the visiting nurse may find no physician willing to modify or provide orders for the medical portion of the plan of care. Visiting nurses spend an inordinate amount of time attempting to arrange ongoing medical care for Medicaid clients receiving home care. In the absence of medical supervision, the visiting nurse may have to return a client to the acute care facility to obtain medical orders or prescriptions, which otherwise could be obtained by a telephone call to a primary care physician. Many states regulating home care require a physician's orders at specified intervals, but there is no legislation requiring physicians to provide a continuum of medical care to persons receiving home care. Ironically, the burden of ensuring adequate medical care for the person receiving home care is on the professional nurse. Visiting nurses try to network with clinic staff (especially nurses and social workers) to communicate with physicians and obtain orders, because, unlike the physicians, the clinic staff is a consistent presence with greater knowledge of the clients.

In 1997 the task of maintaining any continuum of care became even more complex when states began drug testing for Medicaid recipients. The cessation of Medicaid benefits for substance-using persons with HIV disease leads to interruption of access to medical care and, in most cases, forced discontinuation of antiretroviral therapy.

Managing client care at home and planning for care are directly related to the individual client's problems, which result from the numerous AIDS-indicator diseases that may develop in a PLWHIV. Chapters 5 and 6 detail specific individual responses to HIV disease and the related health care.

HOME INFUSION THERAPY

With improved therapies and earlier diagnosis and treatment of AIDS-related OIs many PLWHIV have been experiencing increased survival. These treatments can often include infusion therapies. Because of the nature of HIV infection and the resulting severe immunosuppression, many intravenous anti-infective regimens require lifetime suppressive therapy (Ungvarski & Staats, 1995). During the early years of the epidemic, this presented a dilemma to those providing care to PLWHIV disease because continued hospitalization was not warranted, subacute care was limited, skilled nursing facilities generally did not accept clients who were receiving infusion therapy, and the active treatment of these OIs was equivalent to aggressive therapy, precluding admission to hospice care. As a result, alternative sites for care such as the home became necessary. Also, during this time there were many advances in the technology used to administer intravenous therapy, specifically the use of computer programming for electronic pumps and materials that improved the insertion and maintenance of intravenous lines (Corrigan, 1995). Consequently, infusion therapy for HIV/AIDS-related diseases became commonplace in the home.

With the collaboration of infusion pharmacy companies, licensed and certified home care agencies, physicians, and hospitals, clients were discharged to their homes to continue parenteral therapies (Weinstein, 1993). Although initially many believed that home infusion therapy would

actually decrease health care spending by reducing the number and duration of hospitalizations, in many instances the complexity and long hours of infusions and the home care staff required to ensure safe care resulted in costs comparable to those of hospital care.

The availability of home infusion therapy in specific communities is dependent on the resources available as well as the mind set of the physician, hospital, and home care agency staff. For the implementation of a successful home infusion program, it is imperative that an interdisciplinary/interagency team approach be used (Haddad et al., 1993). HCPs for infusion care include the primary care provider (physician, nurse practitioner, physician's assistant), hospital discharge planners, home care agency staff, pharmacy staff, laboratory staff, and insurance company case managers. Regular contact is required among these persons to coordinate the safe administration of infusions in the home setting.

Infusion therapies can be administered in the home by certified home health agencies or licensed agencies providing the nursing staff, with licensed infusion pharmacies providing the drugs, the infusion equipment, and the supplies. In some instances the infusion pharmacy may provide the nursing services as well. Contracts among vendors or with insurance companies will determine which combination of agencies is used.

The infusion therapies that can be administered in the home have expanded over the years for a number of reasons:

- The relative safety of long-term administration of some drugs has been established
- The safety and ease of maintaining intravenous devices and home infusion therapy have been established and communicated
- A greater effort on cost containment and improving the quality of life of PLWHIV has been emphasized by payers, clients, and client advocates (Crespo-Fierro, 1996).

The therapies fall into six basic categories:

1. Anti-infective therapies (antibiotic, antiprotozoal, antifungal, and antiviral)
2. Antineoplastic therapies
3. Hydration
4. Nutritional therapies
5. Pain management

6. Adjuvant therapies (antiemetics, antidiarrheals, anticonvulsants, anti-inflammatories, colony-stimulating factors, etc.)

Clients may be receiving various combinations in multiple daily doses requiring extensive instruction and support by the nursing and pharmacy staff for safe administration.

HIV disease and the AIDS-indicator diseases can have a serious impact on a person's ability to safely and independently administer infusion therapy in the home (Crespo-Fierro, 1996). The home care nurse must constantly assess for the development of these problems and be creative in devising ways in which the client can maximize independence in this endeavor (Crespo-Fierro, 1996; Ungvarski et al., 1994). Table 10–3 lists the symptoms, their impact on independent infusion therapy, and possible interventions to maintain independence.

The need for infusion therapy is changing. For example, oral ganciclovir is now available, and under certain circumstances primary prophylaxis is recommended, decreasing the potential for cytomegalovirus retinitis (CDC, 1997b). Continued development of oral forms of therapy may result in a decrease in the need for long-term infusion therapy in the home setting (Dagg et al., 1996). However, in view of the fact that increased survival of PLWHIV usually results in an increase in the number of diagnosed HIV-related diseases and the development of drug resistance to lifetime suppressive antimicrobial therapies, it is dif-ficult to project the future need for home infusion therapy.

MEDICATION MANAGEMENT

With the introduction of protease inhibitors and their ability to significantly suppress the replication of HIV, the concept of adherence to antiretroviral therapy has assumed immense importance. This development has complicated the treatment of HIV disease and, consequently, medication management in the community and home care settings. Primary care providers are fully aware that sporadic adherence to medication regimens can lead to drug resistance, but providers need to recognize also that their own behaviors, such as prescribing "drug holidays" and suboptimal dosing, may compound the problem (Ungvarski & Rottner, 1997c). There has been a plethora of articles examining the issues of adherence and HIV treatment in the past year (Crespo-Fierro, 1997; Friedland, 1997; Ungvarski, 1997a; Williams, 1997; Williams & Friedland, 1997). Although these evidence-based articles have presented potential interventions, large-scale formal studies examining specific interventions used with PLWHIV disease have yet to be published.

Since medication management occurs in the "real world" of life outside the hospital or institutional setting, community-based interventions to enhance self-medication management have begun to be explored (Ungvarski, 1997a). Al-

Table 10–3 ■ HIV-related Signs and Symptoms that Affect Home Infusion Therapy

Sign and Symptom	Impact	Intervention
Paresthesias	Decreased fine motor skills (difficulty in assembling and starting infusion)	Assistance of care partner or paraprofessional to steady the client's hands
Impaired vision	Decreased ability to visualize labels on equipment or to operate pump	Increase lighting in home (move near a window or use higher-watt light bulb or flashlight) Use a magnifying glass Large lettering on labels
Impaired cognition	Decreased retention of information; incorrect sequencing of steps	Coaching by care partner or paraprofessional Assigning responsibility for infusion to care partner
Weakness/fatigue	Inability to complete tasks due to lack of strength	Assigning responsibility for infusion to care partner

Data from Crespo-Fierro (1996).

though successful strategies to enhance compliance with tuberculosis (TB) treatment are often cited, directly observed therapy (DOT), in which a health care worker is assigned to watch the client ingest the medication(s) each day, is impractical when numerous drugs to treat ailments associated with HIV/AIDS have to be taken at various intervals throughout the day (Crespo-Fierro, 1997). Day treatment programs and home care services are now being seen as practical options for medication management. However, there are specific criteria for referral to these community resources as well as for reimbursement for these services. Medication management as the sole reason for referral to these services may not meet the preestablished criteria of the insurance payer source. Consequently, inappropriate and unrealistic referrals have been made for clients

who function on a more independent level than most. There is a need for service providers in all settings to understand the scope of services that can be provided by any health care provider. Some agencies and organizations, realizing the limitations of the current reimbursement schedules, have applied for grant funding to provide these services to PLWHIV disease.

In assessing a client for potential problems with adherence to a medication regimen, Stephenson et al. (1993) suggest noting the client's attendance at clinic appointments, assessing the client's responsiveness to the medication regimen, and collecting laboratory data as a direct measure of consumption of medication. When assesssing by interiew, the HCP should use a nonjudgmental, nonthreatening approach in which the diffficulty of taking medications is acknowl-

Table 10–4 ▪ The Transtheoretical and Harm Reduction Models and the Role of the HCP in Medication Management

Stage	Client	HCP
1. Precontemplative	Is aware of problems with medications, not interested in changing behavior	1. Assess behavior in a nonjudgmental, supportive manner 2. Use assessment to point out problems* 3. Discuss the positive aspects of change†
2. Contemplative	Intends to tackle the problem and change behavior in order to better manage medications	1. Reinforce the decision to change, emphasizing the positive aspects of change† 2. Help client weigh the pros and cons of change 3. Provide information as needed
3. Preparation	Expresses serious interest in changing behavior and is willing to accept help	1. Explain different interventions, allowing client to choose those which are suitable in his/her lifestyle 2. Reinforce the positive aspects of change† 3. Discuss the possibility of relapse‡
4. Action	Initiates behavior change by participating in medication management intervention of choice	1. Initiate or assist client to initiate intervention chosen by client 2. Discuss the positive aspects of change†
5. Maintenance	Continues behavior change	1. Discuss goals, praise and support progress, initiate rewards by decreasing visits with HCP 2. Discuss the positive aspects of change†
6. Relapse	Returns to previous behavior (i.e., not taking medications as prescribed)	1. With the client, identify reasons for relapse 2. Use relapse as a learning experience 3. Accept and focus on all that has been achieved 4. Discuss the positive aspects of change 5. Reset goals and start again

*Not taking the medications can result in (1) inadequate drug levels of the antiretrovirals and drug resistance; if this happens, then even if the client takes the drugs properly, they will not work; (2) if they do not take prescribed drugs to prevent infections, they will get sick (e.g., develop an OI); and (3) they may die faster than those persons who take these drugs properly.
†If they take the drugs they will feel better, have less illness, and live longer.
‡The HCP's attitude is pivotal regarding relapse; remember it is not a good or bad issue; it is a normal part of the process of change.
Data from Ungvarski (1997b).

edged. Questions should elicit information on the client's complete medication regimen for all diagnoses, over-the-counter medications, alternative or complementary therapies, cultural beliefs or practices, support systems, family or personal obligations, employment, and adequate home storage and facilities, and necessary utilities in the home such as a refrigerator, stove, bathroom, etc. (Weitzel, 1992; Crespo-Fierro, 1997).

Inherent in the implementation of a medication management program in the community is the adoption of a philosophy that will guide the practice of the providers in working with clients. Of specific note are the Transtheoretical Model of Change (Prochaska et al., 1994) and the Harm Reduction Model (Springer, 1991). Although the Harm Reduction Model was developed specifically to reduce the risk of exposure to HIV in the population using injection drugs, the Transtheoretical Model of Change was initially used with other populations (e.g., smokers, dieters, etc.). The feasibility of applying these models to populations other than those for which they were originally intended has been realized, and their popularity is growing among the health care professions. The similarities of these models is also being recognized (Bradley-Springer, 1996), and they are now being used together in program development (P. Ungvarski, personal communication June 2, 1997).

The Transtheoretical Model is based on the premise that changes in behavior constitute a dynamic, individualized, long-term process. The stages of this process are as follows: precontemplative, contemplative, preparation, action, maintenance, and relapse. Relapse is recognized as an essential component of the process of behavioral change, whereas other philosophies of behavioral change have viewed relapse as failure. On the other hand, the Harm Reduction Model has as its basis the belief that a client engaging in behavioral changes should be approached in an nonjudgmental manner with the acknowledgement that the rights of the individual are of the utmost importance. Table 10–4 lists the stages of the Transtheoretical and Harm Reduction Models in regard to medication management and the corresponding activities of the HCP to support the client in each. Table 10–5 lists possible interventions that can be implemented, during the action stage, specific to medication management.

The conceptualization of medication management as presented here is emerging. The implementation of these theoretical models requires behavioral changes on the part of the HCPs in their interactions with their clients. It would only make sense that HCPs view their own progress in incorporating these models into their practice within the philosophies of the models.

Table 10–5 ▪ Interventions for Use in Medication Management Strategies

Intervention	Definition
Care management	Modality in which a specified provider is responsible for organizing and monitoring the care to assure thoroughness and continuity
Interactive teaching	An educational encounter engaging the individual client or small groups of clients in active discussion of matters regarding health
Written instructions	Educational materials that have been developed to enhance medication compliance
Simplified dosing	A technique used to reduce the complexity of taking numerous medications on a scheduled basis (e.g., a schedule or prepour boxes)
Supervised therapy	Medication therapy that is monitored by a health care professional on a scheduled basis
Reminders	A method influencing the client to comply with the prescribed medication regimen (e.g., an electronic alarm)
Involving clients in self-care monitoring	Activities that encourage proactive efforts in maintaining or improving self-medication management (e.g., a medication diary, pill counts)
Outreach and home visits	Recontacting a client to assure continued assessment of succes of medication self-care management, or to detect problems, or to provide support

Data from Ungvarski (1997a, 1997b).

DRUG UNDERGROUND AND BUYERS' CLUBS

Providers in the community may discover that clients are taking medications not approved by the U.S. Food and Drug Administration (FDA). Because they were discouraged by the slow pace of FDA research in the 1980s, consumer groups set up ways to access medications not yet approved in the United States (Abrams, 1990). These groups publish newsletters and offer information through hotline numbers. Home care nurses may find medications in the home with handwritten labels, or they may find drug information that is written in a language other than English (Schmidt, 1992). As with any medication, the home care nurse needs to notify the primary health care provider and monitor the client for side effects; however, because these medications are not approved in this country, it may be difficult to find information. The National AIDS Information Clearinghouse maintains a database with information on medications available both in the United States and abroad (telephone number 1-800-458-5231). It can supply information on nonapproved medications, known side effects, and available clinical trials.

It is important for nurses to distinguish the drug underground and buyers' clubs from expanded drug access. Expanded drug access may be approved by the FDA when a drug has proved beneficial in clinical trials but has not yet received final FDA approval. The FDA will give drug companies authorization to release the medication to physicians who call an "800" number and complete the necessary paperwork. Expanded access gives clients access to trial drugs through a physician when the clients may not meet the eligibility criteria for a clinical trial.

CLIENT PARTICIPATION IN RESEARCH

Research is one of the means by which information regarding certain disease processes and possible treatment modalities is collected. Clinical research trials may study certain drugs or other HIV-related treatments (psychologic, social, or epidemiologic). PLWHIV may be motivated for various reasons to participate in one or more of the many different types of research trials. It is the HCP's responsibility to assist clients in gathering data about the trials so that they may make realistic decisions about participation. Since some HCPs may be involved with research, as principals or coinvestigators, collaborators, or data collectors, it is important that the client not feel obliged to participate in the trial.

A clinical trial is a study that tests new drugs and other treatments to determine their safety and effectiveness (Department of Health and Human Services, 1989). The drug-approval process occurs with the cooperation of the FDA, the National Institutes of Health (NIH), and the pharmaceutical company. The FDA reviews the data supplied by NIH and the pharmaceutical company and requests additional information until it is satisfied that the drug is safe and effective for the indicated disease. NIH consists of 13 institutes, one of which is the National Institute of Allergy and Infectious Diseases (NIAID).

In 1987, NIAID established the AIDS Clinical Trial Group to conduct collaborative clinical trials for AIDS therapies. By 1990 there were 47 group centers, usually located in major medical centers in geographic areas where the incidence of HIV infection is high. In 1989 NIAID created 18 community programs for clinical research on AIDS to test AIDS-related drugs and vaccines. The purpose of these programs is to "reach out to population groups that have been underrepresented in AIDS research" (NIAID, 1990, p. 11).

Since 1987, through the lobbying of activist community groups such as the AIDS Coalition to Unleash Power (ACT-UP), anti-HIV drugs have been moved even more quickly through the FDA approval process. A pharmaceutical company may submit a drug for approval by a fast-track process, in which the FDA will examine the submitted data, sometimes before or during the final phases of study, as a priority. Approval is contingent on evidence of the long-term safety of the drug. In other words, approval may be revoked at a later date if it is found that severe adverse effects have resulted from long-term use. Activists for other life-threatening illnesses, such as cancer, have emulated the ACT-UP example and demanded the same considerations for new treatments.

In some communities there is also a growing movement to test drugs through alternative mechanisms, such as the Community Research Initiative (AIDS Treatment Resources, 1990). This program offers HIV-positive clients access to drugs that may have uncertain effectiveness or have not been tested within the formal FDA system. Drugs with some demonstrated effectiveness can also be made available through a private physician for clients who cannot participate in a clinical trial; this process is considered a parallel track. However, some physicians may choose not to use this option because of the amount of paperwork required. Some clients will obtain these drugs through the drug underground and buyer's clubs.

The development of a new drug involves three stages of research:

1. Preclinical research that focuses on development, information synthesis, and animal testing
2. Human testing divided into phases I, II, and III
3. Postmarketing research

The three phases of clinical research in humans are the most important stages in new drug development. The purpose of phase I trials is to learn more about the safety of the drug. These trials are usually conducted with healthy volunteers, who are paid for their services. The subjects submit to a variety of tests to determine what the drug does in the human body: how it is absorbed, metabolized, and excreted; its effect on different body parts; and the side effects that occur as the dose is increased. A main reason that drugs fail to proceed to phase II is evidence of toxicity at doses too small to produce any beneficial effects (Flieger, 1988).

During phase II trials information is gathered as to whether the drug is effective in treating the disease or condition for which it is intended. These studies recruit a few hundred patients and attempt to determine short-term side effects and risks in persons whose health is impaired. Most of the phase II trials are randomized, controlled trials that are often double-blinded. When this method is used, potential subjects are randomly divided into two groups, with one group (the experimental group) receiving the experimental drug(s) and the other group (the control group) receiving another drug or a placebo. When the research is double-blinded, neither the patients nor the HCPs know which patient is in which group. By the end of phase II trials, the researchers will know whether the drug has a therapeutic effec-

tiveness and its short-term adverse and other side effects (Flieger, 1988). The FDA can quickly terminate phase II trials when there is evidence that the experimental group is receiving a major benefit over the control group. This is what occurred when zidovudine was tested in 1987, and, as a result, the drug was made readily available before phase III testing.

Phase III studies are designed to provide information about optimal dosage rates and schedules. Because thousands of patients are enrolled, more information about the drug's safety and effectiveness is discovered. Although phase III studies are also controlled, they more closely approximate the conditions of ordinary medical practice.

Patients and HCPs have identified five major benefits of clinical trials:

1. Having a chance to help others
2. Obtaining access to top-quality health care
3. Gaining power for oneself by taking positive action
4. Being helped by a new drug
5. Receiving financial assistance or other compensation (most drugs are provided without charge by the pharmaceutical company, and associated laboratory and other diagnostic tests are usually covered by the agency funding the research study).

There are three major risks associated with participation in clinical trials:

1. The treatment may not have benefits
2. It may actually be harmful
3. The drug may have harmful side effects (Department of Health and Human Services, 1989)

In addition, in many studies the participants are not allowed to take other drugs while they are subjects.

After drugs are approved for general use, postmarketing surveillance continues. The FDA and the pharmaceutical firm must monitor adverse reactions to drugs. To help track the performance of their products, many drug firms rely on their sales personnel (Ackerman, 1988). Clinicians should communicate with these salespersons by sharing ideas and seeking information about the drugs. The FDA has an "adverse drug reaction" form that should be completed whenever an HCP notices an unusual or adverse reaction to a drug or treatment. However, physicians or other HCPs are not legally required to report these adverse drug reactions to the FDA. To increase the number of adverse reaction reports, the FDA is educating physicians, pharmacists, and nurses about how reactions should be reported. Reporting has been made easier by the creation of hotlines and more rewarding by the provision of significant information about the drug (Ackerman, 1988).

Many pharmaceutical companies encourage open communication by providing scientific information about their products. Anecdotal reports may result in the discovery of new uses for established drugs. For example, thalidomide, a drug that was banned from use in the United States because of severe teratogenic effects when used in the 1950s and 1960s as a sleeping aid in pregnant women, is now being studied for use in the treatment of HIV-related wasting and aphthous ulcers. It is legal to prescribe a drug for an indication other than that for which it was originally approved by the FDA (Ackerman, 1988). In the case of thalidomide, there has been much publicity over these studies because of the drug's infamy. However, when alternate uses of drugs are not publicized or are part of a formalized study, the resulting information may be lost to PCPs.

INSTITUTIONAL LONG-TERM CARE

Throughout the HIV epidemic, home care has played by far the most significant role, not only because care at home is so often preferred by consumers but also because the service has so much potential for flexibility (Wyatt, 1990). As with any chronic disease, however, variables associated with the life of the affected person may necessitate care in a setting other than the home. These variables range from the lack of a suitable home in which to provide care to the lack of a significant other to provide the needed care. Alternatives to home care include skilled nursing facilities (SNFs), often referred to as nursing homes, day care, and residential care with supportive services. Although the demand for these alternatives has been evident and is increasing, the supply has remained low and, in some areas, nonexistent.

Care in a Skilled Nursing Facility

According to Benjamin and Swan (1989), when case managers explore the option of nursing home care for PLWHIV, they find not a solution but a service gap, because many SNFs are reluctant to provide care to this client population. Reasons frequently cited for refusal of nursing homes to accept PLWHIV include

1. Increased costs of infection-control measures and staffing
2. Poor Medicaid reimbursement levels
3. An unprepared work force
4. A philosophic orientation toward geriatric care
5. Homophobia among administrators or staff members
6. Already high occupancy rates
7. Possible loss of referrals of non-HIV-infected residents (Taravella, 1990).

Linsk and colleagues (1993) surveyed nursing home administrators in Illinois and found that major concerns were the ability to recruit staff members to care for PWHIV and fear and apprehension on the part of staff members.

Gentry et al. (1994) sampled 85 nursing homes in the five U.S. cities with the highest AIDS incidence: New York, Los Angeles, San Francisco, Miami, and Houston. Nearly 86% expressed concerns about their abilities to meet the special care needs of persons living with AIDS (PLWA); costs of providing care and lack of adequate reimbursement were also cited as crucial issues in decisions about whether to admit PLWA. In addition, the majority of the respondents believed that PLWA were best served in an HIV-dedicated facility or a facility with a special HIV care unit.

Taravella (1990) estimated that skilled nursing homes in the United States would have 1513 beds for persons with AIDS by the end of 1993. Current national statistics are difficult to obtain, but regions have attempted to address the need. According to the New York State AIDS Institute, as of 1997, New York City had 1216 nursing home beds for PLWA, with an additional 78 beds scattered troughout the rest of the state (S. Chorost, personal communication, July 25, 1997).

One of the first SNFs in the United States to admit a PWHIV was the Human Resources Health Center located in Dade County, Florida. According to Diana Liebisch, director of nursing at that time, admission of PLWA to the facility was considered part of its mission, and the staff struggled through fear and confusion, changing care regimens as new information became available and adjusting policies to meet the challenge (Harvard AIDS Institute, 1989). By 1989 the facility had served 169 persons with AIDS and had expanded its capabilities.

Kane and Smith (1989) were the first to study the integration of persons with AIDS into nursing homes. The study was conducted in 16 nursing homes in Minnesota, equally divided between eight SNFs willing to take or already having admitted PLWA and eight SNFs that did not have plans to admit PLWA. Kane and Smith (1989) interviewed 100 nursing home residents, 100 family members of residents, and 100 nursing home staff members. They also interviewed the administrator, the director of nurses, and the director of social work at each of the 16 facilities, as well as four people with AIDS who were residents in the SNFs studied.

In facilities receptive to admitting PLWHIV, the staff was more knowledgeable and held more positive attitudes than the staff in comparison homes. The SNFs that had admitted PLWHIV did not encounter negative reactions of residents or family members, and staff members did not resign as anticipated. An interesting finding was the fear among the residents and their families and among the staff members about the reactions of the others. The residents and their families were fearful that the staff would quit, and the staff members were fearful that families would move the residents to other SNFs; neither fear materialized. The universal concerns over HIV contagion and infection-control practices were noted also but were certainly not limited to the nursing home setting.

Glatt and colleagues (1992) reported how a 10-bed AIDS unit was established in Long Island, New York, the suburban area with the highest incidence of AIDS. Before the unit opened, staff members received extensive training and education, and meetings were held with both nursing home residents and their families to address fears and concerns. Since the unit opened, there have been no complaints from the geriatric patients or their families, and the patients interact well with each other.

In interviews with PLWA in nursing homes, Kane and Smith (1989) reported that the most significant concerns were

1. Lack of training or familiarity of some staff members with high-tech equipment

2. Quality of meals
3. Quality of activities
4. Lack of telephones
5. Routines that prohibited sleeping late
6. Concern about the reactions of non-AIDS residents

The concerns of the PLWHIV regarding a lack of skill with particular equipment are understandable, but the same problem can occur in other health care settings as well. Complaints about meals, schedules, and activities are common among elderly nursing home residents as well as PLWA (Kane & Caplan, 1990).

The clinical needs of clients with HIV infection remain the same regardless of the setting. For example, clients with toxoplasmosis will require suppressive therapy to prevent recurrence, assistance with personal care, and physical and occupational therapy, whether they are in a hospital or nursing home or at home. Dementia is the primary clinical condition that requires the supportive and protective environment of an SNF (Benjamin & Swan, 1989; Kator & Cunningham McBride, 1990). The dementia seen in many of the clients with AIDS can result in bizarre behavior, violent acting out, decline in self-care skills, and delusional thinking (Dunn, 1990). Both staff and residents should be informed about these behaviors as a consequence of disease and taught how to respond appropriately.

As with other health care settings, the nursing home staff needs preparation to meet the clinical needs of HIV-infected persons with specific OIs. They must be trained in such techniques as infusion therapy to suppress OIs and prophylaxis to prevent infections. Flexibility must be introduced into a system of care traditionally dominated by exclusionary rules.

On the basis of 8 years' experience in admitting persons with AIDS to the Palm Beach County Home and General Care Facility in Palm Beach County, Florida, Dunn (1990) recommended that planning for SNF care include

1. Developing procedures specific to the needs of persons with AIDS
2. Increasing social services
3. Providing support group therapy
4. Offering addiction recovery therapy or meetings at the facility
5. Developing policies and plans for handling substance abuse in the facility

6. Providing necessary education and support groups for staff

The concerns and needs of the members of the nursing staff in nursing homes are the same as those expressed by their colleagues in other settings. History has demonstrated that, with education and experience, these fears can be decreased. When Wurmser (1995) surveyed nursing homes in New Jersey regarding the admission of PLWA, those with experience offered this advice: "Start the educational process early, before the need is critical."

Day Care

An underdeveloped option for long-term care of PLWHIV is a day care and treatment program. In August 1988 the Village Nursing Home in New York City (now the Village Center for Care) opened the first day care program designed specifically for PLWHIV. The goals of the program are rehabilitation, socialization, and recreation (McNally & Mason-Beck, 1989). The program also provides meals and respite for the families and significant others.

Day care for clients with AIDS-dementia complex can be an important part of the plan of care because of the socialization experience. Inclusion of cognitive stimulation and exercise therapy can also decrease mental and motor dysfunction associated with the neurotropic effects of HIV. Supervision of medications in this type of program can help ensure compliance. Infusion therapy can be provided at a reduced cost because the nurse can care for several clients at one time.

For clients who have no significant others, live in substandard housing, and have difficulty providing for themselves, the day care program can not only function as a coordinator of care and case management for a variety of services but also provide emotional support (Smith et al., 1992; Wyatt, 1990). Combining day care with home care in the evenings and on weekends for clients with high-level care needs is another option for a plan of care.

Residential Care

In July 1983 the gay community and health care professionals in San Francisco opened the world's first AIDS residence, the Shanti Project (Harvard AIDS Institute, 1989). The program's chief goal was to provide high-quality, long-term, low-cost housing for displaced PLWA or persons with severe HIV disease who are able to live independently and cooperatively with needed support services in a group setting. The staff worked closely with other AIDS agencies to provide the medical and social services needed by the residents. Residents who required home care received services from the Hospice of San Francisco and the Visiting Nurse Association.

In New York City in 1983, members of the gay community recognized the need for housing that was supportive of the needs of PLWHIV and formed the AIDS Resource Center, which initially offered donations to persons for rent and food. Today the AIDS Resource Center (now Bailey House) operates two types of supportive housing program for PLWHIV: a congregate living facility and scatter-site apartments.

The congregate living facility, known as Bailey-Holt House, has 44 private rooms for clients. Case management, support groups, and on-site health supervision by a professional nurse and a visiting physician are provided. The scatter-site housing program offers a series of apartments throughout the boroughs of New York City. Services are similar to those at Bailey House except that no on-site health supervision is offered. Clients in both settings who require home care receive services from the Visiting Nurse Service of New York.

According to New York City's Division of AIDS Services, housing is the biggest nonmedical need for PLWA. City officials estimate that they will need 8900 housing units by the year 2000 (Dunlap, 1997). In addition to congregate living facilities and scatter-site housing, New York City houses clients in SROs.

One of the most prevalent case management problems in residential programs is substance use, including alcohol, "crack" and cocaine, "speed," marijuana, and heroin. The problem becomes obvious when the resulting behaviors are property destruction, physical and verbal abuse of residents and staff, and unsafe sex. The problem of substance use is not limited to self-identified drug users. In fact, many of the problems of substance use may not be addressed until after the client takes up residence in the facility. Case management should include nondiscriminatory rules regarding behaviors that are not allowed and clear communication of the consequences of breaking the rules. Above all, the staff must be willing to enforce the prearranged limits and must do so consistently. A practice of vacillation and making exceptions gives mixed messages to the clients and encourages them to test the rules.

When the Visiting Nurses and Hospice (VNH) of San Francisco established its hotel project to provide care to SRO residents who were active substance abusers, they found that their biggest problems were manipulation, team splitting, safety concerns, and continuous requests for money (Robb,1994). The nurse, the social worker, and the home care aide needed to develop a consistent approach to deal with these issues. VNH uses funding and volunteer support to assure that all residents have basic necessities such as dishes, clothing, linens, and laundry supplies, plus meals and groceries, from the local AIDS organization. Because of concerns about staff safety, a decision was made not to provide aide service at night because of the increased potential for violence.

A recurrent issue encountered by clients in congregate living facilities is the constant reminders that they have HIV infection. Clients must deal with grieving, both actual and anticipatory, which in most situations is handled through support groups. Volunteers and a program of recreation, as well as availability of religious and spiritual counseling, are important adjuncts to quality living by the residents. Other case management issues to be considered include

1. Residents' bringing guests to their rooms to have sex
2. Homophobia and fear of injection drug users among residents
3. Management and supervision of clients with progressive dementia
4. Preferential treatment received and given by both staff and residents

HOSPICE CARE

Since the opening of St. Christopher's Hospice in England in 1967, hospice care has received considerable attention worldwide. By 1980 the Health Care Finance Administration had approved 26 hospice demonstration programs to study the efficacy and economics of hospice care in the United States. Since then, hospice care has become integrated into the schema of health care in the United States. As of 1995, there were 2500 hospices across the country, and 72% were Medicare-certified. Medicaid covers hospice in 39 states, and most private insurance companies and HMOs now offer a hospice benefit (Slomski, 1995).

Hospice care in the United States has emerged as a model of home care for terminally ill persons. A prevalent misconception is that a hospice is a place to institutionalize a dying person. Although all certified hospice programs are required to have inpatient beds available, their use is usually limited to short periods for respite care and control of symptoms. This basic lack of understanding led to demands, early in the AIDS epidemic in the United States, that PLWA be placed in hospices.

The major appeal of hospice care is the concept of interdisciplinary and holistic case management as the ideal health care model. Hospice care emphasizes quality of life for terminally ill persons through control of symptoms (palliative care) and expert psychologic and spiritual care. Most clinicians would agree that this ideal approach to care should be applied to all health care settings. If one goes one step further, all health care professionals should emphasize quality-of-life issues through control of symptoms and expert psychologic and spiritual care. Although most health care professionals have formally studied death and dying, few have formally studied, with hospice experts, the basics of symptom control, especially pain control. Therefore they are limited in applying this concept to client care, irrespective of the clinical setting.

Until 1983 the cause of AIDS remained unknown, and until March 1987 no treatment of HIV infection was available. Consequently, in the early years of the epidemic, AIDS was viewed as a rapidly progressing terminal illness. Through clinical research, the development of antiretroviral agents, and improved methods of treating and preventing OIs, the clinical picture has changed dramatically. Today the needs of the HIV-ill person can be more appropriately described as a continuum of care for chronic illness. This is not meant to imply that hospice care is not needed; it should be available to those persons who wish it.

However, barriers to hospice care for PLWHIV remain. First, federally established reimbursement rates do not reflect the actual costs associated with case management and the clinical needs of HIV-infected persons. Second, national, state, and local hospice organizations have had to redefine palliative care as it relates to AIDS. Among the issues are

1. Continuation of intravenous therapy for palliative reasons (for example, ganciclovir or foscarnet to prevent blindness as a result of cytomegalovirus retinitis)
2. Periodic transfusions to correct anemia
3. Continuation of expensive suppressive medicines specific to HIV-related illnesses

Third, hospice staff members usually do not have the technical preparation to provide the high-tech services often needed by this client population.

Hospice care, regardless of the stage of HIV illness, is unacceptable to many PLWHIV because they are young and because they believe that a cure is imminent (Martin, 1991; Ungvarski, 1988). They often choose to pursue aggressive medical treatment and to participate in research protocols (Ungvarski, 1989). Commenting on knowledge, self-determination, and decision making, Derek Hodel (1990), executive director of the People with AIDS Group, summarized: "The truth is, a lot of people with AIDS don't want to be 'self-empowered.' They want to stay alive" (p. 30). Consequently, although the care providers and significant others may clearly see the benefits of and need for hospice care, they should not be surprised if PLWHIV reject this model of care.

Hospice care focuses on the quality rather than the quantity of life. Therefore the foundation of hospice care is symptom control, that is, taking control of a particular symptom and preventing its recurrence rather than allowing the symptom to control the patient's life and detract from it (MacFadden, 1988). Pomerantz and Harrison (1990) identified common symptoms seen in end-stage HIV illness as (1) pain, (2) diarrhea, (3) nausea and vomiting, (4) dehydration, (5) urinary incontinence, (6) fever, (7) respiratory problems, including chest pain, cough, and hypoxemia, (8) decubitus ulcers, (9) delirium and dementia, (10) weight loss, and (11) depression, anxiety, and fear. Chapter 5 includes a detailed discussion of symptom management, and Chapter 7 covers the psychosocial aspects of care, including grief, spirtuality, and bereavement.

Symptom control is an art as well as a science, and health care professionals who lack the necessary education and experience are strongly encouraged to seek consultation for their clients from the hospice staff. This is especially true with pain control. According to Rogers (1989), many studies have demonstrated that patients often suffer needlessly because of undermedication, which occurs because health care professionals have insufficient knowledge of the pharmacology of analgesics and because they fear they may be fostering narcotic abuse. Bohnet (1986) pointed out that, until the symptoms are controlled or managed, no other concern of the client can be realistically addressed by provider assessment or intervention.

HIV RESEARCH IN COMMUNITY-BASED AND LONG-TERM CARE

Research concerning the advanced practice roles of clinical nurse specialists, nurse practitioners, and nurse midwives has not only provided emerging models of care but also validated the effectiveness of nurses in the case management of HIV-infected persons. Clinical nurse specialists have demonstrated flexibility in role functions by serving as direct care providers, consultants, and case managers in both inpatient and community-based settings (Layzell & McCarthy, 1993; McCann, 1991; Sherman & Johnson, 1991). Aiken and colleagues (1993) compared HIV-related primary care service delivered by physicians with that delivered by nurse practitioners and found not only comparable levels of care but fewer problems reported by patients who were receiving care from nurse practitioners. De Ferrari and associates (1993) examined a midwifery model of care for pregnant HIV-infected women and found high levels of continuity of care.

Wright and colleagues (1993) evaluated case management activities performed by nurse case managers in the California Pilot Care and Waiver Projects for HIV/AIDS patients. They found that these programs provide vehicles for the coordination and linkage of community services for PWHIV and function as a service-delivery model using nurse case management for PWHIV with symptoms. This survey validated the interdisciplinary case management model in a community-based HIV population. Sowell and associates (1992) examined the effects of case management on controlling hospital costs of the care of persons with AIDS. They identified not only lower hospital-based charges for case-managed clients but increased survival time between HIV diagnosis and death.

There has been a major emphasis on HIV care in the community and in the home throughout the first decade of the AIDS epidemic in the United States. Salsberry and colleagues (1993), in an ongoing investigation, are studying the problems that this change in health care delivery has engendered for agencies that provide this care, as well as the agencies' responses to these problems. Their preliminary findings suggest that home care agencies may not be well positioned to meet the cyclic needs of HIV patients, that care is becoming increasingly fragmented, with multiple agencies seeking to patch together a program of comprehensive services, and that the policies of home care agencies may limit the number of HIV-infected patients eligible for home care.

Brown and Powell-Cope (1991) studied the social context of AIDS family caregivers in the home. Their findings revealed that uncertainty was a dominant theme, with a core category of transitions through uncertainty as well as subcategories of concern, including managing and being managed by HIV disease, living with loss and dying, renegotiating relationships, "going public," and containing the spread of HIV disease.

Hurley and Ungvarski (1994) conducted a retrospective study of the home health care needs of adults with AIDS. In addition to identifying physiologic and psychologic needs, problems identified included inadequate nutrition, issues related to compliance with taking prescribed medications, inadequate in-home support systems, inadequate facilities and utilities in the home, financial concerns, and lifestyles that included drug or alcohol abuse. The authors concluded that the home health care needs of persons with AIDS are multifaceted in nature and extend well beyond the clinical manifestations of HIV disease.

Nurse researchers have also studied the problem of access to community-based HIV/AIDS services in rural areas of the United States. Gay men often move from rural to urban areas in other states in order to lead an openly gay lifestyle; if they become infected with HIV, they may return home to be cared for by their families. Smith and associates (1990) studied the problem of migrating home for HIV/AIDS care and concluded that, because the disease in these persons is diagnosed and reported in large urban areas in other states, the actual numbers of PLWHIV are underestimated in many states. Ultimately, the result is underfunding of services for HIV-infected persons residing in rural areas. Davis and Stapleton (1991) and Davis and associates (1992a, 1992b) studied the phenomenon of HIV-infected persons in rural areas and identified the fact that many of the persons who move back home are not terminally ill and return home for a variety of reasons. Those authors concluded that nurses in rural areas need to be prepared to care for PLWHIV and PLWA and must begin to educate and prepare local agencies and community groups.

Swan and associates (1992) studied the average number of nursing care hours required by PLWHIV in an SNF. They demonstrated that the needs of PLWHIV require greater nursing care time, which results in higher costs for this population in nursing homes.

Research Needed

Research in the area of community-based and long-term care for PLWHIV and PLWA is needed to identify the psychologic, physiologic, environmental, and health-related behaviors of clients. Areas for further study include

1. Identification of human responses, both physiologic and psychologic, that clients manifest in various community-based settings
2. Congruency studies of health care needs identified by clients through self-reporting, in comparison with those identified by health care providers
3. Development and validation of assessment tools to identify client needs in various care settings
4. Identification of the availability and utilization of community-based resources
5. Identification of the impact of caregiving on family systems
6. Identification of factors that influence access to health care, such as insurance, finances, housing, community safety, and care in rural areas
7. Identification of issues that impede a person's ability to adhere to prescribed therapies, such

as drug and alcohol use and limited education

8. Comparison of the cost of health care in various community-based settings
9. Evaluation of patient outcomes to compare nurse-managed versus non-nurse-managed care
10. Evaluation of the efficacy and costs of alternative or complementary therapies prescribed by various HCPs
11. Evaluation of patient outcomes related to care provided by advanced practice nurses as compared with nurse generalists or physicians
12. Knowledge, attitude, and practices of HCPs regarding noncompliance and adherence
13. Methods and costs of strategies employed to enhance self-care management with respect to medication

SUMMARY

Planning for the long-term care needs of the client with HIV disease ranges from primary care with scheduled follow-up in the early phase of diagnosis to provision of home care, long-term residential care, or hospice care in the later stages. Health care professionals responsible for case management can improve access to these services if they are familiar with the capabilities and limitations of the various service providers.

In August 1990 the National Commission on AIDS submitted its first annual report to the President and Congress. Among their findings were that (1) the belief that Medicaid will pay for health care needs of PLWHIV is a "Medicaid fantasy"; (2) for medically disenfranchised persons and those unable to pay, no system of care exists; and (3) health care in the United States has been unresponsive to the needs of HIV-infected persons. The report emphasized that at the end of the first decade of the HIV/AIDS epidemic in the United States, there was still no national policy or plan and no national voice. Time has not corrected this situation. Although the strategies announced by the White House since 1990 sound admirable, without the legislative agenda and funding to carry out the proposals, it appears to be continuing rhetoric.

Unquestionably, the health care professionals intimately involved in HIV/AIDS education, care, and research have begun to address the clinical needs of this client population and have clearly articulated what needs to be done to address the problems of care. The federal government must take a more active role. "The development of a comprehensive system with linkages to research protocols, existing community-based services, hospitals, drug treatment programs, local health departments, and long-term care facilities, based on a foundation of adequate support, is long overdue and should be a top priority for the federal government" (National Commission on AIDS, 1990, p. 167).

REFERENCES

Abrams, D.I. (1990). Alternative therapies in HIV infection. *AIDS, 4*(12), 1179–1187.

Ackerman, S. (1988). Watching for problems that testing may have missed. In *New drug development in the United States* (DHHS publication No. [FDA] 88-3168) (pp. 51–53). Rockville, MD: U.S. Department of Health and Human Services.

Agency for Health Care Policy and Research, Public Health Service, U.S. Department of Health and Human Services. (1994). *Evaluation and management of early HIV infection.* Clinical practice guideline #7. (Publication 94-0572.) Washington, DC: Author.

AIDS Treatment Resources. (1990). *Deciding to enter an AIDS/HIV drug trial.* New York: AIDS Treatment Resources, Inc.

Aiken, L.H., Lake, E.T., Semann, S., et al. (1993). Nurse practitioner managed care for persons with HIV infection. *Image: Journal of Nursing Scholarship, 25*(3), 172–177.

Allen, S.M., Fleishman, J. (1992). Problems encountered in home health service delivery to persons with AIDS. *Home Health Care Services Quarterly, 13*(1/2), 129–159.

American Nurses' Association. (1988). *Nursing case management.* Kansas City, MO: The Association.

Associated Press. (December 18, 1996). Clinton offers six AIDS goals, topped by cure. *The New York Times,* A15.

Baigis-Smith, J., Gordon, D., McGuire, D.B., Nanda, J. (1995). Healthcare needs of HIV-infected persons in hospital, outpatient, home, and long-term care settings. *Journal of the Association of Nurses in AIDS Care, 6*(6), 21–33.

Balsam, A., Grant, N., Rogers, B.L. (1996). Program characteristics of home-delivered meals programs for persons with HIV and AIDS. *Journal of Community Health, 21*(1), 37–49.

Bayer, R., Stryker, J. (1997). Ethical challenges posed by clinical progress in AIDS. *American Journal of Public Health, 87*(10), 1599–1602.

Benjamin, A.E., Swan, J.H. (1989). Nursing home care for persons with HIV illness. *Generations, 13*(4), 63–64.

Bohnet, N.L. (1986). Symptom control. In M. O'Rawe Amenta, N.L. Bohnet (Eds.), *Nursing care of the terminally ill* (pp. 67–80). Boston: Little, Brown.

Bowen, G.S., Marconi, K., Kohn, S., Bailey, D.M., Goosby, E.P., Shorter, S., Niemcryk, S. (1992). First year of AIDS services delivery under Title I of the Ryan White CARE Act. *Public Health Reports, 107*(5), 491–499.

Bradley-Springer, L. (1996). Patient education for behavior change: Help from the transtheoretical and harm reduction models. *Journal of the Association of Nurses in AIDS Care, 7*(Suppl. 1), 23–33.

Brook, R.H. (1996). Practice guidelines: To be or not to be. *Lancet, 348,* 1005–1006.

Brown, M.A., Powell-Cope, G.M. (1991). AIDS family caregiving: Transitions through uncertainty. *Nursing Research, 40*(6), 338–345.

Burstin, H.R., Lipsitz S.R., Brennan, T.A. (1992). Socioeconomic status and risk for substandard medical care. *Journal of the American Medical Association, 268*(17), 2383–2387.

Centers for Disease Control and Prevention. (1997a). Update: Trends in AIDS incidence—United States, 1996. *MMWR, 46*(37), 861–867.

Centers for Disease Control and Prevention. (1997b). USPHS/IDSA guidelines for the prevention of opportunistic infections in persons infected with human immunodeficiency virus. *MMWR, 46*(no. RR-12).

Cooper, M. (October 13, 1996). Help on HIV roller coaster. *The New York Times,* The city, p. 15.

Corrigan, A.M. (1995). History of intravenous therapy. In J. Terry, L. Baranowski, R.A. Lonsway, C. Hedrick (Eds.), *Intravenous therapy, clinical principles and practice* (pp. 1–5). Philadelphia: Saunders.

Crespo-Fierro, M. (1996). Home infusion therapy and the HIV/AIDS patient. *Infusion, 2*(4), 10–22.

Crespo-Fierro, M. (1997). Compliance/adherence and care management in HIV disease. *Journal of the Association of Nurses in AIDS Care, 8*(4), 43–54.

Dagg, S., Dobson, P., Ferguson, J.K., Groombridge, C., Boyle, M.J. (1996). *Altering demand for home infusions of amphotericin B: Effect of newer antiretrovirals* (abstract no. 98). Annual Conference of the Australian Society of HIV Medicine, 1996 Nov 14–17.

Darbyshire, P. (1992). The core of nursing. *Nursing Times, 88*(36), 44–45.

Davis, K., Cameron, B., Stapleton, J. (1992a). Impact of HIV patient migration to rural areas. *AIDS Patient Care, 5*(5), 225–228.

Davis, K.A., Ferguson, K.J., Stapleton, J.T. (1992b). Moving home to live: Migration of HIV-infected persons to rural states. *Journal of the Association of Nurses in AIDS Care, 3*(4), 42–47.

Davis, K., Stapleton, J. (1991). Migration to rural areas by HIV patients: Impact on HIV-related healthcare use. *Infection Control and Hospital Epidemiology, 12*(9), 540–543.

De Ferrari, E., Paine, L.L., Gregor, C.L., et al. (1993). Midwifery care for women with human immunodeficiency virus disease in pregnancy: A demonstration project at the Johns Hopkins Hospital. *Journal of Nurse Midwifery, 38*(2), 97–102.

Department of Health and Human Services. (1989). *AIDS clinical trials: Talking it over.* Bethesda, MD: National Institutes of Health.

Dunlap, D. (March 30, 1997). Building blocks in the battle on AIDS. *The New York Times,* Section 9, pp. 1, 6.

Dunn, S. (1990). Providing care in a county nursing home AIDS unit. In V.E. Fransen (Ed.), *Proceedings: AIDS prevention and services workshop* (pp. 116–119). Princeton, NJ: Robert Wood Johnson Foundation.

Fee, E., Fox, D.M. (1992). Introduction: The contemporary historiography of AIDS. In E. Fee, D.M. Fox, (Eds.), *AIDS: The making of a chronic disease* (pp. 1–19). Berkeley: University of California Press.

Fee, E., Krieger, N. (1993). Thinking and rethinking AIDS: Implications for health policy. *International Journal of Health Services, 23*(2), 323–346.

Flieger, K. (1988). *Testing in "real people": New drug development in the United States* (DHHS publication No. [FDA] 88-3168) (pp. 13–14, 17). Rockville, MD: U.S. Department of Health and Human Services.

Franks, P., Clancy, C.M., Gold, M.R. (1993). Health insurance and mortality: Evidence from a national cohort. *Journal of the American Medical Association, 270*(6), 737–741.

Friedland, G.H. (1997). Adherence: The Achilles' heel of highly active antiretroviral therapy. *Improving the Management of HIV Disease, 5*(1) 13–15.

Gebbie, K.M. (1989). The President's Commission on AIDS: What did it do? *American Journal of Public Health, 79*(7), 868–870.

Gentry, D., Fogarty, T.E., Lehrman, S. (1994). Providing long-term care for persons with AIDS. *AIDS Patient Care, 8*(3), 130–137.

Glatt, A.E., Risbrook, A.T., Jenna, R.W. (1992). Successful implementation of a long-term care unit for patients with acquired immune deficiency syndrome in an underserved urban area with a high incidence of human immunodeficiency virus. *Archives of Internal Medicine, 152*(4), 823–825.

Grau, L. (1984). Case management and the nurse. *Geriatric Nursing, 5*(8), 372–375.

Haddad, A.M., Keefer, K.R., Stein, J.E. (1993). Teamwork in home infusion therapy: The relationship between nursing and pharmacy. *Home Healthcare Nurse, 11*(1), 40–46.

Hart, L.K., Freel, M.I., Milde, F.K. (1990). Fatigue. *Nursing Clinics of North America, 25*(4), 967–976.

Harvard AIDS Institute. (1989). Alternatives to hospital care for people with HIV infection (Invitational Conference, November 8–10, 1989). Cambridge, MA: Harvard Schoool of Public Health.

Hodel, D. (October 31, 1990). All fired up or just all fired. *Outweek, 70,* 30–31.

Hurley, P.M., Ungvarski, P.J. (1994). Home healthcare needs of adults with HIV disease/AIDS in New York City. *Journal of the Association of Nurses in AIDS Care, 5*(2), 33–40.

Hurley, P.M., Ungvarski, P.J., Rottner, J.E. (1996). Predictors of home care service costs in adults living with HIV/AIDS in New York City. *Journal of Care Management, 2*(5), 3–11.

Imperato, P.J. (1990). Acquired immunodeficiency syndrome: The agenda for the 1990s. *New York State Journal of Medicine, 90*(3), 115–116.

Kane, R.A., Caplan, A.L. (1990). *Everyday ethics: Resolving dilemmas in nursing home life.* New York: Springer Publishing Company.

Kane, R.A., Smith D. (1989). *Multiple perspectives on AIDS and the nursing home: A pilot study and recommendations for research* (report No. PB 90-101320). Rockville, MD: Agency for Health Care Policy and Research.

Kator, M.J., Cunningham McBride, L. (1990). Developing a long-term care facility program for AIDS patients. *Pride Institute Journal of Long-Term Home Health Care, 9*(1), 15–19.

Katoff, L. (1992). Community-based services for people with AIDS. *Primary Care, 19*(1), 231–243.

Kolata, G. (September 15, 1996). AIDS patients slipping through safety net. *The New York Times,* B1.

Layzell, S., McCarthy, M. (1993). Specialist or generic community nursing care for HIV/AIDS patients? *Journal of Advanced Nursing, 18*(4), 531–537.

Leenerts, M.H., Koehler, J.A., Neil, R.M. (1996). Nursing care models increase care quality while reducing costs. *Journal of the Association of Nurses in AIDS Care, 7*(4), 37–49.

Linsk, N.L., Cick, P.J., Gianfrani, L. (1993). The AIDS epidemic: Challenges for nursing homes. *Journal of Gerontological Nursing, 19*(1), 11–22.

Lyne, B.A., Waller, P.R. (1990). The Denver Nursing Project in Human Caring: A model for AIDS nursing care and professional education. *Family and Community Health, 13*(2), 78–84.

MacFadden, D.K. (1988). Symptom control in AIDS. *Journal of Palliative Care, 4*(4), 42–45.

Martin, J.P. (1991). Issues in the current treatment of hospice patients with HIV disease. *The Hospice Journal, 7*(12), 31–40.

Master, R.J., Gallagher, D., Rivard, M., et al. (1993). *An HMO for Medicaid-covered patients with AIDS (PWAs)* [abstract no. PO-B38-2392]. International Conference on AIDS.

McCabe, E. (1992). Ozone therapies for AIDS. *AIDS Patient Care, 6*(6), 254–255.

McCann, K. (1991). The work of a specialist AIDS home support team: The views and experiences of patients using the service. *Journal of Advanced Nursing Practice, 16*(7), 832–836.

McNally, L., Mason-Beck, L. (1989). Day treatment for persons with AIDS. *Generations, 13*(4), 69–70.

Michaels, D., Levine, C. (1992). Estimates of the number of motherless youth orphaned by AIDS in the United States. *Journal of American Medical Association, 268*(24), 3456–3461.

Morrison, C. (1990). Case management and the determination of appropriate care settings. In Agency for Health Care Policy and Resources Conference Proceedings. *Community-based care of persons with AIDS: Developing a research agenda* (DHHS publication No. PHS 90-3456) (pp. 75–82). Washington, DC: U.S. Government Printing Office.

Morrison, C. (1993). Delivery systems for the care of persons with HIV infection and AIDS. *Nursing Clinics of North America, 28*(2), 317–333.

National Commission on AIDS. (1990, August). Annual report to the President and the Congress. Washington, DC: U.S. Government Printing Office.

National Institute of Allergy and Infectious Diseases. (1990). *NIAID AIDS research.* Bethesda, MD: The Institute.

National League for Nursing. (May 13, 1992). *Community nursing centers: A promising new trend in American health care.* New York: The League.

New York City Department of Health. (1989). *HSA/New York City AIDS Task Force Report.* New York: The Department.

Normand, J., Vlahov, D., Moses, L.E. (Eds.). (1995). *Preventing HIV transmission: The role of sterile needles and bleach.* National Research Council and Institute of Medicine. Washington, DC: National Academy Press.

Palella, F.J., Delaney, K.M., Moorman, A.C., et al. (1998). Declining morbidity and mortality among patients with advanced human immunodeficiency virus infection. *The New England Journal of Medicine, 338*(13), 853–860.

Pessin, N., Lindy, D., Stricoff, D.J., et al. (1993). Integrating mental health and home care services for AIDS patients. *Caring, 12*(5), 30–34.

Piette, J.D., Fleishman, J.A., Stein, M.D., Mor, V., Mayer, K. (1993). Perceived needs and unmet needs for formal services among people with HIV disease. *Journal of Community Health, 18*(1), 11–23.

Pomerantz, S., Harrison, E. (1990). End-stage symptom management. *AIDS Patient Care, 4*(1), 18–20.

Prochaska, J., Redding, C., Harlow, L., Rossi, J., Velicer, W. (1994). The transtheoretical model of change and HIV prevention: A review. *Health Education Quarterly, 21,* 471–486.

Robb, V. (1994). The hotel project: A community approach to persons with AIDS. *Nursing Clinics of North America, 29*(3), 521–531.

Rogers, A.G. (1989). Analgesics: The physician's partner in effective pain management. *Virginia Medical, 116*(4), 164–170.

Salsberry, P.J., Nickel, J., O'Connell, M.O., et al. (1993). Home health care services for AIDS patients: One community's response. *Journal of Community Health Nursing, 10*(1), 39–51.

Schmidt, J. (1992). Case management problems and home care. *Journal of the Association of Nurses in AIDS Care, 3*(3), 37–44.

Schroeder, C. (1993). Nursing's response to the crisis of access, costs and quality in health care. *Advances in Nursing Science, 16*(1), 1–20.

Schroeder, C., Maeve, M.K. (1992). Nursing care partnerships at the Denver Nursing Project in Human Caring: An application and extension of caring theory in practice. *Advances in Nursing Science, 15*(2), 25–38.

Sherman, J.J., Johnson, P.K. (1991). Nursing case management. *Quality Assurance and Utilization Review, 6*(4), 142–145.

Slomski, A.J. (September 25, 1995). Doctors' misconceptions about hospice care. *Medical Economics,* 72–88.

Smith, M.Y., Knickman, J.R., Oppenheimer, L.M. (1992). Connecting the disconnected: Adult day care for people with AIDS in New York City. *Health and Social Work, 17*(4), 273–281.

Smith, J., Landau, J., Bahr, R. (1990). AIDS in rural and small town America: Making the heartland respond. *AIDS Patient Care, 4*(3), 17–21.

Smith, M.Y., Rapkin, B.D. (1996). Social support and barriers to family involvement in caregiving for persons with AIDS: Implications for patient education. *Patient Education and Counseling, 27*(1), 85–94.

Snyder, C.M., Kaempfer, S.H., Ries, K. (1996). An interdisciplinary, interagency, primary care approach to case management of the dually-diagnosed patient with HIV disease. *Journal of the Association of Nurses in AIDS Care, 7*(5), 72–82.

Soloway, B., Hecht, F.M. (1997). Managed care and HIV. *AIDS Clinical Care, 9*(9), 67–69, 71.

Sowell, R.L. (1995). Community-based HIV case management: Challenges and opportunities. *Journal of the Association of Nurses in AIDS Care, 6*(2), 33–40.

Sowell, R.L. (1997). Clinical issues: Reconstruction case management. *Journal of the Association of Nurses in AIDS Care, 8*(6), 43–45.

Sowell, R.L., Fuszard, B., Gritzmacher, D. (1990). Services for persons with AIDS [Nurse executives report]. *Journal of Nursing Administration, 20*(7/8), 44–48.

Sowell, R.L., Gueldner, S.H., Killeen, M.R., et al. (1992). Impact of case management on hospital charges of PWAs in Georgia. *Journal of the Association of Nurses in AIDS Care, 3*(2), 24–31.

Sowell, R.L., Opava, W.D. (1995). The Georgia rural-based nurse model: Primary care for persons with HIV/AIDS. *Public Health Nursing, 12*(4), 228–234.

Springer, E. (1991). Effective AIDS prevention with active drug use: The harm reduction model. In M. Shernoff (Ed.), *Counseling chemically dependent people with HIV illness* (pp. 141–157). New York: Haworth Press.

Stephenson, B.J., Rowe, B.H., Haynes, R.B. (1993). Is the patient taking their treatment as prescribed? *Journal of the American Medical Association, 269*(21), 2779–2781.

Stone, V.E., Seage, G.R., Hertz, T., Epstein, A.M. (1992). The relation between hospital experience and mortality for patients with AIDS. *Journal of the American Medical Association, 268*(19), 2655–2661.

Swan, J.H., Benjamin, A.E., Brown, A. (1992). Skilled nursing facility care for persons with AIDS: Comparison with other patients. *American Journal of Public Health, 82*(3), 453–455.

Taravella, S. (1990). Who will provide long-term care for AIDS patients? *Modern Health Care, 20*(12), 38–39.

The Presidential Commission. (1988, June). *Report of the Presidential Commission on the Human Immunodeficiency Virus Epidemic.* Washington, DC: U.S. Government Printing Office.

Ungvarski, P.J. (1987). AIDS and long-term care. *Caring, 6*(10), 44–47.

Ungvarski, P.J. (1988). Testimony on home care. In The Presidential Commission on the Human Immunodeficiency Virus Epidemic, *Hearing on care of HIV-infected persons, January 13–15, 1988.* Washington DC: U.S. Government Printing Office.

Ungvarski, P.J. (1989). Developing long-term plan of care for the HIV epidemic. *Caring, 8*(11), 4–8.

Ungvarski, P.J. (1996). Challenges for the urban home health care provider: The New York City experience. *Nursing Clinics of North America, 31*(1), 81–95.

Ungvarski, P.J. (1997a). Adherence to prescribed HIV-1 protease inhibitors in the home setting. *Journal of the Association of Nurses in AIDS Care, 8*(Suppl.), 37–45.

Ungvarski, P.J. (1997b). A pilot program to promote medication self-care management for clients with HIV infection/AIDS. Unpublished manuscript.

Ungvarski, P.J., Rottner, J.E. (1997c). Errors in prescribing HIV-1 protease inhibitors. *Journal of the Association of Nurses in AIDS Care, 8*(4), 55–61.

Ungavarski, P.J., Schmidt, J., Neville, S. (1994). Planning homecare services for people living with AIDS. *Home Healthcare Nurse, 13*(1), 17–23.

Ungvarski, P.J., Staats, J.A. (1995). Clinical manifestations of AIDS in adults. In J.H. Flaskerud, P.J. Ungvarski (Eds.), *HIV/AIDS: A guide to nursing care* (3rd ed., pp. 81–133). Philadelphia: Saunders.

Weinstein, S.M. (1993). A coordinated aproach to home infusion therapy. *Home Healthcare Nurse, 11*(1), 15–20.

Weitzel, E.A. (1992). Medication management. In G.M. Bulechek, J.C. McCloskey (Eds.), *Nursing interventions: Essential nursing treatments* (2nd ed., pp. 213–220). Philadelphia: Saunders.

Williams, A. (1997). Antiretroviral therapy: Factors associated with adherence. *Journal of the Association of Nurses in AIDS Care, 8*(Suppl.), 18–23.

Williams, A., Friedland, G. (1997). Adherence, compliance and HAART. *AIDS Clinical Care, 9*(7), 51–54, 58.

Wolfe, G. (1997). The case manager's role in adherence. *Journal of the Association of Nurses in AIDS Care, 8*(Suppl.), 24–28.

Wright, J., Bakken H.S., Holzemer, W.L., et al. (1993). Evaluation of community-based nurse case management activities for symptomatic HIV/AIDS clients. *Journal of the Association of Nurses in AIDS Care, 4*(20), 37–47.

Wurmser, T. (1995). Survey cites need for HIV/AIDS education in long term care. *New Jersey Nurse, 25*(2), 1–2.

Wyatt, A. (1990). AIDS and the long-term care continuum. *Pride Institute Journal of Long-Term Home Health Care, 9*(1), 6–14.

11

Alternative and Complementary Therapies

JOYCE K. ANASTASI

Complementary and alternative medicine (CAM) applies to a wide variety of nonconventional healing practices. The practices are quite different, but most share the individualized nature of treatment. Most of the practices tend to focus on the "whole" body, mind, and spirit. The terms *complementary* and *alternative* are frequently used to describe nonconventional medical practices. *Alternative therapy* means replacing or using another form of therapy, *complementary therapy* means in conjunction with other forms of therapy.

The use of CAM therapies in patients with HIV/AIDS has been established by a number of patient surveys (Anderson et al., 1993; Greenblatt et al., 1991; Hand, 1989; Sutherland & Verhoef, 1995; Van Dam et al., 1992). In the noted study by Eisenberg et al. (1993), 1539 persons were polled on consumer usage of CAM in 1990. Thirty-four percent were found to have used alternative medicines. This finding suggests that, with extrapolation to the U.S. population in 1990, approximately 425 million visits were made to alternative practitioners, representing nearly $13.7 billion in expenditures, including $10.3 billion in out-of-pocket expenses.

Over the past few years much has evolved in the area of health insurance coverage and CAM. It is becoming evident that health care plans of the future will acknowledge a variety of treatment and prevention strategies. Stronger evidence supporting the use of alternative-complementary coverage began in the state of Washington when, in 1995, a law was passed that required all health care plans to include "every category of provider." The providers mentioned in the plan included chiropractors, massage practitioners, acupuncturists, naturopathic physicians, and direct-entry midwives. In 1996 the U.S. Public Health Association included a track on complementary medicine at the Association's annual meeting. In 1997 Oxford, a major managed-care HMO, announced that it would begin offering alternative-medicine benefits to its members (Weeks, 1997).

Why are so many people using CAM?

For some, the motivation is that there is no cure or conventional treatment that works or that current treatments which show promise are toxic and in many cases cause dreadful side effects. In addition, some people distrust traditional Western approaches and will assert personal control over their medical affairs by seeking alternative systems of medicine.

How extensive is the research in CAM?

Unfortunately, much of the information concerning efficacy in the use of CAM therapies is either anecdotal or lacks the rigor involved in experimental designs. Some of the problems inherent in CAM research are the individualization of treatments, the use of placebo or sham interventions, blinding, specificity of the disorder, and outcome measures not specific to CAM therapies (Vickers, 1994). This has led much of the medical community (at least in the United States) to discredit CAM (Moran, 1995). According to Moran (1995), safety, efficacy, and cost-effective-

▪ PRACTICAL GUIDELINES FOR
CONSUMERS OF COMPLEMENTARY
OR ALTERNATIVE THERAPIES ▪

1. It is important to do your homework. The Internet has numerous sources on CAM.
2. Claims of cure should be scrutinized. Proof is essential.
3. Document study findings. Was therapy ever studied? Was the protocol peer reviewed? Were there controls?
4. Does your insurance cover alternative and complementary therapies? Some city, state, and HMO health plans do.
5. What are the credentials of the CAM practitioner administering the treatment?
6. Is the CAM practitioner willing to talk with the patient's primary provider?
7. Are fees necessary to obtain treatment? Sometimes this could be an indication that protocol is spurious. Are CAM therapies within the patient's ability to pay?
8. Is foreign travel required?
9. How much of a description is given about the therapy? Is the therapy toxic? What are the risks and benefits?
10. Are all of the patient's questions really answered?

ness need to be established for alternative treatments as they are for conventional medicine.

In 1992 the National Institutes of Health Office of Alternative Medicine (OAM) was established secondary to a mandate from Congress to facilitate the evaluation of alternative medical treatments. The OAM's mission is "to identify and evaluate unconventional health care practices. The OAM supports and conducts research and research training on these practices and disseminates information" (Complementary Alternative Medicine at the NIH, 1997). See Box above for practical guidelines for CAM consumers to follow.

How many fields of CAM are there?

In 1992 the OAM published a report that identified several fields of alternative medicine: mind-body medicine, bioelectromagnetic applications, alternative systems of medical practice, manual healing methods, pharmacologic and biologic treatments, herbal medicine, and diet and nutrition in the prevention of chronic diseases. Within these fields of medicine there are numerous types of therapy. There follows a discussion of the fields of medicine and specific therapies that have been used by people with HIV or that have an application to the disease or symptoms expressed by HIV/AIDS. One should keep in mind that this is an overview of some of the most frequently used therapies—*not* a comprehensive text on all of the complementary and alternative therapies that are currently available.

MIND-BODY MEDICINE

Mind-body medicine is a term used to emphasize the connection and inseparability of the mind and the body. In recent years there has been a quest to explore the mind's capacity to affect the body. Mind-body medicine has been prompted by the growth in incidence of chronic conditions. The devastation and cost of chronic conditions have generated the search for therapies that can help patients acknowledge and alleviate the causes of their stress by calming the mind and using it to facilitate the healing of the body. Mind-body interventions encompass meditation; tai chi, qi gong, and yoga are built on the concept of the power of the mind and the body to affect one another. Some of the other mind-body practices are imagery and biofeedback, which facilitate the mind's capacity to affect the body (Report to the NIH on Alternative Medical Systems, 1992; Gordon, 1996).

Meditation

Meditation is self-directed, focused concentration aimed at withdrawing attention from the vast number of thoughts that tend to go through one's mind and placing attention on the object of meditation. If the meditator's thoughts stray on images of miscellaneous things that have occurred throughout the day, it is necessary to come back into focus. Although this seems simple, it is often difficult.

There are many forms of meditation, most of which can be done in any position. Most people use the crossed-leg seated position with the spine straight. If this position is not comfortable, one can sit in a chair. Once the person is seated comfortably, he or she closes the eyes and focuses on the rhythm and depth of breathing. The ideal breath is slow and quiet. There are usually a series of counted exhalations and inhalations. It is recommended that meditation be performed every day for 20 to 30 minutes. To do this effectively, one must want to meditate.

Some of the benefits of meditation include decreased heart and respiratory rate, lowered blood pressure, increased blood flow, relaxation, and stress reduction (Weil, 1995).

Imagery

Imagery is the use of therapeutic procedures and mental processes to facilitate changes in behavior, attitudes, and physiologic responses. These mental and sensory processes can include all of the senses: tactile, visual, aural, proprioception, kinesthetic, and olfactory (Report to the NIH on Alternative Medical Systems, 1992). Aspects of our personal selves of which we are not aware can be uncovered by imagery. One method of imagery uses a systematic approach. Patients are initially asked to imagine what their cancer cells, white blood cells, medical treatments, and cancer cell amelioration would look like. At the end of the session patients are asked to see themselves as in control and cured (Wanning, 1993). Imagery can be done with or without a facilitator/therapist. When facilitated by a therapist, it is called interactive imagery. This method typically involves imaginary dialogues with images that represent symptoms or illness (Burton Goldberg Group, 1995). For quite some time, imagery has been used in conjunction with traditional approaches to cancer therapy and smoking cessation.

Biofeedback

Biofeedback is a training method that is used to voluntarily control involuntary body functions by using a specialized electronic instrument that provides the person with information about the involuntary activities (Rankin-Box, 1995). This instrument can display and measure involuntary bodily functions. The key element in biofeedback is receiving information and obtaining knowledge that results from training. Obtaining feedback is important in learning the technique that will help the patient who is attempting to control his or her physiologic activity. For example, a patient who wants to regulate his or her heart rate would train with a biofeedback machine adjusted to transmit an audible sound or blinking light with each heart beat. Through biofeedback training, the patient learns how to control the rate of the blinking light and audible sounds to adjust his or her heart rate (Burton Goldberg Group, 1995).

Biofeedback has many applications, including but not limited to insomnia, anxiety, migraines, asthma, cardiovascular disorders, gastrointestinal disorders, muscular dysfunctions, and pain control (Rankin-Box, 1995). The primary provider should be consulted before initiation of this treatment. Biofeedback may be contraindicated for persons who have psychiatric disorders, impaired attention, poor memory, low blood pressure, seizures, and extreme skepticism (Schwartz & Fehmi, 1982).

ALTERNATIVE SYSTEMS OF MEDICINE

Alternative medical practices have been described as those medical practices that are not traditionally practiced in hospitals or taught in conventional U.S. medical school curricula (Eisenberg et al., 1993; Report to the NIH on Alternative Medical Systems, 1992). The practices, techniques, and systems that challenge the viewpoints of U.S. health care systems are considered alternative medicine. Practitioners of alternative medicine frequently use multiple treatment modalities and tend to focus on the patient's constitution (makeup), which has the underlying ability to fight on its own behalf and enhance the natural healing process.

There are numerous systems of medicine that are considered alternative. The most popular systems of alternative medicine include ayruveda, homeopathy, and traditional Chinese medicine.

Ayurvedic Medicine

Ayurveda is a 5000-year-old traditional system of medicine originating in India. The term *ayurveda* means "life knowledge." This system incorporates the prevention and treatment of illness through lifestyle interventions and natural therapies. The theory behind ayurveda is that all disease begins with an imbalance in the consciousness of the individual and that mental stress leads to unhealthy lifestyles that will contribute to ill health. Accordingly, meditation and other mental practices are considered key to the promotion of health and prevention of disease.

According to ayurvedic principles, all physical expressions of disease are due to an imbalance of physiologic principles in the body known as *doshas.* The doshas are thought to control all bodily functions. The ayurvedic practitioner assesses the doshas by carefully examining the patient's pulse. This assessment will determine the type of treatment plan. The treatment plan generally consists of lifestyle interventions and herbs. The lifestyle interventions encompass dietary, sleeping, and exercise programs based on the patient's body type and assessment (Anselmo & Brooks, 1996).

The physiologic effects of body postures and meditation have been well studied. Physiologic changes in heart rate, respiration, blood pressure, muscle tension, improved stress responses, and pain relief have been shown in studies on the practice of meditation (Murphy, 1992). Other ayurvedic practices have also been shown to be beneficial. For example, there are herbal preparations for treating and preventing colon, lung, and breast cancers (Sharma et al., 1990) in addition to infectious diseases (Thyagarajan et al., 1988). Although no specific treatments have been designated for people with HIV, it seems that many of these practices might be beneficial.

Homeopathic Medicine

Homeopathic medicine was developed in the 1700's by Samuel Hahnemann (Rothouse, 1997). The fundamental principle of homeopathy is the law of similars or "like cures like," which means that a substance that can provoke certain symptoms when given to a healthy person can cure those same symptoms in a person who is sick (Weiner, 1996). Another principle important to this practice has to do with the dilution of a substance. Most people would tend to think that the higher the dose of a remedy, the greater the effect. In homeopathic medicine, however, this is not the case. Diluting or "potentizing" a remedy to high dilutions could reduce the therapeutic side effects of the substance. This aspect of homeopathy has been criticized because one would think that, with such extreme dilutions, the remedies are beyond the point of being effective. Yet those who accept this theory have their own theories to explain how the diluted substance has a beneficial action (Davenas et al., 1988; Delinick, 1991).

Homeopathy in HIV/AIDS

Homeopathy is used by persons with AIDS both for prophylaxis and management of opportunistic infections. This is done by addressing the patient's underlying condition(s), which could have predisposed the patient to his or her condition. Other important aspects are hereditary factors, history of family illnesses, and history of sexually transmitted disease (O'Connor, 1995).

The treatment is specific to the individual patient in order to match the composition of symptoms. Therefore no specific lists of remedies for HIV/AIDS are available. There are common symptoms that have become associated with certain remedies. For example, cutaneous Kaposi's sarcoma has been treated with mistletoe, *Phytolacca decandra,* and vinca preparations. Vinblastine (the chemotherapuetic agent) is derived from vinca (periwinkle) (O'Connor, 1995).

Depending on the type of homeopathic remedy that is prescribed, it may be in the form of a liquid, tablet, powder, or granules. Homeopathic pharmacies would instruct the patient to avoid peppermint or menthol and coffee, as these substances can counteract the effect of the remedies (Rankin-Box, 1995). Patients with a lactose intolerance or diabetes should inform their homeopaths, as the tablet base is often made of lactose (Rankin-Box, 1995). As with all CAM therapies, it is wise to advise the patient to consult with his or her primary provider. Generally speaking, homeopathic remedies are safe and should not interfere with Western pharmaceuticals. However, some homeopaths believe that remedies may be less effective if combined.

Traditional Chinese Medicine

Traditional Chinese medicine involves a highly complex collection of techniques and methods based on Asian philosophy and theory. Some of the methods used in Chinese medicine are acupuncture, acupressure, moxibustion, cupping, herbal medicine, oriental medicinal massage, and qi gong. Oriental medicine is philosophically rooted in the beliefs of Tao, Confucius, and Buddha. Asian culture views the person as a whole. The family structure, environmental influences, emotions, and the physical body are interrelated.

In Chinese medicine the balance and smooth flow of energy or "qi" (pronounced "chee") is critical for optimal health. Qi circulates in the 12 major pathways called meridians. Each meridian or energy pathway corresponds to a specific organ system. If qi or energy is blocked, there will be an imbalance of energy and other important elements in the body. This blockage of energy can result in discomfort or pain. The aim of treatment by an oriental practitioner is to restore energy balance and harmony in order to promote health and treat disease. In attempting to harmonize the body, the practitioner uses the eight principles of Chinese medicine to diagnose and treat the patient: yin and yang, excess and deficiency, interior and exterior, and hot and cold. When making a diagnosis, the practitioner will ask many questions regarding the patient's personal or family history, appetite, sleep patterns, thirst, bowel patterns, urination, and, if the patient is a female, menstrual patterns to name a few. The practitioner will also pay close attention to the patient's skin texture and color, color, coating, and shape of the tongue, eyes, fingernails, hair, tone of voice, breathing, and pulses. All of this information will lead the practitioner in making a diagnosis with use of the eight principles. Once the diagnosis is made, the practitioner will apply the principles specific to the patient. The practice of acupuncture involves the use of specific (acupuncture) points in conjunction with special techniques and methods (tonifying, reducing, moxibustion, cupping). In some cases, herbs may also be prescribed.

Acupuncture

Acupuncture involves stimulation of specific points on the energy pathways or meridians based on the larger body of Chinese medicine already discussed. Specifically, very fine needles are inserted into specific points on the body to control the flow of energy in order to remove stagnation or blockages, tonifying or adding energy, reducing or eliminating excess accumulation of energy, thus restoring a balance. Most acupuncturists today use sterile stainless steel disposable needles for one-time use. It is important for the patient to ask the acupuncturist about the type of needles used and to request the disposable type to avoid any bloodborne diseases. The sensation experienced from the needle stimulation is said to be "electric," "numbing," "tingling," or "distending." Most patients say that they feel rejuvenated and relaxed after a treatment. Acupuncture has been

effective in treating arthritis, colitis, nausea, menstrual pain, sciatica, headaches, impotence, acute or chronic neck and back pain, addictions, and fatigue.

HIV/AIDS ACUPUNCTURE. There have been reports of reduction of symptoms, including night sweats, diarrhea, fatigue, nausea, pain, peripheral neuropathy, and skin reactions (Anastasi et al., 1997; MacIntyre, 1997; Sanders, 1989).

MANUAL HEALING/BODY-WORK

Chiropractic

The term *chiropractic* comes from a Greek term that means "done by hand." The vertebra is seen as the backbone of health. When the vertebrae are misaligned because of poor posture, trauma, or tension, increased pressure on the nerves can result in impaired function, discomfort, and illness. Chiropractors use their hands to adjust the patient's misalignments. In addition, they use their fingers to assess the patients by feeling for misaligned vertebrae, muscle tension, musculoskeletal disorders, and neurologic conditions. The actual treatment is aimed at correcting the misalignments through vertebral adjustments. When the misalignments are corrected, there will be improved circulation of blood, energy, and lymph, relief of muscle tension, and improved nerve impulse(s). Adjustments are also thought to be effective for averting everyday wear and tear on the ligaments and joints. The chiropractor treats each patient as an individual, and thus the treatment is tailored for the patient's specific condition. Some of the conditions for which chiropractic treatment has provided benefit are back pain, joint injuries, headaches, and menstrual disorders.

Massage Therapy

Massage therapy is one of the oldest forms of body work. Many writings have noted massage as a healing modality. These writings are from Chinese medical texts of 4000 years ago, Hippocrates' notes from the 4th century BC, Celsus's writings in the De Medicinia, *De Sanitate Tuenda* by Galen (a medieval physician), and the book *Canon of Medicine* by Avicenna (a Persian physician) (Report to the NIH on Alternative Medical Systems, 1992).

Massage therapy is the tactile manipulation of soft tissue aimed at achieving optimal health and well-being (Report to the NIH, 1992). Massage therapy consists of a group of hands-on techniques, which include application of movable or fixed pressure, resulting in movement of or to the body. Although most massage is done by hand, some therapists apply pressure with their forearms, elbows, or feet. The aim of massage is to increase health by promoting circulation, the lymphatics, and the nervous system of the body.

The massage therapist primarily uses touch in this therapy, and touch can be quite individualized. Therefore technique can vary from one therapist to another. The therapist needs to be sensitive to the patient's body and condition and will adjust the degree of pressure on the basis of his or her assessment.

There are several types of massage therapy. Swedish massage, deep-tissue massage, AMMA massage, tuina, and shiatsu (acupressure) are only a few of the forms in use. Massage therapy can provide relief from anxiety, stress, muscular tension, pain, lymphedema, insomnia, and nausea. Research in this area is broad, from the use of massage in preterm infants and weight gain (Field et al., 1986), to reduction of depression in adolescents (Field et al., 1992), relaxation in the elderly (Fakouri & Jones, 1987), to effective lymph drainage in persons who have undergone radical mastectomy (Zanolla et al., 1984). To date there have been no published reports on the use of massage therapy in patients with HIV. However, one can see the potential benefits that can be applied to this population.

Reflexology

Reflexology is a deep and firm massage of the soles of both feet at special areas that coincide with organ zones. It is thought that all bodily parts, glands, and organs are reflected in the feet; thus the firm pressure of the reflexologist's fingers will stimulate reflexes throughout the body. Palpating a certain zone on the foot could elicit a response to the coinciding reflected part of the body (Stanway, 1994). The theory on which reflexology is based was developed by Dr. William H. Fitzgerald. According to this theory, the body is partitioned into 10 longitudinal zones that surge up and down the entire body. Each zone goes from one toe all the way up the body and then down an arm to the coinciding finger. With the body partitioned into these zones, all the bones, organs, and body parts can be plotted accurately. Although no formal research on reflexology is available, there are anecdotal reports of effectiveness of this modality in reducing stress (Trousdell, 1996), releasing muscular tension, and soothing overexcited hyperactive body parts. Reflexology should be used with caution in persons with deep vein thrombosis because, as muscles relax, there is a remote possibility that a clot may be dislodged (Stormer, 1996).

Therapeutic Touch

Therapeutic touch was developed in the late 1960s by Dolores Krieger and Dora Kunz after exploring many cultures for various therapeutic modalities and known healers (Keegan, 1995). It is estimated that nearly 30,000 health professionals practice this technique. Therapeutic touch is the practice of centering intention while the practitioner moves his or her hands through a patient's energy field, usually without actual physical contact, for the purpose of assessing and treating an energy imbalance (Keegan, 1995; Steele, 1996). Five phases are involved in the therapeutic touch process: centering, assessment, unruffling or clearing, treatment, and evaluation. Centering involves an intense focusing and ability to be at complete attention. In assessment the practitioner surveys the entire body from head to feet, using his or her hands approximately 2 to 6 inches from the patient in an even and sweeping manner. During this phase the practitioner assesses the flow of energy and looks for any fluctuation in the patient's energy flow. This will provide the practitioner with clues to the patient's state of health. Unruffling or clearing promotes the even and rhythmic energy flow through the field by using long downward strokes over the patient's body (Steele, 1996). The treatment phase is aimed at reestablishing energetic order. Practitioners guide energy on and off the patient's body to direct and adjust the energy system. The final step in this process is evaluation, in which the practitioner reassesses the patient's energy field. In the optimal situation, the energy field will be even and will flow openly (Mulloney & Wells-Federman, 1996).

Therapeutic touch has been studied in numerous settings. Stress reduction, anxiety reduction, relaxation, wound healing, psychoimmunity, and pain reduction are some of the reported outcomes (Mulloney & Wells-Federman, 1996).

Qi gong

Medical qi gong is an aspect of traditional Chinese medicine and is frequently used in combination with acupuncture, moxibustion, herbs, and massage. There are two types of qi gong methods: internal qi gong and external qi gong (Sancier, 1996). Both internal and external methods use postures, body movements, and breathing techniques. Internal qi gong is self-healing in that the patient can perform it without the physical presence and supervision of the qi gong practitioner (Shih, 1994). There are several types of qi gong exercises. The gou lin form has been used to stimulate the immune system and promote self-healing in patients with cancer (Sancier, 1991). External qi gong is performed by a qi gong master/doctor who emits his or her own energy "qi" to strengthen the vitality of others who are ill. Although this seems far-fetched, there have been reports of benefits from this therapy (Sancier & Hu, 1991). Most qi gong methods emphasize quiet meditation and correction of the patient's spiritual and emotional state in addition to manipulation of the patient's body. As in tai chi and other Asian forms of exercise, the main purpose is to maintain an internal and external balance in order to develop relaxed strength, emotional balance, and health.

RESEARCH STUDIES. According to Sancier (1991), patients who practice internal qi gong exercises, integrating gentle body movement and meditation along with conventional medical therapies, have experienced an improved outcome from the treatment of coronary artery disease, hypertension, and cancer. Although there is no published research on qi gong in HIV/AIDS, qi gong is currently used as a therapeutic exercise program in San Francisco by HIV-positive instructors who attribute extended survival to the practice of qi gong (Qigong for Health, 1997).

HERBAL MEDICINE

Herbal medicine has been in existence for centuries. A large percentage of prescription medications are derivatives of natural botanicals. For ex-

ample, the extract from the foxglove plant *(Digitalis purpurea)* is the well-known drug digoxin and the extract from the opium poppy *(Papaver somniaferum)* is morphine. Many of our current medications are synthetic forms of the actual plant substance.

Although herbal therapies are used throughout the world, the United States has not always been receptive. This is partially due to the economic impact of the sale and marketing of herbs. Herbs cannot be patented, and the exclusive rights cannot be held by an individual or a company. The incentive for investing in the research on herbal remedies is not economically feasible. Thus many herbs that show promise may never be used because of this issue.

In Europe the use and sale of herbs far exceeds that in the United States. Germany leads the Western world in the sale of herbal remedies, ahead of France and the United States. The sales total about $2 billion in Germany, $1.6 billion in France, and $1.5 billion in the United States.

In 1994 the Congress passed a bill that blocked the restriction on the sale and promotion of nutritional supplements. The main provisions of the U.S. Dietary Supplement Health and Education Act 1994* are as follows:

- Herbal remedies are classed as foods, not medicines, but their promoters are allowed to make claims as long as claims can be substantiated and cannot be construed as "therapeutic claims" (that is, do not mention medical symptoms and conditions).
- Herbal remedies are exempt from regulation as food additives and therefore no longer need premarketing approval. (The FDA has been forced to withdraw a notice requiring this.)
- An independent agency, the Commission on Dietary Supplement Labels, must produce new labeling regulations by 1996 that will be binding on the FDA by 1998.
- Books and other literature mentioning or promoting dietary supplements are exempt from the regulations and can be referred to as long as the information is not misleading or a lie, presents a balanced view, and is displayed sep-

---

*An amendment to the Federal Food, Drug and Cosmetic Act, enforced by the FDA.

arately in the shop or outlet and not sold with the supplement.

- A history of use or other evidence of safety will allow a new dietary ingredient onto the market (without risking a FDA ban as an adulterant), provided there is enough supporting documentation.
- The burden of proof that a product is not safe or is adulterated lies with the FDA, and any subsequent ban is subject to immediate review by the U.S. Secretary of Health and Human Services.
- A new Office of Dietary Supplements within the National Institutes of Health must explore and promote "the benefits of dietary supplements in maintaining health and preventing chronic disease."

Anything taken from a plant (meaning the stem, leaf, root, bark, or other part) is considered an herb. Herbs may be used in the form of an ointment, oil, tea, extract, tablet, capsule, or powder. Herbs are usually used by naturopaths, homeopaths, herbologists, practitioners of Chinese medicine, and other wholistic practitioners.

As with all herbal substances, it is important to consult with a qualified herbologist before using such substances. In Chinese medicine the practitioner must make a diagnosis before prescribing herbs. The herbal prescription is fairly complex and takes years to master. It is not recommended that patients go to a health food store or to underground pharmacopeias to order an herbal prescription without seeking a highly trained practitioner. Each patient should be treated as an individual. The subtleties of symptoms can make a huge difference in the herbal prescription. What is beneficial for one patient could be harmful to another. Also, most of the time more than one herb is used in an attempt to balance the body. Certain herbs in combination can also be harmful. Most herbal substances are generally considered to be safe and easy to use. However, there are three types of contraindication in the use of these preparations: prohibited combinations, pregnancy, and dietary incompatibilities (Bensky & Gamble, 1992). Natural therapies are usually less potent as synthetic pharmaceuticals when taken alone. They can, however, produce a potentiating effect when taken in combination with pharmaceuticals (Kaiser & Donegan, 1996).

Hundreds of herbal substances are used for numerous conditions. However, the herbs and herbal formulas that have received most attention regarding their use in the treatment of HIV/AIDS are bitter melon, compound Q, curcumin, astragalus, echinacea, hypericin, milk thistle, Siberian ginseng, SPV30, and aloe vera. These substances are not used exclusively for HIV but may demonstrate some benefit. In addition, some of the popular pharmacologic and biologic treatments are alpha lipoic acid, iscador, NAC, and shark cartilage.

Bitter Melon

Bitter melon *(Momordica charantia)* belongs to the cucurbitacae plant/fruit family. It is from this fruit that compound Q (GLQ223) was derived. In vitro studies have shown this potent extract to destroy macrophages infected with HIV and to inhibit virus replication in T helper lymphocytes (MacIntyre & Holzemer, 1997). Unfortunately, very little information is available on the efficacy of the botanical. There are, however, many positive and negative anecdotal accounts of the use of bitter melon in HIV. Some of the positive accounts refer to sustained or increased CD4+ cell counts or normalization of the CD4/CD8 ratio, weight gain, and improvement in dermatitis. The negative accounts allude to diarrhea, fevers, and lack of benefit (AIDS Project LA, 1994).

Compound Q

Compound Q (trichosanthin, GLQ223) is a protein extract from the Chinese cucumber *Trichosanthes kirilowii* (Frey & Flynn, 1994). In China it has been used to induce abortion and to treat certain forms of cancer (Frey & Flynn, 1994). Recent laboratory studies demonstrated that compound Q had antiviral activity. Studies have shown that compound Q can selectively kill infected macrophages and CD4+ cells (Frey & Flynn, 1994).

Mechanism of Action. A description of the biochemical properties of compound Q was not found in the literature or anecdotally.

Studies. A study conducted in 1993 was designed to evaluate the efficacy of GLQ223 in persons with HIV/AIDS and prior zidovudine (ZDV) therapy (Frey & Flynn, 1994). This study compared GLQ223 with GLQ223 plus ZDV with ZDV alone. One hundred forty-eight subjects participated in this study. Significant differences were not found among the various arms of the study. Today the clinical efficacy of GLQ223 is still unknown.

Notes. Compound Q is administered intravenously. Common side effects include flu-like symptoms, elevated muscle and liver enzyme values, and fluid retention (Frey & Flynn, 1994). Symptoms usually subside 2 to 3 days after infusion and tend to diminish with subsequent use (Frey & Flynn, 1994). Anaphylactic reactions have also been reported to occur in 10% to 12% of recipients within the first six infusions (Frey & Flynn, 1994). Compound Q is legally available. However, because of potential life-threatening reactions, underground sources will dispense compound Q only through a physician or a skilled medical professional (Frey & Flynn, 1994).

Curcumin

Curcumin is classified as an antioxidant. It is also a component of tumeric, a major ingredient in curry powder. Curcumin is the component that gives curry its yellow color. In 1993, researchers at Harvard Medical School reported that curcumin, along with two other substances (topotecan and beta-lapachone), exhibited anti-HIV activity in laboratory studies (James, 1993). Of the three substances, topotecan was the most active agent against HIV and is an investigational treatment for progressive multifocal leukoencephalopathy (AIDS Treatment Data Network, 1996). The third substance, beta-lapachone, has been tested only on animals, but laboratory data suggest that a useful dose for human consumption is a possibility (James, 1993). Although topotecan is the most potent of the three substances, the accessibility and availability of curcumin makes it more practical as a treatment option (Majchrowicz, 1994b).

Mechanism of Action. Curcumin, topotecan, and beta-lapachone belong to a class of anti-HIV compounds called long terminal repeat (LTR) inhibitors. LTR is a sequence of HIV DNA that requires activation to initiate viral replication (Majchrowicz, 1994b). Since LTR maintains viral replication, it has been suggested that inhibiting the LTR could slow or stop viral progression (James, 1993).

Currently, many questions remain regarding the exact mechanism of the LTR. Many substances appear to affect the LTR by inhibiting or promoting the growth and activity of the virus (James, 1993). In addition, the process by which curcumin inhibits the LTR is still unknown.

Studies. Search Alliance, a community-based research organization in Los Angeles, completed a 20-week open-label pilot study using 2.6 g a day of curcumin (doses were taken three times a day). Nineteen participants were enrolled with CD4+ cell counts between 0 and 400 mm^3. Eleven completed the study. Two dropped out because of gastrointestinal complaints. Four developed opportunistic infections during the study, and three of these dropped out of the trial. The others dropped out for personal reasons (Notes from the Underground #25, 1994). The researchers looked at CD4+ cell responses and viral activity as measured by p24 antigen assay and RNA/PCR testing. Significant changes were not found in either CD4+ cells or p24 antigen assays. However, reductions in viral load were noted between weeks 4 and 12 as measured by RNA/PCR testing. At the conclusion of the study, reductions in viral activity were not as significant as in weeks 4 to 12.

It is difficult to draw any conclusions about curcumin on the basis of this study. However, HIV-positive persons of Indian descent living in Trinidad have been reported to have a slower rate of progression than persons of African descent also residing in Trinidad (James, 1993). The difference noted between the two groups is the use of curry in the diets of those of Indian descent. Questions regarding dosage, absorption, and symptoms are just a few of the many questions that need to be answered. Animal studies have shown that curcumin could not be detected in the bloodstream after ingestion. However, chemists speculate that curcumin is transformed into another compound and is detectable when radioactive curcumin is ingested (James, 1993).

Curcumin has been used extensively as a spice and is believed to be safe in moderate doses, although some researchers have reported that large doses in rats caused stomach cancer. At this time, the effects of doses considered moderate or high are not known in humans (Majchrowicz, 1994).

Astragalus

Astragalus membranaceus is an herb frequently used in traditional Chinese medicine (TCM). The Chinese call this herb *yellow leader* (Majchrowicz, 1994a). In China, astragalus is used to boost the immune system and to prevent chemotherapy-related bone marrow suppression and nausea (Greenberg, 1993/1994).

Mechanism of Action. The exact mechanism of action of astragalus is unknown. All that is known about astragalus is its potential to enhance immune responses (Majchrowicz, 1994a).

Studies. In vitro studies suggest that an extract of astragalus, fraction 3 (F3), was demonstrated to be effective in stimulating the immune response (Greenberg, 1993/1994). Reports claim that macrophage and lymphocyte activities increased with F3. At high doses, however, astragalus was shown to be immunosuppressive (Majchrowicz, 1994a). Other reports also discuss the issue of variability among herbal extracts such as F3. It is important to note that herbs from different sources may vary in quality, thus producing different results (Greenberg, 1993/1994).

Note. Side effects associated with astragalus include hypotension and polyuria (Greenberg, 1993/1994).

Echinacea

Throughout history, echinacea has been used by Native Americans as a folk remedy (Beard & Fornataro, 1994). Echinacea is commonly known as the purple cone-flower (O'Connor, 1995). Today echinacea is widely used by persons living with HIV/AIDS to fight cold and flu symptoms, decrease fatigue, and improve their overall health and vitality (O'Connor, 1995). This medicinal herb has been studied in Europe and shown to have antiviral, antibacterial, antifungal, and anticancer properties (Beard & Fornataro, 1994).

Mechanism of Action. Echinacea has been reported to have immunomodulatory properties and to contain a chemical called echinacein. It has been suggested that echinacein helps strengthen cell membranes and may prevent cells from pathogenic invasions, thereby averting infections (Beard & Fornataro, 1994). This is one possible explanation of the usefulness of echinacea in HIV disease.

Studies. According to Beard and Fornataro (1994), a study was conducted in 1986 to test the efficacy of echinacea in women with recurrent candidiasis. The study showed that women treated with echinacea experienced a 16% recurrence of yeast infections, in comparison with 60% in those treated with an antifungal agent. The efficacy against candidiasis was attributed to the properties of echinacea that enhance immune responses.

Note. Some persons living with HIV/AIDS use echinacea on a daily basis, whereas some take echinacea only in response to cold or flu symptoms (O'Connor, 1995). Caution should be applied to the daily use of echinacea, since there is a risk of overstimulation leading to further compromise of the immune system (O'Connor, 1995).

Hypericin

Hypericin is an extract from the plant St. John's wort *(Hypericum perforatum)* (Greenberg, 1993/1994). This extract is believed to have properties that can inhibit viral replication of cells infected with HIV (Greenberg, 1993/1994). In addition, in vitro studies have suggested that hypericin may have activity against the human papillomavirus (HPV), cytomegalovirus (CMV), Epstein-Barr virus (EBV), and herpes simplex-1 virus (HSV-1) (Majchrowicz, 1994c). In Europe hypericin is also used as an antidepressant, as well as for treating minor wounds and burns (Majchrowicz, 1994c).

Mechanism of Action. Laboratory studies suggest that hypericin may have activity against the viral replication of HIV at two points in the replication process (Majchrowicz, 1994c). Supposedly, hypericin can inhibit reverse transcription and prevent the assembly of new virions (Majchrowicz, 1994c). In addition, hypericin is believed to pass the blood-brain barrier; therefore it is potentially effective in controlling damage to the central nervous system by HIV (Majchrowicz, 1994c).

Studies. In 1991 clinical trials were conducted to test the efficacy of intravenous hypericin, manufactured by VIMRx Pharmaceuticals (Greenberg, 1993/1994). The study conducted at New York University, however, was stopped because of significant photosensitivity experienced by participants. Many complained of painful tingling or burning when skin was exposed to light (Synthetic Hypericin Study, 1994). The sensation stopped when the drug was discontinued. Interestingly, it has been suggested that intense light may be needed to enhance the antiviral activities of hypericin and to some extent the skin reaction may be a sign of drug activity (Synthetic Hypericin Study, 1994). Because of the varying periods of time that participants received hypericin (1 to 24 weeks), data collected from this study were inconsistent and inclusive (Majchrowicz, 1994).

Note. Oral preparations of hypericin are available in many health food stores. However, there is no evidence that this compound will have any effects against HIV (Greenberg, 1993/1994).

Milk Thistle

The seeds of milk thistle *(Silybum marianum)* are believed to have liver-protecting qualities (Greenberg, 1993/1994). It has been suggested that silymarin, the extract from milk thistle, is useful in the treatment of cirrhosis, jaundice, hepatitis, and hepatic toxicities from chemicals, such as drugs and alcohol. Silymarin has also been reported to have immunomodulatory properties (Greenberg, 1993/1994).

Mechanism of Action. A description of the biochemical properties of milk thistle could not be found in the literature or anecdotally.

Studies. No studies of the use of silymarin in persons with HIV/AIDS and liver problems were found. However, anecdotal reports from Germany have suggested that silymarin may be useful in the treatment of acute and chronic hepatitis B infections, in terms of normalization of liver function (Greenberg, 1993/1994). It is difficult to draw any conclusions about silymarin, since available reports are incomplete and need further examination.

Note. No toxic effects of silymarin have been reported. However, because of its liver-protecting qualities, some believe that silymarin may affect the absorption of other drugs (Greenberg, 1993/1994).

Siberian Ginseng

The Siberian ginseng *(Eleutherococcus senticosus)* is a member of the ginseng family. It is important to note that the Siberian ginseng belongs to a different genus than the popular varieties of Korean or Chinese ginsengs, which are members of the genus *Panax* (Kaufman, 1994). The fluid extract from the *Eleutherococcus* contains a standardized content of active glycosides, which is the only form that has yielded positive results in enhancing the immune response to viral infections (Kaufman, 1994). In addition, this plant has

been shown to reduce the side effects of radiation and chemotherapy in patients with cancer (Kaufman, 1994).

Mechanism of Action. The exact mechanism of action of the Siberian ginseng is unknown. This herb is sometimes referred to as an adaptogen, because it is believed to have properties that are capable of balancing the body regardless of disease (Kaufman, 1994). It has been suggested that the active ingredients of the Siberian ginseng are concentrated in the adrenal glands, thereby enhancing the glands' function during times of stress (Kaufman, 1994). The benefits of this herb for persons living with HIV/AIDS are based on its reputed potency in restoring energy and combating fatigue (O'Connor, 1995), a symptom commonly experienced in HIV disease.

Studies. German studies suggest that the Siberian ginseng probably reduces the illness from viral infections by enhancing the immune response rather than by stimulating it (Kaufman, 1994). Researchers suggest that lymphocytic activity is increased by the Siberian ginseng (Kaufman, 1994). Nicholas Weger, a German researcher, developed a compound called PCM-4, composed of Siberian ginseng and porcine spleen (Greenberg, 1993/1994). Porcine spleen is also believed to have immunomodulating properties. The combination of the two compounds has been purported to have immunomodulatory activity and the potential to increase CD4+ counts. Currently, no studies have been found to support such claims.

Note. Side effects associated with Siberian ginseng include insomnia, diarrhea, nervousness, depression, and skin rash. No data were found regarding side effects in relation to dosage consumed.

SPV-30

SPV-30, an extract from the boxwood evergreen, is manufactured by a pharmaceutical company in France. In vitro studies have suggested that SPV-30 has natural antiviral activity. In addition, it appears to be safe and efficacious in the treatment of HIV disease, even for those with advanced immunosuppression (Pharo et al., 1996).

Mechanism of Action. The exact mechanism of SPV-30 could not be found in the literature or anecdotally. However, in vitro studies have reported that the boxwood evergreen had many alkaloids that demonstrated strong antiviral activity (SPV-30 Background, 1997). Currently, many questions still remain as to where and how SPV-30 affects viral activity.

Studies. Two studies of SPV-30 and HIV were completed and presented as abstracts at the Eleventh International Conference on AIDS in Vancouver. The first study was completed by a group of French researchers to evaluate the safety and efficacy of the boxwood evergreen in HIV disease. After 6 months of treatment, 63% of the patients experienced a decrease in viral load by RNA/PCR measurements (Pharo et al., 1996). The second was an informal study conducted to examine the effects of SPV-30 when added to a stable treatment regimen (SPV-30 Background, 1997). In this study also, 63% of the participants experienced a decrease in viral load after 6 months. The researchers observed that participants with baseline viral loads greater than 40,000 copies experienced better results overall (SPV-30 Background, 1997). It is important to note that these studies were conducted before the approval of protease inhibitors; therefore results do not reflect their use. According to researchers, most of the participants experienced improvement in appetite, skin conditions, energy, concentration, memory, and the frequency of diarrhea (Pharo et al., 1996).

Notes. Transient side effects noted with SPV-30 include diarrhea and abdominal cramping (Pharo et al., 1996). Significant toxic effects have not been noted with the use of SPV-30. Currently, limited quantities of SPV-30 remain available for purchase. The FDA has recently labeled SPV-30 as a drug instead of a natural herbal preparation. The FDA is currently requiring the manufacturer of SPV-30 to seek a new drug application (NDA) prior to further marketing and distribution (SPV-30 Background, 1997). NDAs are required for all investigational drugs.

Aloe Vera

Aloe extracts have been used for centuries. Most people are familiar with the use of aloe vera for burns, as a moisturizer for skin, or in hair conditioners. There are several hundred species of *Aloe*. Acemannan, the extract from the aloe plant, is currently being studied as a potential remedy in HIV/AIDS, ulcerative colitis, and cancer. In vitro investigation reports have described aloe vera as having many positive properties, such as antibacterial, antiviral, anti-inflammatory, and antifungal. Further studies submit that acemannan may have anti-HIV features in addition to boosting the immune function (Kahlon et al., 1991; Kahlon et al., 1991; Kemp et al., 1990; McDaniel et al., 1990).

PHARMACOLOGIC AND BIOLOGIC TREATMENTS

Alpha Lipoic Acid

Alpha lipoic acid (thioctic acid) is an antioxidant that can indirectly spare, recycle, or regenerate other antioxidants, thus raising levels in the bloodstream (Lands, 1997). Antioxidants are compounds that prevent cellular damage. Some researchers are currently examining the role of antioxidants in the pathogenesis of HIV disease (Lemens & Sterrit, 1993/1994). In addition, alpha lipoic acid has an important role in the metabolic pathway of liver cells and can be rapidly depleted when the liver is under stress, as in multidrug therapy (Lands, 1997).

Mechanism of Action. As an antioxidant, alpha lipoic acid has a natural affinity for free radicals. Free radicals are oxygen-containing molecules that are normally produced in cellular processes, in respiration, and in the destruction of bacterially and virally infected cells by phagocytes (Lemens & Sterrit, 1993/1994). In general, antioxidants exist in abundance and bond with free radicals before damage to cell membranes, proteins, and nucleic acids can occur (Lemens & Sterrit, 1993/1994). It has been suggested that an imbalance between antioxidants and free radicals increases viral replication. However, scientific studies have not shown that antioxidants can delay or halt the progression of disease (Lemens & Sterrit, 1993/1994).

Studies. In Europe, alpha lipoic acid has long been used in the treatment of hepatic disorders. It is believed to have reparative and protective qualities for the liver (Lands, 1997). Anecdotally, alpha lipoic acid in combination with silymarin, has successfully reduced chronically elevated liver enzyme levels. Reductions were enough to allow enrollment in multidrug clinical trials, whereas elevated liver enzyme levels would have otherwise excluded them (Lands, 1997).

In addition, in vitro studies have shown alpha lipoic acid to have potential as an antiretroviral agent. It has been shown to inhibit viral replication in both acutely and chronically infected cells (Lands, 1997). Synergistic effects have also been demonstrated when alpha lipoic acid and AZT were combined in in vitro studies (Lands, 1997).

Note. Alpha lipoic acid is often taken in doses of 100 to 200 mg, three times a day with meals. No toxic effects have been reported; however, thrombocytopenia is a possibility with high doses (Lands, 1997).

Iscador

Iscador is an extract of the European mistletoe *(Viscum album)*. It is manufactured by a Swiss company under the trade name iscador (Smith, 1989). For more than 60 years, this extract has been used in Europe to treat certain tumor-forming cancers (Smith, 1989). Currently, iscador is believed to have immunomodulatory and antiviral activity against HIV (Smith, 1989).

Mechanism of Action. Viscum album is a semiparasitic organism, in which a host tree is required for growth and survival (Smith, 1989). Host trees are often apple, oak, elm, or pine. Interestingly, the chemical properties of the mistletoe may vary according to the host tree (Smith, 1989), but discussions regarding chemical variability among hosts were not found in the literature. Iscador has been observed to block in vitro syncytia formation, which in theory could prevent viral passage from cell to cell, thus limiting cells infected (Smith, 1989).

Studies. One study presented as an abstract at the Eleventh International Conference on AIDS, examined the use of iscador in 40 participants with CD4+ cell counts of less than 200/mm^3 (Greenberg, 1993/1994). Participants injected themselves with 0.01 mg to 10 mg of iscador twice a week for 18 weeks. Researchers reported that 77% had increased CD4+ cell counts greater than 20% of baseline values (Greenberg, 1993/1994). Anecdotally, the benefits of iscador in persons with HIV/AIDS are an increase in CD4+ cells, natural killer cells, and weight and a regression of KS lesions (Greenberg, 1993/1994). It has been suggested that the regression of KS lesions is indirectly related to the enhancement of the immune response (Smith, 1989).

Notes. Toxicity appears to be related to dose (Greenberg, 1993/1994), and persons with opportunistic infections or low CD4+ cell counts seem to have a lower dose tolerance (Smith, 1989). Iscador may be useless or even detrimental in such persons.

Iscador is administered subcutaneously, but many patients experience redness and tenderness at the site of injection. Some reactions to high dosages are fever, insomnia, fatigue, and loss of appetite (Smith, 1989). Discontinuing injections resolves the reactions (Smith, 1989).

NAC (*N*-Acetylcysteine)

In Europe, NAC (*N*-acetylcysteine) is commonly prescribed for chronic bronchitis and acetaminophen overdose (Lemens & Sterrit, 1993/1994). In 1988 a German immunologist realized that NAC could raise the level of a chemical called glutathione, which is abnormally low in people with AIDS. The researcher also observed that low levels of glutathione strongly predicted a poor survival (James, 1989). However, NAC did not receive public attention until October 1989, when a group of scientists from Stanford University reported that it may be useful in the treatment of HIV disease (James, 1989).

Mechanism of Action. NAC is a derivative of the amino acid cysteine, which is found in the proteins of most diets (James, 1997). In the liver, NAC is converted into cysteine and is used for the production of glutathione. Glutathione is an antioxidant that is critical for energy metabolism and cell division and is the primary defender against oxidative stress (James, 1997). In addition, it has been suggested that low levels of glutathione may accelerate HIV replication (James, 1997).

Studies. Several years ago a small National Institutes of Health study reported that orally ingested NAC was not found in the bloodstream and was therefore ineffective (James, 1996). However, a new study conducted at Stanford University reported that oral NAC can raise blood levels of glutathione. The researchers found that persons with CD4+ cell counts under 200/mm^3 and low glutathione levels had an estimated 3-year survival as low as 20% in comparison with 60% to 80% in those with CD4+ cell counts below 200/mm^3 and adequate glutathione levels (James, 1997).

The results of the Stanford study can best be

described as follows: (1) glutathione level is a useful predictor of survival, without reference to NAC or other treatments; (2) a trial shows the bioavailability of NAC; and (3) observations suggest that there may be a survival benefit from taking NAC (James, 1997).

Note. Currently, a consensus has not been reached regarding appropriate dosing. The Stanford study used high doses of NAC (3200 mg to 8000 mg per day, in divided doses), whereas others reportedly use 1000 mg to 2000 mg per day in divided doses. Adverse effects have not been reported with either the National Institutes of Health or Stanford studies.

Shark Cartilage

The skeletons of sharks are composed entirely of cartilage instead of bones (Majchrowicz, 1994). Sharks are reported to have lower rates of cancer than mammals (Majchrowicz, 1994d). Thus researchers have explored the possibility of using shark cartilage for the treatment of cancer, particularly Kaposi's sarcoma (KS) in persons with HIV/AIDS.

Mechanism of Action. Shark cartilage is rich in a protein that is able to inhibit angiogenesis (Greenberg, 1993/1994). The term *angiogenesis* means growth of new blood vessels. Without angiogenesis, tumor-forming cancers could not grow or nourish themselves (James, 1991). In KS, lesions are caused by an abnormal growth of blood vessels. In theory, if an agent could stop angiogenesis, the further growth of existing tumors could be stopped, as in KS. At present, available information about shark cartilage is mostly anecdotal (Majchrowicz, 1994d).

Studies. Search Alliance, a Los Angeles–based community research organization, completed the first and only human study of the use of shark cartilage as monotherapy for KS. Anecdotal reports were disappointing (Greenberg, 1993/1994). Thirteen persons with KS were enrolled, but only six completed the study. Drop-outs were mostly related to the foul taste and nausea associated with therapy. After 2 to 3 months of therapy, regression of KS lesions was not noted (Greenberg, 1993/1994).

Note. According to a manufacturer of shark cartilage preparations, toxic effects have never been reported. However, appropriate dosing is unknown (Majchrowicz, 1994d).

ACKNOWLEDGEMENT: Special thanks to Bernadette Capili, MS, NP, for her assistance in the preparation of this chapter.

REFERENCES

AIDS Treatment Data Network. (1996). *Trials for the treatment of PML* [On-line]. Available: http://www.atdn.org.

Anastasi, J., Dawes, N., Li, Y. (1997). Diarrhea and human immunodeficiency virus: A possible synergy for clinical practice. *The Journal of Alternative and Complementary Medicine, 3*(2), 163–168.

Anderson, W., O'Connor, B., MacGregor, R., Schwartz, J. (1993). Patient use and assessment of conventional medicine and alternative therapies for HIV infection and AIDS. *AIDS, 7,* 561–566.

Anselmo, P., Brooks, J. (1996). *Ayurvedic secrets to longevity and total health.* Upper Saddle River, NJ: Prentice Hall.

Beard, J., Fornataro, K. (1994, June). Echinacea. *Treatment Review, 12,* 5.

Bensky, D., Gamble, A. (1992). *Chinese herbal medicine: Materia medica.* Seattle, WA: Eastland Press.

Burton Goldberg Group (1995). *Alternative medicine: The definitive guide.* Washington, DC: Future Medicine Publishing Inc.

Complementary Alternative Medicine at the NIH. (1997). *Office of Alternative Medicine Clearinghouse/ NIH, 4*(2), 2–8.

Davenas, E., Beauvais, F., Amara, J. (1988). Human basophil degranulation triggered by very dilute antiserum against IgE. *Nature, 333,* 816–818.

Delinick, A. (1991). A hypothesis on how homeopathic remedies work on the organism. *Berlin Journal on Research in Homeopathy, 1,* 249–253.

Eisenberg, D., Kessler, R., Foster, C. Norlock, F., Calkins, D., Delbanco, T.L. (1993). Unconventional medicine in the United States: Prevalence, costs, and patterns of use. *New England Journal of Medicine, 328,* 246–252.

Fakouri, C., Jones, P. (1987). Relaxation Rx: Slow stroke back rub. *Journal of Gerontological Nursing, 13,* 32–35.

Field, T., Morrow, C., Valdeon, C., Larson, S., Kuhn, C., Schanberg, S. (1992). Massage reduces anxiety in child and adolescent psychiatric patients. *Journal of the American Academy of Child Adolescent Psychiatry, 31*(1), 125–131.

Field, T., Schanberg, S., Scafidi, F. (1986). Tactile/kinesthetic stimulation effects on preterm neonates. *Pediatrics, 77,* 654–658.

Frey, M., Flynn, R. (1994, June). New news on Q. *Project Inform Perspective* [On-line]. Available: http://www.projinf.org/pub/pip index.html.

Gold, J., Anastasi, J. (1995). Educational opportunities

in alternative/complementary medicine for nurses. *The Journal of Alternative and Complementary Medicine, 1*(4), 399–401.

Gordon, J. (1996). Alternative medicine and the family physician. *American Family Physician, 54*(7), 2205–2212.

Greenberg, J. (1994). An alternative treatment activist manifesto. *Treatment Issue, 7*(11/12), 7–27.

Greenblatt, R., Hollander, M., McMaster, J.R., Henke, C. (1991). Polypharmacy among patients attending an AIDS clinic: Utilization of prescribed, unorthodox, and investigational treatments. *Journal of AIDS, 4,* 136–143.

Hand, R. (1989). Alternative therapies used by patients with AIDS. *New England Journal of Medicine, 320,* 672–673.

HIV curry—curcumin shows antiviral activity in PWAs. (1994, March/April). *Notes From the Underground* [On-line], 25, 4–5. Available: http://www.aidsnyc.org/pwahg/notes.html.

James, J.S. (December 1, 1989). NAC: New information. *AIDS Treatment News* [On-line], 92, 1–4. Available: http://www.critpath.org/newsletter/atn/atn.html.

James, J.S. (July 5, 1996). NAC: First controlled trial, positive results. *AIDS Treatment News* [On-line], 250, 1–3. Available: http://www.critpath.org/newsletters/atn/atn.html.

James, J.S. (March 7, 1997). Stanford NAC study: Glutathione level predicts survival. *AIDS Treatment News* [On-line], 266, 1–6. Available: http://www.critpath.org/newsletters/atn/atn.html.

James, J.S. (May 7, 1993). New kind of HIV antiviral: Food spice, cancer drug show activity. *AIDS Treatment News* [On-line], 174, 1–4. Available: http://www.critpath.org/newsletters/atn/atn.html.

James, J.S. (September 20, 1991). Angiogenesis inhibitors—New approach to cancer, KS treatments. *AIDS Treatment News* [On-line], 135, 1–7. Available: http://www.critpath.org/newsletters/atn/atn.html.

Kahlon, J., Kemp, M., Carpenter, R., McAnalley, B., McDaniel, H., Shannon, W. (1991). Inhibition of AIDS virus replication in vitro. *Molecular Biotherapy, 3*(3), 127–135.

Kahlon, J., Kemp, M., Yawei, N., Carpenter, R., Shannon, W., McAnalley, B. (1991). In vitro evaluation of synergistic antiviral effects of acemman in combination with azidothymidine and acyclovir. *Molecular Biotherapy, 3*(4), 214–223.

Kaiser, J., Donegan, E. (1996). Complementary therapies in HIV disease. *Alternative Therapies, 2*(4), 42–46.

Kaufman, K. (1994, Spring). Siberian ginseng. *Treatment Education Program.* Los Angeles: AIDS Project Los Angeles.

Keegan, L. (1995). Touch: Connecting with the healing power. In B. Dossey, L. Keegan, C. Guzzetta, L. Kolkmeier (Eds.), *Holistic nursing practice: A handbook for practice* (2nd ed., pp. 539–567). Gaithersberg, MD: Aspen Publishers.

Kemp, M., Kahlon, J., Carpenter, R. (1990). *Concentration-dependent inhibition of AIDS virus replication and pathogenesis by acemannan in vitro* (abstract no. 1007). Presented at VI International Conference on AIDS, San Francisco, California.

Lands, L. (April 4, 1997). NAC, glutamine and alpha lipoic acid. *AIDS Treatment News, 268,* 1–7.

Lemens, C., Sterrit, C. (1993/1994, Winter). Antioxidants, oxidative stress and nac. *Gay Men's Health Crisis: Treatment Issues, 7,* 56–62.

MacIntyre, R., Holzemer, W. (1997). Complementary and alternative medicine and HIV/AIDS. Part II. Selected literature review. *Journal of the Association of Nurses in AIDS Care, 8*(2), 25–38.

Majchrowicz, M.A. (1994a, Spring). Astragalus. *Treatment Education Program.* Los Angeles: AIDS Project Los Angeles.

Majchrowicz, M.A. (1994b, Spring). Curcumin. *Treatment Education Program.* Los Angeles: AIDS Project Los Angeles.

Majchrowicz, M.A. (1994c, Spring). Hypericin. *Treatment Education Program.* Los Angeles: AIDS Project Los Angeles.

Majchrowicz, M.A. (1994d, Spring). Shark cartilage. *Treatment Education Program.* Los Angeles: AIDS Project Los Angeles.

McDaniel, H., Carpenter, R., Kemp, M. (1990). *HIV-1 infected patients respond favorably to oral acemannan* (abstract no. 493). Presented at VI International Conference on AIDS, San Francisco, California.

Moran, J. (1995). Making alternative therapies everyone's issue. *Alternative Therapies, 1*(4), 79.

Mulloney, S., Wells-Federman, C. (1996). Therapeutic touch: A healing modality. *Journal of Cardiovascular Nursing, 10*(3), 27–49.

Murphy, M. (1992). Scientific studies of contemplative experience. In *The future of the body: Exploration into the future evolution of human nature* (pp. 603–611). Los Angeles: J.P. Tarcher.

O'Connor, B.B. (1995). Vernacular health care responses to HIV and AIDS. *Alternative Therapies, 1,* 35–52.

Pharo, A., Salvato, P., Thompson, C., Stokes, D., Mastman, B., Keister, R. (1996). *Evaluation of the safety and efficacy of SPV-30 (boxwood extract) in patients with HIV disease* (abstract Mo.B.180). Presented at XI International Conference on AIDS, Vancouver, British Columbia.

Qigong for Health (1997, July). Up front: POZ Picks. *POZ,* 59.

Rankin-Box, D. (1995). *The nurses' handbook of complementary therapies.* London: Churchill Livingstone.

Report to the National Institutes of Health on Alternative Medical Systems. (1992). *Alternative medicine: Expanding medical horizons.* Washington, DC: U.S. Government Printing Office.

Rothouse, H. (1997). History of homeopathy reveals discipline's excellence. *Alternative and Complementary Therapies, 3*(3), 223–227.

Sancier, K. (1996). Medical applications of qi gong. *Alternative Therapies, 2*(1), 40–45.

Sancier, K. (1991). *Reports from the Qi Gong Institute.* Menlo Park, CA: East West Academy of Healing Arts.

Sancier, K., Hu, B. (1991). Medical applications of qi gong and emitted qi on humans, animals, cell cultures, and plants: Review of selected scientific research. *American Journal of Acupuncture, 19,* 367–377.

Sanders, P. (1989). Acupuncture and herbal treatment of HIV infection. *Holistic Nursing Practitioner, 3*(4), 38–44.

Schwartz, M., Fehmi, L. (1982). *Applications, standards and guidelines for providers of biofeedback services.* Denver, CO: Biofeedback Society of America.

Shih, T.K. (1994). *Qi gong therapy: The Chinese art of healing with energy.* Barrytown, NY: Station Hill Press.

Sharma, H., Dwivedi, B., Satter, H., Gudehitihlu, W., Malarkey, W., Tejwani, G. (1990). Antineoplastic properties of Maharishi 4, against DMBA-induced mammary tumors in rats. *Journal of Pharmacology, Biochemistry, and Behavior, 35,* 767–773.

Smith, D. (December 1, 1989). Iscador: Promising experience to date. *AIDS Treatment News,* Issue 92. www.critpath.org/newsletters/atn/atn.html.

SPV-30 background. (March 15, 1997). *DAAIR* [Online]. Available: http://www.gmhc.org/aidslib/ti/ti.html.

Stanway, A. (1994). *Complementary medicine: A guide to natural therapies.* New York: Penguin Books.

Steele, A. (1996). A touching experience. *International Journal of Alternative and Complementary Medicine, 14*(12), 11–12.

Stormer, C. (1996). *Reflexology.* Chicago: NTC Publishing Group.

Sutherland, L., Verhoef, M. (1995). Alternative medicine consultations by patients attending a multidiscipinary HIV clinic. *AIDS Patient Care, 6,* 106–110.

Synthetic hypericin study. (1994, March/April). *Notes from the Underground* [On-line], *25,* 4. Available: http://www.aidsnyc.org/pwahg/notes.html.

Thomas, R. (1995, July). FDA 'tiger' puts herbals under threat (politics). *International Journal of Alternative and Complementary Medicine,* p. 14.

Thyagarajan, S., Subramanian, S., Thirunalasundari, T., Venkateswaran, P., Blumberg, B. (1988). Effect of phyllanthus amarus on chronic carriers of hepatitis B virus. *Lancet, 2*(8614), 764–766.

Trousdell, P. (1996). Reflexology meets emotional needs. *International Journal of Alternative and Complementary Medicine, 14*(12), 9.

Van Dam, F., De Boer, C. (1996). *The use of remedies and alternative therapies by patients with symptomatic HIV infection* (abstract no. Mo.B.154). Presented at XI International AIDS Conference, Vancouver, British Columbia.

Vickers, A. (1994). An introduction to medical research. Part II: Special problems of clinical research in complementary medicine. *Journal of Alternative and Complementary Medicine, 12,* 10–13.

Wanning, T. (1993). Healing and the mind/body arts. *AAOHN, 41*(7), 349–351.

Weeks, J. (1997). The emerging role of alternative medicine in managed care. *Drug Benefit Trends, 9*(4), 14–28.

Weil, A. (1995). *Natural health, natural medicine.* New York: Houghton Mifflin.

Weiner, M. (1996). *The complete book of homeopathy.* New York: Avery Publishing Group.

Zanolla, R., Monzeglio, C., Balzarini, A., Martino, G. (1984). Evaluation of the results of three different methods of post-mastectomy lymphedema treatment. *Journal of Surgical Oncology, 26,* 210–213.

12

Legal Issues

RONNIE E. LEIBOWITZ ■ STEVEN L. KESSLER ■ WILLIAM D. FRUMKIN

HIV infection is a unique illness that requires a multidisciplinary approach to care since almost every issue involves medical, public health, ethical, moral, and legal considerations. Legal issues and concerns continue to evolve on an ongoing basis. With the introduction of highly active antiretroviral therapy (HAART) in 1996, many persons with HIV disease are living longer and are able to continue to work or to return to work. Consequently, legal concerns have expanded to include maintenance of medical coverage, workers' benefits, medical leave, and access to Medicaid assistance. The outcomes of legal matters vary from state to state and within local jurisdictions; some jurisdictions may take a conservative approach, whereas others may be more liberal. Although it is beyond the scope of this chapter to discuss all the possibilities of the HIV-related legal issues, some of the more common federal provisions are presented with references to some state differences. Health care providers should be aware of local laws and regulations within their own jurisdiction.

ACCESS TO CARE

Although many of the dilemmas faced by persons living with HIV disease (PLWHIV) are common to numerous other persons in society, they are often exacerbated by the physical and mental states that are the consequences of the HIV illness trajectory. The problems include everything from securing and retaining affordable housing to obtaining home health care services and estate planning.

The Health Insurance Portability and Accountability Act of 1996 (HIPAA), commonly known as the Kennedy-Kassenbaum Health Reform Act (H.R. 3103), attempted to address some of the obstacles that may impede a person's access to health care coverage by establishing access, availability, portability, and renewability standards for group health insurers. It intended to restrict the ability of group plans and health insurance issuers to limit coverage through preexisting-condition exclusions.

The portability provisions of HIPAA provide for crediting a person's prior health care coverage against any permissible preexisting-condition limitations in a new plan or contract. In the individual market, they guarantee the issuance of coverage without preexisting-condition limitations for persons who have had prior group coverage. HIPAA requires group health plans and health insurance issuers in the group and individual markets to provide "certification of creditable coverage" at specified times to enable persons who have lost health care coverage to document their prior coverage for a new plan or issuer. The renewability provisions of HIPAA attempted to prevent a plan or an issuer in the group and individual markets from refusing to continue or renew coverage because of health statute–related factors. An investigation by the General Accounting Office, however, found that the HIPAA was not working successfully since people who exercised their rights under the law were being charged premiums higher than the standard rate and some companies discouraged insurance agents from selling policies to people with preexisting medical problems (Pear, 1998).

A little-publicized provision of the HIPAA makes it a federal crime to knowingly and willfully dispose of assets (including any transfer in trust) in order to become eligible for Medicaid assistance. It is unclear whether the crime will be classified as a felony or a misdemeanor. A misdemeanor will be punishable by a fine of up to $10,000, imprisonment of up to 1 year, or both; punishment for a felony violation will be a fine of up to $25,000, imprisonment of up to 5 years, or both.

Until 1997, it was legal to apply for Medicaid benefits by transferring assets and only a temporary period of ineligibility could be imposed on a person transferring such assets and applying for Medicaid-covered nursing home care. Under the new law, applicants penalized because they did not wait until the end of the penalty period before applying for Medicaid-covered nursing home care would be criminally liable and subject to fine, imprisonment, or both. Although the asset transfer by itself is not a criminal act, applying for Medicaid assistance too soon after the transfer can lead to a fine, imprisonment, or both.

The consensus among attorneys is that the new law would not apply to

1. Transfers made before January 1, 1997, since criminal statutes are not retroactive
2. Transfers made for purposes other than to obtain Medicaid eligibility, such as gifts to grandchildren for their education or medical expenses
3. Exempt transfers, such as spousal transfers

It is also the consensus that the statute should not apply to home care, since there are no transfer penalties under the home care program, but that it will apply only to Medicaid-covered nursing home care.

Although unclear, the law may criminalize the acts of persons who act on behalf of those who make transfers and then apply for Medicaid assistance, such as guardians, trustees, co-owners of joint assets, and attorneys acting under a power of attorney. Attorneys counseling individuals and their families may also fall within the scope of this provision. Because of the numerous questions raised by the HIPAA, persons living with HIV infection (PLWHIV) should consult an attorney before transferring assets or applying for Medicaid. State bar associations, together with other advocacy groups and not-for-profit organizations, are currently working for the repeal of or an amendment to this new law.

Providing access to affordable and adequate home health care services may enable the PLWHIV to remain in their homes or in the home of a family member or life partner and will provide a less expensive alternative to hospitalization. Subchapter XXIV-Part B of Title XXVI of the Public Health Services Act (PHSA) provides that states that meet the statutory requirements are eligible for direct grants from the Secretary of Health and Human Services to assist in improving the quality, availability, and organization of health care and support services for individuals and families with HIV disease or AIDS. States may use the grant money to provide home- and community-based care services for PLWHIV. This is defined by the statute as furnishing health services in the home of a person with HIV disease based on a written plan of care determined by a case management team, which must include appropriate health care professionals. These services include providing durable medical equipment, homemaker or home health aid services and personal care services, day treatment or other partial hospitalization services, home intravenous and aerosolized drug therapy, routine diagnostic testing, and appropriate mental health, development, and rehabilitation services.

Amendments added to the Ryan White Comprehensive AIDS Resources Emergency (CARE) Act in 1996 provide that the Secretary of Health and Human Services shall not make grants, under part B of Title XXVI of the PHSA, to states that do not take administrative or legislative action to require that a good-faith effort be made to notify a spouse of a known HIV-infected patient that he or she may have been exposed to HIV and should seek testing. A spouse is defined as any person who is the marriage partner of an HIV-infected person, or who has been the marriage partner of that individual at any time within the 10-year period preceding the diagnosis of HIV infection.

WILLS, TRUSTS, AND ESTATE PLANNING

Estate-planning problems of a PLWHIV are similar to estate-planning problems of any other person, with some differences. The single person whose possessions are not shared with his or her birth family but with a long-term companion (e.g., life partner or lover) or a community of friends needs to assure that his or her property avoids the presumptions of the law of descent and distribution. The PLWHIV whose health status has improved as a result of HAART now faces greater uncertainties about whether his or her savings and benefits will last through his or her life. A person with parental custody may not have favored family members who are willing or able to care for surviving children. Many PLWHIV, acting under an assumption of early demise, may have followed advice that promised to avoid income taxes on payments made to them from viatical settlements or other distributions.

PLWHIV should also be advised to pay particular attention to certain other matters. Some persons may be so estranged from their birth families that they wish to avoid having family members exercise any control over funeral arrangements and disposition of their bodies. Because many PLWHIV are relatively young and without children, they may have a strong desire to leave something here so that they can be remembered. Although there are certain estate-planning concerns that relate to the disease itself (e.g., AIDS-related dementia, a shortened life expectancy of one's life partner and other beneficiaries, an increasing number of minors being orphaned), it remains that most AIDS-related estate problems are related to gay and lesbian concerns. Therefore, to better assist all PLWHIV, regardless of their sexual orientation or marital status, consideration should be given to provisions of state and federal laws that relate to such matters as intestacy, will contests, will executions, testamentary substitutes, incompetency, Medicaid planning, living wills, health care proxies, and powers of attorney.

Intestacy

If a person dies without a will (intestacy) and owns assets individually, those assets will pass to his or her distributees according to the intestacy laws of that person's domicile. The law may or may not be reflective of that person's estate-planning goals.

In New York State, for example, an intestate person's estate is shared by a spouse and descendants or goes to a spouse alone if there are no descendants. In the absence of a spouse or descendants, the entire estate is given to his or her parents, if surviving or, if not, to his or her brothers and sisters or more remote relatives (New York Estates, Powers and Trusts Law [EPTL], 1997).

As in many states, New York law does not recognize a gay or lesbian lover as a distributee, regardless of the length or seriousness of the relationship, and this law has withstood constitutional challenge (*Matter of Cooper,* 1993; *Matter of Petri,* 1994). New York's high court, the Court of Appeals, has refused to sanction inclusion of homosexual partners in the intestacy distribution scheme by means of adoption (*Adoption of Elizabeth S.,* 1986; *Matter of Robert P.,* 1984). It also has been observed that, in the absence of legislation, marriage is not an option at this time either (*Matter of Jacob,* 1995; *Storrs v. Holcomb,* 1984). For federal purposes, the recently passed Defense of Marriage Act restricts the concept of marriage to heterosexual legal unions as husband and wife and further authorizes states to disregard same-sex marriages that were solemnized in other states.

Against this backdrop, a person who wishes to benefit a nonrelated person must take affirmative steps to achieve his or her estate-planning goals. These steps include executing a will or establishing nontestamentary arrangements (referred to as testamentary substitutes) such as pay-on-death accounts, trust accounts, joint bank or securities accounts, custodial accounts, pension plans, lifetime trusts, and designation of life insurance beneficiaries.

Estate planning for a PLWHIV may be complicated by the fact that the designated recipient of the PLWHIV's possessions may also be HIV-positive and therefore have a shortened life expectancy and considerable medical needs. Although the PLWHIV may want his or her life partner to have the use of his or her possessions and assets during the life partner's lifetime, he or she may want to ensure that the assets will not be dissipated by the life partner's medical expenses. To achieve the dual goal of protecting assets and at the same time, making them available for the life partner's use, the PLWHIV may wish to place the assets into a discretionary testamentary trust, which would limit the trustee's access to the funds should the beneficiary become eligible for governmental benefits. The trust vehicle would ensure that the property will end up with those chosen by the PLWHIV, rather than the relatives or friends of his or her life partner. This is of particular concern in those situations in which the life partner may not live much longer than the PLWHIV.

A will is also the common vehicle for a parent to designate someone to serve as the legal guardian of the person and property of his or her minor children. A PLWHIV who is the single parent of a minor child or children may have a difficult time naming a testamentary guardian for his or her children. If the PLWHIV has been alienated from family members and from the other biologic parent, there may not be anyone he or she can nominate. This may be especially true if one or more of the children is HIV-positive. In many states there is an unmet need for adequate foster care and adoption programs for uninfected children of a person with HIV disease or for surviving children who are HIV-positive.

A will also may contain an "in terrorem" clause coupled with a modest gift to any distributee who might be likely to contest the will. Such a clause provides that a beneficiary will lose any interest he or she has under a will if he or she contests the probate of that will. Such clauses obviously have a chilling effect on will contests but still may be questioned.

Testamentary Substitutes

Although a well-drafted will is recommended as part of any estate plan, the role of testamentary substitutes (properties legally designated outside a written will) should not be overlooked. These include, but are not limited to, joint tenancies and beneficiaries designated in pay-on-death accounts, pension and profit-sharing arrangements, lifetime trusts, and life insurance.

A major advantage of these types of (nontestamentary) assets is that they pass outside the will and are not subject to probate (see Intestacy). Thus the designated beneficiary may receive the property on the death of the testator without any statutory obligation to serve process on the testator's distributees. This reduces, although it does not eliminate, the risk that the transfer will be challenged.

Medicaid Planning

Because of the high costs of medical care, a PLWHIV may soon exhaust his or her own funds and have to apply for public assistance (Medicaid) to cover medical expenses. Medicaid is funded in part by the federal government, but recent legislation has reduced the federal funding available and will allow the states greater scope of experi-

mentation in delivery systems. At present, the system is in transition. PLWHIV and health care providers must advocate for formulation of adequate Medicaid managed care plans within their states, including (1) access to HIV-experienced providers and specialists, (2) increased availability of prescribed drugs through the plan, and (3) adequate coverage of pharmaceuticals ("AIDS Advocates," 1996). This is essential as more states shift Medicaid programs to managed care.

Managed care should, in fact, improve health care for the PLWHIV. In 1995, the first Medicaid managed care program for persons with HIV/AIDS opened in Los Angeles. In 1996, it became easier for persons with AIDS and other chronic diseases in New York State to join HMOs and to see specialists without referrals from their primary health care provider. The downside of this increased access to care is that it requires higher premiums and copayments ("AIDS Advocates," 1996).

Before a PLWHIV applies for Medicaid for institutional care, he or she must review any transfers of assets that were made during a 36-month (or 60-month in the case of certain payments to or from a trust) look-back period before the date of application. If any assets were transferred gratuitously during the look-back period, then the PLWHIV may be deemed ineligible for Medicaid for a number of months determined by dividing the amount transferred by the average cost per month of institutional care in the geographic area where the applicant resides (Social Security Law, 1982). The statute permits the transfer of the applicant's primary residence to a spouse, an adult caretaker child who has resided in the home for 2 years, a sibling who has an equity interest in the home and who has resided in the home for 1 year, or a minor or disabled child. The statute also permits the transfer of assets in addition to a home to a spouse, provided the spouse does not retransfer the resources to anyone other than the institutionalized person or a blind or disabled child.

The statute, however, does not accommodate the transfer to a life partner when the PLWHIV is in a long-term gay relationship or the continued use of the home by the life partner after the sole-owning PLWHIV is permanently institutionalized. Life partners have had to rely on a humanitarian enforcement of the act.

Legislation in 1996 (see HIPAA under Access to Care) may have put a cloud on Medicaid planning that involves transfers of assets for less than fair market value. The law arguably makes such transfers criminal. The criminal sanctions are so vaguely drafted that some argue that they may apply both to the person who makes the transfer and to the lawyers who advise on the transfer. Reports on the poorly drafted law have sent panic waves through the elderly, some wondering if they are prevented from even making small birthday gifts to their grandchildren. There is some possibility that the law will be repealed or substantially modified. Until that occurs, any transfer made as part of a program to qualify for Medicaid should be considered to carry some risk for both the transferor and the professional adviser.

Although there are severe restrictions on planning transfers of assets from a potential Medicaid beneficiary, the situation is different with respect to this same person receiving "gifts in trust." The beneficiary of these "gifts in trust" is allowed to continue to qualify for Medicaid. For example, parents or a life partner who planned to make an outright bequest to an adult child or life partner with HIV infection might consider making a gift in trust that would provide only for luxuries and cannot be used for basic needs. On the other hand, if a PLWHIV renounces an inheritance or does not pursue a right of intestate distribution, the act of giving up the inheritance will be a disqualifying transfer for the purposes of Medicaid eligibility (*Matter of Mattei,* 1996).

Federal law mandates that, on the death of a Medicaid recipient, states must file a claim against the estate of any person who was over the age of 55 at the time of payments. Under the federal law, states have the option to redefine the term *estate* to include any asset in which a recipient had any kind of interest, including joint bank accounts, retirement accounts, life insurance, and annuities, but only to the extent of the recipient's interest. Definitions may vary from state to state; for example, in New York State the law interprets the term *estate* to include only those assets that are in the name of the decedent alone.

Incompetency and Disability

Cognitive impairment and HIV encephalopathy are prevalent in HIV disease. Because of this, it is important for HIV-positive persons to take advantage of a durable power of attorney. Powers of attorney that do not specify their continued ef-

fectiveness after incompetency cease to be effective if the PLWHIV becomes incompetent. Those who are granted the power of attorney are known as "attorneys-in-fact." An attorney-in-fact can be given very broad or only limited power to act on behalf of the PLWHIV. In the event the PLWHIV does not wish this power to be effective immediately, many state laws provide for a "springing power of attorney" to take effect at a future date or upon the occurrence of a specific event in the future, such as incompetency or disability of the PLWHIV or the inability to handle his or her personal affairs.

Without a durable power of attorney in place, it may be necessary to have a guardian appointed to take care of the personal needs or to manage the property of an incapacitated person. The petition by a PLWHIV's life partner to act as guardian may spark resistance from family members, especially if the PLWHIV has considerable assets. The execution of a power of attorney before there is any question of incompetence should alleviate this problem. The designation of a guardian can avoid the naming of family members whom the PLWHIV does not wish to control his or her life.

Sometimes an HIV-positive diagnosis may lead to the alienation of even the closest friends and family members of the PLWHIV, making it difficult to find an appropriate person willing either to serve as an attorney-in-fact or to be appointed as guardian. Many state statutes provide a partial solution to that dilemma by permitting certain not-for-profit corporations, public agencies, and social services officials to act as guardians. Another incompetency and disability planning device is to place one's assets in an "inter vivos" trust naming a trusted friend, family member, or bank or trust company as trustee.

Self-Determination Documents

Many PLWHIVs are concerned with preserving their self-determination if they should become incapacitated. Some have been separated from their natural families for long terms or have become estranged for various reasons. The last thing that they may want is for the family to return and take charge of their lives, ignoring the long-expressed wishes of the PLWHIV. This concern extends even into death, including control over the services to be held in connection with the death and the disposition of the body. Giving the PLWHIV greater control early in his or her illness over the actions that others can take for him in the future will help unburden his or her spirit. Depending on the PLWHIV's situation, the documents that help assure his or her self-determination may include

1. A power of attorney
2. A health care proxy
3. A living will
4. A nomination of a guardian
5. Appointment of a standby guardian of the children
6. Pet care arrangements
7. Pre-need funeral arrangements
8. A will
9. A letter of instructions on funeral and burial wishes

PRIVACY, CONFIDENTIALITY, AND DISCLOSURE

The issue of disclosure relates to concerns of privacy and confidentiality. Since the related laws are state specific and extend to both extremes, health care providers should familiarize themselves with the laws of the state or jurisdiction in which they live or work in order to be in compliance. There are, however, some generic issues. At least 39 states have laws providing for the confidentiality of HIV/AIDS–related information. In New York, for example, with several exceptions, the written consent of a PLWHIV is required before HIV-related information can be released to private individuals or employers. At least 28 states have laws that specifically regulate the dissemination of medical records and related information (National Conference of State Legislatures, 1996). Virtually all states allow for disclosure of HIV-related information in certain circumstances. Most states have criminal penalties for the unauthorized disclosure of information (National Conference of State Legislatures, 1996).

As for the physician's duty to maintain the confidentiality of medical records, most states impose such a duty. About half the states extend this duty to other health care providers. Only four states have specific legislation imposing the duty on insurance companies, and only a few impose a similar duty on employers or other non–health

care institutions. Fewer than half the states have specific laws imposing a duty to maintain confidentiality of electronic or computerized medical records (National Conference of State Legislatures, 1996).

In a related matter, many states have recently enacted laws related to the testing of newborn infants. In California, Florida, Iowa, and Rhode Island, the legislatures have adopted laws for the surveillance of or the testing of newborns. California requires that the number of babies born with HIV, drug dependencies, and STDs be reported to the legislature and the governor annually. Florida permits HIV testing of hospitalized infants when necessary to provide medical care and when the parent cannot be contacted to provide consent. Iowa authorizes the Department of Public Health to conduct blinded studies through HIV testing of newborns to determine the prevalence of HIV. Rhode Island empowers its Department of Health to make the rules and regulations to mandate testing of newborns when there is a strong medical suspicion that a child may have HIV and the doctor is unable to obtain the mother's written consent (National Conference of State Legislatures, 1996).

In June 1996, the New York legislature adopted rules that required the testing of all newborns. Previously, although all newborns were tested to track the HIV epidemic in the state, the tests and their results were blinded, revealing only the actual number of infected infants and not their identity. In adopting the new law, the legislators were not persuaded by arguments that most of the HIV antibody–positive infants were eventually found to be HIV-negative.

ASSISTED SUICIDE AND EUTHANASIA

Before 1997 the law relating to assisted suicide was unclear and depended on the jurisdiction (*Compassion in Dying v. Washington,* 1996; *Quill v. Vacco,* 1996). To date, 35 states have banned doctor-assisted suicide and only Oregon has legalized it. In November 1997, Oregon voters reaffirmed their determination to make assisted suicide a choice for the terminally ill in their state.

In June 1997, in two unanimous decisions, the United States Supreme Court unanimously rejected constitutional challenges to laws in Washington and New York that made doctor-assisted suicide a crime. However, a majority of the justices suggested that at least some terminally ill persons in intractable pain might be able to claim in the future that they have a constitutional right to a doctor's assistance in hastening their deaths. This action left the issue open for debate at a later date. The justices did make it clear, however, that the states are obliged to ensure palliative care to relieve the physical and psychologic pain of the dying. Without palliative care, a ban on assisted suicide can be considered cruel and irrational (*Vacco v. Quill,* 1997; *Washington v. Glucksberg,* 1997).

HIV TRANSMISSION RISK IN HEALTH CARE SETTINGS

Risk to Health Care Providers

With the advent of formalized infection-control programs in health care facilities in the late 1960s, medicine and science have effectively reduced the level of risk involved in many activities of health care providers. However, it would be impossible, or even deceptive, to guarantee health care providers a risk-free environment or to assure them that freedom from all risk of harm is possible and attainable. Courts and public health officials have adopted policies or guidelines that seek to protect health care providers against those situations and circumstances that present a significant risk of harm. In adopting a significant-risk standard, it is acknowledged that some degree of risk may be inevitable. Public policy should not be based on the emotional fear of harm. In *School Board of Nassau County v. Airline* (1987) the U.S. Supreme Court held that a disabled person's employment could not be restricted unless the infectious conditions presented an unreasonable risk of harm to others. An important aspect of this case was the Court's adoption of the American Medical Association's argument that certain factors should be considered in determining the reasonableness of the risk including

1. The likelihood of transmission
2. The length of the period of infectivity
3. The nature of the possible transmission
4. The severity of the outcome if transmission occurs.

As a consequence of the health care services they provide, health care providers face the risk of

acquiring HIV infection on a daily basis. They must come to terms with their own feelings and values and thoroughly understand the mechanism of disease transmission. Constant reinforcement of rational infection-control policies or procedures in caring for all patients is essential in helping health care providers deal with this challenging and often, frightening concern.

An irrational fear of HIV infection may result in a person's being refused treatment by a health care provider. There is no common law requiring physicians or nurses to accept any particular patient, and health care providers may refuse to undertake professional responsibility for prospective patients, but there are some statutory limits on this right to refusal. Once a physician has accepted a person for care or treatment, he or she must continue to provide care until the patient discharges the physician, until the care or treatment may be safely and properly discontinued, or until another physician has assumed responsibility for the care or treatment. Federal and state antidiscrimination laws limit health care providers' rights to refuse to treat a patient with HIV/AIDS.

At least 22 states have passed laws prohibiting discrimination in the access to or provision of health services (National Conference of State Legislatures, 1996). For example, emergency health care workers in Maryland are prohibited by law from refusing to treat or transport a person because of his or her HIV status. The person who has been refused care may find protection in the Federal Rehabilitation Act of 1973 or the more recently enacted American with Disabilities Act (1990). The important question in refusing to care for a patient is whether the refusal of care was necessary because of a significant risk to others. Refusal of care is seldom upheld in court bcause a risk to the health care provider or to others is difficult to substantiate (Hancock, 1993).

Risk to Patients

The debate regarding the risk of HIV transmission from health care providers to patients continues. All available epidemiologic data support the fact that the risk of HIV transmission from patients to health care providers greatly exceeds that of transmission from health care providers to patients, since health care providers are more likely to have contact with blood or blood-contaminated body fluids in the health care setting. The risk of transmission of a blood-borne pathogen from a health care provider to a patient is associated with the actual procedures performed, the infection-control precautions used, the titer of the pathogen in the blood, and the medical status of the health care provider. This risk must be placed in perspective relative to other substantially greater risks that are present during invasive procedures, such as (1) infection (other than HIV), (2) hemorrhage, (3) anesthesia reaction, (4) an allergic reaction to the materials or equipment used in the procedure, or (5) death.

There has been only one report of documented transmission of HIV from a health care provider to six patients, and that occurred in a dental practice in Florida, but the precise events resulting in transmission from the HIV-infected dentist remain unclear. At present, no other cases of HIV transmission from health care workers to patients have been documented.

After the first reports of the possible HIV transmission in Florida, at least one court shifted its focus to the severity of the risk and ruled accordingly. In *Behringer v. The Medical Center at Princeton* (1991), the court upheld the hospital's policy of restricting the surgical privileges of health care providers known to be infected with HIV. The court held that the doctrine of informed consent gave rise to an obligation on the part of the hospital to address patients' fear of a surgical accident and their emotional distress concerning possible HIV transmission. The court agreed with the hospital that any risk (even one that may not be significant) of HIV infection posed a reasonable probability of substantial harm to others and that justified suspension of the doctor's surgical privileges. The *Behringer* court focused on the (higher) risk of injury from HIV transmission, rather than on the (lower) risk of transmission from health care providers to patients.

Risk Management

In response to the HIV epidemic, isolation practices in the United States changed in 1985 (CDC, 1985) by the introduction of universal precautions (UP). Since HIV and other blood-borne infections can be transmitted by persons in whom the infection is unrecognized or undiagnosed, emphasis was placed on applying blood and body fluid precautions universally to all patients (and, by inference, to all health care providers) regardless of their infection status. When used correctly, UP prevents bidirectional (patient to health care provider and health care provider to patient) transmission of bloodborne pathogens, including many that are more infectious than HIV, that can result in severe illness or death. UP emphasized prevention of needle stick injury, use of traditional barriers such as gloves and gowns, use of masks and eye coverings to prevent exposure of mucous membranes during certain procedures, use of individualized ventilation devices when the need for resuscitation is predictable and so forth. UP applied to blood, semen, vaginal secretions, and amniotic, cerebrospinal, pericardial, peritoneal, pleural, and synovial fluids. Other body fluids were not included *unless* they were visibly contaminated with blood inasmuch as epidemiologic studies had not implicated them in the transmission of HIV and hepatitis B virus (HBV) infections (CDC, 1988; Edmond & Wenzel, 1995).

In 1987, body substance isolation (BSI) was proposed as an alternative to diagnosis-driven isolation systems (Lynch et al., 1987). This system was based on the premise that all moist body sites and substances from all patients are potentially infectious, and BSI required that gloves be worn for all anticipated contact with moist body substances and that clean gloves be put on before contact with mucous membranes and nonintact skin. Handwashing after glove removal was not required unless hands were visibly soiled, although the efficacy of using gloves as a substitute for hand-washing was not documented. This isolation system also required the use of additional precautions for infections transmitted by the airborne route.

In 1991 the Occupational Safety and Health Administration (OSHA) published the final rule on occupational exposure to bloodborne pathogens in order to improve *occupational safety* in the care of patients infected with bloodborne pathogens (Department of Labor, 1991). This final rule was based largely on Centers for Disease Control and Prevention (CDC) recommendations regarding UP and the use of hepatitis B vaccine. It created many affirmative duties for employers to eliminate or reduce the risks of employee exposure to bloodborne pathogens in the workplace, such as mandating the development of an exposure control plan and postexposure follow-up.

In 1996 the CDC issued a revised guideline for isolation precautions which synthesized the major features of UP and BSI into a singular set of precautions to be used for the care of all patients, regardless of their presumed diagnosis or infection status (Hospital Infection Control Practices Advisory Committee [HICPAC], 1996). The first tier of these precautions, called "standard precautions," is designed to reduce the risk of transmission of microorganisms from recognized and unrecognized infection sources in hospitals and applies to blood and to all body fluids, secretions, and excretions, except sweat, regardless of the presence of visible blood, nonintact skin, or mucous membranes. The second tier of precautions, called "transmission-based precautions," is specifically to be used for patients known or suspected to be infected with highly transmissible or epidemiologically important pathogens spread by airborne or droplet transmission or by contact with dry skin or contaminated surfaces. Transmission-based precautions must be used in addition to standard precautions, and the two tiers may be combined for diseases that have multiple transmission routes.

Prevention of transmission of HIV and other bloodborne pathogens in health care settings needs a multifaceted approach to decrease the frequency of occupational blood exposures among health care workers, engineering controls that do not rely on worker compliance, such as self-sheathing needles, incorporation of safer work practices and techniques into patient care activities, the use of appropriate personal protective equipment, and training (Chamberland et al., 1995). Percutaneous exposure to blood or blood-contaminated body substances poses the highest risk to health care workers, and therefore special attention must be given to design and handling and disposal of needles, scalpels, and other "sharps." A focus on practices that decrease the risk of these injuries would include, for a start, improved instrument and device design, elimination of needle recapping, and sharps-disposal containers located strategically where needles and other sharps are used.

There have been no reported instances in which the environment has been implicated as a reservoir for HIV transmission (Henderson, 1995). Therefore federal regulations or special recommendations or guidelines for environmental cleaning have not been issued.

DISCRIMINATION: WORKER PROTECTION

Employees infected with HIV may be protected from discrimination in the workplace under several federal, state, and city antidiscrimination statutes. The most notable is Title I of the Americans With Disabilities Act (ADA) of 1990, which prohibits discrimination against qualified persons with disabilities by employers with 15 or more employees. Title I also requires that a covered employer provide reasonable accommodation to a qualified person with a disability if it is necessary for the employee to perform the essential functions of his position.

Title II of the ADA (1990) protects qualified persons with disabilities from discrimination on the basis of disability in the services, programs, or activities of all state and local governments. Title III of the ADA (1990) prohibits discrimination by a public accommodation, such as a hospital or commercial building, against a person with a disability in the operation of that place of public accommodation. In addition to requiring reasonable modifications in policies, practices, and procedures of public accommodations, Title III requires the removal of barriers in existing facilities to make places of public accommodation accessible to persons with disabilities.

To be qualified as a person with a disability, and therefore entitled to the protection of Title I of the ADA, a person must have a disability as defined by the ADA and must (1) satisfy the requisite skills, experience, and other job-related requirements of the employment position held or desired and (2) be able to perform the position's essential functions, with or without reasonable accommodations.

A person with a disability under the ADA (1990) is (1) someone with a mental or physical impairment that substantially limits one or more of the major life activities, (2) someone with a record of such an impairment, or (3) someone regarded as having such an impairment. Most courts follow the ADA's legislative history and the U. S. Supreme Court's decision in *School Board of Nassau County v. Airline* (1987), in holding that people with HIV disease are covered by the ADA. In the *Airline* case, the Supreme Court held that an employer could not discriminate on the basis of fear of contagiousness of a disease. Although Airline involved tuberculosis, many courts have extended its holding to cases involving HIV disease.

Nevertheless, some courts have held that HIV disease may not be a covered disability under the ADA. For example, in *Runnebaum v. Nations Bank of Maryland* (1996), the Fourth Circuit Court of Appeals held that asymptomatic HIV infection does not substantially limit procreation or intimate sexual relations for the purposes of the ADA and, thus, is not a disability. Additionally, with the success of combination antiretroviral therapy delaying symptomatic disease and the diagnosis of AIDS, the issue of whether an asymptomatic HIV-infected person has a disability and should be protected by the ADA is increasingly debated (Gostin & Webber, 1998). The Supreme Court, in hearing its first AIDS case, will decide whether and to what extent persons with HIV are protected under the ADA.

A federal statute that provides protections similar to those of the ADA is the federal Rehabilitation Act (1973), which prohibits discrimination in programs by federal agencies and by contractors and those receiving federal financial assistance. As the precursor to the ADA, the Rehabilitation Act shares the ADA's reasonable accommodation requirement for employers. Many states also have laws that prohibit discrimination. For example, the New York State Human Rights Law prohibits disability-based discrimination (HRL, 1951). Health care providers are advised to determine whether such a law exists in the state in which they live and work.

The most common reasonable accommodations for HIV-infected employees as recognized by the ADA and the Rehabilitation Act are flexible work schedules and time off to accommodate treatment schedules or fatigue problems. Some persons with HIV disease develop other impairments, such as visual impairments or mobility impairments. In those situations, the reasonable accommodations designed for persons with visual or mobility impairments would be available for the person with HIV disease (e.g., *Buckingham v. United States,* 1993, transferring a postal employee with AIDS from Mississippi to California to obtain better medical

treatment may constitute a reasonable accommodation, and *EEOC v. Newport News Shipbuilding & Drydock Co.,* 1996, relocating an HIV-positive employee to an office with an air-conditioning unit, placing him on short-term disability leave, and making several alterations and repairs to reduce the presence of allergens, is considered a reasonable accommodation under ADA).

A person with a disability, however, shall not pose a direct threat to the health or safety of others in the workplace. Direct threat is defined in the ADA (1990) as a significant risk to the health or safety of others that cannot be eliminated by reasonable accommodation.

Most cases in which direct threat can be shown concern the employment of HIV-infected health care workers (HCWs). In July 1991, the CDC published new recommendations that included (1) infected HCWs who adhere to universal precautions and who do not perform invasive procedures pose no risk for transmitting HIV or hepatitis B (HBV) and (2) HCWs who are infected with HIV should not perform exposure-prone procedures unless they have sought counsel from an expert review panel and have been advised under what circumstances, if any, they may continue to perform these procedures.

Cases in which a direct threat of infection has been found sufficient to permit discrimination based on HIV disease generally involve the health care industry. For example, in *Doe v. University of Maryland Medical System Corp.* (1995), a hospital properly barred an HIV-positive surgical resident from performing surgical procedures because he posed a significant risk to patients that could not be eliminated by reasonable accommodation. Similarly, in *Bradley v. University of Texas M.D. Anderson Cancer Center* (1993/1994), a hospital was found not to have violated the Rehabilitation Act when it transferred an HIV-positive employee from the position of surgical assistant (where he often came within inches of open wounds) because, while the risk of transmission was small, it was not so low as to nullify the catastrophic consequences of an accident. In *Mauro v. Borgess Medical Center* (1995), the court held that a hospital did not violate the ADA when it laid off a surgical technician who was HIV-positive, since his condition posed a direct threat to the health and safety of others.

Not all cases involving the health care industry result in permissible discrimination against persons with HIV disease. In *Abbott v. Bragdon* (1997), the court held that treating an HIV-positive dental patient in his office does not pose a direct threat if the dentist implements infection-control guidelines issued by the CDC. Similarly, in *Howe v. Hull* (1994), a hospital's refusal to admit and treat an HIV-infected man who was suffering from a severe non-HIV–related reaction to a drug violated the ADA because refusal to admit the patient was unlawfully motivated by the patient's HIV/AIDS status.

Cases in which no direct threat of infection is found generally involve non-health-care-related industries. For example, in *Chalk v. U.S. District Court* (1988), a teacher with AIDS was reinstated to her position because the court agreed that casual contact between children and AIDS-infected persons is not dangerous. In *Doe v. District of Columbia* (1992), the court found that a Washington, D.C., fire department's withdrawal of an offer of employment to an HIV-positive applicant was improper because the risk of transmitting the virus was so small that the applicant's status did not present a direct threat to other firefighters or to the public. Similarly, in *EEOC v. Dolphin Cruise Line* (1996), a cruise ship was found to have violated the ADA when it revoked a job offer to an entertainer after learning he was HIV-positive. The company failed to demonstrate, other than by speculation and stereotyping, that the health risk posed by the entertainer in the particular work setting was significant. In *EEOC v. Prevo's Family Market* (1996), the court held that a food store produce clerk who was discharged after he revealed his HIV-positive status did not pose a direct threat to coworkers or customers.

HIV Testing and Employment

Under the ADA (1990), an employer may not require an applicant for a job to submit to a medical examination or to answer medical inquiries before a conditional job offer has been made to the applicant. After extending a conditional job offer, an employer may require a medical examination and may condition the offer of employment on the results of that examination, provided the examination is related to the job functions. The examination must be required of all appli-

cants for a particular job category, and the information gathered must be kept strictly confidential on separate forms in a separate medical file. Only a limited number of persons may gain access to these records. An employer may require a medical examination of an employee only if the employer proves that the test is job related and consistent with business necessity.

In addition to the ADA requirements concerning medical testing, individual states may have their own laws concerning medical or HIV testing and confidentiality. Health care providers are advised to check their own state's laws with respect to this issue.

Medical Leave

Employees with HIV disease, or with infected family members, may need medical leave for treatment or hospitalization. The federal Family and Medical Leave Act of 1993 (FMLA) guarantees eligible employees the right to take unpaid leave from a job for up to 12 weeks because of a serious health condition of the employee, a child, a spouse, or a parent. A serious health condition is defined as an illness, injury, impairment, or physical or mental condition that involves (1) inpatient care in a hospital, hospice, or residential medical care facility or (2) continuing treatment by a health care provider (U.S. Dept. of Labor Final Rules Implementing the FMLA, 1995). A serious health condition that does not require inpatient care but involves continuing treatment by a health care provider includes (1) a period of incapacity, such as inability to work, attend school, or perform other regular daily activities for more than three consecutive calendar days; (2) any period of incapacity because of pregnancy or for prenatal care; (3) any period of incapacity or treatment for such incapacity caused by a chronic serious health condition. As a result, if an employee, his or her child, parent, or spouse has HIV disease, which fits the definition of a serious health condition, that employee may have rights under the FMLA. The FMLA applies only to private employers of 50 employees or more.

Benefits

HIV-infected persons can face staggering medical costs while combating the effects of their illness. The potential impact of these costs on insurance rates has led some employers to deny insurance coverage to HIV-infected employees or to simply terminate their employment in an effort to avoid these additional costs.

Section 510 of the Employee Retirement Income Security Act (ERISA), prohibits an employer from taking action against an employee that is designed to deprive the employee of benefits under ERISA-protected plans. ERISA is limited in its protection, however, because it applies only to covered plans. Benefits such as pensions, health, severance, and annuity plans are likely to be protected, whereas noncovered plans will be subject to state law.

ERISA also has been limited in its protection of plan participants or beneficiaries subject to AIDS caps or exclusions. In *McGann v. H&H Music Co.* (1990/1991/1992), an HIV-infected employee challenged an employer's right to switch health insurance coverage to a plan that placed a $5,000.00 lifetime maximum cap on HIV-related coverage. The court held that, in the absence of a contractual commitment to the contrary, ERISA does not prevent an employer from altering insurance coverage in response to past financial experience.

Similarly, in *Owens v. Storehouse, Inc.* (1993), the United States Circuit Court of Appeals for the Eleventh Circuit held that ERISA does not prevent an employer from amending its benefits plan to include a cap on AIDS-related claims because it applies to all employees equally, with no evidence of discriminatory intent. The ADA (1990) also offers some protection for the problem of AIDS caps and exclusions.

In June 1993 the United States Equal Employment Opportunity Commission (EEOC) issued an interim policy guide on the ADA and health insurance, suggesting that disease-specific caps would violate the ADA. Since implementation of these guidelines, the EEOC has obtained settlements leading to abolition of AIDS caps in the states of California, Pennsylvania, and Connecticut. Similar AIDS caps suits have been brought in Maryland, Michigan, and Minnesota. In New York the EEOC brought suit against the Mason Tenders (1993) because its welfare fund denied payment of medical expenses for any AIDS-related illness. Reportedly, the case was ultimately settled.

In fact, a health plan may be sued as "a covered entity" under Title I and as a "public accommo-

dation" under Title III for imposing a lifetime limit on benefits for AIDS-related conditions. An employer may also be liable under the ADA for changing insurance carriers to avoid insuring an employee who has AIDS unless it can show that covering the employee would be an undue hardship. In *Anderson v. Gus Mayer Boston Store* (1996), the district court held that, to avoid liability under the ADA, the employer must prove that coverage for a discrete group of disabilities would be so expensive as to cause the plan to become financially insolvent.

Denying an applicant a life insurance policy because he or she lives with an HIV-positive partner may also violate the ADA under the public accommodation provisions of Title III (*Cloutier v. Prudential Insurance Co.*, 1997). Similarly, in *Kotev v. First Colony Life Insurance Co.* (1996), a woman denied life insurance because of her spouse's HIV status was allowed to bring an action under Title III of the ADA. However, an employer and insurer might not be in violation of either Title I or Title III of the ADA when it provides greater benefits in its long-term disability plan to persons with physical rather than mental disabilities (*Parker v. Metropolitan Life Insurance Co.*, 1997). The *Parker* decision indicates that the Sixth Circuit Court would allow an employer and insurer to limit or exclude benefits for persons with HIV disease since the ADA does not mandate equality between persons with different disabilities. Rather, the ADA prohibits discrimination between the disabled and the nondisabled.

Another potential pitfall for HIV-infected employees is the legal doctrine of judicial estoppel. When a person states that he or she is unable to return to work for purposes of obtaining disability benefits, an issue arises as to whether he or she may also claim to be qualified to perform the essential functions of the job.

Although courts are divided concerning whether the person is judicially estopped from pursuing an ADA claim if he or she has sought disability benefits, a recent Third Circuit Court decision involving an HIV-infected employee illustrates the harsh penalties of the doctrine. In *McNemar v. The Disney Store, Inc.* (1996/1997), an assistant store manager was terminated approximately 1 month after notifying his store manager of his HIV-positive diagnosis and approximately 10 days after he was confronted with this fact by the district manager. The employer claimed that McNemar, a 4-year employee, was terminated for taking 2 dollars from the store register to buy a pack of cigarettes. Unemployed, McNemar applied for federal and state disability benefits and stated on his applications that he was totally disabled since the time he was found to be HIV-positive. The Third Circuit Court of Appeals affirmed the District Court's dismissal of McNemar's ADA, ERISA, and New Jersey State Law claims on the basis that he was precluded by judicial estoppel. Notwithstanding the fact that the plaintiff worked at the store for approximately 1½ months after the diagnosis, the court found that his statements in the disability applications judicially estopped him from claiming in his ADA case that he was otherwise qualified to perform the job.

The *McNemar* decision was at variance with a similar case in Illinois (*Smith v. Dovenmuehle Mortgage, Inc.,* 1994, in which a plaintiff with AIDS received disability benefits from the Social Security Administration on the representation that he was disabled and then sued his former employer under the ADA. In holding that the plaintiff was not judicially estopped from arguing that he was qualified under the ADA, the Court reasoned that to hold otherwise would put the plaintiff in the untenable position of choosing between his right to seek disability benefits and his right to seek redress for an alleged violation of the ADA. Also, judicial estoppel frustrates the ADA's purpose of combating discrimination against disabled persons (*Mohammed v. Marriott International, Inc.,* 1996). Although the law is still being developed, HIV-infected employees must be aware that applying for disability benefits may preclude them from proceeding with a claim of discrimination under the ADA.

CONCLUSION

Society strives to balance the often conflicting rights and responsibilities of individuals with those of the public. HIV infection is representative of this ethical dilemma: balancing the rights of HIV-infected persons with the rights of those who are at risk of HIV exposure. Different, although not necessarily incompatible, legal approaches to the HIV epidemic have been proposed. One approach recommends mandatory

screening, punishment for noncompliance, and use of aggressive measures to restrict the rights and mobility of the HIV-infected person. Justification for this approach often refers to what has been perceived as the lack of social responsibility demonstrated by persons infected with HIV.

Another approach to the HIV epidemic focuses on the public health aspects of the disease, recognizing that information, voluntary testing, education, counseling and help of any kind are the most effective methods of assisting HIV-positive persons and for protecting those at risk of HIV infection. In this approach, reducing the risk of transmission may take precedence over confidentiality and privacy.

Yet a third approach to the HIV epidemic focuses on less government monitoring and more safeguards for confidentiality, protection against any discrimination, stigmatization, or ostracism of HIV-infected persons. Justification for this approach argues that if learning one's HIV status has negative or punitive repercussions, public health efforts to reduce the incidence of HIV infection will not be successful.

In the face of the complexity of the HIV epidemic, this chapter has reviewed the relevant federal provisions and referred to some state laws related to persons infected with HIV and those at risk of exposure or infection. Just as the data relevant to the HIV epidemic are evolving daily, so too are the legal precedents, and health care providers should be mindful of this new information.

REFERENCES

Abbott v. Bragdon, 912 F. Supp. 580 (D. Me. 1995), *aff'd,* 107 F.3d 934 (1st Cir. 1997).

Abbott v. Bragdon, 107 F.3d 934, 6 A.D. Cases (BNA) 780 (1st Cir. 1997).

Adoption of Elizabeth S., 509 N.Y.S.2d 746 (Fam. Ct. 1986).

AIDS advocates, caregivers must play major role in managed care debates. (1996, May). *AIDS Alert, 11*(5), 49–52.

Americans With Disabilities Act (ADA), 42U.S.C. §12101, *et seq.* (1990); *See also,* 29 C.F.R. 1630.

Anderson v. Gus Mayer Boston Store, 924 F. Supp. 763, 5 A.D. Cases (BNA) 673 (E.D. Tex. 1996).

Behringer v. The Medical Center at Princeton, 249 N.J. Super. 597, 592 A.2d 1251 (N.J. Super. 1991).

Bradley v. University of Texas M.D. Anderson Cancer Center, 3 F.3d 922, 2 A.D. Cases (BNA) 1297 (5th Cir.

1993), *cert. denied,* 510 U.S. 1119, 3 A.D. Cases (BNA) 192 (1994).

Buckingham v. United States, F.3d, 2 A.D. Cases (BNA) 1009 (9th Cir. 1993).

Centers for Disease Control. (1985). Recommendations for preventing transmission of infection with human T-lymphotrophic virus type III/lymphadenopathy-associated virus in the workplace. *MMWR, 34,* 681–686, 691–695.

Centers for Disease Control. (1988). Update: Universal precautions for prevention of transmission of human immunodeficiency virus, hepatitis B virus, and other bloodborne pathogens in health-care settings. *MMWR, 37,* 377–382, 387–388.

Centers for Disease Control and Prevention. (1991). Recommendations for preventing transmission of human immunodeficiency virus and hepatitis B virus to patients during exposure-prone invasive procedures. *MMWR, 40*(RR-8), 1–9.

Chalk v. U.S.D.C., 840 F.2d 701, 46 Fair Emp. Prac. Cases (BNA) 279, 1 A.D. Cases (BNA) 1210 (9th Cir. 1988).

Chamberland, M.E., Ward, J.W., Curran, J.W. (1995). Epidemiology and prevention of AIDS and HIV infection. In G.L. Mandell, J.E. Bennett, R. Dolin (Eds.), *Principles and practice of infectious diseases,* (4th ed., pp. 1174–1203). New York: Churchill Livingstone.

Cloutier v. Prudential Insurance Co., No. C-96-1166 WHO (N.D. Cal. 1997).

Compassion in Dying v. Washington, 85 F.3d 1440 (9th Cir. 1996).

Defense of Marriage Act, P.L. 104-99, 110 Stat 2419 (1996).

Department of Labor. Occupational Safety and Health Administration (1991). Occupational exposure to bloodborne pathogens: Final rule. *Federal Register, 56,* 64175–64182.

Doe v. District of Columbia, 796 F. Supp. 559, 59 Fair Emp. Prac. Cases (BNA) 363, 2 A.D. Cases (BNA) 197 (D.C.D.C. 1992).

Doe v. University of Maryland Medical System Corp., 50 F.3d 1261, 4 A.D. Cases (BNA) 379 (4th Cir. 1995).

Edmond, M.B., Wenzel, R.P. (1995). Isolation. In G.L. Mandell, J.E. Bennett, R. Dolin (Eds.), *Principles and practice of infectious diseases* (4th ed., pp. 2575–2579). New York: Churchill Livingstone.

EEOC v. Dolphin Cruise Line, 945 F. Supp. 1550, 6 A.D. Cases (BNA) 187 (S.D. Fla. 1996).

EEOC v. Newport News Shipbuilding & Drydock Co., 949 F. Supp. 403, 6 A.D. Cases (BNA) 369 (E.D.Va. 1996).

EEOC v. Prevo's Family Market, 5 A.D. Cases (BNA) 1526 (W.D. Mich. 1996).

Employee Retirement Income Security Act (ERISA), 29 U.S.C. §1140 (1974).

Family and Medical Leave Act (FMLA), 29 U.S.C. §§2601-2654 (1993).

Gostin, L.O., Webber, D.W. (1998) HIV infection and AIDS in the public health and health care systems: The role of law and litigation. *Journal of the American Medical Association, 279*(14), 1108–1113.

Hancock, S.F., Jr. (1993, February). AIDS and the law. *NYS Bar Journal, 65*(2), 8–13.

Health Insurance Portability and Accountability Act (HIPAA), P.L. 104-91 (1996).

Henderson, D.K. (1995). HIV-1 in the health care setting. In G.L. Mandell, J.E. Bennett, R. Dolin (Eds.), *Principles and practice of infectious diseases* (4th ed., pp. 2632–2656). New York: Churchill Livingstone.

Hospital Infection Control Practices Advisory Committee. (1996, February). Guideline for isolation precautions in hospitals. Part I. Evolution of isolation practices. Part II. Recommendations for isolation precautions in hospitals. *Am J Infect Control, 24*(1), 24–52.

Howe v. Hull, 873 F. Supp. 72, 3 A.D. Cases (BNA) 1485 (N.D. Ohio 1994).

Human Rights Law (HRL), N.Y. Exec. Law §296 (1951).

Kotev v. First Colony Life Insurance Co., 927 F. Supp. 1316 (C.D. Cal. 1996).

Lynch, P., Jackson, M.M., Cummings, M.J., Stamm, W.E. (1987). Rethinking the role of isolation practices in the prevention of nosocomial infections. *Ann Intern Med, 107,* 243–246.

Mason Tenders District Council Welfare Fund v. Donaghey, 2 A.D. Cases (BNA) 1745 (S.D.N.Y. 1993).

Matter of Cooper, 187 A.D.2d 128, 592 N.Y.S.2d 797 (2d Dep't 1993).

Matter of Jacob, 86 N.Y.2d 651, 669, 636 N.Y.S.2d 716, 725 (1995) (Bellacosa, J., dissenting).

Matter of Mattei, 169 Misc.2 989, 647 N.Y.S.2d 415 (Sup. Ct. Nassau Co. 1996).

Matter of Petri, New York Law Journal (p. 29, col. 1), April 4, 1994 (Sur. Ct. N.Y. Co.).

Matter of Robert Paul P., 63 N.Y. 2d 233, 481 N.Y.S.2d 652 (1984).

Mauro v. Borgess Medical Center, 886 F. Supp. 1349, 4 A.D. Cases (BNA) 737 (W.D. Mich. 1995).

McGann v. H&H Music Co., 742 F. Supp. 392 (S.D. Tex. 1990), *aff'd,* 946 F.2d 401 (5th Cir. 1991), *cert. denied,* 506 U.S. 981 (1992).

McNemar v. The Disney Store, Inc., 91 F.3d 610 (3rd Cir. 1996), *cert. denied,* 117 S. Ct. 958 (1997).

Mohammed v. Marriott International, Inc., 994 F. Supp. 277 (S.D.N.Y. 1996).

National Conference of State Legislatures. (February). *HIV/AIDS facts to consider: 1996.* Denver, CO: Author.

New York Estates, Powers and Trusts Law (EPTL), §4-1.1(a), *et seq.* (McKinney Supp. 1997).

Owens v. Storehouse, Inc., No. 91-8696 (11th Cir. 1993).

Parker v. Metropolitan Life Insurance Co., 21 E.B.C. (BNA) 1369 (6th Cir. 1997).

Pear, R. (March 17, 1998). High rates hobble law to guarantee health insurance. *The New York Times,* pp. Al, Al6.

Public Health Services Act (PHSA), 42 U.S.C. §300ff-21, *et seq.* (1990).

Quill v. Vacco, 80 F.3d 716 (2d Cir. 1996).

Rehabilitation Act, 29 U.S.C. §791, et seq. (1973).

Runnebaum v. NationsBank of Maryland, 95 F.3d 1285 (4th Cir. 1996).

Ryan White Comprehensive AIDS Resources Emergency (CARE) Act Amendments of 1996, P. L. 104-146 (effective October 1, 1996).

School Board of Nassau County v. Arline, 480 U.S. 273 (1987).

Smith v. Dovenmuehle Mortgage, Inc., 1994 WL 275028 (N.D. Ill. 1994).

Social Security Law, 42 U.S.C. §1396p (1982).

Storrs v. Holcomb, 168 Misc.2d 286, 482 N.Y.S.2d 201 (Sup. Ct. N.Y.Co. 1984).

U.S. Dept. of Labor Final Rules Implementing the Family and Medical Leave Act, 29 C.F.R. §825.114(a)(2) (April 6, 1995).

Vacco v. Quill, 117 S.Ct. 2293, 138 L.Ed. 2d 834 (U.S. June 26, 1997).

Washington v. Glucksberg, 117 S.Ct. 2258, 138 L.Ed. 2d 772 (U.S. June 26, 1997).

13

Ethical Concerns

JUDITH SAUNDERS

Ethical controversies within the context of HIV/AIDS have been influenced by the nature of the stigmatized population in the United States most affected by this disease: gay men, injection drug users, people of color, and people of poverty. Controversy has permeated discussions of HIV/AIDS since the first case of HIV/AIDS was diagnosed in 1981, and very often the controversy has been rooted in claims about whose perspective was morally correct and whose rights should be preserved or violated. The controversies have been evident in bitter, often polarized, positions as individuals and groups affected by HIV/AIDS took stands on the right way to respond to this world pandemic, with one group advocating mandatory testing, followed by isolation of HIV-positive persons, while other groups advocated education and voluntary testing.

This disease occurred after scientific and technologic advances in medicine already had fueled debate about moral or ethical choices regarding the circumstances of life, death, and reproduction; initiation and withdrawal of treatment; genetic manipulation of personal traits; and scientific integrity (Harron et al., 1983). No aspect of health care has been left untouched by these controversies regarding values and rights of human life, issues about life and death, allocation of public funds for research and treatment, mandatory testing for HIV antibodies, informed consent, profits versus treatment, duty of health care workers to provide care, access of women, children, and minorities to involvement in research, honesty in research endeavors, and rights of patients to specify their own treatment course. Most of the topics were not unique to ethical controversy within the context of HIV/AIDS, but the nature of the illness and its affected population provided an urgency and intensity of debate not commonly encountered in debates before 1981. Walters (1988) cautions that beneficence, justice, and autonomy must all be considered important when public policy that governs society's response to AIDS is examined.

This debate has not been waged in "center ring" by experts who entertained an interested and passive audience in the wings. Not waiting for an invitation, patients and their families voiced their concerns, AIDS activists sat at the conference tables and refused to leave, and health care workers asked hard questions out of fear and concern. New partnerships were formed between clinicians and their patients. Streets became theaters where actors and activists engaged the media to take messages of right and wrong to the public; they defied churches as the source of moral right and demanded new answers to old questions. HIV/AIDS has made many contributions to health care and to the way moral issues are defined and debated.

Although the knowledge base of ethics continues to draw heavily from normative ethics and associated principles, such as autonomy or utility, other views have gained attention. This chapter describes the knowledge base of ethics: principles, rights, situation ethics, feminist ethics, and the ethics of caring. Ethical decision making will be presented after a discussion of these ethical approaches. Together, approaches to ethics and ethical decisions should guide clinicians in their deliberations of ethical problems and encourage reflective responses.

The chapter considers ethical issues within the following topics: HIV/AIDS and the workplace, managed care, access to treatment and care, deciding to accept or refuse treatments, and suicide and assisted dying. Case illustrations will clarify specific ethical problems or demonstrate the complexity of some dilemmas. A final section will consider research and ethics, with specific suggestions for research that is needed.

MAJOR ETHICAL APPROACHES

Moral reasoning, or ethics, is that body of philosophical knowledge that deals with moral human conduct. All people struggle to weigh right from wrong in a given situation. Our deliberations reflect personal values that provide a sense of the right way to behave in ordinary human interaction; as health care workers (HCWs) we learned these values from our families, our teachers, our religions, and our own experiences, observations, and judgments about what is right and wrong. These values form the basis of our personal and traditional codes of conduct.

The terms *ethics* and *moral reasoning* will be used interchangeably in this chapter to refer to a body of knowledge that has evolved from moral philosophy and applies analytical and critical approaches to moral problems and judgments (Beauchamp, 1994; Davis & Aroskar, 1991). Ethics invites a person to use reasoning rather than emotions in the process of forming judgments about what is right or wrong in the situation being considered. Table 13–1 defines terms that are important in ethical discussions.

Principles of Ethics

Normative ethics is applied ethics—i.e., the application of moral reasoning to determine which course of action is most acceptable. The two major theories that provide the basis of most moral reasoning are deontology and utilitarianism. Utilitarianism (also called teleology) gauges the worth of actions by assessing the short-term and long-term consequences of the actions for society. Deontology is concerned with duty and considers how actions are accomplished and not just their consequences. Whereas utilitarians assert that the principle of utility justifies the other principles of ethics, deontologists consider an array of principles, even if they cannot always specify which principle is most important. For example, when considering whether or not to tell a patient that she has terminal-phase lung cancer, the physician-deontologist would believe that telling the truth is most important whereas the physician-utilitarian would base the decision on the consequences of telling the truth versus concealing the prognosis.

To understand what is at stake in problem situations, such as keeping confidential a patient's plan of suicide, the HCW examines the principles most involved in the situation. This understanding will help point the way to actions that are morally correct in the situation, but individuals may perceive different principles as having priority in the situation, so controversy may exist. Table 13–2 presents a brief definition of principles and rules of ethics and provides an accessible, quick reference to these terms.

AUTONOMY. Perhaps the U.S. heritage of rugged individualism has contributed to the high value society places on self-regulation or the right to autonomous behavior. The autonomous person makes decisions and determines actions to follow after selecting a plan. A person is a free agent—free to choose actions that either benefit or harm the self without constraint from others. Being free to choose among alternatives is rele-

Table 13–1 ▪ Common Terms and Their Definitions

Table Term	Definition
Normative ethics	Application of moral reasoning to determine what ought to be done in a specific situation
Dilemma	Moral reasoning indicates choice between equally unappealing solutions
Rights	Justified claims that individuals/groups hold, i.e., their just due
Principle	Fundamental source of justification of judgements reached in situations
Rule	Specific guidelines to actions for ethical principles and values; professional codes contain rules
Value	What an individual feels is important that provides a basis for ethical decisions

Table 13–2 ▪ Definitions of Often Cited Principles and Rules of Ethics

Principle or Rule	Definition
Autonomy	Self-governance: the autonomous person determines his/her own course of action in accordance with a plan chosen by self, with the capacity to understand consequences of the action
Beneficence	Duty to help others further their important and legitimate interests
Justice	Fair distribution of benefits and burdens in society; justice requires a fair distribution of scarce resources, or a balance of claims and needs
Nonmaleficence	Duty to prevent harm, remove harm, and provide benefit
Utility	Balances benefits and harms and looks to the short-term and long-term consequences of the actions
Paternalism	Duty to act for another person, when qualified, when the action is for the other person's good and she or he is unable to act for self; used when autonomy is compromised
Confidentiality	A rule that imposes duties to not disclose certain information; person who discloses confidential information has the burden of proof to justify the conditions of disclosure
Fidelity	Loyalty between humans, often in the context of voluntary relationships
Sanctity of human life	Human life has an inherent value; a moderate interpretation is the usual practice, and this allows refusal of life-saving treatments
Truth telling or veracity	Duty to tell the truth and not lie

vant only when the choices are meaningful to the individual (Agich, 1990). However, not everyone qualifies to act as an autonomous agent. Those who cannot clearly understand the situation and the potential consequences of the chosen action are often termed "ineligible" to act as autonomous agents. This ineligibility may be temporary, such as when one's thinking is clouded by trauma or medications. In some cases, the ineligibility may be more durable, such as during childhood or when severe and enduring confusion prevents simple problem solving.

Because people are social beings, their individual actions occur within a social context, so effects of their actions on others and on their community must also be considered. Regard for others automatically implies that certain circumstances might warrant constraints on personal autonomy. For example, when the action can harm others, then arguments that constraints are justified are advanced.

Autonomy is an important principle in many health care situations. For example, autonomy is important when a HCW determines whether a person

1. Needs a guardian or conservator.
2. Can provide informed consent for a procedure.
3. Has the ability to refuse treatments.
4. Should have involuntary suicide-prevention interventions.

BENEFICENCE. The moral principle of beneficence calls forth the duty to provide benefit to others—that is, to help others when we are in a position to do so. Determining when doing good becomes a duty (moral obligation), rather than a commendable but not obligatory act (moral option), is difficult. Most ethicists recognize that there are limitations on the duty of people to take positive actions to promote good, but they debate how to decide the nature and degree of these limitations. Beauchamp (1994) argues that, in general, person A has a duty of beneficence toward person B when each of the following circumstances is present:

1. Person B is at significant risk of loss or damage.
2. Person A needs to act to prevent this loss.
3. Person A's action is likely to prevent loss or damage.
4. Person A incurs no significant risk in taking the action.
5. Person B will likely gain more than the potential harms to person A through action taken.

Beneficence is especially important in health care in

1. Assessing the HCW's or clinician's duty to provide care.
2. Informing others that they have been exposed to harmful substances or conditions.
3. Informing others that a person plans to harm them.

JUSTICE. The principle of justice is concerned with a fair distribution of society's burdens and benefits. Justice centers around deciding what should be distributed and what reasoning will guide those actions. Giving people their just due means, first of all, that a legitimate claim exists for the benefit being awarded; the benefit is not awarded to someone who does not deserve it, and those who deserve it receive their reward. This simple guideline still leaves room for argument about how that deserving claim should be established. Is a person deserving

1. Because of equal stature with others who have a claim?
2. Because he or she can establish a need for the benefit?
3. Because of the amount of work extended?
4. Because he or she has made significant contributions to society?
5. Because he or she is particularly meritorious (Beauchamp, 1994)?

For example, let us suppose that gene therapy is available for early HIV intervention. This therapy can effectively stop disease progression, but it is delivered through bone marrow transplant. How will we qualify people to receive this therapy? Who will not be allowed access to this treatment? Who will make the decision?

Distributive justice is important when the resource (material, procedure, etc.) is particularly scarce or costly, or when the competition is great, as for gene therapy or phenotyping. Another example involved Bob, a 30-year-old man who lived in the Northwest. Bob said his physician had informed him that he would die if he did not receive either a heart transplant or an artificial heart. He was also informed that he would not be given a high priority for either of these procedures because he did not have a family, was gay, and did not have insurance.

The principle of distributive justice informs public policy on the distribution of budget allocations among research, prevention, and treatment efforts. A less macro level of distributive justice in health care is determining which staff members will be assigned to specific patients, such as assignment of more experienced and competent staff to sicker or more prominent patients.

NONMALEFICENCE. The principle of nonmaleficence calls for preventing harm and undoing harm. This principle is not absolute, and ethicists recognize that temporary suffering might be inflicted to cause a subsequent remedy or to prevent worse harm. Inflicting harm, however, always requires a moral justification. Even a risk of harm is to be avoided if possible, and actions that carry with them potential harm should be considered carefully. Some ethicists restrict their interpretation of nonmaleficence to not inflicting harm while using the principle of beneficence broadly to include preventing harm and removing harm (Beauchamp, 1994). The principle of nonmaleficence is important in considering diverse issues such as assisted dying, implementing clinical trials of a new drug, or refusing to care for patients with AIDS.

UTILITY. The principle of utility examines the anticipated consequences of an action to judge its merit. This principle seeks actions that accomplish the greatest good for the largest number or the least harm for the greatest number. Utility, then, weighs benefits against harm in a situation and tries to determine actions that will maximize benefits while minimizing harm. An action that is perceived as being too harmful in its long-term or short-term consequences will be rejected.

Those whose ethical stances are guided by utilitarianism give greater weight to the principle of utility than do those whose ethical stances are guided by deontology, situation ethics, or some other ethical approach. Outside of utilitarianism, the principle of utility carries no greater or lesser weight than other ethical principles. As a principle, utility is one among many, not the supreme principle as used by utilitarians; i.e., it does not have greater priority than any other principle. The principle of utility does not always weigh the interest of society against the interests of an individual, but the ethicist or clinician may call on other principles (autonomy, beneficence, and nonmaleficence) in considering the interests of the individual.

The principle of utility is pivotal in examining the costs and benefits of any particular action. Costs are often considerations of financial consequences, whereas the term *risk* is used when the potential for human harm is being considered. The cost-benefit approach is important in the examinination of research proposals as well as considerations of public health measures, such as mandatory testing for HIV.

PATERNALISM. Paternalism involves acting on behalf of another person to prevent or restrict harm in circumstances in which the person is unable to act for himself or herself. If person A has person B's permission to act in that situation, then person A's behavior is not considered paternalistic. In paternalistic behavior, person A intends to look out for the good, general welfare of person B and cannot be self-serving. Paternalism *always* needs to be justified because it always violates an existing moral rule. Typically, the justification for paternalistic action arises because person B is perceived as being unable to act for himself or herself—because something compromises person B's autonomy. Paternalism is important in the durable power of attorney or conservatorship where person B, who has the legal right to act, may not always know what person A would have wanted in particular situations that arise.

TRUTH TELLING. The duty to tell the truth seems to be a simple and clear responsibility appropriately associated with a morally right action. Is this duty unconditional? Or are there instances in which telling the truth could be harmful to others? Telling the truth is sometimes confused with how the truth is told. For example, it has been argued that telling someone that he or she has a terminal illness, such as end-stage cancer or AIDS, takes hope away from the person, so telling only a "partial truth" has been advocated. E.H. Shneidman (personal communication, 1980), on the other hand, has pointed out that this argument (removal of hope) has been offered to protect the teller more than the patient, and he advocates that physicians, nurses, and other health care workers be taught how to be attentive to "what to tell whom, under what circumstances,

and to what end." Shneidman explained that the truth should not be used as a weapon of attack but should be delivered with sensitivity to what the person could manage and use at the time, and perhaps continued another day when the person was ready to hear and use more information.

Shneidman, unlike Collins (1981) and his paternalistic stance, did not advocate withholding truth from patients for their own good. Both withholding truth and telling such a partial truth that meaning is distorted are considered tantamount to lying, and both are common practices between physicians, nurses, or other HCWs and their patients. Consider the patient who has said on many occasions, "When I progress to AIDS, I will kill myself, rather than witness my own costly deterioration." Will the truth of his diagnosis of AIDS do more harm than good? Specifically, will the truth trigger a premature death through suicide or cause this man to end his life saddened and without hope?

Whereas many people agree that truth telling is not an absolute duty (i.e., a duty without any constraints), fewer people agree on the criteria for determining when truth telling can be or would be harmful. First of all, the nature of truth is not always clearly agreed upon, especially in the context of illness and its treatment. Second, predicting an individual's response to specific information is not a science, and many would argue that, as an art form, it is fairly primitive.

A different arena for considering issues and problems associated with truth telling has been labeled *whistle-blowing*. Whistle-blowing refers to making public another's unethical or illegal practices and often pits an individual against a corporation or a government agency. Telling the truth in these situations also has overtones of disloyalty to those being accused of unethical or illegal practices. The whistle-blower often has much to risk, such as job loss and personal credibility, in coming forward with the truth.

In health care, truth telling involves decisions about delivering bad news to patients or their families. Another issue in truth telling in health care has involved informing the patient or research study participant of risks involved with specific procedures or medication.

CONFIDENTIALITY. The rule of confidentiality imposes a duty on specific persons to not disclose certain information. There is an issue of privilege between the person and the information; for example, HCWs are privileged to have certain information about patients in order to deliver effective care, and they are responsible for safeguarding that information to assure that it does not go to unprivileged persons. Confidentiality is a duty to the person and is not assigned to the information itself outside of the person or persons who hold the information. For example, the HCW has confidential information about the results of John's HIV test. The slip of paper with that information blows out of the HCW's car window and is retrieved by another person, Belinda. Belinda, who knows John socially, does not necessarily have a duty of confidentiality to John. HCWs who discuss their patients in public places, such as the cafeteria, elevator, or bus, risk violating their duty to hold privileged information in confidence.

Nurses, physicians, and other health care workers have a responsibility to keep the patient's information private, but there are times when keeping information confidential could pose risks for others and the staff's duty to keep information confidential is in conflict with the duty to protect others. For example, in the 14 months since James's diagnosis of AIDS, he had been in and out of hospitals and was again an inpatient. His condition was steadily deteriorating. James had been divorced for 4 years, and he had two children (7 and 6 years of age) whom he saw often. He and his former wife were friendly. Only his wife knew that he was gay. His parents live in the city and they visit often. All the family believe that James has leukemia. James has refused to tell his wife that he has AIDS. Staff members are uncertain about what they should do—whether they should maintain James's privacy or whether they should respect James's former wife and the right of the former gay lover to know of exposure to HIV infection.

FIDELITY. Fidelity is the duty to keep an agreement or a promise. This rule is important in considering agreements not only between HCWs and their patients but also between HCWs and their employers. For example, fidelity is broken in a situation in which the employer learns that an employee has tested positive for HIV antibodies and terminates that employee solely because he or she

is HIV-positive. HCWs undermine the patient's confidence in their care when they promise something they cannot or do not deliver, such as returning promptly with requested pain medicine.

SANCTITY OF LIFE. Sanctity of life, also referred to as respect for life, holds the view that there is an intrinsic value to life and that each person is valuable and unique (The Hastings Center, 1987). A strong commitment to sanctity of life would give priority to this over other duties. If sanctity of life were valued absolutely over all other values, then patients or clients could not refuse lifesaving treatments and suicide would never be an acceptable option. In a society where sanctity of life was an absolute duty, then the most abhorrent crime would be a crime in which a life was taken and capital punishment would be unthinkable. In most societies, sanctity of life is not held to such a rigid standard. The strongest view of sanctity of life is a religious conviction that life is sacred and that therefore individuals may not dispose of it as they choose. Even this view allows persons in life-threatening circumstances to refuse treatment that would save their lives but does not allow them to commit suicide.

Today, we honor the individual's right to use or to forego life-sustaining treatment. Less agreement exists on the circumstances, if any, under which a person has a right to deliberately seek personal death by his or her own independent actions or with the active assistance of another person. Sanctity of life is a major consideration in shaping these judgments. The moral argument about the circumstances that allow or forbid a person to deliberately seek personal death often turns on interpreting sanctity of life as length of life versus quality of life (Daly et al., 1997).

SITUATION ETHICS. Proponents of situation ethics reject ethical rules that are applied to situations. Instead, they look to the situation for moral action guides and deny that any guide to decision making can be universally applied. Rules and guides for past actions provide examples of how similar situations have been handled in the past, but they do not impose an obligation for the person to act in a similar way in the current situation. For example, one nurse addressed the issue of when suicide is acceptable by asserting, "It depends on each case. There are no rules for when suicide is acceptable. You must judge each situation on its own merits" (Valente et al., 1993).

In considering the merits of situation ethics, one has to ask whether any moral rules are absolute and universal. Beauchamp (1994) offers several examples of rules that might be absolute and, if they are correct, would therefore preclude the usefulness of situation ethics: (1) be a caring physician and (2) avoid murder, when murder is defined as unjustified killing. Even these situations cannot always command agreement about actions that constitute caring or circumstances that do or do not justify killing. Situation ethics has not gained strong support as an approach to ethical knowledge.

Rights and Responsibilities

Discussions of ethics often include assertions of individual and group rights, e.g., all humans have a right to respect, he has a right to voice his own opinion, or her right to privacy is greater than his right to know. Many times these discussions reflect strong feelings but may not reflect positions that have been thoughtfully considered. Sometimes, when discussions surrounding moral rights cannot be resolved easily, people turn to legal experts for guidance; yet the two types of rights are not the same. Curtin and Flaherty (1982, p. 4) define a human right as "a person's just due." Other ethicists have asserted that there are no universally accepted human rights (Beauchamp, 1994). Nonetheless, this language—the language of rights—persists and has proved useful in the examination of some ethical issues. Beauchamp (1994) speaks of a moral right as a claim that is justified by ethical principles and rules and points out that rights can be either negative or positive (i.e., one can have the right to something or the right to refuse something). Not all claims will be considered a moral right, and it can be difficult to establish whether or not a claim is truly a moral claim. Determining whether this is a moral claim instead of a want may influence how responsibility to respond to that claim is assigned.

When someone has a claim, or a right, to a form of conduct, a parallel responsibility or obligation is usually inferred. For example, if everyone has a moral right to health care, then who has the responsibility or duty to provide access to that care? For example, if patients have a right to privacy, then HCWs have a responsibility for protecting patient confidentiality. The ethical codes of some health care professionals charge them with this obligation to their patients (Brown, 1987). Other claims cannot be linked so easily with obligations; nor can responsibility be attached so easily to specific groups or individuals. When there is a shared belief of a moral right (e.g., rights of citizens and legal immigrants to immunizations) and a moral responsibility (e.g., various levels of government), disagreement about practical and political means may block implementation of a program to deliver the service that satisfies the rights and responsibilities.

Because all individuals and groups have some rights, these rights will compete or conflict with each other on some occasions. HCWs have a right to pursue their own religious beliefs; however, even though these beliefs may condemn the lifestyles of some of their patients, these patients also have a right to respect. In other instances, HCWs may find their values in conflict with circumstances in the work setting. For example, HCWs have the right to adequate resources to deliver safe care for themselves and their patients and may disagree with their employers about what resources are adequate for accomplishing this. For example, trauma nurses may believe that their work requires puncture-resistant gloves for adequate protection. The hospital administration may believe that the added margin of safety is too small to warrant such a large increase in costs for the gloves. Typically, most HCWs learn more about their responsibilities than they learn about their rights as HCWs. Even when there is a shared belief in a moral right, such as a right to health care, and a moral responsibility, as at various levels of government, disagreement about practical and political means may block implementation.

Level of knowledge and society's attitudes may shape how individual rights, personal and professional responsibilities, and public health practices are enacted to balance individual rights with the public good. Bayer (1994) discussed how advances in technology of detection, treatment methods, and access to therapeutic resources have shifted HIV care from voluntary stances that favored individual rights to mandatory stances that favor the public good.

Curtin (1990) described health care as a moral art that encompasses professional obligations derived from the covenant that it has with the public to provide care and to improve quality of life among those seeking health care. Meeting this covenant requires HCWs to be proactive and involves both individual and collective obligations.

Ethics of Caring and Feminist Ethics

As interest in moral reasoning has strengthened during the recent decades, concerns have also surfaced about the adequacy of ethical principles in guiding our understanding and responses to current problems. Gilligan's (1982) study of female moral development and reasoning helped to focus the criticism that principle-based current approaches to moral reasoning devalued relationship issues while overemphasizing logic. Noddings (1984) developed an ethics of caring ideal that emphasized relationship (how we meet each other morally) and human affect and rejected the universality of principle-based ethics. In ethics of caring, one does not assess a situation by considering autonomy, beneficence, and justice; instead, one considers commitment, reciprocity, grasping the other's reality, and self-maintenance. Others have added to our understanding of the concept of caring, our knowledge of caring as an ethical model, and the relationship between caring and practice (Benner & Wrubel, 1989; Bishop & Scudder, 1987; Condon, 1992; Dunlop, 1994; Hallorsdottir, 1997; Neil & Watts, 1991; Northrup, 1993; Watson, 1985, Woods, 1989).

Questions about caring as an ethical ideal to help us interact effectively with ethical problems have emerged. Hoagland (1991) argued that Nodding's (1984) formulation of caring does not allow an adequate analysis of oppression and does not support a vision of change.

Women's experiences with oppression, indifference, and hostility parallel the experiences of those with HIV infection. Because of these experiences, feminist ethicists criticize traditional ethical approaches as being ineffective in addressing such oppression (Card, 1994). Jaggar (1991) asserted that feminist ethics ensure that the moral experiences of men and women are regarded respectfully. Jaggar (1991) also set the agenda of feminist ethics as examining issues such as domination, control, domestic and international inequities, gender privilege, public and private realms, and the actual as well as the hypothetical.

Both ethics of caring and feminist ethics move from the universal to the contextual and both place a priority on understanding and preventing domination. These emerging ethical approaches may provide insights and useful new formulations of moral action.

RESOLVING ETHICAL DILEMMAS

HCWs confront ethical problems each day in their personal and professional lives, and they recognize that definitions of principles will not, by themselves, be sufficient for ethical problem solving. An ethical problem or dilemma occurs when the HCW is aware of a conflict among competing rights, such as

1. The patient is seeking assistance in deciding the "right" course of action.
2. Staff members disagree about the right actions.
3. The patient and family want one course of action, whereas the staff advocates another.
4. Conflict exists among legally sanctioned family members and life partners or friends who are close enough to be considered family about the best course of action for a patient who cannot make decisions for himself or herself.

Many resources exist to help people resolve these conflict situations: available literature, specialists (such as ethicists), or ethics committees at a hospital or organizational level. Legal solutions to ethics problems are not always satisfactory resolutions, since legal actions are rooted in different traditions than are ethical concerns; i.e., what is legally sanctioned is not always right. For example, unlike the laws of most states, California law permits coroners to harvest corneas without the permission or knowledge of families of the person who died. Reports have indicated that the Los Angeles Coroner's Department has established a common practice of not seeking family permission to remove the cornea, even when the family is easily accessible (Harvest of Corneas at Morgue Questioned, Nov. 2, 1997). Although these practices are legally sanctioned in California, purposely bypassing the family for this decision is simply not a good or just practice.

Resources to Help in Formulating Actions

ETHICS COMMITTEES. Some hospitals, long-term agencies, and ambulatory care resources have formed interdisciplinary ethics committees to assist staff, patients, and families in deciding actions for ethical problems and dilemmas (Albrizio et al., 1992; American Hospital Association, 1985; Bandman & Bandman, 1995; Schultz & Moore, 1993; and Stoll & Mason, 1993). If your agency or organization does not have a resource (such as an ethicist or an ethics committee), you may want to explore the possibility of establishing one. Exploring various options helps you choose the type of resource that best matches your own agency. One of the most comprehensive ethics programs is at Mt. Sinai Hospital in New York City and includes the following features: a full-time ethicist; an ethics committee; monthly ethics seminars; regularly scheduled meetings between the AIDS center clinicians and the ethicist; and inclusion of ethics in grand rounds on AIDS (Stoll & Mason, 1993). Most resources are less extensive but include an educational program on ethics for staff and routine meetings to discuss ethical concerns that arise in the care of patients with HIV disease.

OTHER RESOURCES. Professional organizations at both the national and state levels address topics that concern HCWs as they respond to clinical issues of ethics and human rights. Several professional organizations have established ethics committees and may offer members direct consultation for ethical problems. Some have published position papers on common ethical problems that HCWs encounter. Organizations also have published position statements or papers to guide HCWs in their care of persons affected by HIV disease or who are struggling with issues of assisted dying (American Hospital Association, 1985; American Nurses Association, 1992; CDC, 1991, 1993; Young et al., 1997).

Models of Ethical Decision Making

Cameron (1993) described the model of decision making for ethical problems that people living with AIDS used. This three-step model included the following three questions:

1. What should I believe?
2. Who should I be?
3. What should I do?

Most HCWs use models based on principles to formulate action plans and to resolve clinical dilemmas. These models include the following steps (Aroskar, 1980; Curtin, 1978; Winters et al., 1993):

1. Describe the situation, including who was involved (and what were their roles), when the major events occurred, and the setting(s).
2. What ethical principles (values, rules, etc.) are involved?
3. What solutions are proposed, and what are the solutions trying to accomplish?
4. What alternative actions are available?
5. What are the possible outcomes of these actions, including identification of how moral principles would be affected?

Gadow (1990) recommended that a decision-making model be based on advocacy, where advocacy is directed toward assisting patients in their own actions and not in doing for them. This decision-making model is more accurately described as advocacy for patient autonomy. The decision-making process includes the following five steps:

1. Assessing the patient's ability for self-determination
2. Determining the nature of the HCW-patient relationship
3. Disclosing the HCW's views on the situation
4. Determining the patient's values
5. Other, individual values that have an impact on the patient in considering the situation

This decision-making model emerges from autonomy and focuses on the individual in context, similar to the ethics of caring.

Most groups develop operating rules to facilitate their discussions. Often the first rule is aimed at reducing pressure on individuals to arrive at a consensus. Operating rules will encourage disagreements to surface and be heard. At the same time, operating rules will encourage individuals to examine consequences of their own proposed actions while also hearing others' concerns. As the groups examine specific problems, they often discover unresolved clinical issues rather than ethical problems or dilemmas.

CHOOSING TO ACCEPT OR REFUSE TREATMENTS

Although making choices about medical treatment has grown more complex each year, the right of the individual to choose an unpopular or harmful procedure has grown more acceptable. Freedom of choice remains so highly valued in American society that autonomy seems to be the cornerstone principle against which other principles are measured. Conflict is most apparent in examining consequences of harmful choices (autonomy versus utility), when one person's autonomy negatively affects another or when one person's autonomy interferes with another's rights and responsibilities. Determining whether a person can act autonomously is challenging when that person has an intermittent diminished capacity demonstrated by forgetfulness, a short attention span, confusion, or disorientation. Agich (1990) cautions that respecting autonomy in long-term care of chronically ill and elderly patients means offering meaningful options from a limited array of actions. Giving the appearance of autonomous choice when the available choices are not meaningful to the person has received scant attention in ethics. For example, offering a choice between care in a skilled nursing facility or a residential care setting will not be acceptable to the person who is adamant about continuing to live in his or her own home. Finally, what is the HCW's role in advising patients about their choices? These issues will be discussed under the following headings: (1) accepting and refusing recommended treatments; (2) gaining access to treatments; (3) determining the staff's role in patient choice.

Accepting and Refusing Recommended Treatments

Usually, patients are free to accept or to refuse those medical treatments recommended by their physicians and other health care staff. The person's right to determine whether treatments match personal values does not necessarily cease when that person is no longer able to choose. For example, advance directives and durable power of attorney are two procedures that solicit choice from the able person in anticipation that she or he might not always remain able. These directives allow the person to make personal preferences known.

Ideally, the patient, without constraint, chooses options in partnership with the physician and nurse, who share their expert knowledge with the patient and who know the patient as a person.

Conflicts arise because many situations fall outside this ideal situation and force caregivers to struggle with conditions that limit autonomy.

Gaining Access to Treatments

Example Jake believed that once a problem emerged and had been identified as "serious," he should fight it vigorously. He firmly believed that this attitude had been instrumental in keeping him alive during the 14 years since he become HIV-positive in 1978. It was not surprising, then, after Jake had 10 to 15 Kaposi sarcoma lesions, that he asked his physicians to treat them with radiation. All his lesions were visible, with several on his face, and Jake had noticed people staring at him when he was standing in line at the grocery store. Jake kept himself well informed and was aware of the possibility of developing internal lesions that were more difficult to detect and treat. He was surprised when his physician refused to treat the Kaposi's because "You don't meet the protocol criteria [note: hospital treatment protocol, not a research protocol]. When you develop many more lesions, or when they have coalesced, we can treat you." Jake persisted and finally issued an ultimatum: "Either you treat the Kaposi's, or you stop all treatment." His physician, a resident, consulted with the staff physician, who had known Jake longer and who was aware of Jake's treatment philosophy, and she helped to convince the resident to make an exception so that Jake could be treated.

Issues Related to Example HCWs are not required to prescribe or participate in treatments that they believe will be harmful or ineffective. The physician or nurse has many issues to consider in responding to a patient's request. One issue is the patient's challenge of the stance that the HCW is the expert and should know what is best for him or her. Another issue is consideration of the consequences of participating in an activity perceived as ineffective or harmful. The nurse and the physician might participate in a treatment that is judged harmful so that they can provide safety by monitoring for adverse effects. Preserving a long-standing and effective relationship with the patient might be another consequence that influences a decision to participate, and this seemed to be a major consideration in making radiation treatment available to Jake earlier in the course of Kaposi's sarcoma than was customary. Another issue is recognizing that quality of life is a subjective judgment, and quality-of-life concerns might convince staff members to participate in treatments that they otherwise would refuse; this was a concern in Jake's situation, in which he felt embarrassed when he carried out activities of daily living, such as grocery shopping, because people stared at his Kaposi lesions.

The balance of power and control within a patient-HCW relationship is a dynamic force that varies according to the issue being considered and the resources of the persons involved. The HCW will exert more control when safety and ethical wrongdoing are perceived but can afford to soften influence when less is at stake in the situation. When quality-of-life issues are prominent in the situation, the power and control might be shifted to the patient.

Determining the Staff's Role in Patient Choice

In Gadow's (1990) model of ethics and decision making, the HCW is an active participant and the HCW's view of the situation is offered to patients for them to use in choosing their course of action. To be an effective partner to the patient, the HCW may need to learn about treatment choices outside the usual scope of practice, such as alternative therapies, e.g., qi gong or acupuncture (Cohen & Doner, 1996). This is a major departure from the typical practice of trying to present information objectively to patients, and with the perspective that the HCW is always the expert, Gadow (1990) has stated that her recommendation is based on autonomy as pivotal in health care action. In some situations the duty of HCWs to protect patients may necessitate actions that seem to limit patient autonomy.

Example Rosa and her husband, Claude, had used drugs throughout their 3 years of marriage when Claude was found to have AIDS. He died within a few weeks of the diagnosis, and Rosa found herself both widowed and pregnant. She already had two other young children. She agreed to be tested and was found to be HIV-positive. She entered a drug rehabilitation program and has been clean and sober for 2½ years. She is proud of being a good mother to her three healthy children, despite the challenges of her failing health, severe fatigue, and repeated episodes of infections. On her last visit, the home health nurse was distressed about Rosa's deteriorated condition and questioned whether Rosa was able to provide a safe environment for her children. The nurse wondered whether to initiate proceedings to have the children placed in foster care. The home health nurse had not discussed her concerns and recommendations with Rosa, as she wanted consultation from her team first.

Issues Related to This Example The nurse acted out of beneficence. Aware that Rosa neglected her own needs to provide what her children needed, the nurse was concerned with protecting both Rosa and the children. A major issue in the team discussion was Rosa's capacity to make informed decisions herself, since problems with her attention span and forgetfulness were great. The team also considered the importance to Rosa of being a good parent and the excellent relationship she had with her children.

The team finally decided on the following plan of care:

1. The physician would initiate a neurobehavioral assessment of Rosa.
2. The home health aid would be increased to 5 days per week.
3. The social worker would work with Rosa to see whether she had family or friends who could help her with shopping and during evenings and weekends.
4. The nurse would encourage Rosa to start planning for the placement for her children once she became too sick.
5. The nurse would help Rosa keep an energy log to allocate her limited energy to activities that mattered to her.

What had seemed initially to be a recommendation for paternalistic action from staff revealed a complex situation requiring actions that attended to both clinical and ethical domains. The final plan tried to include meaningful options for Rosa and her children.

THE HEALTH CARE AND WORK SETTING AND HIV/AIDS

For many HCWs, the workplace not only provides a source of income necessary for personal and family needs but also reinforces our self-perceptions and our worth. For HCWs who are HIV-infected, the workplace and the setting of health care are fused into one. At work we do not have free choice of colleagues or of activities. We have expectations of our workplace—expectations that we will be able to work in an environment of mutual respect with adequate resources to complete our tasks. We expect to work within a safe environment, just as patients expect to receive their care in a healthful and safe environment. Patients also have the right to receive care without undue worry that they might be the source of infection to their health care providers; patients can expect that our everyday practices provide mutual safeguards for the HCWs and their patients.

Health care settings have all the expectations and obligations of other types of work settings; in addition, they are expected to be safe for all and healing environments for patients. The public expects those who work in health care settings to provide an environment in which fears can be stilled, not intensified, and in which illness can be cured, not contracted.

The ethical issues surrounding HIV and the workplace encompass questions of how to establish and maintain a safe environment for patients and HCWs and of how to safeguard rights when the rights of nurses and other HCWs conflict with patient rights. Addressing these issues encompasses the scope of ethical knowledge and pits clinical knowledge against public fears and concerns. This discussion of HIV and the workplace is organized around protection of HCWs, protection of patients, other work setting ethical issues, and managed care. Increasingly, the setting for health care involves managed care. The setting of managed care offers elements that are advantageous and elements that are problematic for HIV/AIDS.

Protecting Healthcare Workers

Example In 1985, Barbara Fassbinder, RN, was on duty in the emergency room of a small Wisconsin hospital when a patient was brought in by two people who did not seem to know the patient very well. The patient was in acute distress and soon went into respiratory arrest. During the unsuccessful attempt to resuscitate the patient, Ms. Fassbinder disconnected an arterial line and held a pressure bandage in place for 10 minutes. She noticed blood on her finger and wiped it away, but it was about 45 minutes before she was free to wash her hands. Neither she nor other staff members wore gloves during this procedure because they were not performing sterile procedures and the urgency of the situation had not allowed time for staff members to put on clean gloves for self-protection. A few months later, Ms. Fassbinder was confirmed as the first HCW to have a work-related HIV infection that was not secondary to a percutaneous exposure (Fassbinder, 1993).

Scope of Risk of HIV Infection to HCWs in Hospitals

By June 1996, the CDC had reported a total of 51 documented cases of occupational HIV transmission (CDC, 1996). The risk rate for nonpercutaneous exposures, such as Ms. Fassbinder's, is lower than the risk rate for needle-stick exposures. Although the risks are small, the stakes are high because the disease is life-threatening, and it is these stakes that have fueled HCWs' fears. Combination therapy and a recommended change in protocol that calls for antiviral therapy to be initiated within hours of exposure have the potential to reduce the risk per exposure to almost zero (Porche, 1997).

ETHICAL ISSUES. The health care agency has a responsibility to provide its employees with a reasonably safe work environment that includes access to adequate equipment and supplies for nurses to use in barrier precautions. This responsibility has the weight of law, as the Occupational Safety and Health Administration (OSHA) requires health care settings to implement universal precautions and to provide infection-control plans along with personal protective equipment, worker training, and postexposure follow-up (Porche, 1997; U.S. Office of Technology Assessment, 1992).

During the first decade of the AIDS epidemic, the types of exposure that posed risk of HIV infection in the workplace were well documented. Universal precautions and safe management of "sharps" provided adequate protection to HCWs. It is the HCW's responsibility to be aware of this body of knowledge and to apply reasonable precautions to situations. For example, hepatitis is much easier to contract after exposure than is HIV and a vaccine is available to protect HCWs from hepatitis A and B, but many HCWs fail to be vaccinated.

HCWs must use reasonable precautions to protect themselves as they provide care to patients. To determine precautions needed, the HCW has to assess the circumstances of the HCW–patient care situation. For example, although HIV can be contracted only if the virus enters the bloodstream of the HCW, tuberculosis is spread through droplets from sneezes and coughs. Since persons with AIDS have a very high incidence of tuberculosis and hepatitis, HCWs need to use adequate barriers to protect themselves and other patients from AIDS, tuberculosis, hepatitis, and other infectious illnesses. The health professional's general moral responsibility is to provide knowledge-based care and to take responsibility for his or her own judgments and actions.

TESTING OF PATIENTS IN ACUTE-CARE SETTINGS. A practice with popular support is not necessarily a morally supportable practice. The Oncology Nursing Society's Position Paper on HIV-Related Issues (Halloran et al., 1988, p. 214) stated: "Before there can be restriction of an individual's autonomy, it must be demonstrated that such restrictions will result in an overriding benefit to the cause of a larger societal good." The CDC (1993) has recommended that voluntary, confidential testing be offered to patients and cautioned that testing was not a substitute for universal precautions and other infection-control programs. Their recommendations emphasized conditions of voluntary testing that had been identified by Walters (1988):

1. Counseling to help people understand the test results
2. Establishment of an environment of nondiscrimination
3. Protection of the confidentiality of test results

While HCWs' risk of infection from patients is minimal, it is greater than the risk patients have of becoming infected from their HCWs. Clinicians have a right to safety, so they must have access to the protective devices (masks, gloves, gowns, soap) needed for their own safety and to reassure their HIV-infected patients that HCWs have the resources they need to provide mutual protection. Clinicians must exercise adequate professional judgment about the protection required for the specific situation.

TESTING OF WOMEN OF CHILDBEARING AGE OR OF NEWBORN INFANTS. The rapid increase of HIV/AIDS among women and the demonstration of the effectiveness of AZT in preventing vertical transmission to infants in a placebo-controlled, clinical trial have raised the clinical stakes in access to care for women and their children and in pitting women's rights against those of their babies. The U.S. Public Health Service has recommended routine HIV counseling and voluntary testing for all pregnant women (MMWR, 1995). When pregnant women comply with the recommendations of testing and medical treatment with AZT, ethical issues are less apparent. Some clinicians have recommended mandatory screening of pregnant women for HIV (Wilfert, 1994) or of high-risk babies, regardless of mater-

nal consent (Bhushan & Cushman, 1995). Treatment with AZT is the standard for reducing perinatal transmission. If the pregnant woman has been treated with combination therapy that should not be interrupted, the clinician may still advise that therapy be discontinued in favor of AZT with the health of the infant in mind and without evidence of the potential harm to the pregnant woman. Sacrificing the rights of women in favor of their unborn children through mandatory universal screening of pregnant women for HIV infection is justified by some because they believe this would result in enormous overall savings for the health care system (Wilfert, 1994). Mandatory screening of pregnant women or high-risk babies for HIV infection is simply the first step toward mandatory treatment with AZT, the only protocol tested so far. The long-range consequences of treating women with AZT as a single drug, even if combination therapy might be called for clinically, have not been addressed; for this reason, many clinicians report that they decide on treatment appropriate for the woman despite the limited recommendations of the CDC. Dumois (1993) argued elegantly about the dangers to women and their babies if mandatory, routine testing is initiated for infants. These dangers included denial of privacy to women, increased harm to women, potential harm to infants from denial of treatments, and lack of established benefits to infants for proposed early intervention. Some authors, however, have called for a shift in policy that has emerged from a consideration of individual rights to policies and practices that emphasize a more traditional stance of protecting common interests (Bayer, 1994; Tuohey, 1995).

Protecting Patients in Health Care Settings

Example Bob is an obstetrician/gynecologist who shares a practice with six other physicians. His practice is varied and includes occasional gynecologic surgery. His colleagues and his patients have been aware of his homosexuality. When Bob learned that he was HIV-positive, he told his colleagues but not his patients. He developed *Pneumocystis carinii* pneumonia, responded well to treatment, and soon felt well enough to resume practice. While Bob was ill his colleagues met and decided that it was not wise for him to resume practice unless he limited his activities and obtained an informed consent from his patients. Bob disagreed, saying that he had a right to privacy, that he posed no danger to his patients, and that his partners were being unreasonable and greedy.

Should any constraints be placed on Bob's activities? Which activities should he continue, and which should he curtail or stop? Should he obtain informed consent from his patients? If this is justified in Bob's case, is it justified for all HCWs? Who should decide these issues, since Bob and his partners all have something to gain or lose with almost any decision made?

Scope of Risk of HIV Infection for Patients.

Before 1985, when routine screening of all blood donations was introduced, patients' main risk of HIV infection in health care settings was from blood transfusions. Studies have confirmed that the risks of patients being infected with HIV from health care workers are very low (CDC, 1993; El-Mallakh, Simmons, Forman, & D'Souza, 1993; Lo & Steinbrook, 1992; The U.S. Office of Technology Assessment, 1992). Despite the low risk of patient infection from their HIV-positive HCWs, public and political action has been noteworthy through media coverage, bills introduced in Congress, and recommendations about HCW-patient contacts from government agencies. Many nurses and physicians agree with the general public that patients' risk of infection from HIV-positive HCWs justifies mandatory testing of HCWs, contrary to scientific recommendations (Colombotos et al., 1991).

These two perspectives place respect for HCW autonomy in conflict with the patient's right to be protected from infected HCWs (El-Mallakh et al, 1993). The nature of the contract that physicians and nurses have with their patients requires them to promote well-being among their patients and to prevent their patients from harm. Fear of infection might prevent some patients from seeking care or from using recommended remedies, such as surgery, if they cannot trust their physicians and nurses to be safe. Still, compulsory testing of all HCWs would be too expensive for the small margin of safety that might conceivably be added.

CDC's current recommendations for voluntary testing and minimal restrictions on HCW activity that involves exposure-prone invasive procedures represent a compromise between recognition of differential risk assessment, political expediency, awareness of public fear, and respect for HCWs' autonomy (Lo & Steinbrook,

1992). The principle of nonmaleficence supports voluntary HIV testing and restriction of exposure-prone invasive activities to protect patients from harm. An exposure-prone activity presents a risk of percutaneous HCW injury that is likely to bring the HCW's blood in contact with the patient's body cavities, subcutaneous tissues, or mucous membranes, such as the use of fingers or a sharp object in a confined or poorly visualized site (Lo & Steinbrook, 1991). The recommendations of the CDC do not include any other restrictions on professional practice. All HCWs who perform invasive procedures are advised to know their HIV status and to seek counsel from expert panels about clinical activities (The U.S. Office of Technology Assessment, 1992). Some HCWs are less likely than physicians, under current guidelines, to be in a position where their autonomy and right to privacy are in conflict with activities required to protect patients (Table 13–3).

Other Ethical Issues in the Work Setting

When hospitals curtail the hiring of unmarried male HCWs as a method of reducing the possibility of hiring HIV-positive staff members, they engage in unethical and unacceptable discrimination against a group. What are the ethical issues, if any, involved in having an HIV-infected HCW staff? Specific problems identified have included the following:

1. Public fear that they may be infected if they receive care at hospitals, clinics, long-term care facilities, or home care agencies that employ HIV-positive staff may lead patients to seek care elsewhere.
2. Group insurance rates are increased by a small number of staff members who use their insurance at a much higher rate than other employees.
3. HIV-infected nurses cannot carry a full workload, so work is distributed unevenly.

These problems have in common an economic concern that is rooted in fear more than in ethical concerns. Staff members with HIV/AIDS should not be treated differently from staff members with other chronic, life-threatening illness in terms of using insurance benefits appropriately to access health care that is covered in the insurance policies. The Americans With Disabilities Act protects people from job denial or loss because of

Table 13–3 ▪ Preventing HIV Transmission in Health Care Settings

National Commission on AIDS	CDC Recommendations
Universal precautions	Universal precautions
Improve infection control, including equipment	HCWs who do not perform invasive procedures should not limit clinical activity
Monitoring and education regarding OSHA regulations	HCWs who perform exposure-prone procedures should know HIV status
Acknowledge public fears and address them without allowing rational judgment to be overwhelmed	HIV-positive HCWs who perform exposure-prone procedures should seek counsel from an expert review panel on these activities
Use least restrictive alternatives to reduce/eliminate risk of HIV infection for patients/HCWs	
No mandatory HCW testing for HIV	No mandatory HCW testing for HIV

Adapted from National Commission on AIDS. (1993). *AIDS: An expanding tragedy.* The Final Report of the National Commission on AIDS. Washington, DC: Author.

their disability, such as HIV infection, but extending hospital privileges to physicians is not included in this act. Barbara Fassbinder (1993) reported that she was reassigned to "paper-shuffling tasks" after she contracted HIV infection on the job, and she advocated that nurses get involved with their own agencies to determine the policies already in place to protect HIV-infected HCWs or to initiate needed policies.

With the success of combination therapy and protease inhibitors, some HCWs who had been on disability leave are now healthy enough to resume work. The decision to give up one's disability status to return to work is as complex and anxiety-provoking as was the earlier decision to stop working and to apply for disability. Employers also may be wary of hiring staff members who are trying to exit from their disability status.

MANAGED CARE. The shift from retrospective payment for health care to prospective payment was given a major boost in 1983 when Medicare began paying hospitals on the basis of a prospectively established rate (Davis, 1984). Managed care has led to many changes in health care: formation of patient-HCW partnerships, limitations in patient choices of primary care provider, controlled patient access to designated specialists, increased emphasis on health maintenance and disease prevention, integration of care across the continuum of health care resources from acute care settings to home care settings, and an increased diversity of HCWs who are primary care

providers. Central to managed care are HCWs who function as case managers and HCWs who form a collective organization to function as an integrated network of health care providers.

Ethical problems can arise in managed care settings because the parent organization or insurance company, in order to contain costs, restricts the HCW's ability to use diagnostic tests or specific treatments appropriate to the patient. Case management is defined as a process that augments and coordinates existing care systems from a client-centered perspective (AHCPR, 1994). This definition is broad and does not provide a clear set of expectations for how the role should be enacted or what outcomes are expected (Sowell, 1995). Conflicts sometimes arise because the case manager acts as an advocate for the patient while also serving as a gatekeeper for services from the employing agency (Browdie, 1992). Many primary care providers do not have the expertise or access to knowledge about rapidly changing standards of care for patients with HIV disease; yet managed care is organized around the primary care provider as the major decision maker and organizer of care. Saulo and Wagener (1996) have recommended that case managers use ethical principles, values, and mediation in resolving ethical conflicts.

ACCESS TO CARE

Access to care involves several important dimensions that blend together into an integrated mosaic:

1. Health care facilities and workers must be willing to provide care for people with HIV/AIDS.
2. Individuals must have means to pay for their health care, such as medical insurance, independent wealth, or government funds.
3. Health care resources must exist to care for HIV/AIDS patients in rural or urban areas locally and abroad.
4. Health care must meet minimal standards for competence and quality for managing acute episodes and monitoring the course of illness and palliative care.
5. The nature of the health care delivery system, such as managed care, must provide a context conducive to care.

Standards should demand the delivery of care that is culturally sensitive to the populations being served. Eliason (1993) points out that ethical health care practice requires that the culture and beliefs of the client be considered. Embedded in issues of access to care are individual rights versus public good, distribution of society's benefits and burdens, and examination of consequences or outcomes of decisions. As treatment choices proliferate and become more complex, the issues surrounding access to care also increase in complexity. For example, no clear protocol exists for determining who has access to complex combination therapy for persons with HIV and chemical dependency when there is concern that the patient might not follow the treatment regimen (HIV Care for Substance Users, 1997).

Duty to Provide Care

The following is an excerpt from a letter addressed to the author of an article about AIDS. The letter was from a registered nurse and a writer, and he asserted:

> Yes, I am still a bedside-care nurse, and in keeping with considering myself a true professional, I choose not to care for AIDS patients on a selective basis. If it is an intravenous drug abuser, I'll care for them without any qualms. You may ask, why? I blame our own permissive society for it's [sic] permissiveness to run amok, insofar as drugs are concerned. These poor ignoramoues [sic] have "made their bed" out of ignorance, addiction and naivety [sic]. If a homosexual pt. tells me (convincingly) "I know I've sinned and been wrong," I'll take care of him.

The nurse who wrote this letter will be acting contrary to ethical guidelines for professional HCWs if he bases his refusal to care for persons with HIV/AIDS on his view that homosexuality or drug use is sinful. He also would be subject to legal action. Refusal to care for patients with HIV/AIDS is not common, as was true earlier in this epidemic, but when it does occur, both educators and administrators have a responsibility to examine their policies and practices to ensure that students and clinicians have the information they need. Numerous professional organizations have taken unequivocal stands that their clinicians have a duty to care for patients with HIV/AIDS (ANA, 1992; Halloran et al., 1988). Under what circumstances, if any, can a HCW refuse to care for a person with HIV/AIDS?

Health care workers comprise a service profession whose members have a responsibility to use their professional knowledge and skills for the benefit of society. Most HCWs work as employees in health care agencies and form a contract with those agencies. This differs from a contract formed directly with patients, which is the traditional model for physicians. For employed HCWs, the duty to provide care emerges both from a contract with their employing agency to care for assigned patients and from the accepted tradition that membership in the health professions entails the acceptance of risks involved in caring for patients (Huerta & Oddi, 1992).

Support for this accepted tradition for HCWs to accept necessary risk to provide care comes from many sources. Downes (1991) points out that the legal duty to provide care is not determined by ethical issues but that ethical standards contribute to the standards of care. She expects health care professions to provide leadership to other groups and to the public in setting the tone of coping with conflicts between balancing individual rights with public well-being. For example, the ANA position paper (1988) states that the nurse is morally obligated to care for HIV-infected patients if the care presents only minimal risk and further suggests that a nurse can exercise a moral option of not caring for the HIV-positive patient only if the nurse's risk exceeds the responsibility to the patient. The ANA position is justified by nursing's responsibility to benefit others and to not cause harm, since the patient could be harmed by being denied care. In addition, when a HCW refuses to care for a patient, that patient's care is assigned to other staff members, and this places an undue burden on one's colleagues. Even though it was feared that requiring HCWs to care for HIV/AIDS patients would cause them to leave the profession and impede the recruitment of new health care professionals, this fear has not been realized.

Means to Pay for Health Care

Americans with HIV infection are drawn from groups who are most likely to be uninsured for health care: young adults, the unmarried, blacks, Latinas, and families without a working adult (Short, Monheit, & Beauregard, 1989). As HIV/AIDS has become a chronic illness, people live longer and they require more medications to prevent and treat their associated opportunistic infections and illnesses. Medications are costly, and some are excluded from insurance coverage. Costs of supplemental therapies, such as nutritional supplements and Chinese herbs, usually are not covered by private or government payers. Hence, costs of treating this illness far outdistance most people's resources to pay. As a result, people are not receiving the health care they want and need. America continues to struggle in allocating resources for adequate care when a national health plan is not in effect to guide fair distribution of services.

When money from traditional sources has not been available to help people access the medical care they need, some communities have worked to create resources through political pressure and community action. The gay and lesbian communities united early in the AIDS epidemic to develop resources for people with HIV/AIDS to access medical care and to meet their everyday living needs, such as housing and groceries. Resources included support groups for people to share approaches they found effective in managing their daily lives and the emotional toll of the disease.

Some populations now affected by HIV/AIDS do not have effective resources; nor have they developed strategies for uniting to gain needed resources. HIV infection is burrowing more decisively into communities composed of people of color and women—communities in which effective medical, everyday living, and social support programs are again challenged. Not only do limited income and lack of health insurance coverage impede access to health care among women and people of color, but efforts have been limited in developing culturally sensitive programs of care or educational programs about the benefits of early treatment (National Commission on AIDS, 1992). Our society continues to struggle with the question of whether we will regard access to health care as a basic right or a privilege, but economic concerns have driven access to health care increasingly toward a privileged status.

The concept of American health care is misleading, since services are offered primarily for illness rather than for health promotion. Although a national comprehensive health care plan has not been enacted, many changes in health care have been enacted during recent years, most notably an expansion in managed care practices. Still, public policy questions that affect access to health or illness care for those affected by HIV/AIDS persist. How should money be divided among competing claims for treatment and prevention? Which forms of treatment are most deserving? If treatments that are effective but expensive are developed, how should these treatments be distributed? Is it fair that medications and, it is hoped, vaccines soon, will soon be available to Americans but not to others in the world with HIV/AIDS?

Payment for HIV/AIDS care is increasingly challenged as people think of AIDS as a chronic illness and feel less urgency to allocate funds to finance research, treatment, and prevention. As AIDS spreads to communities without cohesion and political clout, such as injecting drug users and diverse communities of people of color, political pressure may diminish. Many groups are competing for scarce resources, instead of creating coalitions to service their populations and to increase their power. How can programs competently serve culturally diverse communities without also increasing separation?

Adequate Quality of Care

Example Jimmy, a 30-year-old man, has usually said he was Mexican-American, but he really is also half American Indian. When sober, he has a shy grin that masks his characteristic violent reactions when he is using drugs and drinking. He had applied to drug-detoxification and rehabilitation programs, but nearly all refused to honor his Medicaid coverage. One program accepted Medicaid but required that he telephone every day between 9 and 10 AM for a week before they would consider admission. Without an alarm clock, this task proved insurmountable. Now he has been evicted. All the shelters are full, so he sleeps on a park bench. He has been coughing for a month and has night sweats but has not taken his tuberculosis or other medications for 3 to 4 months. He has not seen his physician for about 6 months. His AIDS was diagnosed about 2 years ago, and he is totally discouraged. His case worker told him, "I can't help you until you stop drugs and drinking" and would not suggest other solutions for health care or housing.

ISSUES OF QUALITY OF CARE. Several difficult questions concern quality of care. What is an acceptable quality of care? Is it adequate to diagnose and treat opportunistic illnesses and infections while not offering treatment for the person's substance abuse problems? Is it adequate treatment if we cannot tend to the living context of the sick person to make sure that adequate housing and food are available? Can a person learn how to avoid re-infection if the class is given in an unfamiliar language or when the person is hungry? Do we blame people for their drug addiction and offer punishment instead of help? Standards do not exist to help patients or HCWs determine what is acceptable palliative care, nor are there specialty programs for training HCWs in palliative care measures. Attending to the patient's comfort level is important at all stages of HIV disease but becomes pivotal as the disease progresses and fewer interventions are available to retard progression of the disease.

SUICIDE, ASSISTED SUICIDE, AND EUTHANASIA

Example Richard, who had AIDS, and his lover, Bret, had talked about Richard's death but mostly in terms of managing insurance, household belongings, and other property. Richard made out his will and durable power of attorney and told his family that Bret would manage his estate and be his major beneficiary. Richard regretted his limited vision and had finally conceded that none of the regimens he had tried slowed his rapidly approaching blindness. His diarrhea was worse, and his headaches were unrelenting. Richard had tentatively talked with his nurse about reading *Final Exit* (Humphrey, 1991) and wondered if suicide might be something he would consider when he became sicker. Without warning,

Richard became very confused, had trouble walking without stumbling, and was very forgetful. He wandered outside in the middle of the night and once almost fell into a ravine by the woods adjacent to their house. Soon, though, Richard's energy faded and he lay in bed fairly motionless, unless someone could help him walk to the bathroom or sit with him. He rarely spoke, and his words often made no sense. Bret hired an aid for 12 hours a day Monday through Friday, while he and friends shared Richard's care at night and on the weekends. Bret's law partners were understanding of his situation and covered for Bret when they could.

Bret spoke with Richard's nurse when she came to see Richard. Once Bret talked with her of how painful it was to see Richard reduced to a shadow of his personhood, for Richard had been such a proud and independent man. Bret wondered about Richard's headaches because he held his head often. Bret wistfully said that he and Richard had never spoken about suicide, and he did not know how Richard felt about this. The nurse struggled with her duty of confidentiality to Richard versus her duty to act as his advocate and spokesperson, since Richard could no longer speak for himself. She told Bret that Richard had begun to explore suicide but that he had not seemed to resolve this; indeed, his grasp of the issues involved seemed naive in comparison with the rest of his knowledge about treatments for AIDS. Bret wondered if it was his responsibility, as Richard's lover, to do for him what he was unable to do for himself—specifically, should Bret assist Richard's dying? The nurse helped Bret to explore his sense of duty, the practical issues, and his spiritual and existential views about this.

Definitions and Ethical Issues Involved

During the past three decades, laws and attitudes about suicide have changed in America. Now only a few states have laws against suicide, and one state (Oregon) has successfully survived a court challenge and another voter referendum to legalize physician-assisted suicide. Changes in laws have allowed a person to seek help after attempting suicide without fear of encountering fines or incarceration. There are complex reasons for the shift in attitudes toward a greater tolerance of suicide and euthanasia. Reasons such as consumerism and technologic advances in maintaining and reproducing life are factors often cited (Daly et al., 1997; Saunders & Hughes, 1998).

A concise discussion of ethical issues around suicide, assisted suicide, and euthanasia requires that terms be defined and used consistently. The presence of suicidal thoughts and actions does not imply that a person has any psychiatric disorder. Although suicidal persons are often depressed, HCWs must recognize that suicide and depression can occur without each other (Saunders & Buckingham, 1988; Valente & Saunders, 1998). Suicide is defined as an intentional death that results from injuries or acts by the person who dies. Assisted suicide is defined as a suicide in which the person kills himself or herself but needs significant help from someone else. Significant help could include providing the gun and ammunition or giving the person access to a lethal dose of pills to use. *Rational suicide* is a popular but unfortunate term, as it incorrectly implies that suicide is either a rational or an irrational act. Rational suicide is defined as a self-inflicted, self-intended death under the following circumstances (Siegel, 1986):

1. Unclouded sensorium—i.e., without significant depression or mood-altering drugs
2. Capacity to comprehend consequences
3. Circumstances acceptable to society

Finally, euthanasia refers to person A causing person B's death and is usually differentiated into voluntary (killing for the individual's own benefit) and involuntary (killing for society's benefit).

The ethical issues that dominate discussion of these approaches to dying include autonomy, confidentiality, sanctity of life, utility, paternalism, and slippery slope. All these terms except the concept of slippery slope were defined earlier in the chapter (see Table 13–2). The slippery slope argument, or the wedge argument, refers to the concern that if a limited action is allowed, that action will expand to broader conditions with fewer limitations. Generally, the slippery slope argument has two dimensions:

1. Support for one type of action logically implies support for another because the dissimilarities between the actions are too subtle for the underlying principles to differentiate.
2. Social forces might, over time, change the rules from voluntary to involuntary euthanasia.

Ethical Issues

The first issue that must be addressed is differentiation between clinical and ethical issues. Quill (1993) argued that transient death wishes among persons with progressive and incurable illnesses, such as AIDS, are often associated with complex meanings involving untreated physical symptoms, emerging psychosocial problems, spiritual or existential crises, clinical depression, or suffering from any of many sources. An HIV-positive patient's request to talk about death, suicide, rational suicide, or assisted suicide may be a way of exploring control issues, especially after the patient has been found to be HIV-positive. A patient's comments about death or suicide must be met with an open mind by a HCW who is willing to assess the patient's experience and concerns. The HCW should listen to the patient's whole message and avoid responding to a fragment of it (Quill, 1993; Saunders & Buckingham, 1988; Valente & Saunders, 1998).

The HCW who is a strong supporter of patient autonomy and advocates the easing of society's barriers to suicide and euthanasia may miss as many clinical clues as does the HCW from the opposite perspective that suicide violates sanctity of life and is never defensible. By operating from their own narrow perspectives, both HCWs will fail to understand the patient's viewpoint or to assist the patient to clarify his or her underlying concerns.

A second issue is deciding how the ethical obligations that guide your professional actions differ from those ethical duties toward family and friends when you are not functioning within a HCW-patient relationship. In AIDS care, this is even more complex since our professional and personal relationships are sometimes mixed. In both situations, it is painful to see persons lose a meaningful quality of life, but your roles and resources may differ in personal and professional situations. The American Nurses' Association Position paper on suicide (1988) clearly states that nurses do not abandon the care of their suicidal patients; neither can HCWs, in their health care role, deliberately act to help patients commit suicide. A HCW who would never think of assisting the suicide of a patient might have different responses if an aunt or a grandparent requested help to commit suicide.

Responses to persons who are contemplating suicide because of a terminal illness and to requests for assisted suicide should be carefully thought through. Approaches to considering the issues that have been discussed in the literature can provide useful guidelines for practice (Battin, 1991; Saunders & Valente, 1993; Valente & Saunders, 1996). Similarly, Jamison (1993) has developed a list of questions for the person who is considering assisting another person to die.

Assisting with a suicide is a serious act and one that may have traumatic consequences for those who assist (Jamison, 1996). In addition to painful personal responses, the HCW may fear the loss of professional credentials to practice.

Patients often request confidentiality from the HCW when they discuss their fears and concerns surrounding suicide. The HCW who has promised to keep a patient's suicide plan secret may encounter conflicting obligations that are difficult to resolve. The HCW may wonder whether the patient would benefit from further consultation or treatment but have no way to help the patient access that without breaking a promise and thereby potentially damaging the trust in the HCW-patient relationship.

In a society that has demonstrated an increased acceptance of suicide in certain circumstances, many ethical and practical problems remain unresolved, and these have prompted discussions designed to promote consensus about comprehensive care of the terminally ill (Young et al., 1997). Will increased access to euthanasia or assisted suicide reduce efforts to relieve suffering? Should the same persons who are responsible for helping people have an acceptable quality of life during illness also be responsible for euthanasia and assisted suicide, or should different groups be constituted for this? If voluntary euthanasia is sanctioned to meet the person's request, what conditions might emerge to expand euthanasia to those who do not request death but whose death would benefit society, such as comatose patients or the severely retarded?

Nurses are divided in their beliefs about appropriate responses to suicide and euthanasia. Interviews with 50 oncology nurses found variation in comfort levels in exploring these topics with their patients and divergent views on what is acceptable (Valente et al., 1993). When asked about when suicide was acceptable, nurses responses varied: "Patient has to make own decisions about suicide." "If patient wants to commit suicide, no one can stop him." "Nurses should attempt to prevent ALL suicides." One nurse responded, "If he was really serious about suicide, I'd assist the patient." Other reports have indicated that a fairly large number of nurses have participated in actions related to euthanasia or assisted suicide, although questions have been raised about the quality of research methods used for these reports (Asche, 1996).

HCWs seem to have reached no consensus about suicide, assisted suicide, and euthanasia in American society; nor have they decided appropriate professional roles. The ethical issues underlying choices about suicide and euthanasia are among the most complex and compelling that we face.

ETHICAL ISSUES AND RESEARCH

Current Research

Discussions of patients' rights in research have paralleled the evolution of research in the health professions, yet ethics as a topic of research efforts is very recent. By the mid-1980s, articles that examined ethics in the context of HIV/AIDS from many perspectives emerged. Now studies of ethics and AIDS are emerging. One of the first to emerge is a descriptive, qualitative study of 25 persons living with HIV (PLWH) and five noninfected persons who were significant to the PLWH (Cameron, 1993). The sample included women (37%) and people of color (53%). Cameron (1993, p. 8) asked her study participants, "What situation involving AIDS has caused you the most conflict about the right thing to do?" Their stories reflect a scope of concerns that expand the more narrowly conceived boundaries of principle-based (normative) ethics, situation ethics, or ethics of caring. All the stories disclosed a struggle to determine the right way to live with AIDS, not classroom discussions of abstract or impersonal situations. These stories capture the realness of the struggle and the immediacy of the consequences. Cameron (1993) reported ten major categories of ethical concerns that her analysis revealed for these 30 men and women: alcohol and drugs, chronic illness, death, discrimination, finance and business, health care, personhood, relationships, service, and sexuality. Cameron also discusses strategies that she says will lead to ethical living and believes that health care professionals grapple with how to live ethical lives themselves and with how to help our patients resolve whatever is bothering them.

Although HCWs have been at the forefront of research into patient and family responses to HIV/AIDS, few studies have focused on inherent moral or ethical problems. Many discussions of ethical problems can be found in the literature, but few of these discussions are based on evidence.

Research Needed in Ethics and HIV/AIDS

So little research has been reported in the literature on ethics and HIV/AIDS that studies can be justified in every aspect of ethics. Especially needed are studies that examine the impact of existing and emerging policies and practices on the PLWH. For example, mandatory involuntary testing has been the policy for military recruits and some prisoners, and studies need to compare issues of autonomy, privacy, and utility with persons who have been tested in voluntary programs.

We need a better understanding of what HCWs, in the context of AIDS care, consider moral problems and how they resolve them. Is the current generation of HCWs concerned about a different set of moral issues than was true in the past? What are the moral obligations of the health care professions in this pandemic? And what goals and strategies will help meet those obligations? How does the moral approach used in resolving moral problems affect the process or outcome for HCWs? Does health care practice differ when the HCW is guided by ethics of caring versus principle-based ethics? What are the barriers to clinicians using universal precautions or other self-protective measures?

Dumois (1993) expressed concern that HIV-positive babies do not receive the lifesaving measures, such as forced feeding, that they need as often as do uninfected babies, and this concern is one that warrants full attention. Since testing of infants automatically reveals the mother's HIV status, moving from an autonomous testing program to one in which identities are known has many potential consequences, and this research should be given high priority.

What is the cost to HCWs in AIDS care situations in which their personal ethics conflict with their professional responsibilities? Where do they find support for themselves when they have made tough decisions or have been unable to act as they desired? How do administrators and educators provide support for staff members and students who are grappling with ethical problems that they encounter with their patients who have HIV/AIDS and their families?

HCWs need a better understanding of how PLWH decide that their quality of life is unacceptable and irreparable. We could benefit from learning how HCWs assist patients in issues surrounding their quality of life. What health care interventions are used when patients broach the topic of suicide or euthanasia? And how do the interventions reflect ethical values? What costs (complicated grief, depression) are incurred by people who do assist their loved ones or their patients with suicide?

Since HIV infection is not distributed evenly across the United States, researchers have difficulty giving people access to studies in some areas or including women or people of color in their studies. This uneven distribution leads to some persons being involved in several studies concurrently, whereas others are never approached about participating in research. Consequently, most of our knowledge about health care and AIDS may be informed disproportionately by a less diverse core of volunteer study participants than is needed to guide policy or to develop interventions. American HCWs need to form collaborative studies with colleagues in other nations for a better understanding of human responses to HIV/AIDS within a global perspective. Ethical concerns about participant involvement in research must reach beyond informed consent, autonomous participation, and confidentiality. We should encourage collaboration among researchers that allows comprehensive and broad studies.

AIDS activists have changed the manner of conducting clinical trials research by questioning how long it takes to approve drugs that may mean the difference between life and death for PLWH. Before these changes, participation in clinical trials was viewed as a burden for patients. This burden was justified because of the public good, and precautions were used to reduce individual risk. Increasingly, HIV-infected persons regard participation in research as a right and have challenged the practice of excluding women, infants, and people of color as discriminatory rather than not protective. Research is needed to determine the effects of these changes and to assess current research review processes for adaptation to these changes.

Finally, HCWs have been in the forefront of providing direct care to persons with AIDS, supporting health-promotion efforts of patients, and developing disease-prevention strategies. HCWs have provided some leadership at national or international conferences but all too often seem invisible as leaders and appear as passive consumers. If the health care professions have ethical obligations to work for better resources for our HIV-infected patients and their families, how can we find our voice to participate in local and international programs to speak of the inequities and injustices that we witness among patients in our clinical practice?

REFERENCES

Agency for Health Care Policy and Research, Public Health Service, U.S. Department of Health and Human Services. (1994). *Evaluation and management of early HIV infection.* Clinical practice guideline No. 7 (publication No. 94-0572, 95-100). Washington, DC: Author.

Agich, G.J. (1990). Reassessing autonomy in long-term care. *Hastings Center Report,* (1), 12–17.

AIDSline. (1992). Women vs. their infants in HIV testing debate. *The Robert Wood Johnson Foundation, 4*(4), 1–4.

Albrizio, M.A., Ozuna, J., Mattheis, R., et al. (1992). A nursing bioethics program. *Clinical Nurse Specialist, 6*(2), 97–103.

American Hospital Association. (1985). *Values in conflict: Resolving ethical issues in hospital care. Report of the Special Committee on Biomedical Ethics.* Chicago: Author.

American Nurses Association. (1985). *Code for nurses with interpretative statements.* Kansas City, MO.

American Nurses Association. (1988). *Committee on Ethics. Ethics in nursing: Position statements and guidelines.* Washington, DC: Author.

American Nurses Association. (1992). *Compendium of HIV/AIDS positions, policies and documents.* Washington, DC: Author.

American Nurses' Association Committee on Ethics. (1985). *Code for nurses with interpretive statements.* Kansas City, MO: Author.

Americans with Disabilities Act of 1990. (1990). Pub. L. No. 101-336, 104 Stat 3 27.

Aroskar, M. (1980). Anatomy of an ethical dilemma. *American Journal of Nursing, 80*(4), 658–663.

Asche, D.A. (May 23, 1996). The role of critical care nurses in euthanasia and assisted suicide. *New England Journal of Medicine, 334,* 1374–1379.

Bandman, E.L., Bandman, B. (1995). *Nursing ethics through the life span* (3rd ed.). Norwalk, CT: Appleton & Lange.

Battin, M.P. (1991). Rational suicide: How can we respond to a request for help? *Crisis, 12*(2), 73–80.

Bayer, R. (February 15, 1994). AIDS: Human rights and responsibilities. *Hospital Practice,* 155–163.

Beauchamp, T.L. (1994). *Principles of biomedical ethics* (4th ed.). New York: Oxford University Press.

Benner, P., Wrubel, J. (1989). *The primacy of caring.* Menlo Park, CA: Addison-Wesley.

Bhushan, V., Cushman, L.F. (1995). Paediatric AIDS: Selected attitudes and behaviours of paediatricians in New York City hospitals (1995). *AIDS Care, 7*(1), 27–34.

Bishop, A., Scudder, J. (1987). Nursing ethics in an age of controversy. *Advances in Nursing Science, 9*(3), 34–43.

Browdie, R. (1992). Ethical issues in case management from a political systems perspective. *Journal of Case Management, 1,* 87–89.

Brown, M.L. (1987). AIDS and ethics: Concerns and consideration. *Oncology Nursing Forum, 14*(1), 69–73.

Cameron, M.E. (1993). *Living with AIDS: Experiencing ethical problems.* Newbury Park, CA: Sage Publications.

Card, C. (Ed.). (1994). *Adventures in lesbian philosophy.* Bloomington, IN: Indiana University Press.

Centers for Disease Control. (1991). Recommendations for preventing transmission of human immunodeficiency virus and hepatitis B virus to patients during exposure-prone invasive procedures. *Morbidity and Mortality Weekly Report, 40*(RR-8).

Centers for Disease Control. (1993). Recommendations for HIV testing services for inpatients and outpatients in acute-care hospital settings. *Morbidity and Mortality Weekly Report, 42*(RR-2), 1–6.

Centers for Disease Control. (1996). HIV/AIDS surveillance report. *Morbidity and Mortality Weekly Report, 8*(1), 15.

Cohen, M.R., Doner, K. (1996). *The Chinese way to healing: Many paths to wholeness.* New York: Berkley Publishing.

Collins, J. (1981). Should doctors tell the truth? In T.A. Mappes, J.S. Zembaty (Eds.), *Biomedical ethics* (pp. 64–67). New York: McGraw-Hill.

Colombotos, J., Messeri, P., Burgunder, M., et al. (1991). *Physicians, nurses and AIDS: Preliminary findings from a national survey.* Washington, DC: Agency for Health Care Policy and Research.

Condon, E.H. (1992). Nursing and the caring metaphor: Gender and political influences on an ethics of care. *Nursing Outlook, 40*(1), 14–19.

Curtin, L., Flaherty, M.J. (1982). *Nursing ethics: Theories and pragmatics.* Bowie, MD: Robert J. Brady Co.

Curtin, L. (1978). A proposed model for critical ethical analysis. *Nursing Forum, XVII*(1), 17–27.

Curtin, L. (1990). The commitment of nursing. In T. Pence, J. Cantrall (Eds.), *Ethics in nursing: An anthology* (pp. 283–286). New York: The National League for Nursing.

Daly, B.J., Berry, D., Fitzpatrick, J.J., et al. (1997). Assisted suicide: Implications for nurses and nursing. *Nursing Outlook, 45,* 209–214.

Davis, A.J., Aroskar, M.A. (1991). *Ethical dilemmas and nursing practice* (3rd ed.). Norwalk, CT: Appleton & Lange.

Davis, C.K. (1984). The status of reimbursement policy and future projections. In C.A. Williams (Ed.), *Nursing research and policy formation: The case of prospective payment.* Kansas City, MO: American Academy of Nursing.

Downes, J. (1991). Acquired immunodeficiency syndrome: The nurse's legal duty to serve. *Journal of Professional Nursing, 7*(6), 333–340; 4(5), 331–336.

Dumois, A.O. (1993, October). *Social and political strategies for the HIV epidemic.* Paper presented at HIV Sixth National AIDS Update Conference, San Francisco, California.

Dunlop, M.J. (1994). Is a science of caring possible? In P. Benner (Ed.), *Interpretative phenomenology: Embodiment, caring and ethics in health and illness.* Thousand Oaks, CA: Sage.

Eliason, M.J. (1993). Ethics and transcultural nursing care. *Nursing Outlook, 41*(5), 225–228.

El-Mallahk, P.I., Simmons, C., Forman, L., et al. (1992). Mandatory HIV testing of health care workers: A review. *AIDS Patient Care, 6*(4), 164–168.

Fassbinder, B. (1993). *My personal story of occupational HIV infection.* Panel presentation, Sixth Annual Conference, Association of Nurses in AIDS Care, Century City, California.

Frammolino, R. (November 2, 1997). Harvest of corneas at morgue questioned. *Los Angeles Times,* column one, pp. 1, 28–29.

Gadow, S. (1990). A model for ethical decision making. In T. Pence, J. Cantrall (Eds.), *Ethics in nursing: An anthology* (pp. 52–55). New York: The National League for Nursing.

Gilligan, C. (1982). *In a different voice: Psychological theory and women's development.* Cambridge, MA: Harvard University Press.

Hallosdottir, S. (1997). Implications of the caring-competence dichotomy. In S.E. Thorne, V.E. Hayes (Eds.), *Nursing praxis: Knowledge and action* (pp. 105–124). Thousand Oaks, CA: Sage.

Halloran, J., Hughes, A., Mayer, D.K. (1988). Oncology Nursing Society position paper on HIV-related issues. *Oncology Nursing Forum, 15,* 206–210.

Harron, F., Burnside, J., Beauchamp, T. (1983). *Health and human values: A guide to making your own decision.* New Haven, CT: Yale University Press.

The Hastings Center. (1987). *Guidelines on the termination of life-sustaining treatment and the care of the dying.* Bloomington, IN: Indiana University Press.

HIV care for substance users. (1997, May/June) *HIV Frontline. A Newsletter for Professionals Who Counsel People Living with HIV, 28,* 1–3.

Hoagland, S.L. (1991). Some thoughts about "caring." In C. Card (Ed.), *Feminist ethics* (pp. 246–263). Lawrence, KS: University of Kansas Press.

Huerta, S.R., Oddi, L.F. (1992). Refusal to care for patients with human immunodeficiency virus/acquired immunodeficiency syndrome: Issues and responses. *Journal of Professional Nursing, 8*(4), 221–230.

Humphrey, D. (1991). *Final exit.* Eugene, OR: The Hemlock Society.

Institute of Medical Ethics Working Party on the Ethical Implications of AIDS. (1992, June). AIDS and the ethics of medical care and treatment. *Quarterly Journal of Medicine,* New Series 83(302), 419–426.

Jaggar, A.M. (1991). Feminist ethics: Projects, problems, prospects. In C. Card (Ed.), *Feminist ethics.* Lawrence, KS: University of Kansas Press.

Jamison, S. (1993, July). Helping to die: Some practical questions. *Hemlock Quarterly, 7,* 5–7.

Jamison, S. (1996). When drugs fail: Assisted deaths and not-so-lethal drugs. In M.P. Battin, A.G. Lipman (Eds.), *Drug use in assisted suicide and euthanasia.* New York: Haworth Press.

Lo, B., Steinbrook, R. (1992). Health care workers infected with the human immunodeficiency virus. *Journal of the American Medical Association, 267,* 1100–1105.

National Commission on AIDS. (1993). *AIDS: An expanding tragedy. The final report of the National Commission on AIDS.* Washington, DC: Author.

National Commission on AIDS. (1992). *The challenge of HIV/AIDS in communities of color.* Washington, DC: Author.

Neil, R.M., Watts, R. (Eds.). (1991). *Caring and nursing: Explorations in feminist perspectives.* New York: National League for Nursing.

Ninth National Conference on Women and HIV. (1997, July/August). *HIV Frontline: A Newsletter for Professionals Who Counsel People Living with HIV, 29,* 1–3, 8.

Noddings, N. (1984). *Caring: A feminine approach to ethics and moral education.* Berkeley, CA: University of California Press.

Northrup, D.T. (1993). Self-care myth reconsidered. *Advances in Nursing Science, 15*(3), 59–66.

Porche, D.J. (1997). Treatment review: Postexposure prophylaxis after an occupational exposure to HIV. *Journal of the Association of Nurses in AIDS Care, 8*(1), 83–87.

Quill, T.E. (1993). Doctor, I want to die. Will you help me? *Journal of the American Medical Association, 270*(7), 870–877.

Saulo, M., Wagener, R.J. (1996). How good case managers make tough choices: Ethics and mediation. *The Journal of Care Management, 2*(1), 8–15, 53–55.

Saunders, J.M., Buckingham, S.L. (1988). When the depression turns deadly. *Nursing, 88,* 60–64.

Saunders, J.M., Hughes, A. (1998). Nurses and assisted

dying: Taking our roles to heart and mind. *Journal of the Association of Nurses in AIDS Care, 9*(2), 15–17.

Saunders, J.M., Valente, S.M. (1993). Nicole: Suicide and terminal illness. *Suicide and Life-Threatening Behavior, 23*(1), 76–82.

Schultz, M., Moore, L. (1993). *Bioethics Committee: A subacute model.* Paper presented at the Sixth Annual Conference of the Association of Nurses in AIDS Care, Los Angeles, California.

Short, P., Monheit, A., Beauregard, K. (1989). *A profile of uninsured Americans* (DHHS Publication No. [PHS] 89-344). National Medical Expenditure Survey Research Findings 1. National Center for Health Servces Research and Health Care Technology Assessment. Rockville, MD: Public Health Service.

Siegel, K. (1986). Psychosocial aspects of rational suicide. *American Journal of Psychotherapy, 40*(3), 405–418.

Sowell, R.L. (1995). Community-based HIV case management: Challenges and opportunities. *Journal of the Association of Nurses in AIDS Care, 6*(2), 33–40.

Stoll, J., Mason, P.K. (1993). *Ethics education for nurses in AIDS care.* Paper presented at the Sixth Annual Conference of the Association of Nurses in AIDS Care, Los Angeles, California.

Tuohey, J.F. (1995). Moving from autonomy to responsibility in HIV-related healthcare. *Cambridge Quarterly of Healthcare Ethics, 4,* 64–70.

U.S. Office of Technology Assessment. (1992). HIV in the healthcare workplace: A background paper. *AIDS Patient Care, 6*(4), 169–185.

U.S. Public Health Service. (1995). Recommendations for human immunodeficiency virus counseling and voluntary testing for pregnant women. *Morbitity and Mortality Weekly Report (MMWR), 44*(EE-7), 1–15.

Valente, S.M., Saunders, J.M. (1996). Assisted suicide and euthanasia: Cases and commentaries. *Journal of Pharmaceutical Care in Pain and Symptom Control, 4*(1/2), 291–344.

Valente, S.M., Saunders, J.M. (1998). Suicide and HIV disease. In W. Wolford, S.L. Buckingham (Eds.), *A mental health practitioner's guide to the neuropsychiatric aspects of HIV/AIDS* (pp. 263–293). New York: Guilford Press.

Valente, S.M., Saunders, J.M., McIntyre, L., et al. (1993). *Qualitative analysis of oncology nurses' attitudes toward suicide.* Poster session. Paper presented at the Sixth Annual Conference of the Association of Nurses in AIDS Care, Los Angeles, California.

Walters, L. (1988). Ethical issues in the prevention and treatment of HIV infection and AIDS. *Science, 239,* 597–603.

Watson, J. (1985). *Nursing: Human science and human care.* Norwalk, CT: Appleton-Century-Crofts.

Wilfert, C.M. (1994). Mandatory screening of pregnant women for the human immonodeficiency virus. *Clinical Infectious Diseases, 19,* 664–666.

Winters, G., Glass, E., Sakurai, C. (1993). Ethical issues in oncology nursing practice: An overview of topics and strategies. *Oncology Nursing Forum, Supplement, 20*(10), 21–34.

Woods, N. (1989). Conceptualizations of self-care: Toward health-oriented models. *Advances in Nursing Science, 12*(1), 1–13.

Young, E.W.D., Marcus, F.S., Drought, T., et al. (1997). Report of the Northern California Conference for guidelines on aid-in-dying: Definitions, differences, convergences, conclusions. *Western Journal of Medicine, 166,* 381–388.

14

Personal Perspectives on Policy Issues of the HIV/AIDS Epidemic

Helen M. Miramontes

Policy is the matrix by which a society identifies, defines, and addresses the issues that affect that society. Policy includes the boundaries, the limitations, the focus, and the direction to be taken to address a specific issue. My belief is that policy development is a predictable and natural outcome of advocacy that evolves out of the needs of people and communities. Policy development and implementation do not occur within a vacuum; policy evolves within a social and political context. In addition to the social and political institutions, this context includes the values, beliefs, attitudes, norms, cultures, and current statutes and regulations of the larger society. The social and political context will even determine whether or not an issue is considered important enough to be addressed. HIV/AIDS is a glaring example of an issue that has frequently been marginalized and minimized by many societies worldwide. When AIDS was first identified in the United States in 1981, it was immediately defined as a gay disease, gay-related immune deficiency (GRID), or the gay plague (Burkett, 1995; Shilts, 1987), and shortly afterward as a disease of intravenous drug users (IVDUs). Both populations have been and are still significantly stigmatized and marginalized by the larger society and, as many of us remember, there was minimal mobilization within the federal government to address the evolving epidemic. The mobilization efforts to address the needs of sick and dying men came primarily from the affected community of gay men and a few committed public health officers and health care professionals. Since those early years, we have had to continually battle the stigma, the discrimination, the denial, and the misinformation that have influenced our responses to the epidemic. This stigma and discrimination have also been prevalent worldwide—in all societies.

The evolving policies and legislation that have been generated since the early 1980s, have been produced within this political and social context. Some of the most abusive proposals have been defeated because of the community activists and their ongoing vigilance in monitoring federal, state, and local governmental entities. It is understandable that the social and political context of abusive proposals, stigma, marginalization, discrimination, and alienation has created a pervasive environment of distrust, suspicion, and cynicism. The downside of this climate of distrust is that there has been some legislation enacted aimed at protecting persons from the effects of discrimination that encumbers our efforts to stop the epidemic. This perspective will be expanded, and examples will be provided later in this chapter.

One of the questions that we need to continually ask ourselves as we attempt to establish sound policy on HIV/AIDS issues is, How do we balance the community's rights and the rights of the individual? In our society, with the strong emphasis on individual rights, the balancing is much more difficult than in some other societies. Unfortunately, what sometimes evolves is infringement on a segment of society by the enactment of protective laws for another segment of the society.

My goal in writing this chapter is to challenge us to learn to examine issues from more than one perspective, to identify our assumptions and biases, to ask ourselves the hard questions about the benefits and consequences of policy enactment, and then collectively to act to address the extremely complex policy issues of the HIV/AIDS epidemic.

PERSONAL JOURNEY

My personal journey to this epidemic began a long time before the first cases of *Pneumocystis carinii* pneumonia (PCP) were reported to the Centers for Disease Control (CDC) in 1981. Previous to my entry into nursing, I had been involved in volunteer advocacy in several arenas, including the peace movement, the civil rights movement, and the farm workers' movement. I graduated from a community college nursing program in 1972, the same year that my oldest child graduated from high school. I began working full-time as a registered nurse in an acute care facility and eventually became active in the California Nurses Association (CNA). I was elected to the CNA Board of Directors in 1981 and served for 6½ years as director, president-elect, and president. My position as a leader of the statewide nursing association placed me in an excellent position to become involved in HIV/AIDS policy issues. One of the major difficulties at the time was that many practicing nurses were lobbying the Association to support restrictive legislation that would mandate routine testing of all hospitalized patients and placing test results in patients' charts. In fact, after one particular Republican state assemblyman was lobbied about his proposed discriminatory legislation, he and two other Republican legislators wrote nurses in their districts to inform them of what the nursing leadership in California was doing about the epidemic and that we were not representing their best interests. Fortunately, I had developed credible relationships with the membership of CNA, and their trust in my leadership was demonstrated by their acceptance and backing of my positions on HIV/AIDS legislation.

I also have two gay sons and, therefore, during the early 1980s attempted to learn everything I could about this new disease. I lived and worked in a large community 50 miles south of San Francisco, and about 1983 we began to see patients in the acute care facility with severe cases of PCP. I

worked in the intensive care unit (ICU), and it was not unusual to have 34 patients with PCP on respirators at one time. During this time I also attempted to educate my peers about what was known about this disease. To my dismay, many nurses were as discriminatory, prejudicial, and fearful as the general public. Some even refused to care for patients with AIDS. These dehumanizing issues of discrimination and stigmatization, both within my profession and in the larger society, were the very determinants that catapulted me into AIDS activism in the early years of the epidemic.

In the 1985–86 California state legislature there were 150 proposed bills on numerous HIV/AIDS issues. Some were excellent proposals addressing testing and counseling, confidentiality and HIV antibody test results, research, mental health, and care issues; many other proposals were about similar issues, but from a negative perspective. I spent a great deal of my time in the state capitol testifying against and for many of these legislative proposals, as well as trying to educate the legislators about HIV/AIDS. During this time I worked with various committed advocates, such as Steve Morin, PhD. Steve currently works for Congresswoman Nancy Pelosi of San Francisco, who is one of the leaders in Congress on HIV/AIDS issues. I also worked with Stan Hadden, aide to Senate President Pro Tem David Roberti, Larry Bush, aide to Art Agnos, assemblyman from San Francisco, and Bruce Decker, a political consultant active in gay/lesbian and HIV/AIDS politics. Bruce, a Republican, had worked in the Ford White House. Bruce, Stan, and Larry were actually three of the persons who worked to establish California's HIV/AIDS political agenda, which formed the foundation for the state's effective and compassionate response to the epidemic. Their efforts also helped develop the infrastructure that provided the means for mobilizing communities and organizations statewide to defeat several initiatives that were designed to address HIV/AIDS in very abusive and destructive ways; these discriminatory initiatives, of course, reflected the misinformation, the false beliefs, and the fears and hysteria of the times. As president of CNA, I was on the Statewide Steering Committee to defeat Proposition 64/Stop LaRouche Initiative Campaign and worked with many other political leaders to defeat the initiative. Over the years it has been rewarding to meet and work with many persons committed to making a difference in this epidemic and, in the larger society, to address the issues of discrimination and injustice. During these years I was also a founding member of an HIV/AIDS community-based organization (CBO) located in Santa Clara County and, as a board member, assisted in the development of an infrastructure in the community to carry out the mission of the organization. An enlightened County Board of Supervisors not only funded the development of the CBO but also established an AIDS Task Force to advise the Board of Supervisors on relevant HIV/AIDS issues. I became chair of the Task Force in 1987 and served in that capacity until I moved to San Francisco in 1991. While still living in Santa Clara County, I served as vice-chair of both the United Way HIV/AIDS Advisory Committee and the Health Resources Services Administration (HRSA) AIDS Planning Grant. I also chaired an AIDS Task Force for the American Nurses Association (ANA) and testified for the ANA before congressional committees and the first AIDS Commission during the Reagan Administration on HIV/AIDS issues. In 1989 I worked with the U.S. Department of Labor, Occupational Safety and Health Administration (OSHA), in Washington, D.C., as an expert witness on the development of and testimony for the proposed bloodborne pathogen rule.

After moving to San Francisco, I worked on several boards and task forces, including a statewide group established by the California State Department of Health, to explore and develop policy to address the issue of provider-to-patient HIV transmission after the dental case in Florida. Currently, I am a member of the statewide Advisory Committee to the Office of Women's Health, Department of Health Services, State of California. This advisory committee is an excellent arena in which to identify and address the HIV/AIDS issues for women in California. The Office of Women's Health and the Advisory Committee have become fairly well known, and input has been solicited from other offices within state government and also from the legislature concerning specific health issues important to women, including HIV/AIDS.

In December 1995 I was appointed by President Clinton to serve on the Presidential Advisory Council on HIV/AIDS (PACHA). In this position, I serve on the Research Subcommittee, the International Task Force, the Committee on Adolescent Issues, and the Process Committee. I continue to be fortunate in having opportunities to work with dedicated and talented people. I have learned much over the years and will share my perspectives on some of the controversial issues that continue to impact us as we respond to the needs of people infected and affected by HIV.

HISTORICAL PERSPECTIVE

Before I focus on some specific policy issues, I want to reflect briefly on several broad attempts to develop sound policy and, as part of that reflection, share with you some information about PACHA. In this country we have had a very unflattering and inconsistent history of responding to this epidemic, but I also believe that we have had some very successful policy strategies that have provided resources and support for persons living with HIV (PLWH) and persons at risk of infection. Certainly, the Ryan White (R/W) legislation has greatly assisted communities and states to respond more aggressively to the needs of PLWH. The AIDS Drug Assistance Program (ADAP) of the R/W Act alone has benefited many persons with drug treatment that was not available before the R/W legislation. Also, Title 111, the Early Intervention Program, of the R/W Act has provided significant resources to establish the infrastructure necessary to meet the outpatient treatment and care needs of PLWH. Housing Opportunities for People with AIDS (HOPWA) has provided for the residential needs of many PLWH. The Centers for Disease Control and Prevention (CDC) has also funded many CBOs and public health departments to establish and conduct prevention education and behavioral change programs and testing and counseling programs. The Federal Drug Administration (FDA) has attempted, with some success, the fast tracking of experimental drugs through the approval process in order to increase the number of drugs available for infected persons. Certainly, there have been problems with some aspects of these programs, and there are still tremendous unmet needs of PLWH and those at risk of HIV infection, but we need to stop and reflect on where we would be today without these resources.

As many of you may remember, there have been two previous commissions established by the Presidential Office to address HIV/AIDS. The first AIDS Commission was established by President Reagan in the late 1980s. The Presidential Commission on the HIV Epidemic consisted of a chair, Admiral James D. Watkins (Retired), and 12 other members. Two nurses, Colleen Conway Welch, PhD, RN, FAAN, and Kristine M. Gebbie, RN, DrPH, FAAN, were members of this Commission. The report from this commission was released in July 1988. It was comprehensive, addressing the issues that we continue to struggle with today. The second commission, the National Commission on AIDS established during George Bush's administration, was chaired by June Osborn, MD, and had 12 other members. The chair and members reflected expertise in HIV and leadership in the broader society. The commission's final report was released in 1993. This report was also comprehensive and reflected the best thinking of the time. Some of the recommendations were implemented, and many were not. The lack of movement on either of the commissions' reports does not lie with the appointed commissions, but with the broader society and with the federal government. Neither President Reagan nor President Bush used his position to advocate a rapid, comprehensive response to this epidemic. The reasons for this lack of response have been extensively discussed elsewhere, so I will not rehash the various opinions but will acknowledge that the reasons are probably more complex then we would like to think.

During President Clinton's first term, two additional strategies were implemented to focus on the epidemic. The first was the establishment of a national AIDS policy coordinator. During the presidential campaign, the promise was made that an "AIDS czar" would be appointed and that AIDS funding would be increased. The expectation was that the AIDS czar would have authority and resources to lead the nation, including government, in our response to HIV. As we know, the position established was less than that of a czar. It became a national AIDS policy coordinator position without adequate staff or sufficient resources; the mission and purpose were unclear, and the position of the coordinator in the White House structure was unclear. Kristine Gebbie was appointed, and it soon became apparent that many

in the AIDS community were not pleased with the appointment. There was also significant disappointment about the lack of resources and prestige allocated to the position. The attacks from the community quickly focused on the person appointed rather than on the lack of support, authority, and resources for the office and the position. By mutual agreement, Dr. Gebbie resigned in 1994. Recently Dr. Gebbie (1996) published an article about her perspective on this experience. She describes the process and the factors that influenced the negative reaction to the office and the position, including her own mistakes, that led to the controversy and her eventual resignation. I recommend that anyone interested in the politics of this epidemic read Dr. Gebbie's article.

A short time later Patsy Fleming was appointed to the position. I believe that Ms. Fleming, with extensive experience in the Washington political arena, has served well in the position, bringing some prestige and stability to the office. Jeff Levy, an astute long-time national political activist, served as deputy director. In April 1997 the third policy coordinator, Sandra Thurman, was appointed. Ms. Thurman has been a member of PACHA and had also been an executive director of a large CBO in Atlanta. Her appointment was supported by many AIDS activists and organizations. Ms. Thurman also has very good access to both the President's and the Vice-President's offices. The Office of National AIDS Policy (ONAP) and the position still lack adequate authority and resources, but more support and attention have been promised by the administration. Only time will tell to what extent these promises will or can be fulfilled.

A second strategy instituted by President Clinton was the establishment of a third advisory group, the Presidential Advisory Council on HIV/AIDS (PACHA). This council differs from the previous two commissions in several areas. The two earlier commissions were established to make recommendations to the nation. PACHA was established to advise the President and the Administration on HIV/AIDS, not to advise the nation. The structure of the council is also significantly different from the previous two commissions. The council reflects the experience and the expertise of those most impacted by the epidemic. PACHA is much larger than the previous commissions, with 35 members. Forty percent of the members are infected with HIV. Fifty percent are lesbian, gay, or bisexual. One third of the members are people of color, and all council members have been personally affected by the epidemic. The council also has much greater access to the President and top-level White House and administrative staff and officials than the previous commissions.

A third area of difference is in the process by which we do our work. PACHA has several working committees on research, prevention, services, and discrimination. Several task forces have been added to concentrate on prisons, people of color, adolescents, and international issues. Another committee, the Process Committee, was established to accomplish our work. The council is funded to meet three times a year for several days, so that much of our work is done by means of committee conference calls. Recommendations are developed within the committee structure and submitted to the full council several weeks before a scheduled meeting. Our goal is not to have long lists of recommendations but to fully explore an issue and to submit recommendations that address the issue. As an example, the Research Committee submitted to the full council three recommendations during our April 1997 meeting on HIV vaccine development (see Box below).

■ PACHA RESEARCH COMMITTEE'S RECOMMENDATIONS ON HIV VACCINE DEVELOPMENT ■

Development of a successful HIV/AIDS vaccine is clearly feasible and should be considered of the highest priority by our government. In order to succeed, we suggest the following recommendations:

1. The President must declare an urgent goal of developing a vaccine to prevent HIV/AIDS within a decade in order to mobilize public opinion, political will, and international collaboration and to assign high priority to this effort within each of the governmental agencies involved in HIV/AIDS vaccine research and development. As the HIV/AIDS epidemic has no borders, and a successful vaccine will require international collaboration, the President should work with the leaders of other nations in a global effort to achieve an HIV/AIDS vaccine for all the world.

2. A significant and sustained increase in funds must be made available for HIV/AIDS vaccine research and development. These funds must be derived from *new* sources from both government and industry and must not be taken from existing programs aimed at prevention, research, care, services, or treatment for persons with HIV/AIDS. Innovative use of such funds is essential, as seed money to initiate new and creative hypotheses in vaccine research, to support product development, to expand the proportion of successfully funded grant applications, and to bring additional entities into the HIV/AIDS vaccine field.

3. Development of an effective HIV/AIDS vaccine will require expertise in many areas, including basic science, applied research, public health policy, and legal, ethical, industrial, and international issues. Dr. David Baltimore has recently been chosen to provide advice and leadership for the NIH HIV/AIDS vaccine effort, and the Council is highly supportive of this appointment. In addition,

   a. Participation by nongovernmental sectors and organizations is also essential to achieve the goal of expedited vaccine research, product development, and use. The Vice-President should convene a public-private HIV/AIDS vaccine consultative forum, composed of senior representatives to encourage communication between sectors, to address gaps in the field, and to speed progress towards the President's goal. Participation on this HIV/AIDS vaccine forum should include representation from U.S. government agencies, industry, the international community, academia, the World Bank and other funding agencies, the insurance industry, ethicists, and communities most affected by the epidemic.

   b. To achieve the goal of a more comprehensive vaccine development effort within the government, *all* relevant agencies within the U.S. government—including NIH, CDC, DOD, Department of Veterans Affairs (DVA), FDA, United States Agency for International Development (USAID) and relevant offices within these agencies, especially those relating to minority and women's health—must be substantively involved in the vaccine effort. The agencies must regularly communicate with one another and share information.

▪ PACHA RECOMMENDATION II.D.2. MICROBICIDE RESEARCH AND DEVELOPMENT ▪

The priority for funding by the OAR for microbicide research and development, as well as such funding within CDC, must be increased substantially, with a concomitant increase of full-time equivalents (FTEs) allocated for this priority.

Administration's Response

NIH funding for research on microbicides has increased over the past several years and will continue to increase. The priority accorded to this important area of research has been determined through the OAR planning process, which included consultation with NIH and nongovernment scientists, clinicians, academicians, industry representatives, and AIDS community advocates. These experts reached a consensus on the scientific priorities included in the consolidated NIH Plan and Budget Request. OAR anticipates that this research will continue to receive high priority for funding.

At CDC, the Epidemiology Branch, Division of HIV/AIDS Prevention (DHAP), in collaboration with the Division of Reproductive Health, the Division of STD, and the Women's Health Program Office, coordinated a meeting in mid April to discuss policy, research, and program issues concerning microbicide research relative to CDC's mission of HIV prevention. This meeting was attended by CDC researchers, outside consultants, and representatives from NIH and FDA. Regarding ongoing research, the CDC HIV/AIDS Epidemiology Branch, in collaboration with the Division of Viral and Rickettsial Diseases, is currently conducting a 3-year prospective study of HIV in secretions from the female genital tract. Studies are also being conducted within the Epidemiology Branch to examine women's interpretation of HIV-prevention messages as a function of relevant beliefs and goals concerning close relationships and potential biases in message interpretation due to contextual framing of information and the hierarchical presentation of message content.

Assessment of the Response

The Administration is certainly moving in the right direction regarding this area, although these concrete increases have not yet been seen. The President has used his leadership to emphasize the importance of this area to the public. Two meetings have been held: one by the National Center for HIV, STD, and TB Prevention, CDC, 4/15/96, with Patsy Fleming, Director, Office of National AIDS Policy, and others in attendance, and the other by the International Working Group on Microbicides in Virginia, 4/11/96.

Follow-up Action Recommended

The Administration should require each relevant agency and NIH institute to provide, on an annual basis, information on specific funding and FTE allocations being applied for microbicide research. Tracking of this information should include the specific types and nature of the research being conducted.

Current efforts should be continued, and overall funding for microbicide research must significantly increase.

The committee had been working on this issue for the past 8 months, with scheduled conference calls with more then 24 scientists reflecting diverse views on the issue. We discussed the vaccine issue at several of our meetings and with the full council during the April meeting. We also had a distinguished panel of scientists, again reflecting diverse views, testify before the full council during the meeting. This process is used by all of the committees. On issues that require a much more rapid response and input, conference calls are initiated by Chairman Scott Hitt, an HIV physician and long-time HIV and gay and lesbian activist.

The issue is discussed and frequently a letter or position statement is quickly developed and sent to the President or the appropriate department within the Administration.

The other critical issue is the monitoring of the Administration as to the implementation of PACHA's recommendations. The Process Committee, through ONAP, requests responses from the various administrative offices to which we have sent recommendations. The responses are reviewed and evaluated with respect to the appropriate implementation. Recommendations that are not implemented are revised with stronger language to urge implementation and to reflect the most current knowledge. Basically, what we are doing is giving the President and the Administration a report card that includes areas that need improvement. For an example of this process, see the Box on page 454, PACHA's recommendation II.D.2 on microbicide research. It was approved during our December 1995 meeting and is part of our first report, which was released on July 8, 1996. We are currently beginning the process of reviewing the responses to all recommendations and of writing our second report.

President Clinton has initiated other mechanisms since beginning his second term. In addition to reendorsing the continuation of the Advisory Council, the President has issued the White National AIDS Strategy document (1997). For the first time in this epidemic, a President has taken a direct approach to respond to this epidemic. President Clinton directed ONAP to develop a comprehensive document that would delineate the federal government's long-term plan to address the epidemic. The strategic plan addresses prevention, care and services, research, translation of research advances into practice, civil rights, and international issues. There are some gaps in the document, particularly around the issues of needle exchange as part of the overall strategy to decrease viral transmission in the injection drug–using population, but many other issues are addressed.

I need to acknowledge the ambiguous, sometimes hostile, feelings and perspectives within some activists' groups about both ONAP and the Advisory Council. Frequently, the Council and ONAP are viewed as being only a political ruse on the part of the White House in addressing the issues that are important to many of us. The Council is thought to be a collection of political appointees without expertise or commitment to ending this epidemic. I disagree unequivocally with that perspective. I believe that the Council members reflect the same commitment, the same concern, and the same passion of many activists, but we may disagree significantly in the process of facilitating change. Many of the Council members have been politically active in other arenas, as well as in this epidemic. They have developed finely tuned skills and expertise in the political process to bring about change. Sometimes the process seems very slow, and Council members

become as frustrated with the process as some of the activists, but democracy is a process that requires cooperation, collaboration, and sometimes compromise to secure a desired goal. Compromise may be necessary to maintain open channels of communication. Nothing can change if individuals and groups are not listening and talking to each other. Demonstrating this perspective, I want to share with you an example of the Council's effectiveness in addressing a very important issue, and yet we reached a compromise based on discussion and negotiation with the White House leadership.

Some of you may remember that, during the difficult 1996 federal budget process, a revised version of the Department of Defense (DOD) Reauthorization Act, which President Clinton had originally vetoed, was again on the floor of Congress for a vote. Unfortunately, Robert Dornan, a congressman from Orange County in southern California, had added an amendment to the bill that would have an adverse impact on any Armed Services personnel infected with HIV. Dornan's amendment passed and would require that all HIV-infected military personnel be discharged without benefits, including health care and job retraining. The Council again took a strong position and urged the President to again veto the bill. Members of the Council began to hear rumors that the President was thinking of signing the bill. A conference call to the White House was initiated. The conference call was with Chief of Staff Leon Panetta and White House Legal Counsel Jack Quinn. The White House was concerned that if the bill was again vetoed the support to oppose the Dornan amendment would be withdrawn. The Administration had gained unanimous support to oppose the amendment from the Joint Chiefs of Staff and the Pentagon; also, there was a concerted effort by the White House to obtain commitment by both Democrats and Republicans in Congress to oppose the amendment when the bill came up for a vote. Because of the strong position that the Council had taken earlier on the amendment, the White House was seriously developing the support necessary to defeat the amendment. The President also ordered the Administration to explore methods to ensure appropriate health care coverage for military personnel and their families and to provide job retraining as necessary if any personnel were actually discharged. The final strategy of the President was to order the Justice Department not to defend the amendment if it was passed by Congress and if a court challenge followed. This decision was based on President Clinton's assessment that the amendment was unconstitutional. I do not believe that many people understood the implication of this presidential order to the Justice Department. The normal process for any federal law is for the Justice Department to automatically defend the law in court. This strategy used by President Clinton has been used only once before by a President. The strategies worked. The amendment was repealed and, as many of you may know, Dornan was defeated in the last election. See the Box below for the Council's recommendation and assessment.

One final thought that I want to share with you before I review specific policy issues is that, as many long-time workers in the epidemic know, the knowledge base about HIV/AIDS continues to change, sometimes very rapidly. We are continually "pushing the envelope" with HIV. Policy development depends on current knowledge and understanding. Policies developed and implemented on the basis of 1985–1987 knowledge may not work for us today. The problem is that

policy perspectives are much more difficult to change. Many of us, because of our lived experiences, have very strong beliefs about what are the appropriate methods of responding to this epidemic—"what will work and what will not work"; "what affects my peer group or constituency." It is difficult to "live out there in the unknown," staying open to the possibility of a different perspective, but if we are going to best serve the people in need, we must attempt to live in that place of uncertainty.

SPECIFIC POLICY ISSUES

Testing, Contact Tracing, and Partner Notification

Ten years ago I wrote an article (Miramontes, 1988) about the need for effective national policies on HIV/AIDS. Some of the issues that were controversial then are still controversial today. Testing issues certainly continue to plague us in a variety of ways and arenas. In many states in the mid 1980s we were able to put into place fairly strong policies and regulations that protected the confidentiality of HIV antibody test results and restricted the use and distribution of test results.

■ PACHA RECOMMENDATION II.E.3. THE DORNAN AMENDMENT TO THE DOD REAUTHORIZATION ACT ■

The Administration should oppose any congressional efforts to require that otherwise qualified military service personnel who test positive for HIV be discharged, including a veto of the Department of Defense Reauthorization Act if such a provision is included. The Council recommends that in his veto message, the President state that the veto is, in part, due to the inclusion of this provision.

Administration's Response
The President and the Administration strongly opposed enactment of the so-called "Dornan Amendment." Through the coordinated efforts of the White House, the Department of Defense, the Department of Veterans Affairs, and the Department of Justice—along with the advocacy of many community groups—repeal of this provision was accomplished before any member of the Armed Forces had to be discharged. The Administration will continue to oppose efforts to reimpose this provision.

Assessment of the Response
The Council strongly advised the President to veto for the second time the DOD Reauthorization Act because it still contained the Dornan Amendment. While we opposed his decision to sign the bill, we commend the Administration's vocal opposition to the Dornan Amendment, its bold decision not to defend the law in court, and its leadership in obtaining legislative repeal of this law.

Follow-up Action Recommended
Continued vigilance will be required as similar amendments have been introduced in Congress.

We also defeated numerous proposals to implement mandatory and routine testing programs. Eventually, on the federal level, HIV came under the jurisdiction of the Americans with Disabilities Act (ADA), passed in 1990, which protects individuals from discriminatory practices due to HIV status. The perception during the mid 1980s was that any coercive policies about testing would drive the epidemic underground and people would avoid seeking health care. There also was no or very little treatment at this time. Zidovudine (ZDV/AZT), clinical trials of which were initiated in 1987, was the only antiretroviral treatment available. Persons were encouraged to be tested voluntarily at anonymous testing sites, if possible, in order to know their HIV status and, it was hoped, change their risk behaviors. Another rationale was that mandatory or routine testing would be expensive and require resources that could be used more effectively in the epidemic. Some of those rationales against mandatory or routine testing are still valid today, but some of the reasoning is outdated. Treatment is much more effective today, and the treatment guidelines that have just been released advocate aggressive treatment initiated much earlier then a few years ago (Department of Health and Human Services [DHHS], 1997a, 1997b). Second, research studies have been implemented to study the effects of treatment within the acute infection phase with the hope that very early treatment will prevent infection. Knowledge of HIV status is essential today if people are to receive appropriate treatment, but diverting resources to initiate mandatory or routine testing is still not appropriate, although there are some who would disagree (Burr, 1997).

A particular domain within the testing issue that I have been reevaluating over the last few years is the area of contact tracing and partner notification. Early in the epidemic, when the majority of the identified cases of AIDS were in gay men, many of us decided that, because of the significant discriminatory practices as well as the sexual culture of the gay community and the high prevalence of HIV infection within that community, contact tracing and partner notification would not yield very effective results. In fact, it was believed that such procedures would create significant barriers to prevention and treatment efforts within this specific community by driving the epidemic underground. However, as the epidemic has shifted to other populations and confidentiality laws and nondiscrimination laws have become stronger over time, we may need to rethink some of the restrictions that were put into place a decade ago. Often infected women have verbalized that they had been unaware that they were at risk of HIV infection. They were unaware that their sexual partners were injecting drug users (IDUs) or had engaged in unprotected sex with men. We have encouraged and also urged people to inform their sexual partners of their HIV status and to practice safer sex, but studies show that the majority of the time this does not happen. Toomey of CDC found, in her 6-year study of partner-notification behaviors, that 70% of the people studied failed to inform their sexual partners of their HIV-positive status, and most of these unaware partners were women (cited in Burkett, 1995). We cannot assume that these women may have already been infected. In addition, if a woman becomes pregnant and is infected and unaware of her status or of the treatment options that are available to her, she may deliver an infected infant. The question needs to be asked: "Does the woman's sexual partner have a greater right to protection of HIV status then the woman's right to know she is at risk?"

The potential for vertical transmission of HIV from mother to infant and for the treatment protocol for ZDV (AZT) intervention to reduce vertical transmission has triggered a plethora of legislative initiatives, on both the federal and state levels, aimed at either mandatory testing of all pregnant women or mandatory testing of all infants without consent of the mother. Neither option considers the rights of the woman. The focus is only on the prevention of vertical transmission to the infant. Women have often been viewed as vectors of infection in this epidemic, vectors of infection to men and to infants, without considering that women are frequently infected by someone else, usually their male sexual partners. Women have the right to information and access to testing, counseling, and health care provided in a nondirective, nonjudgmental, supportive environment. Mandatory testing protocols are not effective strategies for decreasing vertical transmission. Knowledge of risk factors and available options is certainly of greater benefit in decreasing viral transmission to infants.

I am not advocating major policy changes, but I am suggesting that we need to consider the impact of potential policies and legislation on other groups. We must understand that it is probably impossible to implement policies that address the issues for all people. The issues must be examined from more than one perspective. As an example, contact tracing and partner notification may not be advantageous for a woman who is infected with HIV if she is at risk of domestic violence or of having her children taken from her (Rothenberg & North, 1991; Rothenberg & Paskey, 1995). Currently, many public health departments do engage in contact tracing and partner notification with appropriate maintenance of confidentiality. Successful contact tracing and partner notification are dependent on the cooperation of the infected person to voluntarily disclose his or her sexual and needle-sharing partners. An infected person may be willing to disclose the names of contacts but unwilling or unable to disclose HIV status directly to his or her contacts. Testing, contact tracing, and partner notification are very complex issues and cannot be addressed through responses that may provide protection for only one group of people.

Needle Exchange

Another topic that has triggered extensive controversy is the issue of distributing clean needles to injecting drug users to prevent the transmission of HIV. Needle exchange is one component of the Harm Reduction Model, a strategy for managing drug use and HIV transmission, that was developed in Liverpool, England, during the mid 1980s (Newcombe & Perry, 1988). HIV seroprevalence among IDUs in Liverpool has remained very low. Soon some other countries adopted the model. The primary conceptual framework of the Harm Reduction Model is that, even if drug users may choose to continue to use drugs, there are strategies that may decrease the harm of substance use and also may decrease the risk of HIV transmission. A comprehensive harm reduction program includes treatment on demand, residential and nonresidential programs, methadone maintenance, and needle exchange. The ideal situation would be to have a comprehensive program. In the United States, though, our philosophy has been zero tolerance for any drug use. Our society equates drug use with drug

abuse. Our society has also defined drug use or abuse as a moral issue rather than a health issue. Consequently, most of the resources targeted in the "War on Drugs" have been spent on law enforcement, prison terms, and police work, and very little has been spent on drug treatment and health care.

In 1990, while I was in Australia consulting on provider HIV/AIDS training, I spent some time with the staff of the needle-exchange program in Sydney. Most of the street outreach personnel were nurses who used a mobile unit each night to provide not only needle exchange but also some nursing/medical interventions, support, counseling, and referrals as needed. The services were user friendly, nonjudgmental, and relevant to substance users' lives. Sydney's HIV seroprevalence rate among IDUs also is low.

A comprehensive program would be ideal, but implementation of needle-exchange programs can provide an effective mechanism for reducing HIV transmission. Such programs serve as a bridge to public health services, including drug-treatment programs. Certainly, there has been significant research that demonstrates that clean-needle exchange does prevent viral transmission (Lurie & Reingold, 1993). These studies have also demonstrated that needle exchange does not increase drug use in the community. Needle-exchange programs have been implemented in many communities across the United States. Local public health departments have the authority to implement emergency measures to protect the health of the community, and needle-exchange programs have been defined as emergency measures in these communities (Burris et al., 1996). In 1995 CDC (*San Francisco Chronicle*, 1995) endorsed needle exchange and called for the repeal of state laws impeding such programs, and a needle-exchange program was started in the nation's capital, Washington, D.C., in 1996 (*Washington Post*, 1996). In a nationwide poll conducted in 1996 (*San Francisco Chronicle*), two out of three families surveyed supported needle-exchange programs to decrease the rate of HIV transmission. Recently the United States Conference of Mayors approved a needle-exchange resolution that called for the Department of Health and Human Services (DHHS) to immediately eliminate current restrictions on the use of federal funds for needle exchange (San Francisco AIDS Foundation, 1997).

Even with all this support and research evidence, we have yet to have a national policy to implement needle-exchange programs, and in 1998 the Secretary of the DHHS announced that the federal government would not fund needle-exchange programs. Furthermore, most states (47) have drug paraphernalia laws, some more restrictive than others, and only five states have exception clauses for needle-exchange programs. In some states local ordinances regulate issues of drug paraphernalia (Gostin et al., 1997). According to the research evidence, it is time for the federal government to address this issue up front and support needle-exchange programs. The concern that many of us have is that if the President issued an executive order today to support needle exchange, restrictive legislation would be proposed in the Senate and similar legislation in the House of Representatives, which would prevent the implementation of resource allotment for needle-exchange strategies. As many of you may remember, a similar bill, the Defense of Marriage Act (DOMA), was quickly passed to prevent same-sex marriages in response to the Hawaiian Supreme Court case. I hope that we will be able to finally address this issue without restrictive legislation from the Congress.

Prevention Issues

Prevention issues is a generic term that encompasses the whole continuum of disciplines and strategies to prevent HIV transmission and infection. These strategies include education, behavioral change, microbicides, barriers (such as condoms), and vaccines. I am targeting this discussion on prevention education and will address some of the other prevention strategies in a later section.

Some people have defined testing and counseling as prevention strategies, and for years the majority of the CDC prevention funds were funneled into counseling and testing programs. The underlying assumption of testing and counseling is that enhancement of knowledge about the risks will have a significant effect on attitudes and beliefs which, in turn, will precipitate behavioral change. What we have found is that much of this type of prevention education has not worked. High levels of risk behaviors in specific populations have continued. The context in which behavior occurs has not been cycled into the behavioral change paradigm. Even within the gay

community that took on the task of educating its members, we see risk behaviors continuing in some subpopulations of the community (Gold & Phil, 1995; Odets, 1995). Of course, some of this behavioral education has influenced some people to change their risk behaviors, but certainly not to the extent that we would like.

The basis for much of the thinking about prevention education evolves out of theoretical research on health promotion and behavioral change, which was developed long before the onset of HIV. These early models emphasized a cognitive approach to individual behavioral change, and the focus was on changing or modifying the individual's behavior. The approach was to help the individual to perceive his or her behavior that was unhealthy, to be able to define the consequences of the behavior, to accept the benefits of changing the behavior, to develop skills to change the behavior, and then to change the behavior. Little or no attention was paid to the social, economic, political, and cultural context of the behavior. With the onset of the HIV epidemic, these models were examined for integration into HIV-prevention programs (Chesney & Coates, 1990; Jemmott & Jemmott, 1991, 1992). Since those early years of HIV prevention, there has been a plethora of ongoing research into development of more effective behavioral change models and programs (Coates et al., 1995; Van Gorder, 1995). Cultural issues and the way they influence behavioral change have been studied (Bayer, 1994; Gomez, 1995; Nyamathi et al., 1993; Peterson et al., 1992). The Report of the National Institute of Health (NIH) AIDS Research Program Evaulation Working Group of the Office of AIDS Research (OAR) Advisory Council reviewed current behavioral research and made extensive recommendations to not only expand the research but to closely link it with biomedical research (NIH, OAR, 1996). New journals have been established that focus only on HIV/AIDS prevention and education in order to disseminate the results of many ongoing studies. In addition to the research funded out of NIH, OAR, CDC, and private foundations have also funded prevention research. Traditionally, our society has never adequately funded prevention interventions or prevention research, but there appears to be a shift in priorities. More people and groups are advocating the targeting of more resources to projects and research that demonstrate prevention. The lack of effective vaccines or microbicides probably has added to the push for effective prevention strategies.

In addition to some of the barriers noted here, the lack of consensus about what should be taught and to whom has been extremely controversial. As an example, there has been a significant lack of agreement in many communities concerning the education of adolescents about sexual behavior. There has been a massive effort by many of a more orthodox religious tradition to teach only abstinence of any sexual behavior, which seems to ignore the well-documented reports of the actual sexual behavior of our youth. The report to the White House on Youth and HIV/AIDS: An American Agenda urged ongoing age-appropriate approaches to HIV prevention and their integration into education about other sexually transmitted diseases (STDs), pregnancy , substance use, sexuality, and self-esteem (ONAP, 1996). A comprehensive adolescent program would include abstinence or delaying onset of sexual activity, but this certainly would not be the only option taught. Accurate information and support for healthy, responsible decisions are more useful to youth. Young persons need a place where they can ask questions, where they can be heard, and where they can be supported; otherwise, we are in danger of losing more of our children to this epidemic.

Microbicides and Vaccines

I had two agenda issues—microbicides and vaccines—when I was appointed to PACHA. My rationale for focusing on these issues was that many people were advocating therapeutic and basic research, prevention education, treatment, care, and services, and only a few were advocating either microbicides or vaccines. Very few resources have gone into research in either field. Without highly effective prevention strategies, such as vaccines and microbicides, we will never stop this epidemic. The priority of many activists had been treatment research. This priority is understandable, considering that many of our activists are HIV-infected or have AIDS.

The lack of attention to microbicides is also understandable when we consider that most of our infected population during the 1980s were men and that microbicides were products that women would use. Besides, we had condoms, and the emphasis on prevention education was consistent with the use of condoms. The problem for women is that women do not use condoms; men use condoms. For many women, even in our society, lack of power and lack of control in relationships hinders negotiation about condom use, and women are always dependent on the cooperation of male sex partners to consistently use condoms. In other societies there are frequently greater gender differences for women in roles, control, power, and ability to control their sexual life than we see in this society. Microbicides are controlled by women and could be a very effective method for prevention of HIV infection. Microbicides would be fairly inexpensive and could be made available for developing countries. If microbicides that were effective in disease prevention but not spermicidal could be produced, some of the cultural barriers would be eliminated or minimized.

During PACHA's December 1995 meeting, several microbicide researchers met with the Research Committee to discuss the need for a greater effort in microbicide research. At that time only about $10 million to $12 million was being spent on microbicide studies. During the 1996 International AIDS Conference in Vancouver, British Columbia, Donna Shalala, Secretary of Health and Human Services, announced that the United States would spend $100 million on microbicide research over the next 4 to 5 years. That is not much more than is currently spent on this research. PACHA made a recommendation in December 1995 (see Box, p. 454) about increasing the resources for microbicide research. That was only a preliminary recommendation, and much more needs to be done. The Research Committee plans to address this issue again later this year after assessment of current efforts.

We are also beginning to see other women and women's groups take on this issue. There is a Microbicide Research Advocacy Project jointly sponsored by the Center for Women's Policy Studies and the Reproductive Health Technologies Project. This joint project is located in Washington, D.C.

The last issue I want to discuss, and one that is a top priority for me, is the issue of vaccines. This is probably one of the most controversial issues in this epidemic. It certainly has been difficult to obtain support for resources aimed at vaccine research. The controversy involves not only the scientific community but many activists as well. A simplified version of the controversy is that the basic scientist perspective is that we do not have sufficient information to develop a vaccine, but vaccine researchers believe that a vaccine is possible and that vaccine research is dependent on both knowledge gained from basic science and knowledge gained from empirical research by conducting clinical trials. Even the failures in clinical trials provide needed information. Most of the non-HIV vaccines that we have today were developed through the use of basic scientific research and empirical research. Vaccine researchers, such as Margaret Johnston, Max Essex, Philip Russell, Jerald Sadoff, Don Francis, and others, stated that a vaccine is possible, but the development of a vaccine must be a priority and resources must be allocated to do the research and development (B.P. Dorman, personal communication, November 22, 1995; Esparza et al., 1996; Essex, 1995; Gallagher, 1997; Johnston, 1996).

Early in the epidemic, some scientists thought that a vaccine might not be possible because of the rapid mutation of the virus; later others stated that a live attenuated virus vaccine or a whole killed virus vaccine could not be used because either would be too dangerous. As a result, much of the vaccine research focused on components of the virus, such as the gp120 and gp160. Both of these components are surface glycoproteins of the virus. Other barriers, in addition to lack of resources for vaccine research, were the inability to identify an appropriate animal model in which to conduct the vaccine research; the disinterest among many pharmaceutical companies to engage in vaccine research; and the lack of broad community advocacy. The lack of interest on the part of pharmaceutical companies stems from the low return on investment and the issue of product liability. Vaccines must be effective, safe, inexpensive, and widely available, which explains why pharmaceutical companies would not be interested in vaccine research. When the polio vaccine was developed, the federal government assumed liability for the vaccine; also, there was significant pressure from the larger society and from President Roosevelt to develop a vaccine. Every mother perceived that her child was at risk of polio. We do not see that advocacy from the larger society in this epidemic.

Most AIDS activists have not advocated a vaccine; in fact, some of the activists have attempted to block development of a vaccine. Some of this opposition is based on social and political considerations and should be reviewed and discussed. A document by the AIDS Action Foundation (1994) delineates some of these issues. Other opposition appears to be more self-serving, holding that resources would be taken from therapeutic issues for treatment of those already infected to fund vaccine research (Cohen, 1994b; Francis, 1995; Francis & Kennedy, 1994; Green, 1995; Schoofs, 1995).

In 1994, on the basis of the preliminary data from Phase I and Phase II trials, a vaccine working group at NIH voted to enlarge and extend Phase II studies on two gp120 vaccines (National Institute of Allergy and Infectious Diseases [NIAID], NIH, 1994). Two months later, during a joint meeting of the AIDS Subcommittee of the National Advisory Allergy and Infectious Diseases Council and the AIDS Research Advisory Committee at NIAID, NIH, the committee voted to stop the clinical trials of the gp120 vaccines. The rationale for stopping the trials, as stated in the minutes of the meeting, was based not on the science of the trials but on other factors. There were nine abstentions in the vote, with 17 "yes" votes (Altman, 1994; NIAID, NIH, 1994). According to Jon Cohen (1994a), writing in *Science,* "A flier from New York's AIDS Coalition to Unleash Power (ACT UP) distributed at the meeting threatened 'a massive boycott' of efficacy trials" (p. 1839).

During this time the Rockefeller Foundation was beginning to focus on the HIV vaccine issue. In March of 1994 the Health Sciences Division of the Foundation held an international meeting of 24 participants, representing 12 countries, to discuss the current status of HIV vaccine research and explore possible avenues for accelerating the research. In October 1994 a second meeting was held to develop recommendations on HIV vaccine research; a third meeting was conducted in October 1995 to identify the financial and structural issues and to make recommendations to move the vaccine issue ahead. Out of this combined effort, the International AIDS Vaccine Initiative (IAVI) was established. IAVI's "first priority is to launch a directed vaccine research and development program . . . which will support promising research efforts that are currently underexplored. A second priority is to undertake a series of activities aimed at reducing key uncertainties and risks associated with private industry investment in AIDS vaccine development" (FitzSimons, 1996, p.8).

I believe that there has been a shift in attention to HIV vaccine research and that this shift and interest, coming from multiple groups, will enhance the efforts to develop a vaccine. The announcement by President Clinton about developing a vaccine within the decade and the President's advocacy at the recent international economic meeting in Denver with the G-7 countries has placed the vaccine issue at the top of the HIV/AIDS agenda. The work of PACHA, IAVI, NIH, and the United Nations AIDS Program has facilitated the move forward, and those of us who are committed to making it happen will continue to advocate and unceasingly monitor the efforts.

In closing, I want to reiterate the need for all of us to be involved in policy development and to carry out our roles in advocacy with responsible, thoughtful consideration, demonstrating critical thinking and sensitivity to the complexity of the issues and the necessity to examine all proposals from multiple perspectives.

REFERENCES

AIDS Action Foundation. (1994). *HIV preventive vaccines: Social, ethical, and political considerations for domestic efficacy trials.* Washington, D.C.: OAR, NIH.

Altman, L.K. (June 18, 1994). Panel rejects wider testing to develop AIDS vaccine. *The New York Times*, p. 6.

Bayer, R. (1994). AIDS prevention and cultural sensitivity: Are they compatible? *American Journal of Public Health, 84*(6), 895–898.

Burkett, E. (1995). *The gravest show on earth.* New York: Houghton Mifflin.

Burr, C. (1997). The AIDS exception: Privacy vs. public health. *The Atlantic Monthly, 279*(6), 57–61, 64–67.

Burris, S., Finucane, D., Gallagher, H., Grace, J. (1996). The legal strategies used in operating syringe exchange programs in the United States. *American Journal of Public Health, 86*(8), 1161–1166.

Chesney, M.A., Coates, T.J. (1990). Putting the models to the test. In S. Petrow, P. Franks, T.R. Wolfred (Eds.), *Ending the HIV epidemic* (pp. 48–62). Santa Cruz: Network.

Coates, T.J., Faigle, M., Koijane, J., Stall, R.D. (1995). *Does HIV prevention work for men who have sex with men?* Washington, D.C.: Office of Technology Assessment, Congress of the United States.

Cohen, J. (1994a). U.S. panel votes to delay real-world vaccine trials. *Science, 264,* 1839.

Cohen, J. (1994b). Are researchers racing toward success, or crawling? *Science, 265,* 1373–1376.

DHHS. (1997a). *Report of the NIH panel to define principles of therapy of HIV infection.* Washington, D.C.: NIH Panel on Principles of Therapy of HIV Infection.

DHHS. (1997b). *Guidelines for the use of antiretroviral agents in HIV-infected adults and adolescents.* Washington, D.C.: Panel on Clinical Practices for Treatment of HIV Infection.

Esparza, J., Heyward, W.L., Osmanov, S. (1996). HIV vaccine development: From basic research to human trials. *AIDS, 10,* S123–S131.

Essex, M. (1995). The HIV-1 vaccine dilemma: Lessons from the cat. *The Journal of NIH Research, 7,* 37–42.

FitzSimons, D. (1996). International AIDS vaccine initiative launched. *IAVI Report, 1*(1), 7–8.

Francis, D.P. (1995). Why AIDS vaccine development is taking longer than it should. *Current Issues in Public Health, 1,* 181–185.

Francis, D.P., Kennedy, D. (July 19, 1994). A private-sector AIDS vaccine? Don't hold your breath. *The Washington Post,* p. 19.

Gallagher, J. (February 18, 1997). Experts agree an AIDS vaccine is doable. *The Advocate, 35,* 38.

Gebbie, K.M. (1996). National health policy: Lessons from a hot seat. *Nursing Administration Quarterly, 20*(3), 9–18.

Gold, R.S., Phil, D. (1995). Rethinking HIV prevention strategies for gay men. *Focus, 10*(3), 1–4.

Goldstein, A. (September 23, 1996). D.C. to use needles in AIDS fight. *The Washington Post,* p. B1.

Gomez, C.A. (1995). Cultural and sexual behavior. *Focus, 10*(4), 5–8.

Gostin, L.O., Lazzarini, Z., Jones, T.S., Flaherty, K. (1997). Prevention of HIV/AIDS and other blood-borne diseases among injection drug users: A national survey on the regulation of syringes and needles. *Journal of the American Medical Association, 277*(1), 53–61.

Green, J. (March 26, 1995). Who put the lid on gp120? *The New York Times Magazine,* pp. 50–57, 74, 82.

Jemmott, L.S., Jemmott, J.B. (1991). Applying the theory of reasoned action to AIDS risk behavior: Condom use among black women. *Nursing Research, 40*(4), 228–234.

Jemmott, L.S., Jemmott, J.B. (1992). Predicting intentions to use condoms among African-American adolescents: The theory of planned behavior as a model of HIV risk-associated behavior. *Ethnicity Disease, 2,* 371–380.

Johnston, M. (1996). Why an HIV vaccine is scientifically possible. *IAVI Report, 1*(1), 1–2, 11.

Lurie, P., Reingold, A.L. (1993). *The public health impact of needle exchange programs in the United States and abroad.* San Francisco: Institute for Health Policy Studies, University of California, San Francisco, and School of Public Health, University of California, Berkeley.

Miramontes, H. (1988). Needed: Effective national policy on AIDS/HIV infection. *Nursing Outlook, 36*(6), 262–263, 296.

National Commission on AIDS. (1993). *AIDS: An expanding tragedy.* Rockville, MD: CDC National AIDS Clearinghouse.

NIH, NIAID, Division of AIDS. (April 21–22, 1994). *HIV vaccine working group meeting.* Bethesda: Author.

NIH, NIAID, Division of AIDS. (June 17, 1994). *Joint meeting of the AIDS Subcommittee of the National Advisory Allergy and Infectious Diseases Council and the AIDS Research Advisory Committee.* Bethesda: Author.

NIH, OAR Advisory Council. (March 13, 1996). *NIH AIDS research program evaluation working group.* Bethesda: Author.

Newcombe, R., Parry, A. (October 22, 1988). *The mersey harm-reduction model: A strategy for dealing with drug users.* Presented at the International Conference on Drug Policy Reform, Bethesda, Maryland.

Nyamathi, A., Bennett, C., Leake, B., Lewis, C., Flaskerud, J. (1993). AIDS-related knowledge, perceptions, and behaviors among impoverished minority women. *American Journal of Public Health, 83*(1), 65–71.

Odets, W. (1995). The fatal mistakes of AIDS education. *Harper's, 290*(1740), 13–17.

Peterson, J.L., Coates, T.J., Catania, J.A., Middleton, L., Hilliard, B., Hearst, N. (1992). High-risk sexual behavior and condom use among gay and bisexual African-American men. *American Journal of Public Health, 82*(11), 1490–1494.

PACHA. (July 8, 1996). *Progress report: Implementation of advisory council recommendations.* Washington, D.C.: ONAP.

Presidential Commission. (1988, June). *Report of the Presidential Commission on the Human Immunodeficiency Virus Epidemic.* Washington, D.C.: Author.

Rothenberg, K.H., North, R.L. (1991). The duty to warn "dilemma" and women with AIDS. *Courts, Health Science & the Law, 2*(1), 90–98.

Rothenberg, K.H., Paskey, S.J. (1995). The risk of domestic violence and women with HIV infection: Implication for partner notification, public policy, and the law. *American Journal of Public Health, 85*(11), 1569–1574.

Russell, S. (March 8, 1995). CDC endorses needle swaps. *San Francisco Chronicle,* p. B1.

Russell, S. (March 27, 1996). Strong backing in poll on steps to prevent AIDS. *San Francisco Chronicle,* p. A13.

San Francisco AIDS Foundation (SFAF). (June 24, 1997). U.S. conference of mayors urges Secretary of Health and Human Services Shalala to end federal restriction on needle exchange. Press release, 1–3.

Schoofs, M. (September 12, 1995). We could have an AIDS vaccine so why don't we? *The Village Voice, 40*(37), 20–24.

Shilts, R. (1987). *And the band played on.* New York: St. Martin's Press.

Toomey, K. (1995). In E. Burkett, *The gravest show on earth.* New York: Houghton Mifflin.

Van Gorder, D. (1995). Building community and culture are essential to successful HIV prevention for gay and bisexual men. *AIDS & Public Policy Journal, 10*(2), 65–74.

The White House. (1997). *The national AIDS strategy.* Washington, D.C.: ONAP.

The White House. (1996). *Youth & HIV/AIDS: An American agenda.* Washington, D.C.: ONAP.

I

Health Teaching for the Client with HIV Infection

WALTER R. WEISS

Topic	Encourage	Discourage	Rationale
Stress	A proactive response style to HIV disease Identifying stressor categories (Pivar & Temoshok, 1990): 1. HIV diagnostic testing 2. Severe symptom or illness episodes 3. Treatment issues 4. Complications with family, work, school (or finances) 5. Physical and psychologic limitations or losses 6. Concerns about future Psychoeducational support groups to reduce stress and improve coping (Moulton et al., 1990; Perry et al., 1991) Individual strategies to reduce and manage stress, such as: 1. Exercise 2. Meditation 3. Use of visualization 4. Relaxation techniques 5. Therapeutic touch Seeking factual information related to HIV disease from knowledgeable health care professionals	Passive attitude or self-destructive behaviors	Stress may negatively affect the immune response and favor progression of HIV-related disease (Evans et al., 1991; Flescher et al., 1992; Hassan & Douglas, 1990). Stress management may buffer illness-related psychologic distress (McCain et al., 1996). Lower CD4+ cell count associated with higher levels of stressful experiences (McCain et al., 1995).

Topic	Encourage	Discourage	Rationale
Exercise	A daily schedule of exercise activities	Continuing or adapting a sedentary lifestyle	Exercise may be physiologically, immunologically, and psychologically beneficial to HIV-infected persons and may favorably influence the course of HIV disease (LaPerriene et al., 1990, 1991, 1994a, 1994b; MacArthur et al., 1992; Rigsby et al., 1992; Schlenzig et al., 1992; Smith et al., 1996).
Sexual practices	Safer sexual practices with partners who are HIV-positive and HIV-negative	Unsafe sex	Emerging trend for HIV-positive persons to have unprotected intercourse (Signorile, 1997).
	Proper use of male condoms, including:	Improper use of a male condom, including:	Use of latex condom reduces the risk of gonorrhea, herpes simplex, genital ulcers, and pelvic inflammatory disease and provides a barrier to HIV, hepatitis B virus, and *Chlamydia trachomatis* (Centers for Disease Control and Prevention [CDC], 1993).
	1. Using a latex condom only	1. Using natural-membrane condoms	
	2. Using a new condom for each sexual act or partner	2. Reusing condom or using same condom for insertive sex when having sex with multiple partners at the same time	
	3. Carefully handling the condom	3. Damaging condom with fingernail, teeth, or other sharp objects	
	4. Putting on the condom before genital contact with partner and when penis is erect	4. Using condom only for vaginal or anal penetration or attempting to apply condom to a flaccid penis	
	5. Ensuring that no air is trapped in tip of condom	5. Leaving air bubble at tip of condom	
	6. Ensuring adequate lubrication during vaginal or anal intercourse	6. Engaging in "dry" intercourse	
	7. Using only water-based lubricants (e.g., K-Y jelly, glycerine) with latex condom	7. Using oil-based lubricants (e.g., petroleum jelly, shortening, mineral oil, massage oils, body lotions, or cooking oil), which can weaken latex	
	8. Holding the condom firmly against base of penis during withdrawal and withdrawing penis while still erect	8. Allowing slippage or spillage when withdrawing	
	9. Storing of condoms in cool, dry place, away from direct sunlight	9. Using damaged condoms, as evidenced by brittleness, stickiness, or discoloration	
	10. Checking expiration date	10. Using outdated condoms	

Table continued on following page

Topic	Encourage	Discourage	Rationale
Sexual practices *Continued*	Proper use of the female condom; second choice to male latex condom	Improper use of the female condom	Data regarding the efficacy of female condoms are incomplete, but these devices should be considered as a reduction strategy (CDC, 1997).
	Use of nonoxynol-9 (a nonionic surfactant spermicide); no studies have shown that the use of nonoxynol-9 with a condom increases the protection provided by use of a latex condom alone (CDC, 1993)		
	Use of barrier protection for fellatio, anal-oral sex, and cunnilingus (condoms and dental dams)	Performing fellatio, anal-oral sex, or cunnilingus without a barrier	
	Using latex gloves for digital insertive manipulative practices	Inserting finger(s) into vagina or rectum without a barrier	
Procreation	Providing unbiased information regarding HIV disease so that client can make informed reproductive decisions, including (Berman, 1993; Smeltzer & Whipple, 1991): 1. Illness may occur in the mother during pregnancy, and choices regarding treatment will have to be made that may be toxic to the fetus 2. Either the child or the mother, or both, may become ill and die.	Negating the fact that the client does have reproductive options	Through counseling, the client may gain sufficient knowledge to make informed choices about procreation (Berman, 1993).
	Viral load testing of mother and antiretroviral therapy (Brandt et al., 1996; Sperling et al., 1996).	Delaying diagnostic testing and treatment	Transmission of HIV to infant is related to viral levels of mother and can be decreased with antiretroviral therapy (Bryson, 1996).
	Viral load testing of infant and antiretroviral therapy (Bush et al., 1996; Shearer et al., 1997).	Delaying diagnostic testing and treatment	
	Smoking cessation	Continued smoking	Cigarette smoking during pregnancy associated with an increased risk of maternal-child HIV transmission (Turner et al., 1997).
	Increased intake of calories and protein during pregnancy	Poor nutrition	Nutritional needs are increased during pregnancy (U.S. Department of Health and Human Services, 1996).

Topic	Encourage	Discourage	Rationale
Procreation *Continued*	Formula feeding of infant Additional considerations 　1. Possible illness and death of the father 　2. Finances 　3. Support systems 　4. Guardianship and adoption Choices including 　1. Contraception 　2. Abortion	Breast-feeding	Transmission of HIV possible through breast milk (Nicoll et al., 1996).
Nutrition	Increased intake of protein (fish, chicken, meat, eggs, milk, cheese, dried beans, nuts, and tofu)	Diets that are inadequate in protein intake	Nutritional counseling and support can improve the nutritional status of people (Beach, 1992; Bradley-Springer, 1991; Kotler, 1992).
	Increased intake of carbohydrates as a source of calories (bread, cereals, rice, macaroni, noodles, potatoes, dried beans, plantain, fruits, cakes, cookies, and candy)	Diets that are calorically sparse	High nutrient intake is associated with higher CD4+ T-cell counts and can reduce the rate of AIDS development (Abrams et al., 1993).
	Limiting intake of fat (butter, margarine, oils, mayonnaise, salad dressing, cheese, sour cream, whole milk, sausages, salami, bacon, bologna, and other high-fat meats and cold cuts)		May increase potential for lipodystrophy, especially when protease inhibitors are prescribed (Henry et al., 1998).
	Increased vitamin and mineral intake by taking a multivitamin daily and eating the above-mentioned foods as well as fruits and vegetables	Inadequate intake of vitamins and minerals	
	Increased intake of water and juices on a daily basis		
	Eating small amounts of food throughout the day (U.S. Department of Health and Human Services, 1996)	Limited number of meals	
	Participation in meal programs for people with HIV disease as an opportunity to learn more about nutrition as well as to socialize		
	Building on the client's current dietary patterns	Introduction of an entirely new menu or standardized menus that may be irrelevant to the client	
Food safety	Prevention of foodborne diseases (CDC, 1989a, 1997; Life Sciences Research Office, 1990) by: 　1. Eating and drinking pasteurized dairy products (only) 　2. Cooking meats, fish, and poultry to "well done"	The nine factors most often implicated in bacterial food poisoning (Nadakavukaren, 1990, p. 219) 　1. Eating raw protein foods, such as uncooked eggs, rare meat, and sushi	Infectious complications can be prevented by avoiding ingestion of contaminated food (Filice & Pomeroy, 1991).

Table continued on following page

Topic	Encourage	Discourage	Rationale
Food safety *Continued*	3. Considering all animal-derived foods as contaminated, and: a. Washing hands immediately after handling b. Using meat thermometer to ensure thorough cooking c. Cooking to achieve internal temperatures of 165° F (73.8° C) for poultry and meats (Nadakavukaren, 1990) d. Using separate cutting boards for raw and cooked foods 4. For microwave cooking, following directions carefully, especially standing time, which allows heat to fully penetrate food 5. When barbecuing, precooking meat first (especially chicken) 6. Washing utensils used for meats before reuse or before use for other foods 7. Wearing disposable gloves if there are cuts or abrasions on hands 8. Washing all fruits and vegetables thoroughly before eating a. Placing raw meat or poultry into plastic bags to prevent juices from leaking onto other foods b. Reading expiration or "sell by" dates and pasteurized labels c. Refrigerating perishables as soon as possible 9. Thawing frozen meat and poultry by microwave or in refrigerator (U.S. Department of Health and Human Services, 1996) 10. Eating leftovers in less than 3 days	2. Failure to refrigerate foods properly 3. Preparing food a day or more before it is to be served 4. Failure to cook foods thoroughly 5. Poor personal hygiene when handling food 6. Improper "hot" holding (keeping foods in heating trays at temperatures under 140° F) 7. Inadequate reheating of cooked foods 8. Failure to avoid moldy or spoiled foods 9. Use of foods after labeled expiration date	

Topic	Encourage	Discourage	Rationale
Water safety	At home, use of boiled water for drinking or boiling of unsafe water for 10 minutes to sterilize it (CDC, 1990)		Infectious complications can be prevented by avoiding ingestion of contaminated water (Filice & Pomeroy, 1991).
	When away from home, drinking bottled or canned carbonated water or soft drinks	Adding ice cubes to drinks	Waterborne diseases continue to occur from relatively sophisticated water systems (CDC, 1991; Gold, 1993).
	After using swimming pools, hot tubs, or whirlpools, showering well and using an antimicrobial soap		Waterborne diseases can occur as a result of surface contact with or swallowing contaminated water (CDC, 1991).
Skin care	Keeping skin moist and intact (Hardy, 1992; CDC, 1997)		Secondary skin infections or transfer of infections from one part of the body to another can be prevented and the effects of xerosis (dry skin) and ichthyosis (rough, thick, scaly skin), the most common dermatoses seen in HIV infection, can be minimized (Duvic, 1991).
	Showering daily for at least 1 minute	Tub baths	
	Maintaining water temperature of 90° to 105° F		
	Using a superfatted soap	Using drying, perfumed soap	
	Patting skin dry and, while damp, applying an emollient cream	Using creams and lotions that have a high alcohol content and are drying	
Hair care	Washing hair infrequently	Washing hair daily	Hair loss related to telogen effluvium (decreases in number of hair follicles), caused by severe stress, recurrent infections, and high fevers can be minimized (Cockerell, 1991).
	Using mild soap	Using drying, perfumed shampoo	
	Using conditioner		
	Covering head while in bed		
	Combing hair	Brushing hair	
Mouth care	Using a soft toothbrush	Using firm or hard toothbrush	The incidence or severity of secondary oral infections, especially thrush, can be reduced.
	Using nonabrasive toothpaste (or baking soda)	Using abrasive toothpaste	
	Brushing surface of teeth only		
	Using Toothettes for mucosal surface cleaning	Brushing mucosal surfaces	
	Performing mouth care three times a day	Performing mouth care only once or twice a day	
	Dental examinations every 6 months	Ignoring dental examinations	
Hand washing	Washing frequently after activities of daily living	Using hot water	Secondary infections related to poor hand-washing practices can be prevented.
	Using soap in a pump dispenser	Using bar soap	
	Rinsing well		
	Applying emollient cream to protect the skin		
	Wearing rubber or latex gloves when cleaning		
	Demonstrating hand-washing	Teaching hand-washing without demonstrating correct method	

Table continued on following page

Topic	Encourage	Discourage	Rationale
Environmental cleaning and safety	Using household bleach (5.25% sodium hypochlorite) diluted: ¼ cup of bleach per gallon of tap water (CDC, 1989b)	Using expensive ineffective (for disinfection) household detergents	Secondary infections related to unclean environment and contamination of environment with HIV can be prevented.
	Discarding solution daily and remixing when necessary	Using cleaning solutions more than 24 hours after mixing	
	Cleaning up blood or body fluids with this solution		
	Using household bleach for laundry soiled with blood or body fluids		
	Using securely fastened plastic bags to discard disposable items contaminated with blood or body fluids	Discarding soiled disposable items without using secured bags	
	Placing used needles and "sharps" in puncture-resistant containers such as detergent containers or coffee cans (United States Environmental Protection Agency, 1990)	Throwing used needles and sharps directly into household garbage	
	Cleaning or changing air-conditioner filters frequently		
Pet care	Education about the risks of acquiring infections from pets		Persons may weigh the risks against benefits of pet ownership (Conti et al., 1996).
	Having pet care performed by someone other than person with HIV disease	Handling pet excreta or cleaning litter boxes, bird cages, or aquariums	Certain infectious complications that are zoonotic can be prevented (Filice & Pomeroy, 1991).
	When necessary, wearing gloves and washing hands when finished		
	Always washing hands, face, etc., after having direct contact with body secretions or excretions from pets or when scratched		
	Keeping domestic pets, especially cats, indoors		
	Feeding only commercially prepared canned or dry pet food and meats that are cooked thoroughly	Feeding raw meat or poultry to domestic animals	
	Ownership of healthy pets	Exotic, wild, sickly pets, particularly cats with feline leukemia and turtles (Downing, 1995)	
	Deworming, vaccinating, and neutering of pets (Florida Department of Health and Rehabilitative Services, 1996)		
	Veterinary care should be sought for pets that develop diarrhea		To detect *Cryptosporidium*, *Salmonella*, or *Campylobacter*.

Topic	Encourage	Discourage	Rationale
Alcohol drinking	Abstinence or modification	Regular consumption of alcohol	Although Kaslow and colleagues (1989) found no effect on the progression of HIV disease, Bagastra and associates (1993) found that alcohol intake did increase HIV replication. Pol and associates (1996) found improvement of CD4+ cell count after alcohol withdrawal in HIV-positive alcoholic patients.
Smoking	Reduction in smoking Avoidance of smoking Starting a smoking cessation program	Continued smoking Returning to smoking as a means of coping with stress	Smoking may negatively influence the course of HIV disease and increase the propensity for development of pulmonary opportunistic infections, oral mucosal lesions, and periodontal disease (Burns et al., 1996; Buskin et al., 1992; Clarke et al., 1993; Conley et al., 1996; Forthal et al., 1992; Hirschtick et al., 1995; Nieman et al., 1993; Palacio et al., 1997; Royce & Winkelstein, 1990; Swango et al., 1991).
Intravenous drug use	Cessation of drug use and referral for treatment Not sharing drug paraphernalia with others Disinfecting drug paraphernalia before sharing equipment (if client persists in sharing) Open dialogue regarding continued drug use Referral to needle-exchange program (if locally available)	Sharing of contaminated drug paraphernalia Client and health care professional avoiding discussion of drug use	Prevent transmission of bloodborne disease. Cessation of intravenous drug (Weber et al., 1990).
Travel	Travel planning	Travel to middle, central, and south central United States, including the Ohio and Mississippi river basins, as well as the Caribbean and South America (to avoid histoplasmosis); travel to Arizona, California, Nevada, New Mexico, Utah, and western Texas, as well as Mexico and Central and South America (to avoid coccidiomycoses)	Prevent opportunistic infections (Jewett & Hecht, 1993).

Table continued on following page

Topic	Encourage	Discourage	Rationale
Travel *Continued*	Nutrition safety 1. Cooking all meat, fish, poultry, and eggs well done and serving hot 2. Eating only fresh fruits and vegetables that can be peeled 3. Drinking only bottled water or canned carbonated water or soft drinks 4. Purchasing food in restaurants or hotels Planning for special needs 1. Requesting in advance a room with a refrigerator (for medication storage), honored by most hotels 2. Requesting a wheelchair in advance for movement into and out of airports, as well as for transfers between connecting flights Consulting with a health care provider before traveling to discuss the possible need for chemoprophylaxis for traveler's diarrhea Hepatitis A vaccine (CDC, 1996)	1. Eating undercooked or raw meat, fish, poultry, or eggs 2. Eating prepared fruits and vegetables that are not cooked (e.g., salads) 3. Adding ice cubes to drinks (even to alcoholic drinks) 4. Buying food from street vendors 1. Waiting until checking in to request the special need 2. Waiting until arriving at the airport to request wheelchair transport	 Prevent gastrointestinal infection (DuPont & Ericsson, 1993).
Health care follow-up	Establishing a pattern for health care follow-up (e.g., physician, nurse practitioner, physician assistant, visiting nurse, clinic) Establishing a relationship with health care professional knowledgeable about HIV disease Watching for signs and symptoms indicating secondary complications for HIV disease, including but not limited to: 1. Skin lesions, rashes, itching, lumps, or bruising 2. Lesions or exudate in mouth 3. Persistent fever, night sweats 4. Extreme fatigue even when getting plenty of rest 5. Weight loss 6. Changes in digestion, difficulty in swallowing, and diarrhea 7. Shortness of breath, persistent coughing	Changing patterns of health care follow-up Seeking health care from professional with knowledge deficits of HIV disease Ignoring warning signs	 Increased survival associated with the level of experience of health care provider (Kitahata et al., 1996). Patients with CD4+ T-cell counts greater than 500/mm^3 and stable, low viral loads are at the same risk of developing any pathologic condition as HIV-negative person and can handle most minor symptomatic problems without professional consultation. Patients with declining CD4+ counts less than 500/mm^3 and increasing viral loads should be taught signs and symptoms that may indicate serious disease (Hecht & Soloway, 1993; Donovan et al., 1996).

Topic	Encourage	Discourage	Rationale
Health care follow-up *Continued*	8. Headache, visual changes, numbness in arms and legs, forgetfulness, dizziness, seizures 9. Unusual bleeding (e.g., bleeding gums)		
Additional considerations	Receiving influenza vaccination annually		
	Using own personal care items (e.g., razors, toothbrushes, make-up)	Sharing personal care items	
	Refraining from donating blood or organs	Donating blood or making plans to donate body organs	
	Informing health care professional responsible for primary care that the client has HIV disease	Withholding information about HIV disease from health care professionals responsible for coordinating care	Preventing transmissions and withholding information on current HIV diagnosis could result in a delay in diagnosing and treating problems related to HIV disease.
	Planning financially	Waiting until a crisis occurs to access entitlements	
	Completion of advance directives	Waiting until a crisis to make decisions	

REFERENCES

Abrams, B., Duncan, D., Hertz-Picaotto, I. (1993). A prospective study of dietary intake and acquired immune deficiency syndrome in HIV seropositive homosexual men. *Journal of Acquired Immune Deficiency Syndromes, 6*(8), 949–958.

Bagastra, O., Kajdacsy-Balla, A., Lischner, H.W., et al. (1993). Alcohol intake increases human immunodeficiency virus type I replication in human peripheral blood mononuclear cells. *Journal of Infectious Diseases, 167*(4), 789–797.

Beach, R.S. (1992). Nutrition and people with HIV/AIDS: A summary for data presented at the VII International Conference on AIDS. *Nutrition and HIV/AIDS, 1*(1), 107–108.

Berman, N. (1993). Family and reproductive issues: Reproductive counseling. *AIDS Clinical Care, 5*(6), 45–47.

Bradley-Springer, L. (1991). Nutrition and support in HIV infection: A multilevel analysis. *Image: Journal of Nursing Scholarship, 23*(3), 155–159.

Brandt, C.D., Sison, A.V., Rakusan, T.A., et al. (1996). HIV DNA blood levels in vertically infected pediatric patients: Variations with age, association with disease progression, and comparison with blood levels in in-fected mothers. *Journal of Acquired Immune Deficiency Syndromes and Human Retrovirology, 13*(3), 254–261.

Bryson, Y.J. (1996). Perinatal HIV-1 transmission: Recent advances and therapeutic interventions. *Journal of Acquired Immune Deficiency Syndromes and Human Retrovirology,* Suppl. 3, S33–S42.

Burns, D.N., Hillman, D., Neaton, J.D., et al. (1996). Cigarette smoking, bacterial pneumonia, and other clinical outcomes in HIV-1 infection. *Journal of Acquired Immune Deficiency Syndromes and Human Retrovirology, 13*(4), 374–383.

Bush, C.E., Donovan, R.M., Manzor, O., et al. (1996). Comparison of HIV type 1 RNA plasma viremia, p24 antigenemia, and unintegrated DNA as viral load markers in pediatric patients. *Journal of Acquired Immune Deficiency Syndromes and Human Retrovirology, 12*(1), 11–15.

Buskin, S.E., Hopkins, S.G., Farizo, K.M. (1992). Heavy smoking increases the risk of *Pneumocystis carinii* pneumonia (PCP) (abstract no. WeC1030). *International Conference on AIDS, 8*(1), We50.

Centers for Disease Control. (1989a). *Eating defensively: Food safety advice for persons with AIDS* (videorecording). Atlanta: CDC.

Centers for Disease Control. (1989b). Guidelines for prevention of transmission of human immunodeficiency virus and hepatitis B virus to health care and public safety workers. *Morbidity and Mortality Weekly Report, 38*(S-6), 1–37.

Centers for Disease Control. (1990). *Health information for international travel* (HHS Pub. No. CDEC 90-8280). Washington, DC: US Government Printing Office.

Centers for Disease Control. (1991). Waterborne-disease outbreaks. *Morbidity and Mortality Weekly Report, 40*(SS-3), 1–13.

Centers for Disease Control and Prevention. (1993). Update: Barrier protection against HIV infection and other sexually transmitted diseases. *Morbidity and Mortality Weekly Report, 42*(30), 589–591, 597.

Centers for Disease Control and Prevention. (1996). Prevention of hepatitis A through active or passive immunization: Recommendations of the advisory committee in immunization practices. *Morbidity and Mortality Weekly Report, 45*(RR-15), 1–30.

Centers for Disease Control and Prevention. (1997). 1997 USPHS/IDSA guidelines for the prevention of opportunistic infections in persons infected with human immunodeficiency virus. *Morbidity and Mortality Weekly Report, 46*(RR-12), 1–46.

Clarke, J.R., Taylor, I.K., Fleming, J. (1993). The epidemiology of HIV-1 infection in the lung in AIDS patients. *AIDS, 7*(4), 555–560.

Cockerell, C.J. (1991). Noninfectious inflammatory skin diseases in HIV-infected individuals. *Dermatologic Clinics, 9*(3), 531–541.

Conley, L.J., Bush, T.J., Buchbinder, S.P., et al. (1996). The association between cigarette smoking and selected HIV-related medical conditions. *Journal of Acquired Immune Deficiency Syndromes and Human Retrovirology, 10*(10), 1121–1126.

Conti, L., Lieb, S., Liberti, T., Kertesz, C. (1996). The need for information about Zoonoses among the immunocompromised: Promoting a healthy human-animal bond (abstract no. TH.C.4561). *International Conference on AIDS, 11*(2), 342.

Donovan, R.M., Bush, C.E., Markowitz, N.P., et al. (1996). Changes in virus load markers during AIDS-associated opportunistic diseases in human immunodeficiency virus-infected persons. *Journal of Infectious Diseases, 174*(2), 401–403.

Downing, D. (1995). HIV and pet ownership. *Step Perspective, 7*(1), 18–20.

DuPont, H.L., Ericsson, C.D. (1993). Prevention and treatment of traveler's diarrhea. *The New England Journal of Medicine, 328*(25), 1821–1827.

Duvic, M. (1991). Papulosquamous disorders associated with human immunodeficiency virus infection. *Dermatologic Clinics, 9*(3), 523–530.

Evans, D.L., Lesserman, J., Perkions, D.O., et al. (1991). Stress related reduction of natural killer cells in HIV (abstract no. TH.B.91). *International Conference on AIDS, 7*(2), 79.

Filice, G.A., Pomeroy, C. (1991). Preventing secondary infections among HIV-positive persons. *Public Health Report, 106*(5), 503–517.

Flescher, M., Watkins, L.R., Lockwood, L.L., et al. (1992). Specific changes in lymphocyte subpopulations: A potential mechanism for stress-induced immunomodulation. *Journal of Neuroimmunology, 41*(2), 131–142.

Florida Department of Health and Rehabilitative Services. (1996). Companionship outweighs disease risk from pets. *AIDS Alert, 11*(1) (Suppl. 1-2).

Food and Drug Administration. (1993). Female condom approval. *FDA Medical Bulletin, 23*(2), 4.

Forthal, D., Gordon, R., Larsen, R. (1992). Cigarette smoking increases the risk of developing cryptococcal meningitis (abstract no. PoB 3172). *International Conference on AIDS, 8*(2), B115.

Gold, D. (1993). Treatment briefs: Risky drinking water. *Treatment Issues: The Gay Men's Health Crisis Newsletter of Experimental AIDS Therapies, 7*(7), 6.

Hardy, M.A. (1992). Dry skin care. In G.M. Bulechek, J.A. McCloskey (Eds.), *Nursing interventions: Essential nursing treatments* (2nd ed., pp. 34–47). Philadelphia: Saunders.

Hassan, N.F., Douglas, S.D. (1990). Stress-related neuroimmunomodulation of monocyte-macrophage functions in HIV-1 infection. *Clinical Immunology and Immunopathology, 54*(2), 220–227.

Hecht, F.M., Soloway, B. (1993). Identifying patients at risk for HIV infection. In D.J. Cotton, G.H. Friedland (Eds.), *HIV infection: A primary care approach* (rev. ed., p. 307). Waltham, MA: Massachusetts Medical Society.

Henry, K., Melroe, H., Huebsch, J., et al. (1998). Severe premature coronary artery disease with protease inhibitors. *Lancet, 351,* 1328.

Hirschtick, R.E., Glassroth, J., Jordan, M.C., et al. (1995). Bacterial pneumonia in persons infected with the human immunodeficiency virus. *New England Journal of Medicine, 334*(3), 195.

Jewett, J.F., Hecht, F.M. (1993). Preventive health care for adults with HIV infection. *Journal of the American Medical Association, 269*(9), 1144–1153.

Kaslow, R.A., Blackwelder, W.C., Ostrow, D.G., et al. (1989). No evidence for a role of alcohol or other psychoactive drugs accelerating immunodeficiency in HIV-1 positive individuals: A report from the Multicenter AIDS Cohort Study. *Journal of the American Medical Association, 261*(23), 3424–3429.

Kitahata, M.M., Koepsell, T.D., Deyo, R.A., et al. (1996). Physicians' experience with the acquired immunodeficiency syndrome as a factor in patients' survival. *New England Journal of Medicine, 334*(11), 701–706.

Kotler, D.P. (1992). Nutritional effects and support in the patient with acquired immunodeficiency syndrome. *Journal of Nutrition, 122*(Suppl. 3), 723–727.

LaPerriere, A.R., Antoni, M.H., Schniederman, N., et al. (1990). Exercise intervention attenuates emotional distress and natural killer cell decrements following notification of positive serologic status for HIV-1. *Biofeedback and Self Regulation, 15*(3), 229–242.

LaPerriere, A.R., Fletcher, M.A., Antoni, M.H., et al. (1991). Aerobic exercise training in an AIDS risk group. *International Journal of Sports Medicine, 12*(Suppl. 1), 553–557.

LaPerriere, A.R., Antoni, M.H., Ironson, G., et al. (1994a). Effects of aerobic exercise training on lymphocyte subpopulations. *International Journal of Sports Medicine, 15*(Suppl. 3), S127–S130.

LaPerriere, A.R., Ironson, G., Antoni, M.H., et al. (1994b). Exercise and psychoneuroimmunology. *Medicine and Science in Sports and Exercise, 26*(2), 182–190.

Life Sciences Research Office, Federation of American Societies for Experimental Biology. (1990, November). *Nutrition and HIV infection* (FDA No. 223-88-2124). Washington, DC: Center for Food Safety and Applied Nutrition, Food and Drug Administration, Department of Health and Human Services.

McCain, N.L., Cella, D.F. (1995). Correlates of stress in HIV disease. *West J Nursing Research, 17*(2), 141–155.

McCain, N.L., Zeller, J.M., Cella, D.F., et al. (1996). The influence of stress management training in HIV disease. *Nursing Research, 45*(4), 245–253.

MacArthur, R.D., Levine, S.D., Birk, T.J., et al. (1992). Cardiopulmonary, immunologic and psychologic responses to exercise training in individuals seropositive for HIV (abstract no. PuB 7327). *International Conference on AIDS, 8*(3), 103.

Miles, S.A., Balsen, E., Megpantay, L., et al., (1993). Rapid serologic testing with immune-complex-dissociated HIV p24 antigen for early detection of HIV infection in neonates. *New England Journal of Medicine, 328*(5), 297–302.

Moulton, J.M., Gurbuz, G., Sweet, D., et al. (1990). Outcome evaluation of eight-week educational support groups: Validating the model using control group comparisons (abstract no. S.B. 400). *International Conference on AIDS, 6*(3), 186.

Nadakavukaren, A. (1990). *Man and environment: A health perspective* (3rd ed.). Prospect Heights, IL: Waveland Press.

Nieman, R., Fleming, J., Coker, R.J., et al. (1993). The effect of cigarettes on the development of AIDS in HIV-1 seropositive individuals. *AIDS, 7*(5), 705–710.

Nicoll, A., Newell, M.L. (1996). Preventing perinatal transmission of HIV: The effect of breast feeding [Let-

ter]. *Journal of the American Medical Association, 276*(19), 1552–1553.

Palacio, H., Hilton, J.F., Canchola, A.J., Greenspan, D. (1997). Effect of cigarette smoking on HIV-related oral lesions. *Journal of Acquired Immune Deficiency Syndromes and Human Retrovirology, 14*(4), 338–342.

Perry, S., Fishman, B., Jacobsberg, L., et al. (1991). Effectiveness of psychoeducational interventions in reducing emotional distress after human immunodeficiency virus antibody testing. *Archives of General Psychiatry, 48*(2), 143–147.

Pivar, I., Temoshok, L. (1990). Coping strategies and response styles in homosexual symptomatic seropositive men (abstract no. S.B. 382). *International Conference on AIDS, 6*(3), 181.

Pol, S., Artru, P., Thepot, V., et al. (1996). Improvement of the CD4 cell count after alcohol withdrawal in HIV-positive alcoholic patients [Letter]. *Journal of Acquired Immune Deficiency Syndromes and Human Retrovirology, 10*(11), 1293–1294.

Rigsby, L.W., Dishman, R.K., Jackson, A.W., et al. (1992). Effects of exercise training on men seropositive for the human immunodeficiency virus-1. *Medicine and Science in Sports and Exercise, 24*(1), 6–12.

Royce, R.A., Winkelstein, W. (1990). HIV infection, cigarette smoking and CD4+ T-lymphocyte counts: Preliminary results from the San Francisco men's health study. *AIDS, 4*(4), 327–333.

Schlenzig, C., Jaeger, H., Wehrenberg, M., et al. (1992). Physical exercise favorably influences the course of illness in patients with HIV and AIDS (abstract no. PoB 3401). *International Conference on AIDS, 8*(2), B153.

Shearer, W.T., Quinn, T.C., LaRussa, P., et al. (1997). Viral load and disease progression in infants infected with human immunodeficiency virus type 1. *New England Journal of Medicine, 336*(19), 1337–1342.

Signorile, M. (1997). Bareback and reckless. *Out,* No. 45, 36–39.

Smeltzer, S.C., Whipple, B. (1991). Women and HIV infection. *Image: Journal of Nursing Scholarship, 23*(4), 249–256.

Smith, B.A., Neidig, J., Nickel, J., et al. (1996). Effects of aerobic and resistive exercise on symptoms, immune status, and viral load in HIV+ men and women (abstract no. B. 304). *International Conference on AIDS, 11*(1), 23.

Sperling, R.S., Shapiro, D.E., Coombs, R.W., et al. (1996). Maternal viral load, zidovudine treatment, and the risk of transmission of human immunodeficiency virus type 1 from mother to infant. Pediatric AIDS Clinical Trials Group Protocol 076 Study Group. *New England Journal of Medicine, 335*(22), 1621–1629.

Swango, P.A., Kleinma, P.V., Konzelman, J.I. (1991). HIV and periodontal health: A study of military personnel with HIV. *Journal of the American Dental Association, 122*(8), 49–54.

Turner, B.J., Hauck, W.W., Fanning, T.R., Markson, L.E. (1997). Cigarette smoking and maternal-child HIV transmission. *Journal of Acquired Immune Deficiency Syndromes and Human Retrovirology, 14*(4), 327–337.

United States Environmental Protection Agency. (1990, January). *Disposal types for home health care* (EPA/530-SW-90-014A). Washington, D.C.: United States Environmental Protection Agency.

U.S. Department of Health and Human Services, Public Health Service, Health Resources Administration. (1996). *Health care and HIV. Nutrition Guide for Providers and Clients.* Rockville, MD: The Author.

Weber, R., Ledergerber, B., Opravil, M., et al. (1990). Progression of HIV infection in misusers of injected drugs who stop injecting or follow a program of maintenance treatment with methadone. *British Medical Journal, 301*(6765), 1362–1365.

Pharmacologic Treatment of HIV/AIDS

ROBERT J. KIZIOR

Generic Name (Trade)	Indications	Dosage
abacavir (Ziagen)	HIV infection	**Adults (PO):** 300 mg bid
acetaminophen (Tylenol)	Pain, fever	**Adults (PO):** 325–650 mg q4–6h (maximum: 4 g/d) **Children (PO): 11 y:** 480 mg per dose; **9–10 y:** 400 mg per dose; **6–8 y:** 320 mg per dose; **4–5 y:** 240 mg per dose; **2–3 y:** 160 mg per dose; **1–2 y:** 120 mg per dose; **4–11 mo:** 80 mg per dose; **0–3 mo:** 40 mg per dose
acyclovir (Zovirax)	Herpes simplex virus (HSV) infection, varicella zoster virus (VZV) infection (herpes zoster, shingles) Epstein-Barr virus (EBV) infection (oral hairy leukoplakia)	*Treatment of HSV* **Adults (PO):** 400 mg tid up to 800 mg 5 times daily; **(IV):** 15–30 mg/kg/d in divided doses q8h **Children (PO):** maximum 80 mg/kg/d in 3–5 doses; **(IV):** 250 mg/m^2 q8h *Treatment of Herpes Zoster, EBV* **Adults (PO):** 800 mg 5 times daily; **(IV):** 10 mg/kg q8h **Children (PO):** 20 mg/kg up to 800 mg per dose; **(IV):** 10 mg/kg q8h *Secondary Prophylaxis for HSV Infection* **Adults (PO):** 200 mg tid or 400 mg bid **Children (PO):** maximum 80 mg/kg/d in 3–4 divided doses *Topical (Ointment)* **Adults, children:** apply q3h 6 times daily
adefovir (Preveon)	HIV infection	**Adults (PO):** 120 mg PO once a day
alprazolam (Xanax)	Anxiety, panic disorders	**Adults (PO):** 4–10 mg/d in 3 divided doses
amikacin (Amikin)	*Mycobacterium tuberculosis* (TB)	**Adults, children (IM/IV):** 5 mg/kg q8h or 7.5 mg/kg q12h (maximum: 1.5 g/d) **Neonates (IM/IV):** initially, 10 mg/kg; then 7.5 mg/kg q12h
amitriptyline (Elavil, Endep)	Depression, neuropathic pain	*Depression* **Adults (PO):** initially 25 mg bid or qid; may increase to 150 mg/d **Children (PO):** 10–30 mg/d in 2 divided doses *Neuropathic Pain* **Adults (PO):** initially 10–25 mg hs; may increase to 75 mg hs **Children (PO):** initially, 0.1 mg/kg hs; may increase to 0.5–2 mg/kg hs
amoxicillin (Amoxil, Trimox)	Bacterial infection (sinusitis, otitis media, bronchitis, pneumonia)	**Adults (PO):** 250–500 mg q8h **Children (PO): 9–20 kg:** 6.7–13.3 mg/kg q8h; **6–8 kg:** 50–100 mg q8h; **<6 kg:** 25–50 mg q8h
amphotericin B (Fungizone)	Aspergillosis, esophageal or disseminated candidiasis, coccidioidomycosis, cryptococcosis, histoplasmosis	**Adults, children (IV):** 0.25 mg/kg initially; then gradually increased to maintenance dose of 0.25–1 mg/kg/d (maximum daily dose) **Test dose should be administered first**

Side Effects	Comments
Headache, malaise, abdominal pain, diarrhea, rash, elevated liver function tests, and a significant hypersensitivity reaction Rarely hypersensitivity reactions	1. May be taken with or without food. 2. Once a hypersensitivity reaction is noted, the drug should never be restarted since severe and potentially fatal reactions have been noted upon rechallenge.
PO: nausea, diarrhea, vomiting, abdominal pain, headache **IV:** pain, swelling, or redness at injection site; loss of appetite, nausea, vomiting, lightheadedness	1. Maintain adequate hydration and urine output. 2. Oral forms may be taken with or without food. 3. Capsules and tablets should not be crushed or opened. 4. IV infusion should be administered over at least 1 hour.
Nausea, vomiting, anorexia, diarrhea, malaise, elevated liver function tests, reductions in serum carnitine levels	Since adefovir depletes the body's store of L-carnitine (which is necessary for breaking down fats and protein), it should be taken with L-carnitine supplements, which can be purchased over-the-counter.
Allergic reactions, extrapyramidal symptoms, muscle weakness	1. Avoid alcohol or other CNS depressants. 2. Rapid withdrawal can cause seizures, delirium.
Greatly altered frequency and amount of urination, increased thirst, loss of appetite, nausea, vomiting, twitching, numbness, seizures, tingling, loss of hearing, ringing or buzzing in ears, fullness in ears, dizziness, nausea, vomiting, clumsiness, itching, redness, rash, or swelling	1. Inject deep IM into large muscle mass. 2. Must be diluted for IV administration. 3. Report loss of hearing, ringing, or roaring in ears or feeling of fullness in ears.
Blurred vision, constipation, dizziness, drowsiness, headache, increased appetite, altered taste, nausea, vomiting	1. May be taken with food to decrease gastric irritation. 2. Avoid alcohol. 3. May cause drowsiness, dry mouth. 4. Avoid discontinuing abruptly.
Mild diarrhea, nausea, vomiting, headache, sore mouth and tongue, vaginal itching or discharge, skin rash, hives, itching	May take without regard to food.
Unusual fatigue or weakness, irregular heartbeat, muscle cramps or pain, fever or chills, nausea, vomiting, diarrhea, headache, altered urination, pain at injection site, loss of appetite, stomach pain	1. Infuse at rate of 0.2–0.4 mg/kg/h. 2. Premedication usually given to reduce side effects (agents used include ibuprofen, acetaminophen, hydrocortisone, diphenhydramine, or meperidine).

Table continued on following page

Generic Name (Trade)	Indications	Dosage
amphotericin B colloidal dispersion (Amphotec)	See amphotericin B	**Adults (IV):** 3–4 mg/kg/d, increasing to 6 mg/kg/d **Test dose should be administered first**
amphotericin B lipid complex (Abelcet)	See amphotericin B	**Adults, children (IV):** 2.5–5 mg/kg as single daily infusion **Test dose not required**
amphotericin B liposome (AmBisone)	See amphotericin B	**Adults (IV):** 3–5 mg/kg/d **Children (IV):** 1–3 mg/kg/d **Test dose should be administered first**
ampicillin (Omnipen, Principen)	Bacterial infections (sinusitis, otitis media, bronchitis, pneumonia)	**Adults (PO):** 250–500 mg q6h **Children (PO):** 12.5–25 mg/kg q6h
aspirin	Pain, fever	**Adults (PO):** 325–650 mg q4h as needed (maximum: 4 g/d) **Children (PO):** 10–15 mg/kg q4h as needed (maximum: 60–80 mg/kg/d)
atovaquone (Mepron)	*Pneumocystis carinii* pneumonia (mild to moderate; A–a gradient <45 mm Hg; PaO_2 >60 mm Hg)	**Adults (PO):** 750 mg tid for 21 days Safety and efficacy in children not established
azithromycin (Zithromax)	*Mycobacterium avium-intracellulare* complex (MAC), sinusitis, bronchitis, pneumonia, *Chlamydia trachomatis*	***Primary Prophylaxis for MAC*** **Adults (PO):** 1200 mg weekly **Children (PO):** 5 mg/kg/d (maximum: 250 mg) ***Treatment of MAC*** **Adults (PO):** 500 mg/d **Children (PO):** 10–20 mg/kg once daily (maximum: 40 mg/kg) ***Secondary Prophylaxis for MAC*** **Adults (PO):** 500 mg/d in combination with ethambutol or rifabutin or both
bleomycin (Blenoxane)	Kaposi's sarcoma	Refer to individual protocols
buprenorphine (Buprenex)	Pain	**Adults (IM/IV):** 0.15–0.6 mg q6h as needed **Children 2–12 y (IM/IV):** 2–6 μg/kg q4–6h as needed
bupropion (Wellbutrin)	Depression	**Adults (PO):** 75 mg bid, increasing to 100 mg tid over 3 days
capreomycin	*Mycobacterium tuberculosis*	**Adults (IM):** 1 g/d for 60–120 d; then 1 g 2–3 times per week
carbamazepine (Tegretol)	Seizures, neuropathic pain	***Seizures*** **Adults (PO):** initially, 100 mg qid; increase to maintenance dose of 800–1200 mg/d **Children (PO): 6–12 y:** initially, 50 mg qid; increase to maintenance dose of 400–800 mg/d; **<6 y:** initially, 10–20 mg/kg/d in 2–3 divided doses; increase to maintenance dose of 250–350 mg/d ***Neuropathic Pain*** **Adults (PO):** initially 100 mg bid, increasing to 800 mg/d

Side Effects	Comments
Fever, chills, headache, nausea, vomiting, diarrhea, loss of appetite, unusually tired or weak, sore throat, unusual bleeding or bruising	Infuse at rate of 1 mg/kg/h.
Fever, chills, headache, nausea, vomiting, diarrhea, loss of appetite, unusually tired or weak, sore throat, unusual bleeding or bruising	Infuse at a rate of 2.5 mg/kg/h.
Chills, diarrhea, nausea, vomiting, renal toxicity	Infuse at a rate of 2.5 mg/kg/h.
Mild diarrhea, nausea, vomiting, headache, sore mouth and tongue, vaginal itching or discharge, skin rash, hives, itching	Take on empty stomach.
Mild stomach pain, heartburn, indigestion, nausea, vomiting, allergic reaction (itching, trouble breathing, rash)	1. Chewable tablets may be chewed, crushed, dispersed in liquid, or swallowed whole. 2. Enteric coated tablets to be swallowed whole; do not crush or chew. 3. Do not use in children with fever (may be associated with development of Reye's syndrome).
Skin rash, fever, cough, headache, inability to sleep, nausea, vomiting, diarrhea, increased liver enzymes	1. Store in cool, dry place (avoid freezing). 2. Take with food (increases absorption).
Abdominal pain, nausea, vomiting, diarrhea	1. Capsules should be taken 1 hour before meals or 2 hours after meals; powder packet may be taken without regard to food. 2. Tablets may be taken without regard to food.
Fever, chills, cough, shortness of breath, sores in mouth and on the lips, skin rash, itching, vomiting, loss of appetite, loss of hair	Give IV slowly over at least 10 minutes.
Sedation, dizziness, headache, hypotension, nausea, vomiting, sweating, unusually slow breathing, lightheadedness	
Seizures, agitation, insomnia, anorexia, nausea, vomiting, weight loss, psychosis	1. Antidepressant effects may take 4 weeks to appear. 2. Avoid alcohol and other antidepressants.
Large increase or decrease in urination frequency, increase in thirst, nausea, vomiting, loss of appetite, skin rash, itching, redness, swelling, fever, muscle cramps, unusually tired or weak, altered hearing, fullness in ears, dizziness, pain, hardness, unusual bleeding at injection site	
Blurred vision, skin rash, itching, hives, diarrhea, confusion, clumsiness, nausea, vomiting, loss of appetite, dry mouth, irritation of tongue and mouth, unusually tired, weak	1. Take with food (decreases gastrointestinal [GI] irritation). 2. Avoid alcohol. 3. May cause drowsiness. 4. Avoid sun; increases sensitivity of skin to sunlight.

Table continued on following page

Generic Name (Trade)	Indications	Dosage
chloral hydrate (Noctec)	Insomnia	**Adults (PO):** 1 g hs
chlorhexidine (Peridex)	Gingivitis	**Adults, children (PO):** 15 ml bid (after brushing and flossing teeth)
chlorpromazine (Thorazine)	Nausea, vomiting	**Adults (PO):** 10–25 mg q4h **Children >6 mo (PO):** 0.5–1 mg/kg q4–6h
cidofovir (Vistide)	Cytomegalovirus retinitis	**Adults (IV):** induction dose is 5 mg/kg once a week for 2 weeks; maintenance dose is 5 mg/kg every other week; **(intraocular):** 20–40 μg by injection
ciprofloxacin (Cipro)	*Mycobacterium avium-intracellulare* complex, Mycobacterium tuberculosis, respiratory infections, salmonellosis	**Adults (PO):** 500–750 mg q12h **Children (PO):** 20–30 mg/kg/d in 2 divided doses (maximum: 1.5 g/d)
cisplatin (Platinol AQ)	Cervical cancer	Refer to individual protocols
clarithromycin (Biaxin)	*Mycobacterium avium-intracellulare* complex, pharyngitis, sinusitis, otitis, pneumonitis, skin and soft tissue infections	***Primary Prophylaxis for MAC*** **Adults (PO):** 500 mg bid **Children (PO):** 7.5 mg/kg bid (maximum: 500 mg) ***Treatment of Infection*** **Adults (PO):** 500 mg bid **Children (PO):** 15–30 mg/kg/d in 2 divided doses (maximum: 1 g/d) ***Secondary Prophylaxis for MAC*** **Adults (PO):** 500 mg bid plus ethambutol or rifabutin or both **Children (PO):** 7.5 mg/kg bid (maximum: 500 mg) plus ethambutol or rifabutin or both
clindamycin (Cleocin)	Toxoplasmosis, *Pneumocystis carinii* pneumonia	***Treatment of Disease*** **Adults (IV):** 900–1200 mg q6h; **(PO):** 300–450 mg q6h **Children (IV):** 25–40 mg/kg/d in 3–4 divided doses; **(PO):** 10–30 mg/kg/d in 3–4 divided doses ***Secondary Prophylaxis for Toxoplasmosis*** **Adults (PO):** 300–450 mg q6–8h plus pyrimethamine and leucovorin **Children (PO):** 20–30 mg/kg qid plus pyrimethamine and leucovorin
clofazimine (Lamprene)	*Mycobacterium avium-intracellulare* complex	**Adults (PO):** 100 mg 1–3 times a day (combination) **Children (PO):** 1–2 mg/kg/d (maximum: 100 mg/d)

Side Effects	Comments
Nausea, diarrhea, dependence, tolerance	
Change in taste, increased tartar in teeth, increased staining of teeth, mouth, tooth fillings, or dentures; swollen glands on side of face or neck; irritation to mouth and tip of tongue	1. Use after brushing and flossing, rinsing toothpaste completely from mouth before using. 2. Do not eat or drink for several hours after using. 3. Swish in mouth for 30 seconds; then spit out; do not swallow. 4. Causes change in taste; may cause staining and increase in tartar.
Constipation, dizziness, drowsiness, dry mouth, nausea, vomiting, stomach pain, decreased sweating	1. Take with food (decreases GI irritation). 2. Take extended release capsules whole; do not chew.
Nausea, vomiting, fever, asthenia (generalized weakness), rash, diarrhea, headache, loss of hair, chills, loss of appetite, dyspnea, abdominal pain, renal failure, infection, unusually tired or weak, pneumonia, decrease in intraocular pressure	1. Should not be given if serum creatinine is >1.5 mg/dl. 2. Probenecid 2 g PO taken 3 hours before and the 1 g at 2 and 8 hours after infusion (antihistamines, acetaminophen, or antiemetics may be given to reduce probenecid hypersensitivity). 3. Must infuse 1 L of normal saline over 1–2 hours before administration of cidofovir. 4. Should not be given with other drugs with potential renal toxicity (foscarnet, amphotericin, pentamidine, NSAIDs).
Dizziness, lightheadedness, headache, insomnia or drowsiness, nausea, vomiting, diarrhea, stomach or abdominal pain or discomfort, increased sensitivity to sunlight	1. May give without regard to food (best if 2 hours after meals). 2. Antacids delay absorption.
Unusual fatigue or weakness, fever, chills, cough, hoarseness, painful urination, severe nausea, vomiting, joint pain, loss of appetite, numbness and tingling in fingers and toes, trouble hearing	1. Avoid immunizations unless approved by physician. 2. Notify physician of unusual bleeding, bruising, or red spots on skin.
Abnormal taste, nausea, vomiting, diarrhea, abdominal pain, headache	1. Avoid crushing or breaking tablets. 2. May take without regard to food. 3. May take with milk.
Severe abdominal or stomach cramps or pain, abdominal tenderness, diarrhea (watery or severe), fever, nausea, vomiting	1. May take without regard to food. 2. Best taken with full glass of water. 3. Watch for increasing diarrhea.
Loss of appetite, diarrhea, nausea, vomiting, dry or rough or scaly skin, discoloration of skin (pink to brownish black), itching, skin rash, discoloration of sweat, tears, sputum, urine	1. Take with meals or milk (increases absorption). 2. Rarely used to treat MAC because of limited efficacy.

Table continued on following page

Generic Name (Trade)	Indications	Dosage
clonazepam (Klonopin)	Anxiety, panic disorders, seizures	**Adults (PO):** 0.5 mg tid up to 1 mg tid **Children (PO):** 0.01–0.03 mg/kg/d in 2–3 divided doses up to 0.1–0.2 mg/kg/d
clorazepate (Tranxene)	Anxiety, seizures	***Anxiety*** **Adults (PO):** 7.5–15 mg bid to qid ***Seizures*** **Adults (PO):** 7.5 mg tid up to 90 mg/d **Children 9–12 y (PO):** 7.5 mg bid up to 60 mg/d
clotrimazole (Mycelex, Gyne-Lotrimin)	Vulvovaginal candidiasis, oropharyngeal candidiasis	***Vulvovaginal Candidiasis*** **Adults, children >12 y (vaginal):** *tablet:* one tablet (100 mg) hs for 7 days, *or* 2 tablets (200 mg) hs for 3 days, *or* 1 tablet (500 mg) once; *cream:* one full applicator hs for 7–14 days ***Oropharyngeal Candidiasis*** **Adults, children >3 y (buccal):** 10 mg troches 3–5 times daily for 7–14 days
codeine	Pain	**Adults (PO/SC/IM):** 30 mg q4–6h (range: 15–60 mg) **Children (PO/SC/IM):** 0.5–1 mg/kg q4–6h (maximum dose: 60 mg)
cyanocobalamin (Nascobal)	Vitamin B$_{12}$ deficiency	**Adults (intranasal):** 500 µg (metered dose) once a week
cycloserine (Seromycin)	*Mycobacterium tuberculosis*	**Adults (PO):** 250 mg q12h for 2 weeks; then increase up to 250 mg q6–8h (maximum: 1 g/d) **Children (PO):** 10–20 mg/kg/d in divided doses
cytarabine (Cytosar)	Non-Hodgkin's lymphoma	Refer to individual protocols
dacarbazine (DTIC)	Kaposi's sarcoma	Refer to individual protocols
dapsone (Avlosulfon)	*Pneumocystis carinii* pneumonia (PCP), toxoplasmosis	***Primary Prophylaxis for PCP*** **Adults (PO):** 50 mg bid or 100 mg once daily with pyrimethamine and leucovorin **Children ≥1 mo (PO):** 2 mg/kg/d (maximum: 100 mg) ***Primary Prophylaxis for Toxoplasmosis*** **Adults (PO):** 50 or 100 mg daily with pyrimethamine and leucovorin **Children ≥1 mo (PO):** 2 mg/kg or 15 mg/m^2 once daily with pyrimethamine and leucovorin ***Treatment for PCP*** **Adults (PO):** 100 mg/d for 21 days with trimethoprim

Side Effects	Comments
Confusion, depression, clumsiness, dizziness, drowsiness, change in vision, irritability, nausea, vomiting	1. Give with food or water. 2. Avoid alcohol (may cause drowsiness). 3. Limit caffeine. 4. Avoid abrupt discontinuation following prolonged use.
Confusion, depression, clumsiness, dizziness, drowsiness, change in vision, irritability, nausea, vomiting	1. Give with food or water. 2. Avoid alcohol (may cause drowsiness). 3. Limit caffeine. 4. Avoid abrupt discontinuation following prolonged use.
Vaginal: Vaginal burning, itching, vaginal discharge **Oral:** Abdominal or stomach cramping or pain, nausea, vomiting, diarrhea	1. Vaginal tablet or cream: use vaginal applicator, inserting high into vagina. 2. Troches: Dissolve in mouth over 15–30 minutes and swallow saliva.
Confusion, constipation, decreased blood pressure, increased heart rate, sweating, redness, flushed face, trouble breathing, decreased urination, stomach pain or cramps, dizziness, lightheadedness, unusual fatigue or weakness, drowsiness, dry mouth, headache	1. Avoid getting up suddenly. 2. Lie down if nausea, vomiting, dizziness, lightheadedness occur. 3. Use sugarless gum or candy for relief of dry mouth. 4. Avoid alcohol.
Asthenia, headache, nausea, paresthesia, rhinitis	Nasacobal is indicated for maintaining the hematologic status of patients with vitamin B_{12} deficiency who have been stabilized with injection therapy.
Anxiety, confusion, dizziness, drowsiness, restlessness, depression, muscle twitching, trembling, nightmares, mood changes (including psychosis), skin rash, numbness, burning, pain, weakness in hands and feet, seizures, headache	1. Take after meals (decreases GI irritation). 2. Avoid alcohol. 3. Give with pyridoxine.
Loss of appetite, nausea, vomiting, headache, dizziness, drowsiness, itching, loss of hair, fever, chills, painful urination, sores in mouth or on lips, unusual bleeding, bruising, pinpoint red spots on skin, unusual fatigue, numbness and tingling in fingers, toes, and face, joint pain; swelling of feet or lower legs	May give IV or SC.
Pain, redness, swelling at injection site, fever, chills, cough, lower back pain, painful urination, unusual bleeding, bruising, pinpoint red spots on skin, nausea, diarrhea, loss of appetite, loss of hair, joint or muscle pain	1. Refrigerate; protect from light. 2. May give IV push or IV infusion. 3. Avoid exposure to sunlight. 4. Try to restrict food intake for 4–6 hours before administration (decreases vomiting).
Back, leg, or stomach pain, loss of appetite, pale skin, unusual fatigue or weakness, fever, bluish fingernails, lips, or skin, skin rash, difficulty breathing, nausea	1. Store in a cool, dry place. 2. May take with or without food. 3. Do not give with antacids (may decrease absorption). 4. Give 2 hours before or after didanosine.

Table continued on following page

Generic Name (Trade)	Indications	Dosage
dapsone (Avlosulfon) *Continued*		***Secondary Prophylaxis for PCP*** **Adults (PO):** 50 mg bid *or* 100 *or* 200 mg once daily with pyrimethamine and leucovorin **Children ≥1 mo (PO):** 2 mg/kg/d (maximum: 100 mg) ***Secondary Prophylaxis for Toxoplasmosis*** **Adults (PO):** 50 mg daily with pyrimethamine and leucovorin
daunorubicin liposomal (DaunoXome)	Kaposi's sarcoma	**Adults (IV):** 40 mg/m²; repeat q2wk
delavirdine (Rescriptor)	HIV infection	**Adults (PO):** initially, 200 mg tid for 14 days; then 400 mg tid
desipramine (Norpramin)	Depression, neuropathic pain	***Depression*** **Adults (PO):** initially, 75 mg/d in divided doses (maximum: 300 mg/d) **Children (PO): >12 y:** initially, 25–50 mg/d (maximum: 150 mg/d); **6–12 y:** initially, 1–3 mg/kg/d (maximum: 5 mg/kg/d) ***Neuropathic Pain*** **Adults (PO):** initially, 25 mg hs, increasing to 100–150 mg/d (maximum: 300 mg/d)
dexamethasone (Decadron)	Cerebral edema, pneumonia, non-Hodgkin's lymphoma, minimize side effects of cancer chemotherapy	**Adults (PO):** 2 mg bid or tid **Children (PO):** 0.03–0.15 mg/kg daily in 3–4 divided doses
diazepam (Valium)	Anxiety	**Adults (PO):** 2–10 mg bid to qid **Children (PO):** 0.04–0.2 mg/kg q6–8h
diclofenac (Cataflam, Voltaren)	Pain	**Adults (PO):** 100–200 mg/d in 2–4 divided doses
didanosine (ddI) (Videx)	HIV infection	**Adults (PO): >60 kg:** *tablets:* 200 mg q12h; *powder:* 250 mg q12h; **<60 kg:** *tablets:* 125 mg q12h; *powder:* 167 mg q12h **Adult alternative dosing (PO):** 400 mg hs **Children (PO): <90 days old:** 50 mg/m² q12h; **>90 days old:** 90–150 mg/m² q12h
diphenoxylate-atropine (Logen, Lomotil)	Diarrhea	**Adults (PO):** 15–20 mg/d in 3–4 divided doses **Children (PO): 8–12 y:** 2 mg 5 times daily; **5–8 y:** 2 mg qid; **2–5 y:** 2 mg tid

Side Effects	Comments
Fatigue, headache, loss of appetite, abdominal pain, nausea, diarrhea, vomiting, cough, fever, allergic reaction (skin rash or itching), sweating, loss of hair, sores in the mouth and on the lips, fever, chills, cough or hoarseness, lower back pain, painful or difficult urination	1. Infuse over 1 hour. 2. Refrigerate vials (use within 6 hours after reconstitution). 3. Do not freeze; protect from light.
Diffuse, itchy, maculopapular rash, nausea, arthralgia, insomnia, changes in dreams, headache, diarrhea, fatigue, elevated serum liver enzyme levels	1. Store at room temperature. 2. May take without regard to food.
Blurred vision, constipation, dizziness, drowsiness, headache, increased appetite, altered taste, nausea, vomiting	1. Take with food to decrease GI irritation. 2. Avoid alcohol. 3. May cause drowsiness. 4. May increase appetite. 5. May cause urine to be blue-green.
Increased appetite, indigestion, nervousness, restlessness, trouble sleeping, headache, dizziness	1. Take with food (decreases GI irritation). 2. Caution in receiving skin tests, vaccinations, or immunizations.
Confusion, depression, clumsiness, dizziness, drowsiness, change in vision, irritability, nausea, vomiting	1. Take with food. 2. Avoid alcohol (may cause drowsiness). 3. Limit caffeine. 4. Avoid abrupt discontinuation following prolonged use.
Dizziness, drowsiness, mild to moderate headache, abdominal cramps, pain, discomfort; diarrhea, constipation, increased blood pressure, decreased urination, swelling of face, fingers, lower legs; weight gain, nausea, indigestion	Take with food to decrease GI irritation.
Pancreatitis (abdominal pain, nausea, vomiting), peripheral neuropathy (tingling, burning, numbness or pain in the fingertips or feet), anxiety, headache, irritability, inability to sleep, restlessness, dry mouth, nervousness, rash	1. Give on empty stomach (1 hour before or 2 hours after a meal). 2. Tablets chewed, crushed, or dispersed in water (when dispersed, use within 1 hour); powder should be mixed in drinking water only. 3. Pediatric powder is mixed into solution by pharmacist and is stable for 30 days, if refrigerated. 4. Do not give within 2 hours of administration of dapsone. 5. Given in combination with other antiretrovirals, never as monotherapy.
Blurred vision, constipation, dry skin and mouth, fever, loss of appetite, stomach pain, nausea, vomiting, dizziness, drowsiness, depression	1. Avoid alcohol. 2. May give with food (decreases GI irritation).

Table continued on following page

Generic Name (Trade)	Indications	Dosage
doxepin (Adapin, Sinequan)	Depression, neuropathic pain	***Depression*** **Adults, children (>12 y) (PO):** initially, 25 mg tid, increased gradually (maximum daily dose: 150 mg) ***Neuropathic Pain*** **Adults (PO):** initially, 25 mg hs up to 150 mg (maximum single dose: 150 mg)
doxorubicin (Adriamycin, Rubex)	Kaposi's sarcoma	Refer to individual protocols
doxorubicin liposomal (Doxil)	Kaposi's sarcoma	**Adults (IV):** 20 mg/m^2 over 30 minutes, once q3wk
dronabinol (Marinol)	HIV-related weight loss	**Adults (PO):** initially, 2.5 mg bid (before lunch and supper) for a total of 5 mg/d; if not tolerated, decrease to 2.5 mg as single evening or bedtime dose; may increase to 5 mg bid (maximum: 20 mg/d)
efavirenz (Sustiva)	HIV infection	**Adults (PO):** 600 mg hs
EMLA brand name for lidocaine and prilocaine	To prevent procedural pain (starting IV infusions, spinal taps, changing dressings)	**Adults, children (>3 mo) (topical):** apply thick layer to intact skin; cover with occlusive dressing at least 1 hour before procedure
epoetin alfa (Epogen, Procrit)	Anemia related to HIV infection (serum erythropoietin level <500 mU/ml)	**Adults (SC/IV):** initially, 100 U/kg 3 times per week for 8 weeks; then, dose adjusted by 50–100 U/kg to a maximum of 300 U/kg 3 times per week Safety and efficacy in children has not been established
ethambutol (Myambutol)	*Mycobacterium tuberculosis, Mycobacterium avium-intracellulare* complex	**Adults, children (PO):** 15–25 mg/kg as single daily dose (maximum: 2.5 g/d) *or* 50 mg/kg 2 times per week (maximum dose: 2.5 g)
ethionamide (Trecator S.C.)	*Mycobacterium tuberculosis*	**Adults (PO):** 250 mg q8–12h (maximum: 1 g/d) **Children (PO):** 4–5 mg/kg q8h (maximum: 750 mg/d)
etoposide (VePesid, VP-16-213)	Kaposi's sarcoma	Refer to individual protocols
famciclovir (Famvir)	Herpes simplex virus infection, herpes zoster (shingles)	***Herpes Simplex*** **Adults (PO):** 125 mg q12h for 5 days ***Herpes Zoster*** **Adults (PO):** 500 mg q8h for 7 days

Side Effects	Comments
Blurred vision, constipation, dizziness, drowsiness, headache, increased appetite, altered taste, nausea, vomiting	1. May give with food to decrease GI irritation. 2. Avoid alcohol. 3. May cause drowsiness and dry mouth. 4. May increase appetite. 5. Avoid exposure to sunlight.
Fever, chills, cough or hoarseness, lower back pain, difficult urination, sores in the mouth and on the lips, shortness of breath, swelling in feet and lower legs, pain at injection site, unusual bruising or bleeding, nausea, vomiting, diarrhea, loss of hair	1. Give slow IV over 3–5 minutes or IV infusion over 1–4 hours. 2. Transient red-orange urine discoloration. 3. Notify physician if fever, sore throat, bleeding, or bruising occurs. 4. Report any stinging at injection site.
Flushing, shortness of breath, facial swelling, headache, chills, back pain, tightness in chest, throat, hypotension, fever, unusual bleeding or bruising, nausea, vomiting, fever, loss of hair, diarrhea, constipation, fatigue	1. Refrigerate diluted medication and give within 24 hours. 2. Avoid freezing. 3. Infuse over 30 minutes. 4. For IV use only.
Dizziness, abnormalities in thinking, drowsiness, nausea, vomiting, changes in mood, fast or pounding heartbeat, altered vision	1. Use caution in performing hazardous tasks. 2. Avoid alcohol. 3. May cause drowsiness and dry mouth.
Dizziness, lightheadedness, nightmares, diarrhea, rash	Should not be used in pregnant women because of potential birth defects
At application site, burning feeling, swelling, itching, skin rash, very white or red skin	1. Avoid contact with eyes, lips, or mouth. 2. Do not apply to open wounds, burns, or broken or inflamed skin. 3. Apply thick layer; do not spread; cover with occlusive dressing.
Chest pain, swelling of face, fingers, ankles, and feet, weight gain, headache, increased blood pressure, altered vision, bone pain, muscle weakness, nausea, diarrhea, fatigue, dizziness	1. May give SC or IV. 2. Do not shake vial. 3. Single use vial (1 ml per vial) must be discarded (does not contain a preservative). 4. Multidose vial (2 ml per vial with preservative) must be refrigerated.
Optic neuritis, acute gouty arthritis (chills, pain and swelling of joints, especially the toes, ankle, or knee; hot skin over affected joint), confusion, disorientation, abdominal pain, nausea, vomiting, loss of appetite, headache	1. Take with food to prevent GI irritation. 2. Report any visual changes, numbness, tingling in hands or feet, rash, fever, and chills.
Hepatitis (yellow eyes, skin), numbness, tingling, pain, burning in hands and feet, confusion, depression, change in mental status, loss of appetite, metallic taste, nausea, vomiting, sore mouth, dizziness	1. Give as single daily dose (after evening meal or at bedtime). 2. Take with food to decrease GI irritation.
Fever, chills, cough or hoarseness, lower back pain, painful or difficult urination, unusual bleeding or bruising, nausea, vomiting, loss of appetite, loss of hair	1. IV administered over at least 30–60 minutes. 2. Notify physician of fever, sore throat, painful or burning urination, bruising, bleeding, or shortness of breath.
Headache, nausea, vomiting, diarrhea, fatigue	1. May take with or without food. 2. Give with food to decrease GI irritation. 3. Only recommended for immunocompetent individuals; use in immunosuppressed persons is under study.

Table continued on following page

Generic Name (Trade)	Indications	Dosage
fentanyl (Duragesic)	Management of chronic pain	**Adults, children (topical):** individualized (depends on desired therapeutic effects, patient's weight, and existing opiate tolerance)
filgrastim (Neupogen)	Neutropenia (absolute neutrophil count [ANC] <500–750/mm^3)	**Adults, children (IV/SC):** 5–10 µg/kg as single daily dose for up to 14 days; then titrated to maintain ANC >1000–2000/mm^3
fluconazole (Diflucan)	Oropharyngeal, esophageal, vaginal candidiasis, cryptococcosis, histoplasmosis	***Primary Prophylaxis (Not Routinely Recommended; Indicated for Use Only in Unusual Cases)*** **Adults (to prevent candidiasis, cryptococcosis) (PO):** 100–200 mg daily **Children (to prevent cryptococcosis) (PO):** 3–6 mg/kg daily ***Treatment of Oropharyngeal Candidiasis*** **Adults (PO):** 200 mg on first day; then 100 mg/d (maximum: 400 mg/d) **Children (PO/IV):** 6–12 mg/kg daily (maximum: 200 mg/d) ***Treatment of Esophageal Candidiasis*** **Adults (PO/IV):** 200 mg on first day, then 100 mg/d (maximum: 400 mg/d) **Children (PO/IV):** 6–12 mg/kg daily (maximum: 200 mg/d) ***Treatment of Vaginal Candidiasis*** **Adults (PO):** 150 mg one time dose ***Treatment of Cryptococcal Meningitis*** **Adults (PO/IV):** 400 mg on first day; then 200–400 mg daily until cultures are negative **Children (PO/IV):** 6–12 mg/kg daily (maximum: 200 mg/d) ***Secondary Prophylaxis*** **Adults (PO)** **For cryptococcosis:** 200 mg daily **For coccidioidomycosis, histoplasmosis:** 400 mg daily **For vaginal or esophageal candidiasis in severe cases:** 100–200 mg daily **Children (PO)** **For cryptococcosis, histoplasmosis:** 3–6 mg/kg daily **For coccidioidomycosis:** 6 mg/kg daily **For candidiasis in severe cases:** 3–6 mg/kg daily
flucytosine (Ancobon)	Severe candidiasis, cryptococcosis	**Adults, children (PO):** 12.5–37.5 mg/kg q6h
fluoxetine (Prozac)	Depression	**Adults (PO):** 10–40 mg daily, usually as a single dose in morning
flurazepam (Dalmane, Durapam, Apo-Flurazepam)	Insomnia	**Adults (PO):** 15–30 mg hs

Side Effects	Comments
Difficulty breathing, seeing, hearing, decrease in volume or frequency, anxiety, confusion, dizziness, drowsiness, weakness, loss of appetite, diarrhea, abdominal pain, headache, vomiting, nausea, sweating, itching	1. Avoid getting up suddenly. 2. Lie down if nausea, vomiting, dizziness, lightheadedness occur. 3. Use sugarless gum or candy for relief of dry mouth. 4. Avoid alcohol. 5. Apply to nonhairy area of intact skin of upper torso. 6. Rotate sites of application. 7. Variable absorption, depending on patient's fat stores.
Redness or pain at injection site, pain in joints, muscles, lower back, or pelvis, headache, skin rash or itching	1. If ANC does not rise appreciably after the first 7 days, the drug should be discontinued. 2. Unused portion of medicine may be drawn from vial into a syringe and refrigerated for later use.
Fever, chills, rash, itching, dizziness, drowsiness, headache, constipation or diarrhea, nausea, vomiting, loss of appetite, abdominal pain	1. May administer PO or IV. 2. Report any unusual bleeding or bruising, yellowing of skin or eyes, severe skin rash. **PO:** may take without regard to food and may take with milk. **IV:** infuse over 1–2 hours.
Unusually tired or weak, yellow eyes or skin, skin rash, redness, or itching, fever, sore throat, unusual bruising or bleeding, increased sensitivity of skin to sunlight, abdominal pain, diarrhea, loss of appetite, nausea, vomiting, headache, drowsiness, dizziness or lightheadedness	1. Take over 15 minutes to decrease nausea, vomiting. 2. Used with amphotericin B (not used as monotherapy).
Anorexia, weight loss, nausea, anxiety, agitation, insomnia, sexual dysfunction, drowsiness, dry mouth, sweating, tremors, headache, chills, rash, fever	1. Take with food to minimize gastric irritation. 2. May take up to 4 weeks to achieve antidepressant effects.
Daytime sedation, drowsiness, impairment of dexterity	Useful for intermittent treatment of insomnia.

Table continued on following page

Generic Name (Trade)	Indications	Dosage
foscarnet (Foscavir)	Cytomegalovirus infection, acyclovir-resistant herpes simplex virus infection, and herpes zoster infection	***Treatment of CMV Retinitis and (Other Sites)*** **Adults, children (IV):** initially, 60 mg/kg q8h or 90 mg q12h for 14–21 days; then, 90–120 mg/kg/d as single daily dose **Children >3 mo (IV):** 2–5 mg/kg q8h or 5 mg/kg q12h ***Treatment of Acyclovir-resistant HSV Infection or Herpes Zoster*** **Adults (IV):** 40 mg/kg q8h or 60 mg/kg q12h up to 3 wk or until lesions heal ***Secondary Prophylaxis*** **Adults, children (IV):** 90–120 mg/kg daily
ganciclovir (Cytovene)	Cytomegalovirus retinitis and CMV disease	***Primary Prophylaxis (Not Routinely Recommended; Indicated for Use Only in Unusual Cases)*** **Adults (PO):** 1 g tid ***Treatment of CMV Retinitis*** **Adults, children >3 mo (IV):** 5 mg/kg q12h for 14–21 days ***Secondary Prophylaxis*** **Adults (IV):** 5 mg/kg daily for 5–7 days per week; **(PO):** 1 g tid **Children (IV):** 5 mg/kg daily
hydrocodone (Hycodan)	Pain	**Adults (PO):** 5–10 mg q4–6h as needed **Children (PO):** 0.15 mg/kg q6h as needed (maximum: 5 mg)
hydromorphone (Dilaudid)	Pain	**Adults, children ≥50 kg (PO):** 2–6 mg q3–4h; **(IM/SC):** 1.5 mg q3–4h **Adults (rectal):** 3 mg q4–8h as needed
hydroxyurea (Hydrea)	HIV infection	**Adults (PO):** 500 to 1000 mg/d
hydroxyzine (Atarax, Vistaril)	Nausea, vomiting	**Adults (PO):** 25–100 mg tid to qid as needed; **(IM):** 25–100 mg per dose **Children (PO):** 0.5 mg/kg q6h as needed; **(IM):** 1 mg/kg as single dose
ibuprofen (Advil, Motrin, Nuprin, Rufen)	Pain	**Adults (PO):** 200–400 mg q4–6h **Children (PO):** 5–10 mg/kg per dose (maximum: 40 mg/kg/d)
imipramine (Tofranil)	Depression, neuropathic pain	***Depression*** **Adults (PO):** initially, 25 mg tid to qid; increase gradually to 300 mg/d maximum **Children (PO):** initially, 1.5 mg/kg/d, increase by 1 mg/kg q3–4d up to maximum of 5 mg/kg/d in 1–4 divided doses ***Pain*** **Adults (PO):** same as for depression **Children (PO):** initially, 0.2–0.4 mg/kg hs, increase by 50% q2–3d up to maximum of 1–3 mg/kg per dose

Side Effects	Comments
Abdominal pain, loss of appetite, nausea, vomiting, anxiety, confusion, dizziness, fatigue, headache, either decreased urination or increased thirst and urination, peripheral neuropathy (tingling, burning, numbness, or pain in fingers or feet), penile ulcers, seizures (related to renal failure or hypocalcemia)	1. Give by IV infusion over 2 hours. 2. Report any symptoms of hypocalcemia: numbness or tingling in extremities, perioral paresthesia. 3. Safety in children not established. 4. May also be administered locally via sustained-release intravitreal implant.
Fever, sore throat, unusual bruising or bleeding, fatigue or weakness, headaches, seizures, confusion	1. Take capsules with food. 2. Administer IV over 2 hours. 3. Neutropenia occurs 25%–40% of the time, requiring coadministration of filgrastim. 4. Zidovudine increases the risk of neutropenia; concomitant use should be avoided.
Confusion, constipation, decreased blood pressure, increased heart rate, sweating, redness, flushed face, trouble breathing, decreased urination, stomach pain or cramps, dizziness, lightheadedness, unusual fatigue or weakness, drowsiness, dry mouth, headache	1. Avoid getting up suddenly. 2. Lie down if nausea, vomiting, dizziness, lightheadedness occur. 3. Use sugarless gum or candy for relief of dry mouth.
Confusion, constipation, decreased blood pressure, increased heart rate, sweating, redness, flushed face, trouble breathing, decreased urination, stomach pain or cramps, dizziness, lightheadedness, unusual fatigue or weakness, drowsiness, dry mouth, headache	1. Avoid getting up suddenly. 2. Lie down if nausea, vomiting, dizziness, lightheadedness occur. 3. Use sugarless gum or candy for relief of dry mouth.
Anemia, erythrocytic abnormalities, leukopenia, stomatitis, thrombocytopenia, diarrhea, drowsiness, anorexia, nausea, vomiting, skin rash, itching	1. Hydroxyurea has been approved by the FDA for the treatment of various forms of cancer and is under study as an HIV antiretroviral agent. 2. Usually taken with didanosine.
Drowsiness, dry mouth, dizziness, headache, thickening of mucus, tremor, convulsions, blurred vision, decreased blood pressure, increased sweating, loss of appetite	1. Take with food to decrease gastric irritation. 2. IM injections given deep into muscle.
Dizziness, drowsiness, mild-to-moderate headache, abdominal cramps, pain, discomfort, diarrhea, constipation, elevated blood pressure, reduced urination, swelling of face, fingers, lower legs, weight gain, nausea, indigestion	Take with meals or food to decrease gastric irritation.
Blurred vision, constipation, dizziness, drowsiness, headache, increased appetite, altered taste, nausea, vomiting, dry mouth	1. Take with food to decrease gastric irritation. 2. Avoid alcohol.

Table continued on following page

Generic Name (Trade)	Indications	Dosage
immune globulin (IVIG) (Gamimune, Gamma-gard, Iveegam, Sandoglobulin, Venoglobulin)	To prevent or modify acute bacterial or viral infections, thrombocytopenia	***To Prevent or Modify Infections*** **Adults, children (IV):** 400 mg/kg once a month ***Thrombocytopenia*** **Adults, children (IV):** 400 mg/kg daily for 5 days, repeated every 10–21 days
indinavir (Crixivan)	HIV infection	**Adults (PO):** 800 mg q8h *or* 1200 mg q12h **Children:** 500 mg/m² q8h
indomethacin (Indocin)	Pain	**Adults (PO):** 50–200 mg/d in 3–4 divided doses
interferon alfa 2a (Roferon-A)	Kaposi's sarcoma, hepatitis, non-Hodgkin's lymphoma	**Adults (IM/SC):** 36 million U/d for 10–12 weeks, then 3 times per week; *or* 20 million U/m²/d for 4 weeks, then 3 times per week
interferon alfa 2b (Intron-A)	Kaposi's sarcoma, cervical cancer, non-Hodgkin's lymphoma	**Adults (IM/SC):** 30 million U/m² 3 times per week
interferon alfa n1 (Wellferon)	Kaposi's sarcoma, hepatitis, non-Hodgkin's lymphoma	**Adults (IM/IV):** 20 million U/m² daily for 2 months
isoniazid (INH, Isotamine, Laniazid, Teebaconin, Nydrazid)	*Mycobacterium tuberculosis*	***Primary Prophylaxis*** **Adults (PO):** 300 mg daily or 900 mg twice a week plus pyridoxine for a total of 12 months **Children (PO/IM):** 10–15 mg/kg daily (maximum: 300 mg) or 20–30 mg/kg (maximum: 900 mg) twice a week plus pyridoxine for a total of 12 months ***Treatment*** **Adults (PO):** 300 mg daily or 900 mg 2–3 times a week **Children (PO/IM):** 10–20 mg/kg daily (maximum: 300 mg) *or* 20–30 mg/kg (maximum: 900 mg) 2–3 times per week

Side Effects	Comments
Trouble breathing, fast or pounding heartbeat, burning sensation in hands, fatigue, wheezing, pain, backache, headache, joint pain, malaise, muscle pain, vomiting, facial flushing, sweating, rash, dizziness	1. For IV use only; should be given in a rate-escalating manner (increasing flow rate gradually) based on vital signs and clinical response. 2. Epinephrine should be available for hypersensitivity reactions. 3. Patient may require premedication with a corticosteroid. 4. May interfere with body's immune response to MMR (measles, mumps, rubella) vaccine.
Kidney stones (blood in urine, sharp back pain), nausea, diarrhea, vomiting, abdominal pain, headache, insomnia, altered taste, dizziness, generalized weakness, asymptomatic hyperbilirubinemia, elevated blood glucose (symptoms include increased thirst, hunger, and urination, weight loss, fatigue, dry skin, itching), elevated triglyceride and cholesterol levels, fat accumulation, buffalo hump	1. Given in combination with other antiretrovirals, never as monotherapy. 2. Store at room temperature. 3. May be taken with a light meal (avoid high-fat, high-calorie, high-protein meal). 4. If indinavir is given with didanosine, give at least 1 hour before or after didanosine. 5. Must drink at least 1.5 L of water daily. 6. Compounded with lactose; lactose-intolerant patients can take LactAid tablets before taking indinavir. 7. Extremely moisture sensitive; should be kept in original container with desiccants; should not be prepoured into medication pill boxes; do not keep in bathroom. 8. Blood glucose, triglyceride, and cholesterol levels should be monitored.
Dizziness, drowsiness, mild-to-moderate headache, abdominal cramps, pain, discomfort, diarrhea, constipation, elevated blood pressure, decreased urination, swelling of face, fingers, and lower legs, weight gain, nausea, indigestion	1. Take with meals or food to decrease GI irritation. 2. Swallow delayed release capsules whole; do not break, chew, or crush before swallowing.
Fever, chills, flulike symptoms, nausea, vomiting, loss of appetite, altered or metallic taste, diarrhea, dizziness, dry mouth, liver toxicity	1. Give IM or SC. 2. Rotate SC injection sites. 3. Do not change brands. 4. Inform physician of any mental status changes. 5. Refrigerate; do not shake. 6. Best given at bedtime because of flulike symptoms after injection.
Fever, chills, flulike symptoms, nausea, vomiting, loss of appetite, altered or metallic taste, diarrhea, dizziness, dry mouth, liver toxicity	1. Give IM or SC. 2. Rotate SC injection sites. 3. Do not change brands. 4. Inform physician of any mental status changes. 5. Refrigerate. 6. Best given at bedtime because of flulike symptoms after injection.
Fever, chills, flulike symptoms, nausea, vomiting, loss of appetite, altered or metallic taste, diarrhea, dizziness, dry mouth, liver toxicity	1. Give by IM or IV injection. 2. Best given at bedtime because of flulike symptoms after injection.
Anorexia, nausea, vomiting, diarrhea, malaise, jaundice, peripheral neuropathy, bleeding, bruising, sore throat, rash, pain at injection site, arthralgia, seizures, depression, blurred vision with or without eye pain	Alcohol ingestion while taking this medication increases potential for hepatitis.

Table continued on following page

Generic Name (Trade)	Indications	Dosage
itraconazole (Sporanox)	Aspergillosis, candidiasis (esophageal, oropharyngeal, vaginal), cryptococcosis, histoplasmosis, dermatophytic infections	*Primary Prophylaxis for Cryptococcosis, Histoplasmosis (Not Routinely Recommended; Indicated for Use Only in Unusual Cases)* **Adults (PO):** 200 mg daily **Children (PO):** 2–5 mg/kg q12–24h *Treatment of Disease:* **Adults (PO)** **Aspergillosis:** 200 mg bid **Esophageal or vaginal candidiasis:** 100–200 mg tid **Thrush:** 100–200 mg bid for 1 day *or* 100–200 mg daily for 2–3 days **Histoplasmosis:** initially, 300 mg q12h for 3 days; then 200 mg q12h **Cryptococcosis:** 200 mg tid for 3 days; then 200 mg bid **Dermatophytic infections:** 100 mg daily *Secondary Prophylaxis to Prevent Recurrent Cryptococcosis, Histoplasmosis* **Adults (PO):** 200 mg bid **Children (PO):** 2–5 mg/kg q12–48h *Secondary Prophylaxis to Prevent Recurrent Coccidioidomycosis* **Adults (PO):** 200 mg bid
kanamycin (Kantrex)	*Mycobacterium tuberculosis*	**Adults, children (IM/IV):** 15 mg/kg once daily (maximum: 1.5 g)
kaolin-pectin (Kaopectate)	Diarrhea	**Adults (PO):** 60–120 ml after each loose bowel movement. **Children (PO): >12 y:** 45–60 ml per dose; **6–12 y:** 30–60 ml; **3–6 y:** 15–30 ml
ketoconazole (Nizoral)	Candidiasis (esophageal, oropharyngeal, vaginal)	*Treatment of Esophageal Candidiasis* **Adults (PO):** 200–400 mg bid **Children (PO):** 5–10 mg/kg/d in divided doses *Treatment of Thrush* **Adults (PO):** 200 mg 1–2 times daily **Children (PO):** 5–10 mg/kg/d in divided doses *Treatment of Vaginal Candidiasis* **Adults (PO):** 200–400 mg/d for 7 days or 400 mg/d for 3 days *Secondary Prophylaxis for Frequent or Severe Episodes* **Adults (PO):** 200 mg daily
lamivudine (3TC, Epivir)	HIV infection	**Adults (PO): >50 kg:** 150 mg bid; **<50 kg:** 2 mg/kg bid **Children (PO): <30 days old:** 2 mg/kg q12h; **>30 days old:** 4 mg/kg q12h
lamivudine-zidovudine (Combivir)	HIV infection	**Adults (PO):** one tablet (contains 150 mg of lamivudine and 300 mg of zidovudine) bid Because of the fixed dose combination, should not be given to children under the age of 12 years

Side Effects	Comments
Fever, chills, rash, itching, dizziness, drowsiness, headache, constipation or diarrhea, nausea, vomiting, loss of appetite, abdominal pain	1. Take with food. 2. Do not give with antacids or H_2 antagonists. 3. Requires gastric acid; best taken with orange juice, cola drinks, ginger ale.
Greatly altered frequency and amount of urination, increased thirst, loss of appetite, nausea, vomiting, twitching, numbness, seizures, tingling, loss of hearing, ringing or buzzing in ears, fullness in ears, dizziness, nausea, vomiting, clumsiness, itching, redness, rash, or swelling	1. IM injection should be deep into large muscle mass. 2. Must be diluted for IV administration. 3. Report loss of hearing, ringing or roaring in ears, or feeling of fullness in ears.
Constipation (usually mild, transient)	1. Do not use if diarrhea is accompanied by fever or by blood or mucus in stool. 2. Notify physician if diarrhea is not controlled within 48 hours.
Fever, chills, rash, itching, dizziness, drowsiness, headache, constipation or diarrhea, nausea, vomiting, loss of appetite, abdominal pain	1. Give with food to minimize GI irritation, nausea, vomiting. 2. Give 2 hours before antacids or H_2 antagonists. 3. Avoid alcohol. 4. Requires gastric acid; best taken with orange juice, cola drinks, or ginger ale.
Peripheral neuropathy (tingling, burning, numbness or pain in the hands, arms, feet, or legs), pancreatitis (nausea, vomiting, severe abdominal or stomach pain), unusual fatigue or weakness, fever, chills, sore throat, skin rash, headache, nausea, malaise, diarrhea, cough, insomnia, dizziness, muscle pain, joint pain, abdominal cramps, dyspepsia	1. Given in combination with other antiretrovirals, never as monotherapy. 2. May be taken without regard to food. 3. Store at room temperature. 4. Avoid alcohol. 5. Report persistent, severe abdominal pain, nausea, vomiting, numbness or tingling.
Headache, malaise, fever, chills, nausea, vomiting, diarrhea, anorexia, abdominal pain or cramps, neuropathy, insomnia, dizziness, nasal signs and symptoms, musculoskeletal pain, rash, neutropenia, anemia	May be taken with or without food.

Table continued on following page

Generic Name (Trade)	Indications	Dosage
leucovorin (folinic acid, Wellcovorin)	Prophylaxis and treatment of toxicity related to use of folic acid antagonists (methotrexate, pyrimethamine, trimethoprim, trimetrexate)	**Adults (PO):** (when taking pyrimethamine) 25 mg weekly except when taking secondary prophylaxis for toxoplasmosis; then up to 10–25 mg qid **Children (PO):** (when taking pyrimethamine) 5 mg every 3 days
levofloxacin (Levaquin)	Bacterial infections (pneumonia, sinusitis, urinary tract infection)	**Adults (PO):** 250–500 mg daily
loperamide (Imodium)	Treatment of diarrhea	**Adults (PO):** initially 4 mg, then 2 mg after each loose bowel movement (maximum: 16 mg/d) **Children 2–11 y (PO):** 0.08–0.25 mg/kg/d in 2–3 divided doses (maximum dose: 2 mg)
lorazepam (Ativan)	Anxiety, tension headaches	**Adults (PO):** 1–3 mg bid to tid
megestrol acetate (Megace)	HIV wasting syndrome, weight loss	**Adults (PO):** 80 mg qid up to 800 mg/d **Children (PO):** 8 mg/kg/d, titrated to achieve weight gain
methadone (Dolophine)	Pain, treatment for opiate addiction	***Pain*** **Adults (PO):** 5–20 mg q4–8h (maximum: 120 mg/d); **(SC/IM):** 2.5–10 mg q6–8h **Children (PO):** 0.2 mg/kg q4–8h; **(IV):** 0.1 mg/kg q4–8h ***Opiate Addiction in Adults*** Individualized
methotrexate (MTX, Folex, Mexate)	Kaposi's sarcoma	Refer to individual protocols
metoclopramide (Reglan)	Nausea, vomiting, symptomatic gastroesophageal reflux (GERD)	***Nausea, Vomiting*** **Adults, children (PO/IV):** 1–2 mg/kg q2–4h ***GERD*** **Adults (PO/IM/IV):** 10–15 mg qid **Children (PO/IV):** 0.2–0.4 mg/kg qid
metronidazole (Flagyl)	Bacterial vaginosis, gingivitis, amebiasis, trichomoniasis, diarrhea due to *Clostridium difficile*	**Adults (PO):** 250–500 mg qid **Children (PO):** 20–35 mg/kg/d divided q6h
miconazole (Monistat)	Vaginal candidiasis	**Adults (vaginal): suppository:** 200 mg/d for 3 days *or* 100 mg/d for 7 days; **cream:** one full applicator hs for 7 days
mitoxantrone (Novantrone)	Non-Hodgkin's lymphoma	Refer to individual protocols

Side Effects	Comments
Dizziness, lightheadedness, headache, insomnia or drowsiness, nausea, vomiting, diarrhea, stomach or abdominal pain or discomfort, increased sensitivity to sunlight	1. May give without regard to food (best if taken 2 hours after meals). 2. Antacids delay absorption.
Rare: skin rash, bloating, constipation, loss of appetite, severe stomach pain, nausea, vomiting, dizziness, drowsiness, dry mouth	1. Do not use if diarrhea is accompanied by fever or blood or mucus in stool. 2. Maintain adequate fluid intake.
Confusion, depression, clumsiness, dizziness, drowsiness, change in vision, irritability, nausea, vomiting	1. Take with food. 2. Avoid alcohol (may cause drowsiness). 3. Limit caffeine. 4. Avoid abrupt discontinuation following prolonged use.
Diarrhea, impotence, rash, elevated blood pressure, generalized weakness, inability to sleep, nausea, headache, possibly drug-induced diabetes	Should not be used when hyperglycemia and weight loss develop as a result of protease inhibitor therapy.
Confusion, constipation, decreased blood pressure, increased heart rate, sweating, redness, flushed face, trouble breathing, decreased urination, stomach pain or cramps, dizziness, lightheadedness, unusual fatigue or weakness, drowsiness, dry mouth, headache	1. Avoid getting up suddenly. 2. Lie down if nausea, vomiting, dizziness, or lightheadedness occurs. 3. Use sugarless gum or candy for relief of dry mouth. 4. Half-life of methadone is 72 hours; cumulative effects may develop.
GI ulceration, bleeding, diarrhea, stomach pain, fever, chills, cough, hoarseness, lower back pain, painful urination, unusual bleeding or bruising, pinpoint red spots on skin, sores in mouth or on lips, loss of appetite, nausea, vomiting, skin rash, itching, loss of hair	1. Avoid alcohol. 2. Report any fever, sore throat, bleeding, bruising, shortness of breath, painful urination.
Diarrhea, drowsiness, restlessness, unusual fatigue or weakness, breast tenderness, swelling, constipation, nausea, skin rash, headache, dizziness, insomnia, dry mouth	1. Give 30 min before meals and at bedtime. 2. May impair ability to perform hazardous tasks requiring mental alertness.
Headache, dizziness or lightheadedness, diarrhea, loss of appetite, nausea, vomiting, stomach pain or cramps, altered taste, metallic or sharp taste, dry mouth, dark urine, numbness, tingling, pain or weakness in hands or feet, seizures (with high doses)	Take with food to decrease gastric irritation.
Vaginal burning, itching	
Cough, shortness of breath, GI bleeding, fever, chills, painful urination, decreased urination, fast or irregular heartbeat, swelling of feet and lower legs, yellow eyes and skin, seizures, unusual bleeding, bruising, pinpoint red spots on skin, diarrhea, nausea, vomiting, headache, loss of hair	1. Must dilute prior to use. 2. For IV use only. 3. May cause urine or whites of eyes to be blue-green.

Table continued on following page

Generic Name (Trade)	Indications	Dosage
morphine (MS Contin, Oramorph, Roxanol)	Pain	**Adults (PO):** 10–30 mg q3–4h (30 mg q8–12h when using extended release); **(SC/IM):** 5–20 mg q4h; **(IV):** 4–10 mg per dose **Children (PO):** 0.3 mg/kg q3–4h; **(IV):** 0.1–1 mg/kg q3–4h
nandrolone (Durabolin)	HIV-related muscle wasting	**Adults (IM):** 25–100 mg/wk
naproxen (Anaprox, Naprosyn)	Pain	**Adults (PO):** initially, 500 mg; then 250 mg q6–8h
nelfinavir (Viracept)	HIV infection	**Adults (PO):** 750 mg tid *or* 1250 mg bid **Children 2–13 y (PO):** 20–30 mg/kg q8h
nevirapine (Viramune)	HIV infection	**Adults (PO):** initially, 200 mg/d for 14 days; then 200 mg bid **Children (PO): ≤3 mo:** start with 5 mg/kg once daily for 14 days, followed by 120 mg/m^2 q12h for 14 days, followed by 200 mg/m^2 q12h; **>3 mo:** start with 120 mg/m^2 once daily for 14 days, increasing to 120–200 mg/m^2 q12h if there is no rash or other untoward effects
nortriptyline (Aventyl, Pamelor)	Depression, neuropathic pain	*Depression* **Adults (PO):** initially, 10–25 mg hs, increasing to 50–100 mg hs or 25 mg tid or qid *Neuropathic Pain* **Adults (PO):** 10–25 mg hs, increasing over a 2–3 week period to a maximum of 75 mg hs
nystatin (Mycostatin, Nilstat)	Oropharyngeal candidiasis	*Solution* **Neonates (PO):** 100,000 units qid or 50,000 units to each side of mouth qid **Infants (PO):** 200,000 units qid or 100,000 units to each side of mouth qid **Adults, children (PO):** 400,000–600,000 units qid *Pastilles (Lozenges)* **Adults, children >5 y (PO):** 200,000–400,000 units qid *Vaginal Tablets* **Adults:** 100,000 units 1–2 times daily

Side Effects	Comments
Confusion, constipation, decreased blood pressure, increased heart rate, sweating, redness, flushed face, trouble breathing, decreased urination, stomach pain or cramps, dizziness, lightheadedness, unusually tired or weak, drowsiness, dry mouth, headache	1. Avoid getting up suddenly. 2. Lie down if nausea, vomiting, dizziness, or lightheadedness occurs. 3. Use sugarless gum or candy for relief of dry mouth.
Chills, diarrhea, feeling of stomach fullness, altered libido, muscle cramps, trouble sleeping; in men: acne, decreased sex ability	Important to have diet high in protein and calories while taking this drug.
Dizziness, drowsiness, mild-to-moderate headache, abdominal cramps, pain, or discomfort, diarrhea, constipation, increased blood pressure, decreased urination, swelling of face, fingers, and lower legs, weight gain, nausea, indigestion	Take with meals or food to decrease gastric irritation.

Diarrhea, flatulence, nausea, abdominal pain, generalized weakness, rash, may elevate blood glucose level (symptoms include increased thirst, hunger, and urination, weight loss, fatigue, dry skin, itching), elevated triglyceride and cholesterol levels, fat accumulation, buffalo hump	1. Given in combination with other antiretrovirals, never as monotherapy.
	2. Loperamide can be given to control diarrhea.
	3. Oral powder may be mixed with a small amount of water, milk, or dietary supplement:
	   a. Do not mix with acidic food (e.g., apple sauce or juice, orange juice); produces a bitter taste.
	   b. Mix with chocolate milk or pudding.
	   c. Once mixed, consume entire contents within 6 hours.
	4. Give with food for optimal absorption.
	5. Blood glucose, triglyceride, and cholesterol levels should be monitored.

Rash, fever, nausea, headache, abnormal liver function tests, stomatitis (sores or ulcers in mouth), numbness, muscle pain, hepatitis (yellow skin, diarrhea, nausea, headache)	1. Given in combination with other antiretrovirals, never as monotherapy. 2. Store tablets at room temperature. 3. May take without regard to food.
Dry mouth, dizziness, blurred vision, constipation, urinary hesitancy, orthostatic hypotension, sedation, decreased libido, weight gain	1. Avoid getting up suddenly. 2. Lie down if nausea, vomiting, dizziness, or lightheadedness occurs. 3. Use sugarless gum or candy for relief of dry mouth.
Stomach pain, nausea, vomiting, diarrhea	1. Shake suspension well prior to administration. 2. Hold suspension in mouth or swish throughout mouth as long as possible before swallowing or spitting out. 3. For neonates or infants: paint suspension into recesses of mouth. 4. All pastilles (lozenges) are to dissolve slowly; do not chew or swallow whole.

Table continued on following page

Generic Name (Trade)	Indications	Dosage
octreotide (Sandostatin)	Diarrhea associated with cryptosporidiosis, micro-sporidiosis	**Adults (SC):** 50–100 µg 1–3 times daily, increasing up to 500 µg tid for 8 weeks (maximum: 1500–3000 µg/d divided into 2–3 doses) **Children (SC):** 1–10 µg q12h
ofloxacin (Floxin)	*Mycobacterium tuberculosis*	**Adults (PO):** 600–800 mg/d
ondansetron (Zofran)	Nausea, vomiting	**Adults, children >11 y (IV):** 4 mg per dose; **(PO):** 8 mg tid **Children 4–11 y (IV):** 0.15 mg/kg per dose; **(PO):** 4 mg tid
oxandrolone (Oxandrin)	HIV wasting syndrome and weight loss	**Adults (PO):** 2.5 mg bid to qid; range: 2.5–20 mg/d **Children (PO):** 0.25 mg/kg/d in 2–4 divided doses
oxycodone (Roxicodone)	Pain	**Adults (PO):** 2.5–5 mg q6h; extended release 10–30 mg q12h
paclitaxel (Taxol)	Kaposi's sarcoma	**Adults (IV):** 135 mg/m^2 q3wk *or* 100 mg/m^2 q2wk
para-aminosalicylate (P.A.S.)	*Mycobacterium tuberculosis*	**Adults (PO):** 3.3–4 g q8h *or* 5–6 g q12h (maximum: 20 g/d) **Children (PO):** 50–75 mg/kg q6h *or* 67–100 mg q8h
paromomycin (Humatin)	Cryptosporidiosis	**Adults (PO):** 500–750 mg qid for 21 days
pentamidine (NebuPent, Pentam-300)	*Pneumocystis carinii* pneumonia	***Primary Prophylaxis*** **Adults (inhalation):** 300 mg once a month via Respirgard II nebulizer **Children ≥5 y (inhalation):** 300 mg once a month via Respirgard II nebulizer; **(IV):** 4 mg/kg q2–4wk ***Treatment*** **Adults, children (IV):** 3–4 mg/kg daily ***Secondary Prophylaxis*** **Adults (inhalation):** 300 mg once a month via Respirgard II nebulizer **Children ≥5 y (inhalation):** 300 mg once a month via Respirgard II nebulizer; **(IV):** 4 mg/kg q2–4wk
prednisone (Deltasone)	Adjunctive therapy in moderate to severe cases of *Pneumocystis carinii* pneumonia (Po$_2$ <70 mm Hg)	**Adults (PO):** 40 mg q12h for 5 days; then 40 mg daily for 5 days; then 20 mg daily until treatment is completed
primaquine	*Pneumocystis carinii* pneumonia	**Adults (PO):** 26.3–52.6 mg (15–30 mg base) daily for 21 days

Side Effects	Comments
Abdominal pain or discomfort, nausea, diarrhea, vomiting, pain, burning, stinging, redness, or swelling at injection site, dizziness, lightheadedness, swelling of feet or lower legs, headache, fatigue, red or flushed face, weakness	1. Give by subcutaneous injection. 2. Rotate injection sites.
Dizziness, lightheadedness, headache, insomnia or drowsiness, nausea, vomiting, diarrhea, stomach or abdominal pain or discomfort, increased sensitivity to sunlight	1. May give without regard to food. 2. Antacids delay absorption (avoid taking one within 2 hours of ofloxacin administration). 3. Take with full glass of water.
Constipation, diarrhea, headache, fever, abdominal pain, stomach cramps, dizziness, drowsiness, dry mouth, rash, unusually tired or weak	Report to physician if vomiting persists.
Chills, diarrhea, feeling of stomach fullness, altered libido, muscle cramps, trouble sleeping (men: acne, decreased sex ability)	Important to have diet high in protein and calories while taking this drug.
Confusion, constipation, decreased blood pressure, increased heart rate, sweating, redness, flushed face, trouble breathing, decreased urination, stomach pain or cramps, dizziness, lightheadedness, unusual fatigue or weakness, drowsiness, dry mouth, headache	1. Avoid getting up suddenly. 2. Lie down if nausea, vomiting, dizziness, or lightheadedness occurs. 3. Use sugarless gum or candy for relief of dry mouth.
Fever, chills, unusual bleeding or bruising, muscle pain, joint pain, numbness in the feet or lower legs, nausea, vomiting, diarrhea, unusual fatigue or weakness	Infused slowly over 3 hours.
Fever, joint pain, skin rash, itching, unusual fatigue or weakness, lower back pain, pain while urinating, abdominal pain, loss of appetite, nausea, diarrhea, vomiting, yellow eyes or skin	Take with or after meals to decrease gastric irritation.
Headache, vertigo, rash, diarrhea, nausea, abdominal cramps, loss of appetite, steatorrhea, ototoxicity, hematuria	1. Take with food. 2. Report ringing in ears, dizziness, loss of hearing.
Aerosol: Chest pain or congestion, cough, difficulty breathing, burning pain or dryness in the throat, difficulty swallowing, skin rash, wheezing, bitter or metallic taste **Parenteral:** Sudden rash or itching, anemia, unusual fatigue, fever or chills, cough or hoarseness, lower back pain, painful or difficult urination, unusual bruising or bleeding, pinpoint red spots on skin, diarrhea, headache, loss of appetite, nausea, vomiting, skin rash	1. Report fever, cough, shortness of breath. 2. Avoid alcohol. 3. Maintain adequate fluid intake. 4. Give IV over 60 minutes. 5. Pentamidine stimulates the release of histamine so hypotension can occur during infusion. 6. Sterile abscess may occur with IM injections.
Increased appetite, weight gain, fluid retention, indigestion, nervousness, restlessness, insomnia, mood swings	1. Taper dose. 2. May mask signs of infection. 3. May result in the appearance of new infections, e.g., thrush, herpes simplex.
Back, leg, or stomach pain, dark urine, loss of appetite, fever, unusual fatigue or weakness, bluish fingernails, lips, or skin, dizziness or lightheadedness, difficulty breathing, nausea, vomiting, abdominal pain	1. Take with meals or antacids to decrease GI irritation. 2. Given with clindamycin to treat PCP for patients who cannot tolerate standard treatment.

Table continued on following page

Generic Name (Trade)	Indications	Dosage
prochlorperazine (Compazine)	Nausea, vomiting	**Adults (PO):** 5–10 mg tid to qid (maximum: 40 mg/d); extended release: 15–30 mg once daily or 10 mg q12h (maximum: 40 mg/d) **Children (PO), syrup: 9–13 kg:** 2.5 mg 1–2 times daily (maximum: 7.5 mg/d); **14–17 kg:** 2.5 mg bid to tid (maximum: 10 mg/d); **18–39 kg:** 2.5 mg tid or 5 mg bid (maximum: 15 mg/d)
pyrazinamide	*Mycobacterium tuberculosis*	**Adults (PO):** 25–30 mg/kg in 3–4 divided doses (maximum: 2 g/d); up to 60 mg/kg/d for drug-resistant TB **Children (PO):** 15–30 mg/kg/d in 2 divided doses (maximum: 2 g/d)
pyrimethamine (Daraprim)	Toxoplasmosis, *Pneumocystis carinii* pneumonia	*Primary Prophylaxis for PCP and Toxoplasmosis* **Adults (PO):** 50 mg weekly with dapsone and leucovorin *Primary Prophylaxis for Toxoplasmosis* **Children (PO):** 1 mg/kg daily with dapsone and leucovorin *Treatment of PCP* **Adults:** 50 mg weekly with dapsone and leucovorin *Treatment of Toxoplasmosis* **Adults (PO):** 100–200 mg loading dose; then 50–100 mg/d with leucovorin and sulfadiazine or trisulfapyrimidine **Children (PO):** 1–2 mg/kg/d for 1–3 days; then 0.5–1 mg/kg/d *Secondary Prophylaxis for PCP* **Adults (PO):** 50 mg weekly with dapsone and leucovorin *Secondary Prophylaxis for Toxoplasmosis* **Adults (PO):** 25–75 mg/d with either sulfadiazine or clindamycin plus leucovorin **Children (PO):** 1 mg/kg/d with either sulfadiazine or clindamycin plus leucovorin
ranitidine (Zantac)	Gastric or duodenal ulcers, hypersecretory syndrome, gastroesophageal reflux disease	**Adults (PO):** 150 mg bid or 300 mg hs **Children (PO):** 2–4 mg/kg bid (maximum: 300 mg/d)
rifabutin (Mycobutin)	*Mycobacterium avium-intracellulare* complex, *Mycobacterium tuberculosis,* (INH-resistant strains)	*Primary Prophylaxis for MAC and TB* **Adults (PO):** 300 mg daily *Primary Prophylaxis for MAC* **Children (PO):** ≥**6 y:** 300 mg daily; <**6 y:** 5 mg/kg/d *Treatment for MAC* **Adults (PO):** 300–600 mg/d **Children (PO):** 10–20 mg/kg/d *Secondary Prophylaxis for MAC* **Adults (PO):** 300 mg daily **Children (PO):** ≥**6 y:** 300 mg daily; <**6 y:** 5 mg/kg/d
rifampin (Rifadin, Rimactane)	*Mycobacterium tuberculosis*	*Primary Prophylaxis* **Adults (PO):** 600 mg daily **Children (PO):** 10–20 mg/kg/d (maximum: 600 mg/d) *Treatment* **Adults (PO):** 10 mg/kg once daily or 2–3 times a week (maximum: 600 mg/d) **Children (IV):** <**1 mo:** 10–20 mg/kg/d or 2 or 3 times per week; ≥**1 mo:** 10–20 mg/kg/d or 2 or 3 times per week (maximum: 600 mg/d)

Side Effects	Comments
Constipation, dizziness, drowsiness, dry mouth, nausea, vomiting, stomach pain, decreased sweating	1. Take with food to decrease gastric irritation. 2. Take extended release capsules whole; do not chew.
Pain or swelling of joints, especially big toe, ankle, and knee, hot skin over affected joints, loss of appetite, unusual weakness or fatigue, yellow eyes or skin, itching, skin rash	1. Store in a cool, dry place. 2. May take without regard to food. 3. Report fatigue, weakness, nausea, vomiting, joint pain or swelling.
Pain, burning, or inflammation of the tongue, change in or loss of taste, fever, sore throat, unusual fatigue or weakness, unusual bruising or bleeding; high doses may cause loss of appetite, nausea, vomiting, or diarrhea	1. Store in cool, dry place. 2. Give with meals to decrease vomiting. 3. Report rash, sore throat, pallor, glossitis (pain, burning, inflammation of tongue, change in taste). 4. Given with folinic acid (leucovorin).
Constipation, diarrhea, dizziness, drowsiness, headache, nausea, vomiting, skin rash	May take without regard to food.
Skin rash, nausea, vomiting, reddish orange to reddish brown discoloration of urine, feces, saliva, skin, sputum, sweat, and tears (may also discolor soft contact lenses)	1. May take on an empty stomach or with food if gastric irritation occurs. 2. Dividing the daily dose will decrease the potential for gastric irritation. 3. May mix contents of capsules with applesauce if swallowing capsule is difficult.
Stomach cramps, diarrhea, reddish-orange to reddish-brown discoloration of urine, feces, saliva, skin, sputum, sweat, and tears (may also discolor soft contact lenses)	1. Best given 1 hour before or 2 hours after meals. 2. Give with food to decrease GI upset. 3. May mix contents of capsules with applesauce.

Table continued on following page

Generic Name (Trade)	Indications	Dosage
ritonavir (Norvir)	HIV infection	**Adults (PO):** initially, 300 mg q12h , increasing by 100 mg q12h to a maximum of 600 mg q12h; when given with saquinavir (400 mg bid) ritonavir dosage is 400 mg bid **Children (PO):** initially, 250 mg/m² q12h, increasing by 50 mg/m² q12h over 5 days to a maximum of 400 mg/m² q12h
saquinavir (Invirase, Fortovase)	HIV infection	**Adults (PO):** Invirase, 600 mg tid; Fortovase, 1200 mg tid
somatropin (human growth hormone, Serostim)	HIV wasting syndrome and weight loss	**Adults (SC): >55 kg:** 6 mg daily; **45–55 kg:** 5 mg daily; **35–44 kg:** 4 mg daily
stavudine (Zerit)	HIV infection	**Adults (PO): >60 kg:** 40 mg q12h; **<60 kg:** 30 mg q12h **Children (PO):** 1 mg/kg q12h (up to weight of 30 kg)
streptomycin	*Mycobacterium tuberculosis*	**Adults (IM):** 15 mg/kg/d (maximum: 1 g) **Children (IM):** 20–40 mg/kg/d (maximum: 1 g)
sulfadiazine	Toxoplasmosis	***Treatment*** **Adults (PO):** 2–8 g/d divided q6h (with pyrimethamine and leucovorin) **Children (PO):** 120–200 mg/kg/d divided q6h (with pyrimethamine and leucovorin) ***Secondary Prophylaxis*** **Adults (PO):** 500–1000 mg qid (with pyrimethamine and leucovorin) **Children (PO):** 85–120 mg/kg/d in 2–4 divided doses (with pyrimethamine and leucovorin)

Side Effects	Comments

Nausea, vomiting, diarrhea, loss of appetite, abdominal pain, taste alterations, headache, dizziness, sleepiness, tingling sensation or numbness around the lips, hands, or feet; fatigue, weakness
May elevate liver enzymes and triglycerides; blood sugar may increase blood glucose (symptoms include increased thirst, hunger, and urination, weight loss, fatigue, dry skin, itching), elevated triglyceride and cholesterol levels, fat accumulation, buffalo hump
	1. Store capsules, solution in refrigerator; protect from light.
	2. Refrigeration of solution not necessary if used within 30 days of reconstitution, but store below 77° F.
	3. Take with food.
	4. Taste of oral solution may be improved by:
	   a. Mixing with vanilla or chocolate milk, pudding, or ice cream within 1 hour of dosing
	   b. Dulling the taste buds before adminstration by chewing on ice, popsicles, or spoonfuls of partially frozen orange or grape juice
	   c. Eating peanut butter to coat the mouth before taking ritonavir
	   d. Chewing gum or hard candies after taking dose
	5. Review other medications before initiating them—many drug interactions.
	6. Tobacco decreases serum plasma levels.
	7. Blood glucose, triglyceride, and cholesterol levels should be monitored.
	8. Given in combination with other antiretrovirals, never as monotherapy.

Nausea, diarrhea, ulcers in mouth, abdominal discomfort, abdominal pain, burning or prickling sensation, skin rash, weakness, headache; may increase blood glucose (symptoms include increased thirst, hunger, and urination, weight loss, fatigue, dry skin, itching), elevated triglyceride and cholesterol levels, fat accumulation, buffalo hump	1. Compounded with lactose; lactose-intolerant patients can take LactAid tablets before taking saquinavir. 2. Take with a full meal. 3. Taking with grapefruit juice increases bioavailability. 4. Photosensitivity can occur; use sunscreen or protective clothing. 5. Blood glucose, triglyceride, and cholesterol levels should be monitored.
Musculoskeletal discomfort, fever, increased tissue turgor, diarrhea, neuropathy, nausea, headache, abdominal pain, fatigue	1. Do not shake. 2. Reconstituted solution should be refrigerated and must be used within 24 hours after reconstituting. 3. Rotate injection sites (abdomen and thighs). 4. Concomitant antiretroviral therapy is required (may potentiate HIV replication).
Numbness, tingling, or pain in the hands or feet, headache, diarrhea, chills, fever, nausea, vomiting, muscle pain, loss of strength or energy, insomnia, anxiety, joint pain, back pain, loss of appetite, nervousness, dizziness	1. Compounded with lactose; lactose-intolerant patients can take LactAid tablets before taking stavudine. 2. May take without regard to food. 3. Avoid alcohol. 4. Report tingling, burning, pain, or numbness of hands or feet.
Greatly altered frequency and amount of urination, increased thirst, loss of appetite, nausea, vomiting, twitching, numbness, seizures, tingling, loss of hearing, ringing or buzzing in ears, fullness in ears, dizziness, clumsiness, burning of face or mouth, itching, redness, rash, swelling, any loss of vision	1. IM injection should be deep into large muscle mass. 2. Do not exceed concentration of 500 mg/ml.
Dizziness, headache, lethargy, nausea, vomiting, diarrhea, loss of appetite, fever, itching, skin rash, increased sensitivity to sunlight	1. Give on an empty stomach with 8 ounces of water. 2. Drink several extra glasses of water daily to prevent kidney stones. 3. Avoid large amounts of vitamin C or acidifying agents (e.g., cranberry juice) to prevent crystalluria. 4. Report rash, sore throat, fever, arthralgia, shortness of breath.

Table continued on following page

Generic Name (Trade)	Indications	Dosage
terconazole (Terazol)	Vulvovaginal candidiasis	**Adults (vaginal):** *tablet:* 1 tablet hs for 3 days; *cream:* 1 full applicator 0.4% cream hs for 7 days *or* 0.8% cream hs for 3 days
testoterone (testosterone cypionate, testosterone enanthate)	Hypogonadism and HIV wasting	**Adult men (IM):** 100–200 mg q2wk **Adult men (transdermal):** 4–6 mg patch changed every day
thalidomide (Synovir)	HIV wasting and weight loss	**Adults (PO):** 100–200 mg daily
thiethylperazine (Torecan)	Nausea, vomiting	**Adults (PO):** 10 mg 1–3 times daily
trimethoprim (Proloprim, Trimpex)	*Pneumocystis carinii* pneumonia, moderate PCP	**Adults (PO):** 15 mg/kg/d
trimethoprim-sulfamethoxazole (Bactrim, Septra, TMP-SMZ)	*Pneumocystis carinii* pneumonia, toxoplasmosis	***Primary Prophylaxis for PCP*** **Adults (PO):** one double strength tablet per day or three times a week, or one single strength tablet per day **Children (PO):** 150/750 mg/m^2/d in 2 divided doses, or three times a week on consecutive days, or three times a week on alternate days ***Primary Prophylaxis for Toxoplasmosis*** **Adults (PO):** one double strength tablet daily **Children (PO):** 150/750 mg/m^2/day in 2 divided doses ***Treatment of PCP*** **Adults, children >2 mo (PO/IV):** TMP 15–20 mg/kg/d + SMZ 75–100 mg/kg/d in 3–4 divided doses ***Secondary Prophylaxis for PCP*** **Adults (PO):** one double strength tablet daily *or* three times a week, *or* one single strength tablet daily **Children (PO):** 150/750 mg/m^2/day in 2 divided doses, *or* three times a week on consecutive days, *or* three times a week on alternate days
trimetrexate (Neutrexin)	*Pneumocystis carinii* pneumonia	**Adults (IV):** 45 mg/m^2 daily
valacyclovir (Valtrex)	Herpes zoster virus infection	**Adults (PO):** 1 g q8h
vinblastine (Velban)	Kaposi's sarcoma	Refer to individual protocols
vincristine (Oncovin)	Kaposi's sarcoma	Refer to individual protocols

Side Effects	Comments
Vaginal burning, itching, discharge or irritation, headache, abdominal or stomach cramps or pain	1. Safety and efficacy not established for children <3 years of age. 2. Use at bedtime.
Bladder irritability, urinary tract infection, edema, nausea, vomiting, diarrhea, acne, irritation at site of injection, gynecomastia, irritation at site of transdermal patch	Patch must be applied to shaved, dry scrotum.
Drowsiness, dizziness, altered mood, constipation, xerostomia, increased appetite, weight gain, headache, decreased libido, swelling of face, hands, and legs, nausea, itching, loss of hair, fever, chills, dry skin, rash, numbness, tingling, and burning of hands and feet	Important for diet to be high in protein and calories while thalidomide is being taken.
Drowsiness, dizziness, constipation, dry mouth, nose, or throat, unusual fatigue or weakness, fever, headache, skin rash	1. Take with food (decreases GI irritation). 2. Avoid alcohol. 3. May cause drowsiness, blurred vision, dry mouth.
Nausea, vomiting, diarrhea, loss of appetite, stomach cramps, headache	1. May give without regard to food. 2. Give with food if stomach upset occurs.
Dizziness, headache, lethargy, nausea, vomiting, diarrhea, loss of appetite, fever, itching, skin rash, increased sensitivity to sunlight	1. May be given PO or IV. 2. Not recommended for infants <1 month or infants up to 6 weeks taking zidovudine. 3. **PO:** Administer on empty stomach with 8 ounces of water; drink several extra glasses of water daily. 4. **IV:** Infuse over 60–90 minutes.
Fever, sore throat, unusual fatigue or weakness, mouth sores or ulcers, skin rash or itching, unusual bruising or bleeding, blood in urine or stool, pinpoint red spots on skin, confusion, nausea, vomiting, stomach pain	1. Infuse IV over 60–90 minutes. 2. Leucovorin (folinic acid) must be given concurrently and 72 hours following last dose trimetrexate.
Nausea, headache, dizziness, fatigue, constipation, diarrhea, loss of appetite, stomach pain, vomiting	1. Take with meals. 2. Only recommended for immunocompetent individuals; use in immunosuppressed persons is under study.
Fever, chills, cough, hoarseness, lower back pain, painful or difficult urination, muscle pain, nausea, vomiting, joint pain, loss of hair, sores in the mouth or on the lips, pain, redness at injection site, swelling of the feet or lower legs	1. For IV administration only. 2. Report fever, sore throat, bleeding, bruising.
Constipation, stomach cramps, dizziness or lightheadedness, joint pain, lower back or side pain, diarrhea, loss of weight, nausea, vomiting, skin rash, loss of hair, pain or redness at injection site, blurred vision or double vision, pain or numbness in the fingers, toes	1. For IV administration only. 2. Report fever, sore throat, bleeding, bruising, or shortness of breath.

Table continued on following page

Generic Name (Trade)	Indications	Dosage
zalcitabine (ddC, Hivid)	HIV infection	**Adults (PO):** 0.75 mg q8h **Children (PO):** 0.005–0.01 mg/kg q8h
zidovudine (ZDV, AZT, Retrovir)	HIV infection	***Prophylaxis for Vertical Transmission of HIV*** **Maternal therapy (after first trimester) (PO):** 100 mg q4h while awake **Intrapartum: IV during delivery:** 2 mg/kg loading dose over 30–60 minutes followed by continuous infusion of 1 mg/kg/hour until the cord is clamped **Newborn (Syrup, PO):** 2 mg/kg q6h; **(IV if NPO):** 1.5 mg/kg over 30 minutes q6h ***Treatment*** **Adults (PO):** 200 mg q8h *or* 300 mg q12h; **(IV):** 1 mg/kg q4h **Children (PO): premature birth to 2 weeks of age:** 1.5 mg/kg q12h, increasing to 2 mg/kg q8h after 2 weeks of age; **neonatal:** 2 mg/kg q6h; **<12 y:** 160 mg/m^2 q8h; **>12 y:** adult dose **Children (IV): neonatal:** 1.5 mg/kg q6h; **<12 y:** *intermittent infusion:* 120 mg/m^2 q6h (maximum: 160 mg/m^2 per dose); *continuous infusion:* 20 mg/m^2/h

Data from

Acute Pain Management Guideline Panel. (1992, February). *Acute pain management: Operative or medical procedures and trauma.* Clinical Practice Guideline. (AHCPR Pub. No. 92-0032). Rockville, MD: Agency for Health Care Policy and Research, Public Health Service, U.S. Department of Health and Human Services.

AIDS Institute. (1997, July). HIV medical evaluation and preventive care. In *Protocols for the medical care of HIV infection* (7th ed.). Albany, NY: New York State Department of Health.

Bartlett, J. (1997). *Medical management of HIV infection.* Available at: http://www.hopkins-aids.edu.

Breitbart, W., McDonald, M.V. (1996). Pharmacologic pain management in HIV/AIDS. *Journal of the International Association of Physicians in AIDS Care, 2*(7), 17–26.

Carpenter, C.C., Fischl, M.A., Hammer, S.C., et al. (1997). Antiretroviral therapy for HIV infection in 1997: Updated recommendations of the international AIDS Society-USA Panel. *Journal of the American Medical Association, 277*(24), 1962–1969.

Carr, D.B., Dubois, M., Luu, M., Shepard, K.V. (1994). Pharmacotherapy of pain in HIV/AIDS. In D.B. Carr (Ed.), *Pain in HIV/AIDS* (pp.18–28). Washington, DC: France-USA Pain Association.

Centers for Disease Control and Prevention. (1993). Recommendations of the Advisory Committee on Immunization Practices (ACIP): Use of vaccines and immune globulins in persons with altered immunocompetence. *Morbidity and Mortality Weekly Report, 42*(RR-4), 1–18.

Centers for Disease Control and Prevention. (1997). 1997 USPHS/IDSA guidelines for the prevention of opportunistic infections in persons infected with human immunodeficiency virus. *Morbidity and Mortality Weekly Report, 46*(RR-12), 1–46.

Deeks, S.G. (1998). Antiretroviral agents: The next generation. *AIDS Clinical Care, 10*(5), 34–36, 39.

Fanning, M.M. (Ed.). (1997). *HIV infection: A clinical approach* (2nd ed.). Philadelphia: Saunders.

Ferris, F.D., Flannery, J.S., McNeal, H.B., Morissette, M.R., Cameron, R., Bally, G.A. (1995). *A comprehensive guide for the care of persons with HIV disease, Module 4: Palliative care.* Toronto: Mount Sinai Hospital and Casey House Hospice.

Henry, K., Melroe, H., Huebsch, J., et al. (1998). Severe premature coronary artery disease with protease inhibitors. *Lancet, 351,* 1328.

Lo, J.C., Mulligan, K., Tai, V.W., et al. (1998). "Buffalo hump" in men with HIV-1 infection. *Lancet, 351,* 867–870.

Miller, K.D., Jones, E., Yanovski, J.A., et al. (1998). Visceral abdominal-fat accumulation associated with use of indinavir. *Lancet, 351,* 871–875.

Reiter, G.S., Kudler, N.R. (1996). Palliative care and HIV, part II: Systemic manifestations and late-stage issues. *AIDS Clinical Care, 8*(4), 27–36.

Sande, M.A., Volberding, P.A. (Eds.). (1997). *The medical management of AIDS* (5th ed.). Philadelphia: Saunders

United States Pharmacopeial Covention. (1997). *USPDI Volume I: Drug information for the health care professional.* Tauton, MA: Rand McNally.

Working Group on Antretroviral Therapy and Medical Management of HIV Infected Children. (1997). *Guidelines for the use of antiretroviral agents in pediatric HIV infection.* Rockville, MD: Health Resources Services Administration, Public Health Service, U.S. Department of Health and Human Services.

Side Effects	Comments
Numbness, tingling, burning and pain in lower extremities, abdominal pain, nausea, vomiting, rash, GI intolerance, fever, sore throat, headache, fatigue, nausea, pruritus, muscle pain, difficulty swallowing, arthralgia	1. Store tablets at room temperature. 2. Best taken on an empty stomach. 3. Swallow tablets whole, drinking plenty of water.
Fatigue, muscle pain, headache, nausea, vomiting, insomnia, anemia (pale skin, unusual fatigue or weakness), neutropenia (fever, chills, sore throat), confusion, mental changes, seizures, bluish-brown bands on fingernails	1. Store capsules and syrup at room temperature. 2. Protect from light. 3. May take without regard to food. 4. Take with food to decrease nausea; avoid high-fat meal, which impairs absorption. 5. Infusion should be given over a minimum of 60 minutes.

Diagnostic Testing in HIV Disease

JOHN K. WEISER

Test Name	Interpretation

HIV DIAGNOSTIC TESTS

HIV antibody test (HIV Ab)
Enzyme-linked immuno-
  sorbent assay (EIA, ELISA)
Western blot
Indirect immunoflourescence
  assay (IFA)

Several assays are commercially available to detect antibody to HIV. The EIA is the most commonly used test to screen blood products, for diagnosing HIV infection, and for epidemiologic purposes. Antibodies are usually detected within 4–12 weeks but may not be detectable for a prolonged period after infection. Consequently a negative EIA does not rule out HIV infection. If reactive, the EIA is repeated. If two of three EIAs are reactive, a confirmation test, usually a Western blot, is done. If reactivity is confirmed by a Western blot, the HIV antibody test is reported as positive. Virtually all patients who are HIV antibody positive have ongoing HIV infection. EIA results can be falsely positive in patients who are rapid plasma reagin (RPR; VDRL) positive or patients who have hemophilia or are on dialysis. In addition, false-positive results occur in multiparous women, in patients recently vaccinated against hepatitis B or influenza, in patients who have had multiple blood transfusions, in those with autoimmune disease, and in some other conditions.

HIV antigen test
  (p24 antigen)

p24 antigen is detected by monoclonal antibody against HIV core. p24 is present in the serum several weeks before seroconversion but may become undetectable as antibody levels rise. Later in HIV disease, as antibody levels decrease, p24 antigen may again become detectable. HIV p24 antibody has largely been replaced by HIV RNA tests.

HIV culture

HIV isolation entails cocultivation of the patient's specimen with stimulated mononuclear white blood cells. The culture is checked weekly for 4 to 6 weeks for viral activity.

TESTS FOR MONITORING HIV DISEASE

HIV nucleic acid detection
  (viral load testing)
Polymerase chain reaction
  (PCR)
Branched chain DNA
  (bDNA)
Nucleic acid sequence based
  amplification (NASBA)

PCR, bDNA, and NASBA can detect minute amounts of HIV nucleic acids. The sensitivity and specificity are equivalent to HIV culture. Quantitative tests are used for prognostic purposes, to monitor disease progression, and to assess the effectiveness of treatment. Viral load testing, considered together with a patient's CD4 count, is highly predictive of long-term outcome. PCR results are generally double those of bDNA results. The threshold of detectability on the commercially available PCR test (Amplicor HIV-1, Roche) and the NASBA (Organon) is 400 copies per microliter. The threshold of the widely available bDNA test (Quantiplex HIV RNA Assay, Chiron) is 500 copies per microliter. The threshold of future tests will be 20–40 copies per microliter (Roche Ultrasensitive, Chiron bDNA Version 3, NASBA Version 2). A threefold to tenfold (0.5–1.0 log) change in viral load level is considered a significant change.

Test Name	Interpretation
VIROLOGIC TESTS	
Cytomegalovirus (CMV) culture	Urine is the best single specimen for CMV recovery. Recovery of CMV from urine, blood, or tissue may reflect either active disease caused by CMV or asymptomatic viral replication. CMV cultures are not invariably positive in patients with CMV disease. Diagnosis of disease caused by CMV should be made by tissue biopsy with histologic evidence of virus-mediated damage. In healthy adults the excretion rate is ≤1%. Up to 90% of people with HIV disease are infected with CMV, and ≥50% of immunocompromised patients excrete the virus by one or more routes.
Cytomegalovirus antibody	CMV antibody prevalence in the population above the age of 30 may range from 40% to 100%. The presence of CMV antibody may indicate primary, quiescent, or reactivation disease. Therefore, it should not be relied on to confirm CMV as the cause of disease. A negative test does not necessarily indicate the absence of infection since the assays are not 100% sensitive.
Hepatitis A virus antibody (anti-HAV) Total anti-HAV (IgG + IgM) IgM anti-HAV	A high percentage of the population has antibody to HAV (total anti-HAV) acquired from clinically unapparent infections. Both IgG and IgM antibodies occur early in the acute infection with IgG persisting for years. Diagnosis of acute hepatitis A requires the presence of IgM anti-HAV. After acute infection, IgM anti-HAV usually disappears after 3–4 months but may persist for up to 10 months. Patients with IgG anti-HAV due to vaccination or natural infection are protected from reinfection.
Hepatitis B core antibody (anti-HBc, HBcAb) Total HBcAb (IgG + IgM) IgM-anti-HBc	HBcAb (total anti-HB) is present in cases of acute, chronic, and resolved hepatitis B. It is important in diagnosing resolving hepatitis B because it may be present after disappearance of HBsAg and before appearance of HBsAb. It is not present in a patient who has been vaccinated for hepatitis B and who has not had natural infection with hepatitis B virus (HBsAb is typically present). IgM-anti-HBc is only present in acute hepatitis B infection and must be positive to document *acute* hepatitis B
Hepatitis B DNA (HBV-DNA)	The presence of HBV-DNA in serum confirms active hepatitis B infection and implies infectivity of serum. Current use of the assay is for confirming active hepatitis B infection in immunosuppressed patients with confusing serologic markers and for monitoring the responses of hepatitis B to therapy such as interferon-alfa.
Hepatitis B surface antibody (anti-HBs, HBsAb)	With naturally occurring hepatitis B infection, anti-HBs usually appears in the serum several weeks after the disappearance of HBsAg. The presence of anti-HBs usually means there is protection against hepatitis B infection. However, convalescent anti-HBs may fall below limits of detection. A qualitative anti-HBs is usually adequate to assess natural immunity, but a quantitative test finding of ≥10 IU/L for postvaccine testing is the accepted concentration that confers immunity.
Hepatitis B surface antigen (HBsAg)	HBsAg is usually the first detectable marker of acute hepatitis B and is usually present in chronic infections. Although rare, hepatitis B infection has been documented in the absence of HBsAg. In this case the presence of the virus can be documented by the presence of HBV-DNA.
Hepatitis B e antigen and antibody (HBeAg, anti-HBe, HBeAb)	HBeAg and anti-HBe should be ordered together and should only be studied in a patient who is HBsAg positive. In general, active viral replication is associated with infective serum that is HBeAg positive and anti-HBe negative. Upon conversion to a nonreplicative state, anti-HBe appears in the serum and HBeAg disappears. The main utility of these tests is to assess the response of hepatitis B infection to therapy such as interferon-alfa.

Table continued on following page

Test Name	Interpretation
VIROLOGIC TESTS *Continued*	
Hepatitis C virus antibody (anti-HCV)	Anti-HCV is present in patients with acute, chronic, and resolved hepatitis C infection. Approximately 85% of patients with detectable anti-HCV have persistent infection. The presence of anti-HCV, therefore, does not confer immunity to infection. Persistent HCV infection in a patient with a positive anti-HCV can be confirmed with a test for HCV-RNA.
Hepatitis C virus RNA (HCV-RNA)	Detection of HCV-RNA confirms the presence of persistent HCV infection in a patient who is positive for anti-HCV. A qualitative test of HCV-RNA can be used to assess the effectiveness of treatment for HCV infection such as interferon-alfa.
Herpes simplex virus (HSV) tests Serologic test for HSV, culture, direct antigen tests	Up to 77% of patients with HIV have serologic evidence of previous HSV infection. Therefore a positive serologic test for HSV does not confirm that HSV is the cause of mucocutaneous or other disease. A culture for HSV obtained during the first week of illness may be positive and is generally confirmatory. Asymptomatic viral shedding has been documented on 1% to 4% of the days on which cultures were obtained in nonimmunocompromised patients. Direct microscopic examination for HSV antigen in specimens is possible by examining for the presence of multinucleated giant cells; however, all herpesviruses, e.g., CMV and VZV, will produce similar morphologies. Amplification by means of PCR is now available in clinical practice.
MICROBIOLOGIC TESTS	
Toxoplasma antibody IgG	Latent infection with the parasite *Toxoplasma gondii* can be identified by the presence of serum antibodies (IgG) to the organism. The test should be done as part of the initial evaluation of an HIV patient and, if negative, should be repeated periodically. Patients who are *Toxoplasma* antibody positive should be offered prophylaxis if the CD4+ cell count is below 100/µl. IgM titers, routinely used to diagnose acute toxoplasmosis in HIV-uninfected patients, are rarely present in patients with HIV.
Mycobacterial culture	Conventional culturing may not be positive for 3–4 weeks. Newer radiometric techniques (Bactec) or other automated technologies (Organon Teknika) may reduce this time. Six to eight weeks are required before cultures can be considered negative for mycobacteria if conventional methods are used. Mycobacterial cultures can be performed on blood, urine, bone marrow, CSF, bronchial or tracheal aspirates, sputum, and tissue.
Acid fast stain for mycobacteria (AFB stain)	The same specimen should be used for AFB smears as for mycobacterial cultures. Smears may be negative as much as 50% of the time, even with positive cultures. Smears may remain positive longer than cultures when patients have been on chemotherapy for mycobacterial infection.

Test Name	Reference Range	Interpretation
HEMATOLOGIC TESTS		
Hemoglobin (Hb)	*g/dl (95% range)* 18–44 y, M: 13.2–17.3 F: 11.7–15.5 45–64 y, M: 13.1–17.2 F: 11.7–16.9 65–74 y, M: 12.6–17.4 F: 11.7–16.1	Low hemoglobin and hematocrit values may be due to neoplasms, infection, HIV, folic acid deficiency, vitamin B_{12} deficiency, hemolytic anemia, hemophagocytic syndrome, thrombic thrombocytopenia, disseminated intravascular coagulation, or drug therapy. Drugs causing mylosuppression include antiretrovirals (zidovudine, lamivudine, stavudine, didanosine), antivirals (ganciclovir, foscarnet), antifungals (amphotericin B, flucytosine), antiprotozoals (sulfonamides, trimethoprim, pyrimethamine, pentamidine), antineoplastics (paclitaxel, vinblastine, doxorubicin [Doxil], daunorubicin [DaunoXome], adriamycin, cyclophosphamide), and immunomodulators (interferon-alfa). Additionally, HIV can cause anemia, e.g., anemia of chronic disease or blunted erythropoietin production or response.
Hematocrit (Hct)	*% (packed erythrocytes)* 18–44 y, M: 39–49 F: 35–45 45–64 y, M: 39–50 F: 35–47 65–74 y, M: 37–51 F: 35–47	
Leukocyte count (white blood cell count, WBC)	*Cells/μl* ≥21 y: 4500–11,000 Blacks 3600–10,200	Elevated WBC counts (leukocytosis) occur in leukemia, most infections, hemorrhage, and after splenectomy. Reduced WBC counts (leukopenia) occur in certain infections, bone marrow infiltration, hematopoietic disorders, and drug therapy (zidovudine, ganciclovir, interferon-alfa, sulfonamides, pentamidine, trimetrexate, and cancer chemotherapy).
Platelet count	150,000–400,000/μl	Elevated counts occur in myeloproliferative disorders, polycythemia vera, some inflammatory disorders, some anemias, some malignancies, and after splenectomy. Reduced counts occur in hereditary disorders and acquired states such as idiopathic thrombocytopenic purpura (ITP), HIV-related immune thrombocytopenia, bone marrow infiltrative processes, vitamin and mineral deficiencies, infections, liver disease, hypersplenism, and drugs such as interferon-alfa, ganciclovir, trimetrexate, and cancer chemotherapy.
IMMUNOLOGIC TESTS		
T-cell subsets	*Marker Cells/μl % Lymphocytes* CD4+ 436–1394 35.9–63.5 CD8+ 166–882 15.2–41.6 Ratio of helper to suppressor cells, CD4+/CD8+: 0.5–3.3	In the absence of cytotoxic therapy, lymphoproliferative disease, a CD4+ cell count <100/μl is strongly suggestive of HIV infection with impending or current opportunistic infection. A CD4+ cell count • <200/μl is associated with increased risk for *P. carinii* pneumonia • <100/μl is associated with toxoplasmic encephalitis and • <50/μl is associated with disseminated *Mycobacterium avium-intracellulare* complex (dMAC). An elevated CD8+ count has been associated with viral infections (HBV, EBV, CMV, HIV).

Table continued on following page

Test Name	Reference Range	Interpretation
GENERAL CLINICAL TESTS		
Alanine aminotransferase (ALT, SGPT)	M: 10–40 U/L F: 7–35 U/L	Elevated levels indicate hepatocellular injury (liver damage) or severe heart or kidney injury. Causes include viral hepatitis, acute or chronic alcohol abuse, obstructive jaundice, severe shock, and extensive myocardial infarction. Elevated levels also occur with hepatic drug toxicity caused by isoniazid (INH), rifampin, rifabutin, sulfonamides, ethambutol, fluoroquinolones (e.g., ciprofloxacin), macrolides (e.g., azithromycin, clarithromycin), pentamidine, nucleoside reverse transcriptase inhibitors (e.g., didanosine, zalcitabine), ganciclovir, foscarnet, and others.
Albumin	3.4–4.8 g/dl	This predominant protein in serum is reduced in acute and chronic inflammation due to infection, autoimmune disorders, and malignancy. Low levels also result from impaired synthesis by the liver, which is seen in hepatitis, malnutrition, and malignancy. Marked decreases can result from body losses of protein as in nephrotic syndrome or hemorrhage. Albumin levels correlate with overall nutritional status and can be used to monitor nutritional therapy.
Alkaline phosphatase	Varies, depending on type of test	Enzyme found in liver, bone, intestine, placenta, and lung. Serum levels elevated in liver disease, particularly disease caused by biliary obstruction as in CMV or *Cryptosporidium* biliary tract disease, gallstones, cholangitis, and cholecystitis. Also increased in liver toxicity caused by drugs.
Aspartate aminotransferase (AST, SGOT)	M: 15–40 U/L F: 13–35 U/L	Found in all body tissues, but highest levels in liver, heart, skeletal muscles, and red blood cells. Used in combination with alanine aminotransferase (ALT); AST and ALT levels are elevated in similar conditions. AST levels are usually higher than ALT levels in liver cell injury due to any cause including cholestatic or obstructive jaundice, drug toxicity, and alcoholic hepatitis. ALT levels are usually higher than AST levels in chronic hepatitis (the reverse indicates a poor prognosis).
Bilirubin	*Total:* 0.3–1.2 mg/dl *Direct:* <0.2 mg/dl	A component of bile and a breakdown product of hemoglobin. Elevated levels are due to hepatocellular (liver) injury, biliary tract obstruction, drugs causing cholestasis, and hemolytic disorders. Elevation in the absence of other liver function test abnormalities may be a normal variant. An elevated direct bilirubin level (the conjugated fraction) is more specific for liver disease.
Blood urea nitrogen (BUN)	6–20 mg/dl	Serum levels are elevated with impaired kidney function as in congestive heart failure, dehydration, shock, and acute or chronic intrinsic kidney disease. Levels also are elevated in cases of renal drug toxicity due to, for example, aminoglycosides, amphotericin B, cidofovir, foscarnet, pentamidine, sulfonamides, or radiographic contrast media. Levels are reduced in low-protein diets.

Test Name	Reference Range	Interpretation
GENERAL CLINICAL TESTS *Continued*		
Cholesterol, total	*mg/dl* *5th–95th percentile* (varies by age and sex) 20–24 y, M: 124–218 F: 122–216 60–64 y, M: 159–276 F: 172–297	Commonly low levels in patients with HIV disease. The causes have not been defined, although the role of gastrointestinal disease, including impaired hepatic synthesis or malabsorption are considered possible contributing factors. Elevations have been noted in association with protease inhibitor therapy, in liver disease, including hepatitis and biliary tract obstruction, and in kidney disease, including nephrotic syndrome.
Creatinine	M: 0.9–1.3 mg/dl F: 0.6–1.1 mg/dl	Serum levels elevated in all causes of kidney dysfunction (see blood urea nitrogen). Low levels in debilitation due to age or decreased muscle mass.
Gamma glutamyltransferase (GGT, γ-GT)	Depends on type of test	Serum levels elevated in all types of liver disease, especially biliary tract obstruction. GGT is also a sensitive indicator of recent alcohol use.
Glucose-6-phosphate dehydrogenase (G6PD)	Depends on type of test	G6PD deficiency is an inherited predisposition to hemolytic anemia following exposure to certain oxidant drugs such as dapsone, pyrimethamine, and less commonly, sulfonamides. G6PD deficiency is most common in men of Mediterranean, South Asian, and Southeast Asian descent.
Protein, total	6.4–8.3 g/dl	Elevated serum levels most commonly reflect an increase in levels of immunoglobulins (one type of serum protein) seen in chronic infection (HIV, hepatitis viruses), autoimmune disorders, sarcoidosis, and chronic liver disease. Elevated levels also are seen in some malignancies. Reduced levels are seen in inherited immunoglobulin deficiency diseases and albumin deficiency (see albumin). The albumin-globulin ratio is often low in patients with HIV due to a combination of increased immunoglobulin levels and decreased albumin synthesis by the liver.
Testosterone	*Total* (ng/dl) M: 265–800 F: 10–40 *Free* (pg/ml) M: 50–210 F: 1–8.5 *Bioavailable* (ng/dl) M: 66–417 F: 0.6–5.0	Circulating testosterone is found in three forms: 1. A non-protein-bound, free form 2. A tightly protein-bound form (bound to sex hormone-binding globulin, SHBG) 3. A loosely protein bound form (bound to albumin). Tightly bound testosterone is not available for biological action in the tissues. Loosely bound testosterone rapidly dissociates from albumin and is available for target-cell entry. Bioavailable testosterone is composed of loosely bound and free testosterone and correlates with a clinical condition better than free testosterone does

Table continued on following page

Test Name	Reference Range	Interpretation
GENERAL CLINICAL TESTS *Continued*		
Triglycerides	*mg/dl* *5th–95th percentile* *(varies by sex and age)* 20–24 y, M: 44–201 F: 36–131 60–64 y, M: 58–291 F: 56–239	With progression from early to advanced HIV disease, triglyceride levels rise. Levels above 500 mg/dl put patients at risk for pancreatitis. This is of added concern for patients on medication that predisposes a person to pancreatitis, such as didanosine, zalcitabine, stavudine, and intravenous pentamidine. Elevations associated with protease inhibitor therapy have been reported. Increased production and decreased clearance of triglyceride is associated with elevated serum levels of interferon-alfa.

Data from

Centers for Disease Control and Prevention. (1997). 1997 USPHS/IDSA guidelines for the prevention of opportunistic infections in persons infected with human immunodeficiency virus. *Morbidity and Mortality Weekly Report, 46*(RR-12), 1–46.

Koelle, D.M., Benedetti, J., Langenberg, A., et al. (1992). Asymptomatic reactivation of herpes simplex virus in women after the first episode of genital herpes. *Annals of Internal Medicine, 116,* 433–437.

Levine, A.M. (1997). Hematological manifestations of HIV disease. *Clinical care options for HIV continuum of care series* (Vol. 10). Available at http://www.healthcg.com/

Siegel, D., Golden, E., Washington, E., et al. (1992). Prevalence and correlates of herpes simplex infections: The population-based AIDS in multiethnic neighborhoods study. *Journal of the American Medical Association, 268,* 1702–1708.

Tietz, N.W. (Ed.). (1995). *Clinical guide to laboratory tests* (3rd ed.). Philadelphia: Saunders.

IV

Postexposure Prophylaxis

PETER J. UNGVARSKI

The assumption underlying postexposure prophylaxis (PEP) is that antiretroviral agents administered immediately after exposure to HIV may prevent cellular infection and propagation of the virus and allow the host immune defenses to eliminate the virus (Katz & Gerberding, 1997). Animal studies have demonstrated that antiretroviral agents can prevent infection with the simian immunodeficiency virus (SIV) or HIV-2 when they are administered within 24 hours of exposure that occurred through intravenous or intrarectal routes (Bottinger et al., 1997; Tsai et al., 1995). Using human cadaver skin specimens, Pope and associates demonstrated that antiretroviral agents could block the dissemination of HIV from dendritic cells to susceptible T cells, which may be critical in the initial pathogenesis of HIV infection (Henderson, 1997; Pope et al., 1995).

Studies in humans have demonstrated that when zidovudine was administered to HIV-infected women and their infants, there was a 67% reduction in perinatal HIV transmission (Connor et al., 1994). The lack of significant decreases in viral load with zidovudine monotherapy in HIV-infected pregnant women further suggests that the protective effects of zidovudine prophylaxis for vertical HIV transmission may be due to preventing HIV transcription in the newborn infant (Melvin et al., 1997; Sperling et al., 1996). Advances in antiretroviral therapy have demonstrated that combination antiretroviral therapy is superior to monotherapy in reducing viral load in HIV-infected persons and may provide an added dimension of protection when used for PEP purposes.

PEP FOR OCCUPATIONAL EXPOSURE

Prospective studies estimate that the risk of HIV transmission to a health care worker (HCW) after percutaneous exposure is 0.03% and after a mucous membrane exposure is 0.09% (Bell, 1997; Henderson et al., 1990; Ippolito et al., 1993; Tokars et al., 1993). The risk of occupationally acquired HIV is increased under the following conditions (CDC, 1995, 1998):

1. The injury to the HCW is deep.
2. There is visible blood on the device causing the injury.
3. The device causing the injury was previously placed in the source-patient's vein or artery.
4. The source-patient was diagnosed as having AIDS and died within 60 days of the exposure (presumably having a high viral load associated with advanced disease).

According to Henderson (1997) a fifth factor for HIV infection in HCWs occupationally exposed may be the lack of PEP when an accident occurs. In a case-control study of 33 HCWs exposed to HIV through needlesticks or sharp objects, the incidence of HIV infection was 81% less among HCWs who used zidovudine for PEP (Cardo et al., 1997; CDC, 1996).

Limited data on the clinical characteristics of seroconversion in HIV-exposed HCWs have shown that 81% experienced a syndrome compatible with primary HIV infection within a median range of 25 to 46 days following exposure (Busch & Satten, 1997; CDC, 1998). In three instances, however, seroconversion was delayed and occurred between 6 and 12 months after exposure (Ciesielski & Metler, 1997; CDC, 1998; Rizdon et al., 1997).

On the basis of these findings the U.S. Public Health Service has published considerations for the rationale and recommendations for PEP (CDC, 1998):

1. Theoretically the initiation of antiretroviral PEP soon after exposure may prevent or inhibit systemic infection by limiting the proliferation of virus in the initial target cells or lymph nodes.

2. Both animal and human studies provide direct evidence of the efficacy of antiretroviral drugs as agents for PEP.

3. Although thus far only zidovudine, a nucleoside analogue reverse transcriptase inhibitor (NRTI), has been shown to prevent HIV transmission, theoretically a combination of drugs with activity at different stages in the viral replication cycle, e.g., adding a protease inhibitor (PI) to an NRTI regimen, could offer additive preventive effect in PEP.

4. At present, antiretroviral agents recommended to be given with zidovudine for PEP

STEP 1: Determine the Exposure Code (EC)

Is the source material blood, bloody fluid, other potentially infectious material (OPIM),[1] or an instrument contaminated with one of these substances?

Yes

No → No PEP needed

OPIM[2] — Blood or bloody fluid

What type of exposure has occurred?

| Mucous membrane or skin integrity compromised[3] | Intact skin only[4] | Percutaneous exposure |

Volume

No PEP needed

Severity

Small (e.g., few drops, short duration)

Large (e.g., several drops, major blood splash, and/or longer duration [i.e., several minutes or more])

Less Severe (e.g., solid needle, superficial scratch)

More Severe (e.g., large-bore hollow needle, deep puncture, visible blood on device, or needle used in source patient's artery or vein)[5]

EC 1

EC 2

EC 2

EC 3

[1]Semen or vaginal secretions; cerebrospinal, synovial, pleural, peritoneal, pericardial, or amniotic fluids; or tissue.
[2]Exposures to OPIM must be evaluated on a case-by-case basis. In general, these body substances are considered a low risk for transmission in health-care settings. Any unprotected contact to concentrated HIV in a research laboratory or production facility is considered an occupational exposure that requires clinical evaluation to determine the need for PEP.
[3]Skin integrity is considered compromised if there is evidence of chapped skin, dermatitis, abrasion, or open wound.
[4]Contact with intact skin is not normally considered a risk for HIV transmission. However, if the exposure was to blood and the circumstance suggests a higher volume exposure (e.g., an extensive area of skin was exposed or there was prolonged contact with blood), the risk for HIV transmission should be considered.
[5]The combination of these severity factors (e.g., large-bore hollow needle *and* deep puncture) contributes to an elevated risk for transmission if the source person is HIV positive.

Figure IV–1 ■ Steps to determine the need for HIV postexposure prophylaxis (PEP) after an occupational exposure. This algorithm is intended to guide initial decisions about PEP and should be used in conjunction with other guidance provided by a specialist or in the report. (Adapted from Centers for Disease Control and Prevention. [1998]. Public Health Service guidelines for the management of health-care worker exposures to HIV and recommendations for postexposure prophylaxis. *Morbidity and Mortality Weekly Report, 47*[RR-7], 1–33.)

include an additional NRTI, including lamivudine, didanosine, or zalcitabine, and, when warrented, a PI, either indinavir or nelfinavir. Most exposures will warrant only a two drug regimen, using two NRTIs, usually zidovudine and lamivudine.

5. For pregnant HCWs, both zidovudine and lamivudine appear safe and well tolerated. No data are available regarding the pharmacoki-

netics, safety, or tolerability of any of the PIs in pregnancy.

6. PEP should be initiated within a few hours rather than days after an exposure. Although animal studies suggest that PEP probably is not effective when started more than 24 to 36 hours after exposure, the interval after which there is no benefit from PEP in humans is undefined.

STEP 2: Determine the HIV Status Code (HIV SC)

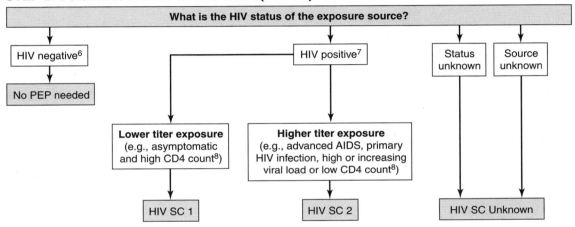

[6]A source is considered negative for HIV infection if there is laboratory documentation of a negative HIV antibody, HIV polymerase chain reaction (PCR), or HIV p24 antigen test result from a specimen collected at or near the time of exposure and there is no clinical evidence of recent retroviral-like illness.
[7]A source is considered infected with HIV (HIV positive) if there has been a positive laboratory result for HIV antibody, HIV PCR, or HIV p24 antigen or physician-diagnosed AIDS.
[8]Examples are used as surrogates to estimate the HIV titer in an exposure source for purposes of considering PEP regimens and do not reflect all clinical situations that may be observed. Although a high HIV titer (HIV SC 2) in an exposure source has been associated with an increased risk for transmission, the possibility of transmission from a source with a low HIV titer also must be considered.

STEP 3: Determine the PEP Recommendation

EC	HIV SC	PEP Recommendation
1	1	**PEP may not be warranted.** Exposure type does not pose a known risk for HIV transmission. Whether the risk for drug toxicity outweighs the benefit of PEP should be decided by the exposed HCW and treating clinician.
1	2	**Consider basic regimen.**[9] Exposure type poses a negligible risk for HIV transmission. A high HIV titer in the source may justify consideration of PEP. Whether the risk for drug toxicity outweighs the benefit of PEP should be decided by the exposed HCW and treating clinician.
2	1	**Recommend basic regimen.** Most HIV exposures are in this category; no increased risk for HIV transmission has been observed but use of PEP is appropriate.
2	2	**Recommend expanded regimen.**[10] Exposure type represents an increased HIV transmission risk.
3	1 or 2	**Recommend expanded regimen.** Exposure type represents an increased HIV transmission risk.
Unknown		If the source or, in the case of an unknown source, the setting where the exposure occurred suggests a possible risk for HIV exposure and the EC is 2 or 3, consider PEP basic regimen.

[9]Basic regimen is four weeks of zidovudine, 600 mg per day in two or three divided doses, *and* lamivudine, 150 mg twice daily.
[10]Expanded regimen is the basic regimen plus *either* indinavir, 800 mg every 8 hours, *or* nelfinavir, 750 mg three times a day.

Figure IV–1 ■ *Continued*

Table IV–1 ▪ Basic and Expanded HIV Postexposure Prophylaxis Regimens

Regimen Category	Application	Drug Regimen
Basic	Occupational HIV exposures for which there is a recognized transmission risk (Fig. IV–1)	4 weeks (28 days) of both zidovudine 600 mg every day in divided doses (i.e., 300 mg twice a day, 200 mg three times a day, or 100 mg every 4 hours) and lamivudine 150 mg twice a day
Expanded	Occupational HIV exposures that pose an increased risk for transmission (e.g., larger volume of blood or higher virus titer in blood (Fig. IV–1)	Basic regimen plus either indinavir 800 mg every 8 hours or nelfinavir 750 mg three times a day[1]

[1]Indinavir should be taken on an empty stomach (i.e., without food or with a light meal) and with increased fluid consumption (i.e., drinking six 8 oz glasses of water throughout the day); nelfinavir should be taken with meals.
Adapted from Centers for Disease Control and Prevention. (1998). Public Health Service guidelines for the management of health-care worker exposures to HIV and recommendations for postexposure prophylaxis. *Morbidity and Mortality Weekly Report, 47*(RR-7), 21.

7. If the source-patient's HIV status is unknown, initiating PEP should be decided on a case-by-case basis, taking into consideration the exposure risk and likelihood of HIV infection in known or possible source patients. If additional information becomes available, decisions about PEP can be modified.

8. Three major activities are recommended for managing PEP: (1) Determine the exposure code (nature of the exposure). (2) Determine the HIV status code (of the source patient). (3) Determine the PEP recommendation (Fig. IV–1). Then the appropriate postexposure prophylaxis regimen can be selected (Table IV–1).

9. HCWs with occupational exposures to HIV should receive follow-up counseling and medical evaluation, including HIV-antibody tests at baseline and periodically for at least 6 months after exposure, scheduled at intervals of 6 weeks, 12 weeks, and 6 months, and should be advised to observe precautions to limit the spread of HIV. Extended follow-up, testing at 12 months after exposure, may be indicated not only for clinical reasons but also to reduce the psychological distress of the exposed HCW. If PEP is prescribed, drug toxicity monitoring should include a complete blood count and renal and hepatic function tests at baseline and 2 weeks after starting

Table IV–2 ▪ HIV Postexposure Prophylaxis Resources and Registries

Resource or Registry	Contact Information
National Clinicians' Postexposure Hotline	Telephone: 888-448-4911
HIV Postexposure Prophylaxis Registry	Telephone: 888-737-4448 (888-PEP4HIV)
	Address: 1410 Commonwealth Drive, Suite 215 Wilmington, NC 28405
Antiretroviral Pregnancy Registry	Telephone: 800-258-4263
	Fax: 800-800-1052
	Address: 1410 Commonwealth Drive, Suite 215 Wilmington, NC 28405
Food and Drug Administration (for reporting unusual or severe toxicity to antiretroviral agents)	Telephone: 800-332-1088
CDC (for reporting HIV seroconversion in health-care workers who received postexposure prophylaxis)	Telephone: 404-639-6425

Adapted from Centers for Disease Control and Prevention. (1998). Public Health Service guidelines for the management of health-care worker exposures to HIV and recommendations for postexposure prophylaxis. *Morbidity and Mortality Weekly Report, 47*(RR-7), 21.

PEP. If subjective or objective toxicity is observed, expert consultation should be requested.

10. Health care providers in the United States should consider enrolling HCWs who receive PEP in an anonymous registry developed by the CDC, Glaxo Wellcome, Inc., and Merck & Co., Inc., to assess toxicity (telephone 1-888-737-4448 [1-888-PEP-4HIV]). Unusual or severe toxicity from antiretroviral drugs should be reported to the manufacturer or Food and Drug Administration (1-800-332-1088). Updated information on HIV PEP is available from the Internet at the CDC's home page (http://www.cdc.gov) (see Table IV–2).

PEP FOR SEXUAL CONTACT OR INJECTING DRUG USE

PEP after sexual exposure is being prescribed by some clinicians (Katz & Gerberding, 1997). According to Katz and Gerberding (1997) the absolute risk of HIV transmission associated with an episode of insertive anal intercourse is similar to vaginal intercourse and the probability of acquiring HIV after using contaminated drug injection equipment is slightly higher than an occupational exposure. Because of the potential for HIV transmission through rape, PEP has been recommended for victims of rape (Foster & Bartlett, 1989; Gostin et al., 1994). Katz and Gerberding recommend initiating PEP within 72 hours in high risk cases such as

1. Unprotected anal or vaginal intercourse
2. Receptive oral intercourse with ejaculation
3. Sharing of needles with an infected partner
4. When the exposure is a single event or involves someone who intends to stop such behavior.

The treatment recommendations, similar to PEP for occupational exposure, include zidovudine and lamivudine, with the addition of a protease inhibitor such as indinavir if the source-patient has AIDS or a high viral load or has been treated with nucleoside analogs. Both Katz and Gerberding (1997) conclude that although there are sufficient data to support the use of PEP in these situations, this type of treatment should be prescribed judiciously and only in the presence of a comprehensive program of prevention.

REFERENCES

Bell, D.M. (1997). Occupational risk of human immunodeficiency virus infection in healthcare workers: An overview. *American Journal of Medicine, 102*(Suppl. 5B), 9–15.

Bottinger, D., Johansson, N.G., Samuelsson, B., et al. (1997). Prevention of simian immunodeficiency virus, SIVsm, or HIV-2 infection in cynomolgus monkeys by pre- and postexsposure administration of BEA-005. *AIDS, 11*(2), 157–162.

Busch, M.P., Satten, G.A. (1997). Time course of viremia and antibody seroconversion following human immunodeficiency virus exposure. *American Journal of Medicine, 102*(Suppl. 5B), 117–124.

Cardo, D.M., Culver, D.H., Ciesielski, C.A., et al. (1997). A case-control study of HIV seroconversion in health workers after percutaneous exposure. *New England Journal of Medicine, 337*(21), 1485–1490.

Centers for Disease Control and Prevention. (1995). Case-control study of HIV seroconversion in health-care workers after percutaneous exposure to HIV-infected blood—France, United Kingdom, and United States, January 1988–August 1994. *Morbidity and Mortality Weekly Report, 44*(50), 929–933.

Centers for Disease Control and Prevention. (1996). Update: Provisional Public Health Service recommendations for chemoprophylaxis after occupational exposure to HIV. *Morbidity and Mortality Weekly Report, 45*(22), 468–472.

Centers for Disease Control and Prevention. (1998). Public Health Service guidelines for the management of health-care worker exposures to HIV and recommendations for postexposure prophylaxis. *Morbidity and Mortality Weekly Report, 47*(No. RR-7), 1–33.

Ciesielski, C.A., Metler, R.P. (1997). Duration of time between exposure and seroconversion in healthcare workers with occupationally acquired infection with human immunodeficiency virus. *American Journal of Medicine, 102*(Suppl. 5B), 115–116.

Connor, E.M., Sperling, R.S., Gelber, R., et al. (1994). Reduction of maternal-infant transmission of human immunodeficiency virus type 1 with zidovudine prophylaxis. *New England Journal of Medicine, 331*, 1173–1180.

Foster, I., Bartlett, J.G. (1989). Rape and subsequent seroconversion to HIV. *British Medical Journal, 299*, 1282.

Gostin, L.O., Lazzarini, Z., Alexander, D., et al. (1994). HIV testing, counseling, and prophylaxis after sexual assault. *Journal of the American Medical Association, 271*, 1436–1444.

Henderson, D.K. (1997). Postexposure treatment of HIV: Taking some risks for safety's sake. (Editorial). *New England Journal of Medicine, 337*(21), 1542–1543.

Henderson, D.K., Fahey, B.J., Willy, M., et al. (1990). Risk for occupational transmission of human immunodeficiency virus type 1 (HIV-1) associated with clinical exposures. A prospective evaluation. *Annals of Internal Medicine, 113*(100), 740–746.

Ippolito, G., Puro, V., DeCarli, G. (1993). The risk of occupational human immunodeficiency virus infection in health care workers. Italian Multicenter Study. The Italian Study Group on Occupational Risk of HIV Infection. *Archives of Internal Medicine, 153*(12), 1451–1458.

Katz, M.H., Gerberding, J.L. (1997). Postexposure treatment of people exposed to the human immunodeficiency virus through sexual contact or injection drug use. *New England Journal of Medicine, 336*(15), 1087–1100.

Melvin, A.J., Burchett, S.K., Watts, D.H., et al. (1997). Effect of pregnancy and zidovudine therapy on viral load in HIV-1-infected women. *Journal of Acquired Immune Deficiency Syndromes and Human Retrovirology, 14*(3), 232–236.

Pope, M., Gezelter, S., Gallo, N., Steinman, R.M. (1995). Low levels of HIV-1 infection in cutaneous dendritic cells promote extensive viral replication upon binding to memory CD4+ T cells. *Journal of Experimental Medicine, 182*(6), 2045–2056.

Ridzon, R., Gallagher, K., Ciesielski, C., et al. (1997). Simultaneous transmission of human immunodeficiency virus and hepatitis C virus from a needle-stick injury. *New England Journal of Medicine, 336*(13), 919–922.

Sperling, R.S., Shapiro, D.E., Coombs, R.W., et al. (1996). Maternal viral load, zidovudine treatment, and the risk of transmission of human immunodeficiency virus type 1 from mother to infant. Pediatric AIDS Clinical Trials Group Protocol 076 Study Group. *New England Journal of Medicine, 335*(220), 1678–1680.

Tokars, J.I., Marcus, R., Culver, D.H., et al. (1993). Surveillance of HIV infection and zidovudine use among health care workers after occupational exposure to HIV-infected blood. *Annals of Internal Medicine, 118*, 913–919.

Tsai, C.C., Follis, K.E., Sabo, A., et al. (1995). Prevention of SIV infection in macaques by (R)-9-(2-phosphonylmethoxypropyl) adeine. *Science, 270*(5239), 1121–1122.

Index

Note: Pages in *italics* indicate illustrations; those followed by a t refer to tables.